Nonprescription Products:

Formulations
& Features
'97-98

Notices

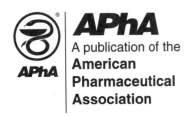

APhA
A publication of the
**American
Pharmaceutical
Association**

Nonprescription Products:

Formulations
& Features
'97-98

Edited by Leroy C. Knodel, PharmD
Director, Drug Information Service
The University of Texas Health Science Center
San Antonio, Texas

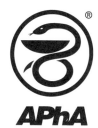

APhA
Published by
American Pharmaceutical Association
The National Professional Society of Pharmacists
2215 Constitution Avenue, NW
Washington, DC 20037

Susan C. Kendall
Product Table Editor

Linda L. Young
Managing Editor

Mary Jane Hickey
Director, Art and Production

Julian I. Graubart
Editorial Assistant

Database Development: Benjamin M. Bluml, Cygnus Systems Development, Inc.

Editorial Services: Publications Professionals, Inc.

Printing: United Book Press, Inc.

Library of Congress Catalog Card Number: 97-072866
ISBN 0-917330-85-4
ISSN 1092-1621

How to Order This Book
By phone: 800-878-0729 (802-862-0095 from outside the United States).
VISA®, MasterCard®, and American Express® cards accepted.

Contents

Nutritional Product Tables

Infant Formula Product Table

Weight Control Product Table

Ophthalmic Product Tables

Contact Lens Product Tables

Otic Product Table

Oral Health Product Tables

Dermatologic Product Tables

Acne Product Table

Introduction

Welcome to the second edition of *Nonprescription Products: Formulations & Features*. New to this edition are APhA's "Products for Patients with Special Needs" (pages 9–28), which formerly was published and sold separately, and four new product tables (pages 30–33)—HIV Test Kits, Urine Test Kits, Drugs of Abuse Test Kits, and Hormonal Supplements.

Some of you have purchased this book separately; others have received it as part of your purchase of the 11th Edition of the *Handbook of Nonprescription Drugs*. If you have opened a copy of any of the first 10 editions of the *Handbook,* you know that tables containing detailed comparative information on nonprescription products were previously incorporated in the textbook. Why have we now split the book into two publications?

The overriding reason is readers' expressed interest in receiving up-to-date nonprescription product information in today's rapidly changing market. Similar to many other comprehensive medical textbooks, a new edition of the *Handbook* is published every 3 to 4 years. In that time, however, the information in *Formulations & Features* will have become dated. To meet our readers' needs, APhA publishes new issues of this title once a year and provides the most current edition of *Formulations & Features* to purchasers of the *Handbook.* The link between product and ingredient information in the two publications is established with cross-references: Each product table (except for the four new ones) contains a cross-reference to the textbook chapter that discusses the pharmacology of the ingredients and therapeutic use of the products; similarly, the textbook chapters cross-reference the appropriate product tables.

A second reason is portability. When the product tables were a part of the large—and growing—textbook, quickly extracting product information became difficult, whereas putting this material in a separate publication provides ready access to the product information. Incidentally, readers told us they preferred the *hardcover binding* used in editions prior to the 10th, but at the same time were concerned that the book was becoming very heavy to carry. With the 11th Edition, the textbook is once again hardbound, but the separate binding of approximately 500 pages of prod-

uct tables actually makes the 11th Edition lighter than the softbound 10th Edition.

A third reason for publishing the product tables separately is simply that we believe the information in *Formulations & Features* is valuable in its own right. Creating a separate book makes this information accessible to many health care professionals whose primary interest or need is the product information.

Current changes in the U.S. health care system have made comparison of nonprescription products an invaluable tool for health care professionals. The more than 500 new product listings from one year ago reflect the current rapid expansion of the nonprescription product market, which is being driven in part by sweeping changes in the U.S. health care system and the pharmaceutical industry. An increased reliance on self-care by the public and the availability of a large number of medications recently reclassified as nonprescription demand that health care professionals be on the leading edge of the self-care movement. Further, the continuing evolution of pharmacy practice from dispensing of medications to management of patients makes this type of information essential to pharmacists in making the most appropriate recommendations to their patients with regard to nonprescription drug use.

APhA's electronic database of nonprescription products—the OTC Product Database—facilitated publication of this book. This database, which is in Microsoft Access format and can be provided for computer applications in standard ASCII or other appropriate media, is available for use by system vendors, software and CD ROM developers, and health care professionals. Interested parties may call 1-800-237-2742, ext. 7561 for more information about the database.

APhA welcomes your suggestions for improving its nonprescription product information and this book. Please write to *Nonprescription Products: Formulations & Features,* American Pharmaceutical Association, 2215 Constitution Avenue, N.W., Washington, DC 20037.

Leroy C. Knodel, PharmD
Editor
June 1997

About the Product Tables

This annual edition of *Formulations & Features* contains the 82 product tables of the previous edition plus 4 new ones. The new tables consist of product categories recently introduced to the marketplace, and all products included are new entries to APhA's OTC Product Database. The titles of the new tables follow:

- HIV Test Kits
- Urine Test Kits
- Drugs of Abuse Test Kits
- Hormonal Supplements

Product Table Features

Some features of the product tables, such as the ingredient/formulation codes and the use of bullets and other codes, pertain to the characteristics or presentation of the product ingredient information. Other features serve as links between the product tables and the *Handbook* chapters.

Ingredient and Formulation Codes

The ingredient and formulation codes, which appear to the left of a product trade name, have been rated as "extremely useful" by past users of the product information. These codes provide guidance in selecting products for patients with special needs. The codes and their definitions are as follows:

AL = alcohol free
AF = aspirin free
CA = caffeine free
CO = cholesterol free
DY = dye free
FL = fluoride free
FR = fragrance free
GL = gluten free
LA = lactose free
PR = preservative free
PU = purine free
SO = dietetically sodium free
SL = sulfite free
SU = dietetically *sucrose* free (product may contain other sugars or artificial sweeteners)
GE = geriatric formulation
PE = pediatric formulation

These codes are supplied by the manufacturers and are not necessarily comprehensive. Because this information could not be independently verified, readers should use the codes only as a guide to help them locate products that might meet special needs. Further, product formulations change frequently; therefore, pharmacists and patients should always carefully check the ingredients listed on product packages.

Other Codes
** = New listing
This code, which also appears to the left of an applicable product trade name, designates products that were not listed in *Formulations & Features* '96-97 or in previous editions of the *Handbook of Nonprescription Drugs*. These products can be either new to the marketplace or new to the OTC Product Database.

• = Bullet
This graphic symbol serves to separate the ingredients listed for each product.

Blank column = No information supplied
If a column for a particular product contains no data, the product may not contain the ingredient(s) pertinent to that column, or the manufacturer may have chosen not to provide the information. In the case of the column Other Ingredients, a blank column usually means the manufacturer did not provide the information.

Cross-References to the *Handbook*
To allow *Handbook* users quick access to the product information, the tables are grouped and ordered according to the chapter discussions of the product ingredients and their therapeutic uses. Each product table (except the four new ones) contains a cross-reference to the *Handbook* chapter that discusses the product ingredients in detail.

Multisource Products
For a small number of products, the manufacturer/supplier is listed as "Multisource." This term is commonly used to designate generic or store-brand versions of trade-name products, which are available from many manufacturers/suppliers. Because of the numerous generic products available, multisource list-

ings in this publication have been limited to products whose dosage forms or strengths differ from those of trade-name products and to widely used products for which no trade-name product is available (e.g., Ipecac, Magnesium Salicylate).

Scope

Formulations & Features presents a broad range of products in each therapeutic category, including national as well as regional products. The numerous products available in some categories preclude listing every product submitted by manufacturers. If a large number of products are available for a particular category, a representative sampling of the dosage forms, strengths, flavors, etc., is presented.

Data Accuracy and Completeness

Every effort has been made to ensure that product data are as accurate and complete as possible. The scope of the product tables, however, makes it impossible to verify all information independently. Some manufacturers listed all ingredient information for their products, whereas others concentrated on providing information for only active or significant ingredients. Pharmacists and patients are encouraged to also check product packages for ingredient information.

Susan C. Kendall
Product Table Editor

New Listings

The 590 products classified here as "new listings" fall into one of the following three categories:

- Products new to the market since publication of *Nonprescription Products: Formulations & Features* '96-97;
- Existing products not recently, or never before, listed in the *Handbook of Nonprescription Drugs*;
- New dosage forms of products that became available after publication of *Formulations & Features* '96-97.

Note: Some brand names of phytomedicinal products include the total weight of the solid dosage forms, not the weight of the active ingredients alone.

A + D Ointment with Zinc Oxide
Schering-Plough Healthcare

A Kid's Companion Wafers
Natrol

A&D UA-702 Manual Inflation Digital B.P. Monitor
A&D Medical

A&D UA-751 Auto-Inflation with Printer Digital B.P. Monitor
A&D Medical

A&D UA-767 One-Step Auto-Inflation Digital B.P. Monitor
A&D Medical

A&D UA-777 One-Step Auto-Inflation Digital B.P. Monitor
A&D Medical

A&D UB-211 Finger Digital B.P. Monitor
A&D Medical

A&D UB-302 Compact Wrist Digital B.P. Monitor
A&D Medical

A&D UB-325 Wrist Digital B.P. Monitor
A&D Medical

Absorbine Arthritis Strength liquid
W. F. Young

Accu-Chek InstantPlus
Boehringer Mannheim

Adeks Chewable Tablets
Scandipharm

Adeks Drops
Scandipharm

Advil, Children's suspension
Whitehall-Robins Healthcare

Advil, Junior Strength tablet
Whitehall-Robins Healthcare

Afrin 4-Hour Extra Moisturizing nasal spray
Schering-Plough Healthcare

Aler-Dryl caplet
Reese Chemical

Aler-Releaf timed-release capsule
Reese Chemical

Alka-Seltzer PM effervescent tablet
Bayer Consumer

Alka-Seltzer, Cherry effervescent tablet
Bayer Consumer

Allercreme lotion
Carmé

Allercreme Moisturizer with Sunscreen SPF 8 lotion
Carmé

Aloe Grande cream
Gordon Labs

Ambenyl-D Cough syrup
Forest Ph'cals

Ammens Extra Medicated powder
Bristol-Myers Products

Anti-Oxidant Take One Capsules or Tablets
Natrol

Aqua Glycolic Hand & Body lotion
Allergan Skin Care

Aqua Glycolic Shampoo & Body Cleanser shampoo; liquid
Allergan Skin Care

Aquafresh Gum Care paste
SmithKline Beecham

Aquaphor Healing ointment
Beiersdorf

Aquaphor Original ointment
Beiersdorf

Arctic pump spray
Systems Design

ArthriCare Ultra gel
Del Ph'cals

Arthur Itis cream or liquid
Stellar Health Products

Ascriptin Enteric Adult Low Strength tablet
Novartis Consumer

Ascriptin Enteric Regular Strength tablet
Novartis Consumer

Aspergel gel
Thompson Medical

Autolet Mini
Owen Mumford

Azo-Cranberry 450 mg capsule
PolyMedica Ph'cals

B-C-Bid Caplets
Lee Consumer

B-D Pen
Becton Dickinson Consumer

B-D Ultra-Fine II Short Needle Syringe
Becton Dickinson Consumer

Baby Gasz drops
Lee Consumer

Baby Gumz gel
Lee Consumer

Bain de Soleil Le Sport lotion
Pfizer Consumer

Bain de Soleil Mademoiselle lotion
Pfizer Consumer

Balance PC
MediLife

Bayer Aspirin Regimen Adult Low Strength with Calcium caplet
Bayer Consumer

Bayer PM Extra Strength Aspirin with Sleep Aid caplet
Bayer Consumer

Bi-Zets lozenge
Reese Chemical

Bilberry capsule
Natrol

Bilberry Extract 60 mg capsule
Nature's Resource/Pharmavite

Bilberry Extract 280 mg capsule
NaturPharma

Bio Sun Children lotion
Playtex Products

Bio Sun Faces lotion
Playtex Products

Bio Sun lotion
Playtex Products

BioShield Facial Sunblock for Normal or for Sensitive Skin lotion
Hawaiian Tropic

Biotène Dry Mouth Toothpaste
Laclede Research Labs

Blue Needle Box Sharps Disposal System
Bio-Oxidation

Born Again Vaginal Moisturizing gel
Alvin Last

Boroleum ointment
Sinclair Pharmacal

Buckley's DM syrup
W. K. Buckley

Buckley's Mixture syrup
W. K. Buckley

Buckley's White Rub ointment
W. K. Buckley

Bufferin Enteric tablet
Bristol-Myers Products

Bug Stuff IPF 20 lotion
Wisconsin Pharmacal

Bull Frog Quik gel
Chattem

CalaGel Medicated Anti-Itch gel
Tec Labs

Calcium and Magnesium with Zinc tablet
American Health

Calcium with Vitamins A&D wafer
American Health

Calicylic Creme cream
Gordon Labs

Cameo Oil bath oil
Medco Lab

Camp Lotion for Kids
Wisconsin Pharmacal

Capzasin-HP cream
Thompson Medical

Capzasin-HP lotion
Thompson Medical

Capzasin-P lotion
Thompson Medical

Carbo Zinc Powder
Nu-Hope Labs

CarePlus condom; spermicide insert
Selfcare

Cayenne 455 mg capsule
NaturPharma

Cayenne capsule
Natrol

Cayenne Pepper 450 mg capsule
NaturaLife

Cayenne Power-Herb 450 mg capsule
Nature's Herbs

Celestial Herbal Extracts Ginseng Plus softgel
Celestial Seasonings

Cepacol Sore Throat Maximum Strength, Cherry lozenge
J. B. Williams

Cepacol Sore Throat Maximum Strength, Cherry pump spray
J. B. Williams

Cepacol Sore Throat Maximum Strength, Cool Menthol pump spray
J. B. Williams

Cevi-Bid Tablets
Lee Consumer

CharcoAid G suspension
Requa

Chaste Tree Berry Extract tincture
Herb Pharm

Chasteberry-Power capsule
Nature's Herbs

Chewy Bears Chewable Calcium wafer
American Health

Chewy Bears Citrus Free Vitamin C Chewable Wafers
American Health

Chewy Bears Complete Chewable Tablets
American Health

Chewy Bears Multi-Vitamins with Calcium Chewable Wafers
American Health

Children's Multi-Vitamin Liquid
Natrol

Chroma Trim gum
GumTech

Chromemate capsule
Natrol

Chromium Picolinate capsule
Natrol

Chromium Picolinate tablet
American Health

Class Act Smooth Sensation latex
Carter Products

Class Act Smooth Sensation with Spermicide latex
Carter Products

Clean & Clear Pore Prep Clarifier liquid
Johnson & Johnson Consumer

Cleanlet
Gainor Medical

Clinical Care Antimicrobial Wound Cleanser pump spray
Care-Tech Labs

Clinical Nutrients for Men Tablets
PhytoPharmica

Clinical Nutrients for Women Tablets
PhytoPharmica

Cloverine Salve ointment
Medtech

Colace Microenema
Roberts Ph'cal

Cold Control timed-release capsule
Reese Chemical

Coldmax timed-release capsule
Reese Chemical

Coldvac Lozenges
Alva-Amco Pharmacal

Colgate Baking Soda & Peroxide Whitening paste
Colgate-Palmolive

Colgate Platinum Whitening with Baking Soda paste
Colgate-Palmolive

ComfortCare GP Comfort Drops
Allergan

ComfortCare GP Dual Action tablets
Allergan

ComfortCare GP Wetting & Soaking solution
Allergan

Compete Tablets
Mission Pharmacal

Compleat Pediatric liquid
Novartis Nutrition

Comply liquid
Mead Johnson Nutritionals

Compound-W Wart Remover pad
Medtech

Comtrex Allergy-Sinus Daytime caplet
Bristol-Myers Products

Comtrex Deep Chest Cold and Congestion Relief liqui-gel
Bristol-Myers Products

Confide HIV Testing Service
Direct Access Diagnostics

Consept 1 liquid
Allergan

Consept 2 solution
Allergan

Consort Hair Regrowth Treatment for Men solution
Alberto Culver

Coppertone Aloe & Vitamin E Lip Balm with Sunscreen stick
Schering-Plough Healthcare

Coppertone Bug & Sun Adult Formula SPF 15 lotion
Schering-Plough Healthcare

Coppertone Bug & Sun Adult Formula SPF 30 lotion
Schering-Plough Healthcare

Coppertone Bug & Sun Kids Formula SPF 30 lotion
Schering-Plough Healthcare

Coppertone Gold Dark Tanning oil
Schering-Plough Healthcare

Coppertone Gold Dry oil
Schering-Plough Healthcare

Coppertone Gold Tan Magnifier oil
Schering-Plough Healthcare

Coppertone Kids Colorblock Disappearing Purple Sunblock lotion
Schering-Plough Healthcare

Coppertone Kids Sunblock stick
Schering-Plough Healthcare

Coppertone Natural Fruit Flavor Lip Balm with Sunscreen stick
Schering-Plough Healthcare

Coppertone Oil-Free Sunblock lotion
Schering-Plough Healthcare

CortiCool Anti-Itch gel
Tec Labs

Cranberry capsule
Natrol

Cranberry Fruit 405 mg capsule
Nature's Resource/Pharmavite

Cranberry-Power capsule
Nature's Herbs

Creamalin tablet
Lee Consumer

Creo-Terpin liquid
Lee Consumer

Crest MultiCare gel/paste
Procter & Gamble

Cruex Prescription Strength AF cream
Novartis Consumer

Cruex Prescription Strength aerosol spray powder
Novartis Consumer

Cutter Backwoods aerosol spray
Spectrum

Cutter Outdoorsman lotion or stick
Spectrum

Cutter Pleasant Protection aerosol spray
Spectrum

Daily Garlic tablet
NaturPharma

Daily Ginseng 495 mg capsule
NaturPharma

Delacort lotion
Mericon

Dentapaine gel
Reese Chemical

Dentemp Temporary Filling Mix liquid; powder
Majestic Drug

Dentlock powder
Lee Consumer

Dentu-Gel
Dentco

Derifil Tablets
Menley & James Labs

Dermatox lotion
Reese Chemical

Dermi-Heal ointment
Quality Formulations

Devko Tablets
Parthenon

DHEA capsule
Natrol

DHEA cream
Young Again

DHEA for Men timed-release caplet
Celestial Seasonings

DHEA for Women timed-release caplet
Celestial Seasonings

DHEA tablet
American Health

DHEA tablet
Breckenridge Ph'cal

DHEA tablet
Natrol

DHEA tablet
Young Again

DHEA Therapeutic cream
Breckenridge Ph'cal

Diabetic Pure Skin Therapy Azulene Night Repair cream
Consumers Choice

Diabetic Pure Skin Therapy Day Protection SPF 15 cream
Consumers Choice

Diabetic Pure Skin Therapy Diapedic Foot Cream
Consumers Choice

Diabetic Pure Skin Therapy Hand & Body cream
Consumers Choice

Diabetic Tussin DM Liqui-Gels gelcap
Health Care Products

Diabetic Tussin DM Maximum Strength Liqui-Gels gelcap
Health Care Products

Diarrid caplet
Stellar Health Products

Dignity Lites pad
Humanicare

Dignity Pads
Humanicare

Dignity Plus Briefmates Guards pad
Humanicare

Dignity Plus Briefmates Pads
Humanicare

Dignity Plus Briefmates Undergarments
Humanicare

Dignity Plus Fitted Briefs
Humanicare

Dignity Plus Liners pad
Humanicare

Dimetapp Cold & Allergy Quick Dissolve tablet
Whitehall-Robins Healthcare

Diostate D Tablets
Lee Consumer

Dolorac cream
GenDerm

Double Cap cream
Breckenridge Ph'cal

Double Tussin DM liquid
Reese Chemical

Doxidan softgel
Pharmacia & Upjohn

Dr. Hand's Teething gel or lotion
Lee Consumer

Dr. Powers Colloidal Mineral Source liquid
American Health

DuoFilm Wart Remover Patch for Kids disc
Schering-Plough Healthcare

Dynafed EX. tablet
BDI Ph'cals

Dynafed IB tablet
BDI Ph'cals

early Ovulation predictor
Selfcare

Echinacea 380 mg capsule
NaturaLife

Emecheck liquid
Savage Labs

Epilyt Concentrate lotion
Stiefel Labs

Epso-Pine Bath Salts granule
Majestic Drug

Ester-C Capsules
Natrol

Ester-C Liquid
Natrol

Ester-C Softgels
Natrol

Eucerin Light Moisture-Restorative lotion
Beiersdorf

Evening Primrose Oil softgel
Natrol

Evening Primrose Oil softgel
NaturPharma

Ex-Lax Stool Softener caplet
Novartis Consumer

ExACT Tinted cream
Premier Consumer

ExacTech R·S·G
MediSense

Excedrin PM geltab
Bristol-Myers Products

EZ-Detect Urine Blood Test
Biomerica

EZ-Let II
Palco Labs

EZ-Let Thin
Palco Labs

Femizol-M cream
Lake Consumer

Feosol caplet
SmithKline Beecham

Feverfew 380 mg capsule
NaturaLife

Feverfew-Power softgel
Nature's Herbs

Fiber Naturale caplet
Alva-Amco Pharmacal

First Teeth Baby Toothpaste gel
Laclede Research Labs

Fixodent Free cream
Procter & Gamble

Flexall Ultra Plus gel
Chattem

Flexcin cream
Breckenridge Ph'cal

Fluoride Foam
Laclede Research Labs

Fototar cream
ICN Ph'cals

Free & Active Pads
Humanicare

Fungi Nail solution
Kramer Labs

Fungoid AF solution
Pedinol Pharmacal

Garlic Enteric Coated tablet
Natrol

Garlic-Power tablet
Nature's Herbs

Ginger-Power capsule
Nature's Herbs

Ginkai 50 mg tablet
Lichtwer Pharma

Ginkgo Biloba capsule
Natrol

Ginkgo Extract 389 mg capsule
NaturPharma

Ginkgo-Power 389 mg capsule
Nature's Herbs

Ginseng Extract 270 mg capsule
NaturPharma

GLUCOchek PocketLab
Clinical Diagnostics

GLUCOchek Visual Blood Glucose Test strip
Clinical Diagnostics

Gold Bond Cornstarch Plus Medicated Baby Powder
Chattem

Goody's PM powder
Goody's Ph'cals

Gordochom solution
Gordon Labs

Gordon's Vite A Creme cream
Gordon Labs

Grape Seed Extract 25 mg capsule
Nature's Resource/Pharmavite

Grape Seed Extract capsule
Natrol

Grape Seed-Power 50 capsule
Nature's Herbs

Grape Seed-Power 100 capsule
Nature's Herbs

Gyne-Lotrimin 3 Combination Pack cream; suppository
Schering-Plough Healthcare

Gyne-Lotrimin 3 Inserts suppository
Schering-Plough Healthcare

Hawaiian Tropic 45 Plus Lip Balm stick
Hawaiian Tropic

Hawaiian Tropic Clear Sense lotion
Hawaiian Tropic

Hawaiian Tropic Clear Sense Sunblock lotion
Hawaiian Tropic

Hawaiian Tropic Dark Tanning with Extra Sunscreen Oil
Hawaiian Tropic

Hawaiian Tropic Dark Tanning with Sunscreen Oil
Hawaiian Tropic

Hawaiian Tropic Golden Tannning lotion
Hawaiian Tropic

Hawaiian Tropic Herbal Tanning lotion
Hawaiian Tropic

Hawaiian Tropic Herbal Tanning Mist pump spray
Hawaiian Tropic

Hawaiian Tropic Just for Kids Sunblock lotion
Hawaiian Tropic

Hawaiian Tropic Protection Plus lotion
Hawaiian Tropic

Hawaiian Tropic Protective Tanning Dry Oil pump spray
Hawaiian Tropic

Hawaiian Tropic Sport Sunblock lotion
Hawaiian Tropic

Hawaiian Tropic Tan Amplifier lotion
Hawaiian Tropic

Hay Fever & Allergy Reiief Maximum Strength tablet
Hudson

HealthCheck Uri-Test Nitrite
Health-Mark Diagnostics

HealthGuard Minoxidil Topical Solution for Men
Bausch & Lomb Ph'cal

HealthGuard Minoxidil Topical Solution for Women
Bausch & Lomb Ph'cal

Healthmate
MedData Interactive

Herb-Lax tablet
Shaklee

Hibistat liquid
Zeneca Ph'cals

High Gear gum
GumTech

Home Access
Home Access Health

Home Access Express
Home Access Health

Humibid GC caplet
Menley & James Labs

Hydrolatum cream
Denison Ph'cals

Icy Hot Arthritis Therapy gel
Chattem

Identi-Find Medic-ID Card
Identi-Find

In Touch
LifeScan

Insta-Char With Cherry Flavor suspension
Frank W. Kerr

Insta-Char With Sorbitol and Cherry Flavor suspension
Frank W. Kerr

Insta-Char, Unflavored suspension
Frank W. Kerr

Insul-Guide
Stat Medical

Iodex Anti-Infective ointment
Lee Consumer

Iodex with Methyl Salicylate ointment
Lee Consumer

IvyBlock lotion
EnviroDerm Ph'cals

Johnson's Baby Lotion
Johnson & Johnson Consumer

Just Lotion
Care-Tech Labs

K-Y Liquid
Advanced Care Products

K-Y Long Lasting gel
Advanced Care Products

Kao Lectrolyte Individual Packets, Flavored or Unflavored
Pharmacia & Upjohn

Kao-Paverin liquid
Reese Chemical

Keri Anti-Bacterial Hand lotion
Bristol-Myers Products

Kira 300 mg tablet
Lichtwer Pharma

Korean Ginseng Power-Herb 535 mg capsule
Nature's Herbs

Labtron 02-959 Automatic Wrist B.P. Monitor
Graham-Field

Lactaid Ultra caplet
McNeil Consumer

Lanacane Maximum Strength cream
Combe

Lemon Balm Extract tincture
Herb Pharm

LifeStyles Extra Strength with Spermicide
Ansell

LifeStyles Lubricated
Ansell

LifeStyles Spermicidally Lubricated
Ansell

LifeStyles Ultra Sensitive
Ansell

LifeStyles Ultra Sensitive with Spermicide
Ansell

LifeStyles Vibra-Ribbed
Ansell

LifeStyles Vibra-Ribbed with Spermicide
Ansell

LifeStyles; Assorted Colors, Form Fitting, or Studded
Ansell

Lip-Ex ointment
Lee Consumer

Lipmagik liquid
Reese Chemical

Lipomul liquid
Lee Consumer

Liquid Ginkgo Biloba drops
Natrol

Listerine Toothpaste Tartar Control, Cool Mint gel or paste
Warner-Lambert Consumer

Loving Lotion
Care-Tech Labs

Lubrex lotion
Allerderm Labs

Lumiscope 1090 Wrist B.P. Monitor
Lumiscope

Magna II Timed-Release Tablets
American Health

Magna One Timed-Release Tablets
American Health

Magnacal Renal liquid
Mead Johnson Nutritionals

Medotar ointment
Medco Lab

Melatonin lozenge
Natrol

Melatonin PM Dual Release tablet
Celestial Seasonings

Melatonin PM Fast Acting chewable tablet
Celestial Seasonings

Melatonin softgel
Natrol

Melatonin tablet or timed-release tablet
Natrol

Melatonin timed-release tablet
Hudson

MG217 for Psoriasis shampoo
Triton Consumer

MG217 Tar-Free for Dandruff shampoo
Triton Consumer

Micatin Cooling Action Spray Liquid aerosol spray
Johnson & Johnson Consumer

Micatin Jock Itch cream
Johnson & Johnson Consumer

Microlipid oil
Mead Johnson Nutritionals

Milk Thistle Extract 540 mg capsule
NaturPharma

Milk Thistle Seed Extract 140 mg capsule
Nature's Resource/Pharmavite

Mineral Complex tablet
Natrol

Mini Thin Diet Aid timed-release capsule
BDI Ph'cals

Minoxidil Topical Solution for Men
Copley Ph'cal

Mitrolan chewable tablet
Whitehall-Robins Healthcare

Monistat 3 Combination Pack cream; suppository
Advanced Care Products

More Than a Multiple Tablets
American Health

Motrin, Children's chewable tablet
McNeil Consumer

Motrin, Children's drops
McNeil Consumer

Motrin, Junior Strength chewable tablet
McNeil Consumer

Multi-Vitamin Liquid
Natrol

My Favorite Multiple Take One Tablets
Natrol

My-B-Tabs Tablets
Legere Ph'cals

Mycelex-3 cream
Bayer Consumer

Mylanta Children's Upset Stomach Relief liquid
Johnson & Johnson·Merck

Mylanta Children's Upset Stomach Relief, Bubble Gum or Fruit chewable tablet
Johnson & Johnson·Merck

Mylanta·AR tablet
Johnson & Johnson·Merck

N'Ice Sore Throat & Cough, Cherry lozenge
SmithKline Beecham

N'Ice Sore Throat & Cough, Herbal Mint or Honey Lemon lozenge
SmithKline Beecham

Nasal Moist gel
Blairex Labs

Nasalcrom nasal spray
Pharmacia & Upjohn

Natural White Baking Soda paste
Natural White

Natural White Fights Plaque paste
Natural White

Natural White Sensitive paste
Natural White

Natural White with Peroxide gel
Natural White

Neutrogena Body Lotion
Neutrogena Dermatologics

Neutrogena Daily Moisture Supply lotion
Neutrogena Dermatologics

Neutrogena Kids Sunblock lotion
Neutrogena Dermatologics

Neutrogena Multi-Vitamin Acne Treatment cream
Neutrogena Dermatologics

Neutrogena Oil Free Sunblock lotion
Neutrogena Dermatologics

Neutrogena Sunblock pump spray
Neutrogena Dermatologics

Neutrogena Sunless Tanning Lotion; Light/Med, Med/Deep, Deep cream
Neutrogena Dermatologics

NicoDerm CQ transdermal patch
SmithKline Beecham

Nicotrol transdermal patch
McNeil Consumer

Nivea Daily Care for Lips stick
Beiersdorf

Nivea Sun Kids lotion
Beiersdorf

Nivea UV Care Lip Balm stick
Beiersdorf

Nose Better gel
Lee Consumer

Nu-Hope Adhesive
Nu-Hope Labs

NuBasics liquid
Nestlé Clinical Nutrition

NuBasics Plus liquid
Nestlé Clinical Nutrition

NuBasics VHP liquid
Nestlé Clinical Nutrition

NuBasics with Fiber liquid
Nestlé Clinical Nutrition

Nutren 1.0 Complete liquid
Nestlé Clinical Nutrition

Nutren 1.0 with Fiber Complete liquid
Nestlé Clinical Nutrition

Nutren 1.5 Complete liquid
Nestlé Clinical Nutrition

Nutren 2.0 Complete liquid
Nestlé Clinical Nutrition

Nutri-Mega Softgels
American Health

Ocurest Redness Reliever Lubricant drops
Ocurest Labs

Ocurest Tears Formula Lubricant drops
Ocurest Labs

Odor-Eaters Antifungal powder
Combe

Odor-Eaters Foot & Sneaker aerosol spray powder
Combe

Off! Deep Woods with Sunscreen liquid or lotion
S. C. Johnson & Son

Off! Skintastic with Sunscreen lotion
S. C. Johnson & Son

Oncovite Tablets
Mission Pharmacal

Ony-Clear spray
Pedinol Pharmacal

Opti-Free SupraClens Daily Protein Remover liquid
Alcon Labs

Orajel Baby liquid
Del Ph'cals

Orajel P.M. gel
Del Ph'cals

Orajel Perioseptic Super Cleaning Oral Rinse solution
Del Ph'cals

Oralbalance Moisturizing gel
Laclede Research Labs

Orchid Fresh II Liquid
Care-Tech Labs

Pain-X gel
B. F. Ascher

Palmer's Aloe Vera Formula Medicated Lip Balm stick
E. T. Browne Drug

Palmer's Cocoa Butter Concentrated Hand Cream SPF 8
E. T. Browne Drug

Palmer's Cocoa Butter cream
E. T. Browne Drug

Palmer's Cocoa Butter Formula Moisturizing Lip Balm stick
E. T. Browne Drug

Palmer's Cocoa Butter lotion
E. T. Browne Drug

Palmer's Medicated Aloe Vera Formula gel
E. T. Browne Drug

Palmer's Skin Success Acne Medication Cleanser liquid
E. T. Browne Drug

Palmer's Skin Success Anti-Darkening cream
E. T. Browne Drug

Palmer's Skin Success Fade Cream, Dry Skin
E. T. Browne Drug

Palmer's Skin Success Fade Cream, Normal Skin
E. T. Browne Drug

Palmer's Skin Success Fade Cream, Oily Skin
E. T. Browne Drug

Palmer's Skin Success Fade Serum liquid
E. T. Browne Drug

Palmer's Skin Success Invisible Acne Medication cream
E. T. Browne Drug

Palmer's Skin Success ointment
E. T. Browne Drug

Pamprin gelcap
Chattem

PDT-90 Personal Drug Testing Service
Psychemedics

Pearl Drops Whitening Toothpolish gel
Carter Products

Pearl Drops Whitening Toothpolish, Icy Cool Mint gel
Carter Products

Pedia Care Cold-Allergy chewable tablet
Pharmacia & Upjohn

Pedialyte Freezer Pops
Ross Products/Abbott Labs

Peptamen Complete liquid
Nestlé Clinical Nutrition

Peptamen Junior Complete liquid
Nestlé Clinical Nutrition

Peptamen VHP Complete liquid
Nestlé Clinical Nutrition

Pete & Pam Toothpaste Pre-measured Strips
Laclede Research Labs

Peterson's Ointment
Lee Consumer

Phade gel
Alva-Amco Pharmacal

Pharmacist's Creme cream
Reese Chemical

Phazyme Gas Relief, Cherry or Mint liquid
Block Drug

Physicians Formula Self Defense Moisturizing SPF 15 lotion
Pierre Fabre Dermatology

Podactin Antifungal cream
Reese Chemical

Poli-Grip Free cream
Block Drug

Polident Double Action tablet
Block Drug

Polident Overnight tablet
Block Drug

Preferred DHEA capsule
Reese Chemical

Preferred DHEA Therapeutic cream
Reese Chemical

Preferred Pycnogenol Plus capsule
Reese Chemical

Pregnenolone cream
Young Again

Pregnenolone tablet
Young Again

Premsyn PMS gelcap
Chattem

Prestige
Home Diagnostics

Pretty Feet & Hands Replenishing Creme cream
B. F. Ascher

Pretty Feet & Hands Rough Skin Remover cream
B. F. Ascher

Primrose-Power softgel
Nature's Herbs

ProBalance Complete liquid
Nestlé Clinical Nutrition

Protac Troches lozenge
Republic Drug

Protain XL liquid
Mead Johnson Nutritionals

Protect Your Life Card
Apothecary Products

Protect Your Life Keychain
Apothecary Products

Protective Barrier Film Wipes
Bard Medical

Proxigel gel
Block Drug

Pycnogenol 30 mg capsule
American Health

Pycnogenol capsule
Natrol

Qwik-Let
Stat Medical

Recofen caplet
Reese Chemical

Rectacaine ointment
Reese Chemical

Rectacaine suppository
Reese Chemical

Red Fox Bottle O'Butter lotion
Majestic Drug

Red Fox Tub O'Butter cream
Majestic Drug

Redacon DX drops
Reese Chemical

Reflect lotion
Wisconsin Pharmacal

Reflect Sun Stick
Wisconsin Pharmacal

Regular One-Piece Colostomy Pouches
Bard Medical

Rejoice Liners
Humanicare

Rejoice Pants
Humanicare

Rekematol Anti-Nausea liquid
Reese Chemical

Releaf Menopause Formula Tablets
Lake Consumer

Releaf Osteoporosis Formula tablet
Lake Consumer

Releaf Stress Formula Tablets
Lake Consumer

Renalcal Diet liquid
Nestlé Clinical Nutrition

Repel 100 pump spray
Wisconsin Pharmacal

Repel Classic Sportsmen Formula Unscented aerosol spray
Wisconsin Pharmacal

Repel Family Formula Scented IPF 18 pump spray
Wisconsin Pharmacal

Repel Natural Citronella Towelettes wipe
Wisconsin Pharmacal

Repel Sportsmen Formula IPF 18 pump spray
Wisconsin Pharmacal

Repel Sportsmen Formula IPF 20 lotion
Wisconsin Pharmacal

Repel Unscented IPF 20, SPF 15 lotion
Wisconsin Pharmacal

Rephenyl caplet
Reese Chemical

Replete Complete liquid
Nestlé Clinical Nutrition

Replete with Fiber Complete liquid
Nestlé Clinical Nutrition

Repose PMS gum
GumTech

ReSource Bar
Novartis Nutrition

ReSource Yogurt Flavored Beverage
Novartis Nutrition

Retre-Gel gel
Triton Consumer

Sarnol-HC lotion
Stiefel Labs

Saw Palmetto Complex 95 mg softgel
American Health

Saw Palmetto Extract softgel
NaturPharma

Saw Palmetto Plus 160 mg capsule
Shaklee

Saw Palmetto-Power 160 softgel
Nature's Herbs

Saw Palmetto-Power 320 softgel
Nature's Herbs

Saw Palmetto-Power softgel
Nature's Herbs

Sayman Salve ointment
Merz Consumer

Scandishake individual packet
Scandipharm

Scandishake (Sweetened with Aspartame) individual packet
Scandipharm

Scope, Baking Soda liquid
Procter & Gamble

Scot-Tussin Diabetes CF liquid
Scot-Tussin Pharmacal

Selsun Blue 2-in-1 Treatment shampoo
Ross Products/Abbott Labs

Selsun Blue Moisturizing Treatment shampoo
Ross Products/Abbott Labs

Sensodyne Original Flavor paste
Dentco

Sensodyne Tartar Control paste
Dentco

Siberian Ginseng 418 mg capsule
MMS Professional

Siberian Ginseng Power-Herb 404 mg capsule
Nature's Herbs

Sinadrin Plus tablet
Reese Chemical

Sindadrin Super tablet
Reese Chemical

Sine-Off Sinus, Cold, and Flu Medicine Night Time Formula gel caplet
Hogil Ph'cal

Skedaddle! for Children SPF 15 lotion
Minnetonka Brands

Skedaddle! lotion
Minnetonka Brands

Skin Magic lotion
Care-Tech Labs

Skin Miracle pump spray
Breckenridge Ph'cal

Sleep-Ettes D caplet
Reese Chemical

Small Drainable One-Piece Pouches
Coloplast

Small Drainable Two-Piece Pouches
Coloplast

Small Urostomy Two-Piece Pouches
Coloplast

Snoopy Sunblock pump spray
Minnetonka Brands

Snoopy Sunblock SPF 15 Plus Insect Protection lotion
Minnetonka Brands

Snug Cushions sponge
Mentholatum

Soft Skin After Bath Oil pump spray
Care-Tech Labs

Soft Touch Lancet
Boehringer Mannheim

Solar Gel SPF 15 Plus Insect Protection lotion
Minnetonka Brands

Solar pump spray
Minnetonka Brands

SOLO·care solution
CIBA Vision/Novartis

St. John's Wort capsule
Natrol

St. John's Wort Extract 150 mg capsule
Nature's Resource/Pharmavite

St. John's Wort Extract 375 mg capsule
NaturPharma

St. John's-Power 0.3% capsule
Nature's Herbs

St. John's-Power capsule
Nature's Herbs

Standard Drainable One-Piece Pouches
Coloplast

Standard Drainable Two-Piece Pouches
Coloplast

Standard Urostomy Two-Piece Pouches
Coloplast

Stevens Lip Cream SPF 15
Stevens Skin Softener

Sudafed Children's Nasal Decongestant chewable tablet
Warner-Lambert Consumer

Sudafed Cold & Sinus liquid-cap
Warner-Lambert Consumer

Summer's Eve Disposable Douche, Ultra liquid
C. B. Fleet

Sun & Bug Stuff IPF 20, SPF 15 lotion
Wisconsin Pharmacal

Sun Ban 30 Moisturizing Lip Conditioner stick
Stanback

Sun Stuff lotion
Wisconsin Pharmacal

Sun Stuff stick
Wisconsin Pharmacal

Sunbeam Model 7624 Manual Digital B.P. Monitor
Sunbeam

Sunbeam Model 7654 Digital B.P. Monitor
Sunbeam

Sunbeam Model 7685 Digital Wrist Unit B.P. Monitor
Sunbeam

Super Sunblock cream
ICN Ph'cals

Supreme II
Chronimed

Sure-Dose Plus Syringe
Terumo Medical

Sure-Dose Syringe
Terumo Medical

SureLac chewable tablet
Caraco Ph'cal Labs

SureStep
LifeScan

Sweedish-Formula Creme cream
Palco Labs

Tagamet HB 200 tablet
SmithKline Beecham

Tempra Quicklet tablet
Bristol-Myers Products

tenderfoot
Biocare

Tenderlett
Biocare

Tetra-Formula lozenge
Reese Chemical

Theracaps caplet
Reese Chemical

Theracof liquid
Reese Chemical

TheraFlu Max. Strength Flu, Cold & Cough Medicine NightTime caplet
Novartis Consumer

TheraPatch transdermal patch
CNS

Thex Forte Caplets
Lee Consumer

TI-Screen Cooling spray
Pedinol Pharmacal

TI-Screen Sunless Tanning Creme cream
Pedinol Pharmacal

Tiseb shampoo
Allerderm Labs

Tiseb-T shampoo
Allerderm Labs

Topifram Age Spot Fade Cream cream
E. T. Browne Drug

Topifram Traitement Dermatologiste Moisturising lotion
E. T. Browne Drug

Torbot Healskin Powder
Torbot

Torbot PeeWees Pediatric Urine Collection bag
Torbot

Total Antioxidant Softgels
Celestial Seasonings

Travasorb HN powder
Nestlé Clinical Nutrition

Travasorb MCT powder
Nestlé Clinical Nutrition

Travasorb STD powder
Nestlé Clinical Nutrition

Tri-Biozene ointment
Reese Chemical

Triple Hormone tablet
Young Again

Trojan Ultra Pleasure latex
Carter Products

Trojan Ultra Pleasure with Spermicide latex
Carter Products

Tums E-X Sugar Free chewable tablet
SmithKline Beecham

Tylenol Children's Flu liquid
McNeil Consumer

Tylenol Cold Severe Congestion Multi-Symptom caplet
McNeil Consumer

Tylenol Junior Strength, Fruit Burst chewable tablet
McNeil Consumer

Tylenol, Children's Fruit Burst chewable tablet
McNeil Consumer

Ultra Active Saw Palmetto 160 mg softgel
PhytoPharmica

Ultra Active Valerian & Passion Flower 495 mg tablet
NaturaLife

Ultra Brite Baking Soda & Peroxide paste
Colgate-Palmolive

Uristat tablet
Advanced Care Products

UroFemme tablet
Kramer Labs

UTI Home Screening
Consumers Choice

Vagistat-1 ointment
Bristol-Myers Products

Valerian Evening Formula capsule
Natrol

Valerian-Power 455 mg capsule
Nature's Herbs

Vaseline Dual Action Alpha Hydroxy Formula cream
Chesebrough-Pond's

Verazinc capsule
Forest Ph'cals

Vicks Chloraseptic Cough and Throat Drops, Cherry or Lemon lozenge
Procter & Gamble

Vicks Chloraseptic Cough and Throat Drops, Menthol lozenge
Procter & Gamble

Vince powder
Lee Consumer

Viractin cream or gel
Schering-Plough Healthcare

Vita ACES+ Gum
GumTech

Vita-Ray Creme cream
Gordon Labs

Vitex Extract capsule
NaturPharma

Wearever Reusable, Washable Briefs (Universal)
Wearever Health Care

Wearever Reusable, Washable Briefs For Men
Wearever Health Care

Wearever Reusable, Washable Briefs For Women
Wearever Health Care

Witch Hazel Hemorrhoidal Pads
T. N. Dickinson

Wondergel Personal Liquid gel
Lake Consumer

XS Hangover Relief liquid
Lee Consumer

Zilactin Baby gel
Zila Ph'cals

Zinc tablet
Natrol

Products for Patients with Special Needs

Note: These special needs designations were provided by the manufacturers and are not necessarily comprehensive. Because the designations have not been independently verified, use this list only to locate products that might meet special needs.

Some brand names of phytomedicinal products include the total weight of the solid dosage forms, not the weight of the active ingredients alone.

ALCOHOL FREE

ANTACID AND ANTIREFLUX PRODUCTS
Phillips' Milk of Magnesia Concentrate, Strawberry

ANTIEMETIC PRODUCTS
Dramamine, Children's
Rekematol Anti-Nausea
Triptone

ASTHMA INHALANT PRODUCTS
Asthma Haler
Asthma Nefrin
Broncho Saline
Sodium Chloride Inhalation Solution USP

COLD, COUGH, AND ALLERGY PRODUCTS
Benadryl Allergy
Benadryl Allergy Decongestant
Benadryl Allergy Dye-Free
Benylin Adult Cough Formula
Benylin Cough Suppressant Expectorant
Benylin Multi-Symptom Formula
Benylin Pediatric Cough Formula
Bromfed
Buckley's DM
Buckley's Mixture
Chlor-Trimeton 4-hour Allergy
Clear Cough DM
Clear Cough Night Time
Codimal
Codimal DM
Codimal PH
Delsym Extended Release
Demazin
Diabe-tuss DM
Diabetic Tussin Allergy Relief
Diabetic Tussin DM
Diabetic Tussin DM Maximum Strength
Diabetic Tussin EX
Diabetic Tussin, Children's
Dimetapp
Dimetapp Allergy, Children's
Dimetapp Cold & Fever, Children's
Dimetapp Decongestant, Pediatric
Dimetapp DM
Dorcol Children's Cough
Double Tussin DM
Guaifed
Hayfebrol
Ipsatol
Naldecon DX, Adult
Naldecon DX, Children's
Naldecon DX, Pediatric

Naldecon EX, Children's
Naldecon EX, Pediatric
Naldecon Senior DX
Naldecon Senior EX
Pedia Care Cough-Cold Formula
Pedia Care Infants' Decongestant
Pedia Care Infants' Decongestant Plus Cough
Pedia Care Night Rest Cough-Cold Formula
Pertussin CS
Protac SF
Redacon DX
REM Liquid
Robitussin
Robitussin CF
Robitussin Night Relief
Robitussin PE
Robitussin Pediatric
Robitussin Pediatric Cough
Robitussin Pediatric Cough & Cold
Robitussin Pediatric Night Relief
Safe Tussin 30
Scot-Tussin Allergy Relief Formula
Scot-Tussin Diabetes CF
Scot-Tussin DM
Scot-Tussin Expectorant
Scot-Tussin Original
Scot-Tussin Senior
St. Joseph Cough Suppressant for Children
Sudafed Children's Cold & Cough
Sudafed Children's Nasal Decongestant
Sudafed Pediatric Nasal Decongestant
Theracof
Triaminic AM, Non-Drowsy Cough & Decongestant Formula
Triaminic AM, Non-Drowsy Decongestant Formula
Triaminic DM, Cough Relief
Triaminic Expectorant, Chest & Head Congestion
Triaminic Infant, Oral Decongestant
Triaminic Night Time
Triaminic Sore Throat, Throat Pain & Cough
Triaminic, Cold & Allergy
Triaminicol Multi-Symptom Relief
Tussar-DM
Tylenol Children's Cold Multi-Symptom
Tylenol Children's Cold Plus Cough
Tylenol Infants' Cold Decongestant and Fever Reducer

Vicks 44e Pediatric Cough & Chest Congestion Relief
Vicks 44m Pediatric Cough & Cold Relief
Vicks DayQuil Children's Allergy Relief
Vicks DayQuil Multi-Symptom Cold/Flu Relief
Vicks NyQuil Children's Cold/Cough Medicine

INTERNAL ANALGESIC AND ANTIPYRETIC PRODUCTS
Acetaminophen Suspension, Children's Flavored
Aspirin Free, Infants'
Liquiprin for Children
Motrin, Children's
Tempra 1
Tempra 2
Tylenol, Children's Bubble Gum Flavor
Tylenol, Children's Cherry
Tylenol, Children's Cherry or Grape
Tylenol; Infants' Suspension, Cherry or Grape

IRON PRODUCTS
Feostat

LAXATIVE PRODUCTS
Fleet Babylax
Fleet Glycerin Rectal Applicators
Fleet Mineral Oil Oral Lubricant
Fletcher's Castoria
Haleys M-O, Flavored or Regular
Kellogg's Tasteless Castor Oil
Liqui-Doss
Phillips' Milk of Magnesia Concentrate, Strawberry
Phillips' Milk of Magnesia; Cherry, Mint, or Original
Senokot Children's
Therevac Plus
Therevac-SB

ORAL DISCOMFORT PRODUCTS
Amosan
Anbesol Baby, Grape
Anbesol Baby, Original
Baby Gumz
Campho-phenique
Dentapaine
Dentemp Temporary Filling Mix
Hurricaine, Wild Cherry or Pina Colada
Hurricaine; Wild Cherry, Pina Colada, or Watermelon
Little Teethers Oral Pain Relief
Orabase Baby
Orabase Lip Cream
Orabase Plain

Orabase-B with Benzocaine
Orajel Baby
Orajel Baby Nighttime Formula
Probax
SensoGARD
Zilactin Baby

ORAL HYGIENE PRODUCTS
Tech 2000 Antimicrobial Rinse
Tom's Natural Mouthwash, Cinnamon or
Spearmint

SORE THROAT PRODUCTS
Vicks Chloraseptic Sore Throat, Cherry
or Menthol

TOPICAL FLUORIDE PRODUCTS
Reach Act Adult Anti-Cavity Treatment,
Cinnamon
Reach Act Adult Anti-Cavity Treatment,
Mint
Reach Act for Kids

VITAMIN PRODUCTS
Adeks Drops
Kenwood Therapeutic Liquid
Kovitonic Liquid
LKV (Liquid Kiddie Vitamins) Drops
Poly-Vi-Sol Vitamin Drops
Poly-Vi-Sol with Iron Vitamin Drops
Theragran High Potency Multivitamin
Liquid
Tri-Vi-Sol Vitamins A,D+C Drops
Tri-Vi-Sol With Iron Vitamin A,D+C
Drops
Vitalize Liquid

ASPIRIN FREE

**ANTACID AND ANTIREFLUX
PRODUCTS**
XS Hangover Relief

CALCIUM PRODUCTS
Os-Cal 500

**COLD, COUGH, AND ALLERGY
PRODUCTS**
A.R.M. Caplet
Actifed
Actifed Allergy Daytime/Nighttime
Actifed Sinus Daytime/Nighttime
Advil Cold & Sinus
Alka-Seltzer Plus Cold & Cough
Medicine Liqui-Gels
Alka-Seltzer Plus Cold Medicine Liqui-
Gels
Alka-Seltzer Plus Flu & Body Aches
Liqui-Gels
Allerest Maximum Strength
Allerest No Drowsiness
Allergy Relief
Benadryl Allergy
Benadryl Allergy Decongestant
Benadryl Allergy/Cold
Benadryl Allergy/Sinus/Headache
Formula
Cepacol Sore Throat Maximum Strength,
Cherry
Cepacol Sore Throat Maximum Strength,
Mint
Cepacol Sore Throat Regular Strength,
Cherry
Cepacol Sore Throat Regular Strength,
Original Mint
Chlor-Trimeton 6-Hour Allergy, Sinus,
Headache

Codimal
Coldonyl
Comtrex Allergy-Sinus
Comtrex Deep Chest Cold and Conges-
tion Relief
Comtrex Maximum Strength
Comtrex Maximum Strength Cold and
Flu Relief
Comtrex Maximum Strength Day & Night
Comtrex Maximum Strength Non-
Drowsy
Comtrex Maximum Strength Non-
Drowsy Cold and Flu Relief
Congestac
Coricidin Cold & Flu
Coricidin D
Dristan Cold Maximum Strength No
Drowsiness
Dristan Cold Multi-Symptom
Dristan Cold Multi-Symptom Maximum
Strength
Dristan Sinus
Drixoral Allergy Sinus
Drixoral Cold & Flu
Efidac/24
Emagrin Forte
Excedrin Sinus Maximum Strength
Hay Fever & Allergy Relief Maximum
Strength
Hytuss
Hytuss 2X
Motrin IB Sinus
Napril
Nasal-D
ND-Gesic
Nolahist
Oranyl
Oranyl Plus
Pedia Care Cough-Cold Formula
Propagest
Pyrroxate
Ricola Cough Drops, Original Flavor
Ricola Sugar Free Herb Throat Drops,
Alpine-Mint
Ricola Sugar Free Herb Throat Drops,
Cherry- or Lemon-Mint
Ricola Sugar Free Herb Throat Drops,
Mountain Herb
Ricola Throat Drops, Cherry-Mint
Ricola Throat Drops, Honey-Herb
Ricola Throat Drops, Lemon-Mint or
Orange-Mint
Ricola Throat Drops, Menthol-Eucalyptus
Scot-Tussin DM Cough Chasers
Sinarest Extra Strength
Sinarest Sinus Medicine
Sine-Aid IB
Sine-Aid Maximum Strength
Sine-Off Sinus, Cold, and Flu Medicine
Night Time Formula
Sinulin
Sinus Relief Extra Strength
Sinutab Non-Drying
Sinutab Sinus Allergy Medication
Maximum Strength
Sinutab Sinus without Drowsiness
Maximum Strength
Sudafed
Sudafed 12-Hour Extended Release
Sudafed Children's Nasal Decongestant
Sudafed Cold & Cough
Sudafed Cold & Sinus
Sudafed Severe Cold Formula

Sudafed Sinus Non-Drowsy Maximum
Strength
Sudafed Sinus Non-Drying Non-Drowsy
Maximum Strength
Tavist-1 Antihistamine
Tavist-D Antihistamine/Nasal Deconges-
tant
TheraFlu Flu and Cold Medicine
TheraFlu Flu, Cold, & Cough Medicine
TheraFlu Max. Strength Flu & Cold
Medicine For Sore Throat
TheraFlu Max. Strength Flu, Cold &
Cough Medicine NightTime
Theraflu Maximum Strength Non-Drowsy
TheraFlu Maximum Strength Sinus Non-
Drowsy
Triaminicin
Tuss-DM
Tylenol Allergy Sinus Maximum Strength
Tylenol Allergy Sinus NightTime
Maximum Strength
Tylenol Children's Cold Multi-Symptom
Tylenol Children's Cold Plus Cough
Tylenol Children's Flu
Tylenol Cold Medication Multi-Symptom
Formula
Tylenol Cold Multi-Symptom
Tylenol Cold No Drowsiness Formula
Tylenol Cold Severe Congestion Multi-
Symptom
Tylenol Cough Multi-Symptom
Tylenol Cough with Decongestant Multi-
Symptom
Tylenol Flu Maximum Strength
Tylenol Flu NightTime Maximum
Strength
Tylenol Flu NightTime Maximum
Strength Hot Medication
Tylenol Infants' Cold Decongestant and
Fever Reducer
Tylenol Severe Allergy Maximum
Strength
Tylenol Sinus Maximum Strength
Vicks 44 Cough, Cold, & Flu Relief
LiquiCaps
Vicks 44 Non-Drowsy Cough & Cold
Relief LiquiCaps
Vicks DayQuil Allergy Relief 12-Hour
Vicks DayQuil Multi-Symptom Cold/Flu
Relief LiquiCaps
Vicks DayQuil Sinus Pressure &
Congestion Relief
Vicks DayQuil Sinus Pressure & Pain
Relief with Ibuprofen
Vicks Nyquil Hot Therapy
Vicks NyQuil Multi-Symptom Cold/Flu
Relief LiquiCaps

**INTERNAL ANALGESIC AND
ANTIPYRETIC PRODUCTS**
Acetaminophen Suspension, Children's
Flavored
Acetaminophen Uniserts
Actamin
Actamin Extra
Actamin Super
Actron
Advil
Advil, Children's
Advil, Junior Strength
Aleve
Alka-Seltzer
Aminofen
Aminofen Max

Anacin Aspirin Free Maximum Strength
Arthriten
Aspirin Free Pain & Fever Relief,
  Children's
Aspirin Free Pain Relief
Aspirin Free, Infants'
Azo-Dine [c]
Azo-Standard [c]
Backache from the Makers of Nuprin
Bromo-Seltzer
Doan's Extra Strength
Doan's Regular Strength
Dyspel
Excedrin Aspirin Free
Feverall Adult Strength
Feverall Junior Strength
Feverall Sprinkle Caps Powder,
  Children's Strength
Feverall Sprinkle Caps Powder, Junior
  Strength
Feverall, Children's
Feverall, Infants'
Haltran
Liquiprin for Children
Midol IB Cramp Relief Formula
Midol Menstrual Regular Strength
  Multisymptom Formula
Mobigesic
Momentum
Motrin IB
Motrin, Children's
Motrin, Junior Strength
Nuprin
Orudis KT
Percogesic Coated
Prodium [c]
Re-Azo [c]
Stanback AF Extra-Strength
Tapanol Extra Strength
Tempra 1
Tempra 2
Tempra 3
Tempra 3, Double Strength
Tempra Quicklet
Tylenol Extended Relief
Tylenol Extra Strength
Tylenol Extra Strength Adult
Tylenol Junior Strength Swallowable
Tylenol Junior Strength, Fruit Burst
Tylenol Junior Strength, Fruit Flavor
Tylenol Junior Strength, Grape
Tylenol Regular Strength
Tylenol, Children's Bubble Gum Flavor
Tylenol, Children's Cherry
Tylenol, Children's Cherry or Grape
Tylenol, Children's Fruit Burst
Tylenol, Children's Fruit Flavor
Tylenol, Children's Grape
Tylenol; Infants' Suspension, Cherry or
  Grape
Ultraprin
Valorin
Valorin Extra
Valorin Super
Valprin
XS Hangover Relief
MENSTRUAL PRODUCTS
Aqua-Ban
Backaid Pills
Diurex MPR
Diurex PMS
Diurex Water Caplet
Diurex-2 Water Pills

Lurline PMS
Midol Menstrual Maximum Strength
  Multisymptom Formula
Midol PMS Maximum Strength
  Multisymptom Formula
Midol PMS Multisymptom Formula
Midol Teen Multisymptom Formula
Odrinil Water Pills
Pamprin MultiSymptom Formula
Premsyn PMS
SLEEP AID PRODUCTS
Anacin P.M. Aspirin Free
Backaid PM Pills
Dormin
Excedrin PM
Melatonin PM Dual Release
Melatonin PM Fast Acting
Midol PM Night Time Formula
Nervine Nighttime Sleep-Aid
Nytol
Nytol Maximum Strength
Sleep Rite
Sleep-eze 3
Sleepinal
Sominex Maximum Strength
Sominex Original
Sominex Pain Relief Formula
Tranquil
Tranquil Plus
Tylenol PM Extra Strength
Unisom Nighttime Sleep Aid
Unisom Pain Relief
SORE THROAT PRODUCTS
Cepacol Sore Throat Maximum Strength,
  Cherry
Cepacol Sore Throat Maximum Strength,
  Cool Menthol
Cepacol Sore Throat Maximum Strength,
  Mint
Cepacol Sore Throat Regular Strength,
  Cherry
Cepacol Sore Throat Regular Strength,
  Original Mint
Ricola Cough Drops, Original Flavor
Ricola Sugar Free Herb Throat Drops,
  Alpine-Mint
Ricola Sugar Free Herb Throat Drops,
  Cherry- or Lemon-Mint
Ricola Sugar Free Herb Throat Drops,
  Mountain Herb
Ricola Throat Drops, Cherry-Mint
Ricola Throat Drops, Honey-Herb
Ricola Throat Drops, Lemon-Mint or
  Orange-Mint
Ricola Throat Drops, Menthol-Eucalyptus
Vicks Chloraseptic Sore Throat, Cherry
  or Menthol

CAFFEINE FREE

**COLD, COUGH, AND ALLERGY
PRODUCTS**
Nasal-D
**ENTERAL FOOD SUPPLEMENT
PRODUCTS**
Criticare HN
**INTERNAL ANALGESIC AND
ANTIPYRETIC PRODUCTS**
Acetaminophen Uniserts

Actamin
Actamin Extra
Aleve
Aminofen
Aminofen Max
Arthritis Pain Formula
Ascriptin Arthritis Pain
Ascriptin Maximum Strength
Ascriptin Regular Strength
Aspercin
Aspercin Extra
Aspergum, Cherry or Orange
Aspermin
Aspermin Extra
Aspirin Free Pain & Fever Relief,
  Children's
Aspirin Free Pain Relief
Aspirin Free, Infants'
Aspirtab
Aspirtab Max
Back-Quell
Backache from the Makers of Nuprin
Bayer 8-Hour Aspirin Extended-Release
Bayer Arthritis Pain Regimen Extra
  Strength
Bayer Aspirin Extra Strength
Bayer Aspirin Regimen Regular Strength
Bayer Aspirin, Genuine
Bayer Children's Aspirin, Cherry or
  Orange
Bayer Plus Extra Strength Buffered
  Aspirin
Bromo-Seltzer
Buffaprin
Buffaprin Extra
Buffasal
Buffasal Max
Bufferin Arthritis Strength, Tri-Buffered
Bufferin Extra Strength, Tri-Buffered
Bufferin, Tri-Buffered
Buffinol
Buffinol Extra
Doan's Extra Strength
Doan's Regular Strength
Dyspel
Feverall Adult Strength
Feverall Junior Strength
Feverall Sprinkle Caps Powder,
  Children's Strength
Feverall Sprinkle Caps Powder, Junior
  Strength
Feverall, Children's
Feverall, Infants'
Liquiprin for Children
Midol IB Cramp Relief Formula
Midol Menstrual Regular Strength
  Multisymptom Formula
Momentum
Motrin IB
Norwich Aspirin
Nuprin
Orudis KT
Percogesic Coated
Prodium [c]
Stanback AF Extra-Strength
Tempra 1
Tempra 2
Tempra 3
Tempra 3, Double Strength
Tempra Quicklet
Tylenol Extended Relief
Tylenol Extra Strength
Tylenol Extra Strength Adult

Tylenol Junior Strength Swallowable
Tylenol Junior Strength, Fruit Flavor
Tylenol Junior Strength, Grape
Tylenol Regular Strength
Tylenol, Children's Bubble Gum Flavor
Tylenol, Children's Cherry
Tylenol, Children's Cherry or Grape
Tylenol, Children's Fruit Flavor
Tylenol, Children's Grape
Tylenol; Infants' Suspension, Cherry or Grape
Ultraprin
Valorin
Valorin Extra
Valprin

MENSTRUAL PRODUCTS
Aqua-Ban
Backaid Pills
Diurex MPR
Diurex PMS
Diurex Water Caplet
Diurex-2 Water Pills
Lurline PMS
Midol PMS Maximum Strength Multisymptom Formula
Midol PMS Multisymptom Formula
Midol Teen Multisymptom Formula
Odrinil Water Pills
Pamprin Maximum Pain Relief
Pamprin MultiSymptom Formula
Premsyn PMS

ORAL DISCOMFORT PRODUCTS
Numzit Teething

VITAMIN PRODUCTS
Circus Chews with Iron

CHOLESTEROL FREE

ENTERAL FOOD SUPPLEMENT PRODUCTS
Citrotein
Comply
Deliver 2.0
Isocal
Isocal HN
Lipisorb
Magnacal Renal
MCT Oil
Microlipid
Moducal
NuBasics
NuBasics Plus
NuBasics VHP
NuBasics with Fiber
Protain XL
ReSource
ReSource Crystals
ReSource Fruit Beverage
ReSource Plus
Scandishake
Scandishake (Sweetened with Aspartame)
Scandishake Lactose Free
Sustacal Basic
Sustacal Plus
Sustacal with Fiber
Tolerex
Ultracal
Vivonex Pediatric

Vivonex Plus
Vivonex T.E.N.

LAXATIVE PRODUCTS
Metamucil Original Texture, Regular Flavor

DYE FREE

ANTACID AND ANTIREFLUX PRODUCTS
Arm & Hammer Pure Baking Soda
Dicarbosil
Gaviscon
Gaviscon Extra Strength
Gaviscon Extra Strength Liquid
Gaviscon-2
Maalox
Maalox Therapeutic Concentrate
Mag-Ox 400
Uro-Mag

ANTIDIARRHEAL PRODUCTS
Percy Medicine

ANTIEMETIC PRODUCTS
Nauzene

ANTIFLATULENT PRODUCTS
Baby Gasz
Charcoal
CharcoCaps
Little Tummys Infant Gas Relief
Phazyme Gas Relief

BLOOD SUGAR ELEVATING PRODUCTS
Glutose

CALCIUM PRODUCTS
Calci-Caps
Calci-Caps Super
Calci-Mix
Calcium Complex
Calcium Magnesium
Citracal
Citracal + D
Citracal Liquitab
Fem Cal
Mag/Cal Mega
Nephro-Calci
Os-Cal 500
Parvacal 500
Super Cal/Mag
Vita-Cal

COLD, COUGH, AND ALLERGY PRODUCTS
BC Allergy·Sinus·Cold
BC Sinus·Cold
Benadryl Allergy Dye-Free
Benadryl Allergy Dye-Free Liqui-gels
Buckley's DM
Buckley's Mixture
Clear Cough DM
Clear Cough Night Time
Codimal DM
Cough-X
Diabe-tuss DM
Diabetic Tussin Allergy Relief
Diabetic Tussin Cough Drops, Cherry
Diabetic Tussin Cough Drops, Menthol-Eucalyptus
Diabetic Tussin DM
Diabetic Tussin DM Liqui-Gels
Diabetic Tussin DM Maximum Strength
Diabetic Tussin DM Maximum Strength Liqui-Gels

Diabetic Tussin EX
Diabetic Tussin, Children's
Dimetapp Allergy, Children's
Hayfebrol
Herbal-Menthol
Nasal-D
Nolahist
Pinex Concentrate
Propagest
REM Liquid
Ricola Cough Drops, Original Flavor
Ricola Sugar Free Herb Throat Drops, Alpine-Mint
Ricola Sugar Free Herb Throat Drops, Cherry- or Lemon-Mint
Ricola Sugar Free Herb Throat Drops, Mountain Herb
Ricola Throat Drops, Cherry-Mint
Ricola Throat Drops, Honey-Herb
Ricola Throat Drops, Lemon-Mint or Orange-Mint
Ricola Throat Drops, Menthol-Eucalyptus
Safe Tussin 30
Scot-Tussin Allergy Relief Formula
Scot-Tussin Diabetes CF
Scot-Tussin DM
Scot-Tussin DM Cough Chasers
Scot-Tussin Expectorant
Scot-Tussin Original
Scot-Tussin Senior
Sudafed Pediatric Nasal Decongestant
TheraFlu Maximum Strength Sinus Non-Drowsy
Triaminic AM, Non-Drowsy Cough & Decongestant Formula
Triaminic AM, Non-Drowsy Decongestant Formula
Triaminic Infant, Oral Decongestant

DENTIFRICE PRODUCTS
Arm & Hammer Dental Care
Arm & Hammer Dental Care Toothpowder
Arm & Hammer PeroxiCare
Crest Sensitivity Protection, Mild Mint
Dr. Tichenor's Toothpaste
Gleem
Pearl Drops Whitening Baking Soda Tartar Control
Pearl Drops Whitening Extra Strength
Pearl Drops Whitening Regular Tartar Control
Pearl Drops Whitening Toothpolish, Spearmint
Rembrandt Whitening Natural
Revelation
Sensodyne Baking Soda
Sensodyne Tartar Control

ENTERAL FOOD SUPPLEMENT PRODUCTS
Casec
Choice dm
Criticare HN
Deliver 2.0
Isocal
Isocal HN
Lipisorb
Magnacal Renal
MCT Oil
Microlipid
Moducal
Protain XL
Respalor
Sustacal

TraumaCal
Ultracal
GASTRIC DECONTAMINANT PRODUCTS
CharcoAid G
HERBAL AND PHYTOMEDICINAL PRODUCTS
Asian Ginseng Complex
Bilberry Extract
Bilberry-Power
Cayenne
Cayenne Extract
Cayenne Pepper
Cayenne Power-Herb
Chaste Tree Berry Extract
Cranberry
Cranberry-Power
Daily Garlic
Daily Ginseng
Echinacea
Echinacea-Power
Evening Primrose Oil
Feverfew
Feverfew Extract
Feverfew-Power
Garlic-Power
Ginger Extract
Ginger Root
Ginger-Power
Ginkgo Extract
Ginkgo-Power
Ginseng Extract
Grape Seed-Power 100
Grape Seed-Power 50
Korean Ginseng Power-Herb
Lemon Balm Extract
Milk Thistle Extract
Milk-Thistle Power
Primrose-Power
Saw Palmetto Extract
Saw Palmetto-Power
Saw Palmetto-Power 160
Saw Palmetto-Power 320
Siberian Ginseng
Siberian Ginseng Extract
Siberian Ginseng Power-Herb
St. John's Wort
St. John's Wort Extract
St. John's-Power
St. John's-Power 0.3%
Super Echinacea Extract
Super Echinacea Liquid Extract
Ultra Active Bilberry
Ultra Active Garlic Enteric Coated
Ultra Active Ginkgo Biloba
Ultra Active Milk Thistle
Ultra Active Valerian & Passion Flower
Ultra Active Vitex
Valerian Extract
Valerian Plus
Valerian-Power
Vitex Extract
HISTAMINE II RECEPTOR ANTAGONISTS
Tagamet HB 200
INFANTS' AND CHILDREN'S FORMULA PRODUCTS
Enfamil
Enfamil Human Milk Fortifier
Enfamil Next Step Soy
Enfamil Premature Formula
Enfamil Premature Formula with Iron
Enfamil with Iron

Gerber Baby Formula Low Iron
Gerber Baby Formula with Iron
Gerber Soy Baby Formula
Kindercal
Lactofree
Lofenalac
MSUD Diet
Nutramigen
Phenyl-Free
Portagen
Pregestimil
ProSobee
INTERNAL ANALGESIC AND ANTIPYRETIC PRODUCTS
Arthriten
BC
BC Arthritis Strength
Goody's Extra Strength
Goody's Extra Strength Headache
Mobigesic
Motrin IB
Supac
IRON PRODUCTS
Feostat
Fer-In-Sol
Iron Plus Vitamin C
Niferex
LAXATIVE PRODUCTS
Ceo-Two
Fiber Naturale
Kellogg's Tasteless Castor Oil
Mag-Ox 400
Metamucil Fiber Wafer, Apple Crisp or Cinnamon Spice
Metamucil Original Texture, Regular Flavor
Metamucil Smooth Texture, Sugar Free Regular Flavor
Uro-Mag
MISCELLANEOUS MINERAL PRODUCTS
Chromium, Organic
Manganese Chelate
Maxi-Minerals
Selenium, Oceanic
Verazinc
Zinc
ORAL DISCOMFORT PRODUCTS
Dent-Zel-Ite Oral Mucosal Analgesic
Dentemp Temporary Filling Mix
Hurricaine, Wild Cherry
Hurricaine, Wild Cherry or Pina Colada
Hurricaine; Wild Cherry, Pina Colada, or Watermelon
Lipmagik
Little Teethers Oral Pain Relief
Probax
Proxigel
Zilactin Baby
ORAL HYGIENE PRODUCTS
Dr. Tichenor's Antiseptic
ORAL REHYDRATION SOLUTIONS
Infalyte
SLEEP AID PRODUCTS
Arthriten PM
Nytol
Tranquil
Tranquil Plus
SORE THROAT PRODUCTS
Entertainer's Secret Throat Relief
Herbal-Menthol
Ricola Cough Drops, Original Flavor
Ricola Sugar Free Herb Throat Drops, Alpine-Mint

Ricola Sugar Free Herb Throat Drops, Cherry- or Lemon-Mint
Ricola Sugar Free Herb Throat Drops, Mountain Herb
Ricola Throat Drops, Cherry-Mint
Ricola Throat Drops, Honey-Herb
Ricola Throat Drops, Lemon-Mint or Orange-Mint
Ricola Throat Drops, Menthol-Eucalyptus
TOPICAL FLUORIDE PRODUCTS
Fluorigard Anti-Cavity
VITAMIN PRODUCTS
A-D-E with Selenium Tablets
Adeks Chewable Tablets
Adeks Drops
C Vitamin Tablets
C Vitamin Timed-Release Tablets
Centrum High Potency Liquid
Clinical Nutrients for Men Tablets
Clinical Nutrients for Women Tablets
Coldvac Lozenges
DiabeVite Tablets
Freedavite Tablets
Fruit C Chewable Tablets
Geri-Freeda Tablets
Gevrabon Liquid
Jets Chewable Tablets
Kovitonic Liquid
KPN (Key Prenatal) Tablets
LKV (Liquid Kiddie Vitamins) Drops
Monocaps Tablets
Natalins Tablets
Nephro-Vite Tablets
Oxi-Freeda Tablets
Parvlex Tablets
Pro-Pep Chewable Tablets
Quintabs-M Tablets
Super A&D Tablets
Super Dec B-100 Coated Tablets
Super Quints-50 Tablets
Theragran High Potency Multivitamin Liquid
Ultra-Freeda Tablets
Unilife-A Gelcaps
Vitalets Chewable Tablets, Flavored or Unflavored
Vitalize Liquid

FLUORIDE FREE

DENTIFRICE PRODUCTS
Tom's Natural Baking Soda with Propolis & Myrrh
Tom's Natural with Propolis & Myrrh
Viadent Original

FRAGRANCE FREE

DRY SKIN PRODUCTS
Allercreme
Allercreme Moisturizer with Sunsreen SPF 8
Alpha Glow Body Care Lotion with SPF 16
Alpha Glow Day Cream with SPF 16
Aveeno Bath Treatment Moisturizing Formula

Aveeno Bath Treatment Soothing
  Formula
Aveeno for Combination Skin
Aveeno for Dry Skin
Aveeno Gentle Skin Cleanser
Aveeno Moisturizing
Aveeno Shower & Bath
Cetaphil Gentle Cleanser
Cetaphil Moisturizing
Complex 15 Therapeutic Moisturizing
Curél Alpha Hydroxy
Curél Therapeutic Moisturizing,
  Fragrance-Free or Scented
Dermal Therapy Extra Strength Body
Dermsol
DiabetiDerm
DML Facial Moisturizer
DML Forte
Gormel
Jergens Advanced Therapy Dual Healing
Jergens Advanced Therapy Ultra
  Healing, Reg. or Frag. Free
Johnson's Ultra Sensitive Baby Cream
Johnson's Ultra Sensitive Baby Lotion
Keri Silky Smooth, Fragrance Free or
  Sensitive Skin
Lac-Hydrin Five
Little Noses Saline Moisturizing
Moisturel
Moisturel Sensitive Skin
Neutrogena Norwegian Formula
  Emulsion
Pen-Kera
Physicians Formula Self Defense
  Moisturizing SPF 15
Plexolan Moisturizing
Shepards Cream Lotion
Shepards Skin Cream
Silk Solution
Soft Sense Alpha Hydroxy Moisturizing
Soft Sense Moisturizing, Fragrance Free
  or Original
Stevens Skin Softener
Theraplex Hydrolotion
U-Lactin
Vita-Ray Creme
FEMININE HYGIENE PRODUCTS
Massengill Medicated Disposable
  Douche
Norforms, Unscented
SUNSCREEN AND SUNTAN PRODUCTS
Banana Boat Maximum Sunblock
Banana Boat Sport Sunblock
BioShield Facial Sunblock for Normal or
  for Sensitive Skin
Dermsol-30
DuraScreen
Nivea Sun Kids
PreSun 46 Moisturizing
TI-Baby Natural Sunblock
TI-Screen Moisturizing
TI-Screen Moisturizing Lip Protectant
TI-Screen Natural Sunblock
TI-Screen Sports
VAGINAL LUBRICANT PRODUCTS
Born Again Vaginal Moisturizing
K-Y Long Lasting
Maxilube

GLUTEN FREE

**ANTACID AND ANTIREFLUX
PRODUCTS**
Almora
Arm & Hammer Pure Baking Soda
Dicarbosil
Gaviscon Extra Strength Liquid
Gaviscon Liquid
Maalox
Maalox Heartburn Relief
Maalox Therapeutic Concentrate
Mag-Ox 400
Phillips' Milk of Magnesia
Tums E-X Extra Strength, Wintergreen or
  Asst. Fruit Flavors
Tums Ultra, Fruit or Mint Flavors
Tums, Peppermint or Asst. Fruit Flavors
Uro-Mag
ANTIDIARRHEAL PRODUCTS
Diar Aid
Diasorb
Kaopectate
Pepto-Bismol
Pepto-Bismol, Cherry
ANTIEMETIC PRODUCTS
Dramamine
Dramamine Original
Nauzene
ANTIFLATULENT PRODUCTS
Charcoal
CharcoCaps
Gas-X
Gas-X Extra Strength
Maalox Antacid/Anti-Gas Extra Strength
Riopan Plus
Riopan Plus Double Strength
Tums Anti-Gas/Antacid
APPETITE SUPPRESSANT PRODUCTS
Acutrim 16 Hour Steady Control
Acutrim Late Day Strength
Acutrim Maximum Strength
Amfed T.D.
Dexatrim Caffeine Free Extended
  Duration
Dexatrim Caffeine Free Maximum
  Strength
Dexatrim Caffeine Free with Vitamin C
Dieutrim T.D.
Protrim S.R.
Thinz-Span
ASTHMA ORAL PRODUCTS
Bronkaid Dual Action Formula
Primatene
BLOOD SUGAR ELEVATING PRODUCTS
Insta-Glucose
CALCIUM PRODUCTS
Calcet
Calci-Caps
Calci-Caps Super
Calci-Caps with Iron
Calci-Chew; Cherry, Lemon, or Orange
Calci-Mix
Calcium Complex
Caltrate 600 High Potency
Caltrate 600 High Potency+ D
Caltrate Plus
Caltrate Plus Nutrient Enriched,
  Spearmint
Citracal
Citracal + D
Citracal Liquitab
Citron

Fem Cal
Florical
Mag/Cal Mega
Nephro-Calci
Os-Cal 250 + D
Os-Cal 500
Os-Cal 500 + D
Oyster Calcium
Oyster Calcium 500 + D
Oystercal 500
Oystercal-D 250
Parvacal 500
Posture
Posture-D
Super Cal/Mag
Tums 500; Asst. Fruit or Peppermint
Vita-Cal
**COLD, COUGH, AND ALLERGY
PRODUCTS**
Actifed
Allerest Maximum Strength
Allerest No Drowsiness
Allergy Relief
Buckley's DM
Buckley's Mixture
Cepacol Sore Throat Maximum Strength,
  Cherry
Cepacol Sore Throat Maximum Strength,
  Mint
Cepacol Sore Throat Regular Strength,
  Cherry
Cepacol Sore Throat Regular Strength,
  Original Mint
Comtrex Allergy-Sinus
Comtrex Deep Chest Cold and Conges-
  tion Relief
Comtrex Maximum Strength
Comtrex Maximum Strength Cold and
  Flu Relief
Comtrex Maximum Strength Day & Night
Comtrex Maximum Strength Non-
  Drowsy
Comtrex Maximum Strength Non-
  Drowsy Cold and Flu Releif
Dristan Cold Maximum Strength No
  Drowsiness
Dristan Cold Multi-Symptom
Dristan Cold Multi-Symptom Maximum
  Strength
Dristan Sinus
Efidac/24
Excedrin Sinus Maximum Strength
Fisherman's Friend, Extra Strong, Sugar
  Free
Fisherman's Friend, Licorice Strong
Fisherman's Friend, Original Extra Strong
Fisherman's Friend, Refreshing Mint,
  Sugar Free
Hay Fever & Allergy Relief Maximum
  Strength
Hayfebrol
Herbal-Menthol
Hytuss
Hytuss 2X
Napril
Nasal-D
ND-Gesic
Nolahist
Propagest
Ricola Cough Drops, Original Flavor
Ricola Sugar Free Herb Throat Drops,
  Alpine-Mint

Ricola Sugar Free Herb Throat Drops,
Cherry- or Lemon-Mint
Ricola Sugar Free Herb Throat Drops,
Mountain Herb
Ricola Throat Drops, Cherry-Mint
Ricola Throat Drops, Honey-Herb
Ricola Throat Drops, Lemon-Mint or
Orange-Mint
Ricola Throat Drops, Menthol-Eucalyptus
Scot-Tussin Allergy Relief Formula
Scot-Tussin Diabetes CF
Scot-Tussin DM
Scot-Tussin DM Cough Chasers
Scot-Tussin Expectorant
Scot-Tussin Original
Scot-Tussin Senior
Sinarest Extra Strength
Sinarest Sinus Medicine
Sine-Off Sinus, Cold, and Flu Medicine
Night Time Formula
Sinus Relief Extra Strength
Tavist-1 Antihistamine
TheraFlu Flu and Cold Medicine
TheraFlu Flu, Cold, & Cough Medicine
TheraFlu Max. Strength Flu, Cold &
Cough Medicine NightTime
Triaminicin
Tuss-DM
Vicks DayQuil Allergy Relief 12-Hour
Vicks DayQuil Multi-Symptom Cold/Flu
Relief LiquiCaps
Vicks DayQuil Sinus Pressure &
Congestion Relief
Vicks Nyquil Hot Therapy
Vicks NyQuil Multi-Symptom Cold/Flu
Relief LiquiCaps

**ENTERAL FOOD SUPPLEMENT
PRODUCTS**
Advera
Boost
Casec
Choice dm
Citrotein
Compleat Pediatric
Comply
Criticare HN
Deliver 2.0
Ensure
Ensure High Protein
Ensure Light
Ensure Plus
Ensure Plus HN
Ensure with Fiber
Forta Drink
Glucerna
Impact
Impact 1.5
Impact with Fiber
Isocal
Isocal HN
IsoSource 1.5 Cal
IsoSource VHN
Isotein HN
Jevity
Lipisorb
Magnacal Renal
MCT Oil
Meritene
Microlipid
Moducal
Nepro
NuBasics
NuBasics Plus

NuBasics VHP
NuBasics with Fiber
Nutren 1.0 Complete
Nutren 1.0 with Fiber Complete
Nutren 1.5 Complete
Nutren 2.0 Complete
Osmolite
Osmolite HN
Peptamen Complete
Peptamen Junior Complete
Peptamen VHP Complete
Perative
Polycose
ProBalance Complete
Promote
Protain XL
Pulmocare
Renalcal Diet
Replete Complete
Replete with Fiber Complete
ReSource Crystals
ReSource Diabetic
ReSource Just for Kids
ReSource Yogurt Flavored Beverage
Respalor
SandoSource Peptide
Scandishake
Scandishake (Sweetened with Aspar-
tame)
Suplena
Sustacal
Sustacal Basic
Sustacal Plus
Sustacal with Fiber
Tolerex
TraumaCal
Travasorb HN
Travasorb MCT
Travasorb STD
Two Cal HN
Vital High Nitrogen
Vivonex Pediatric
Vivonex Plus
Vivonex T.E.N.

**GASTRIC DECONTAMINANT
PRODUCTS**
CharcoAid G

**HERBAL AND PHYTOMEDICINAL
PRODUCTS**
Bilberry Extract
Bilberry-Power
Cayenne
Cayenne Extract
Cayenne Pepper
Cayenne Power-Herb
Chaste Tree Berry Extract
Cranberry
Cranberry-Power
Daily Garlic
Daily Ginseng
Echinacea
Echinacea-Power
Evening Primrose Oil
Feverfew
Feverfew Extract
Feverfew-Power
Garlic-Power
Ginger Extract
Ginger Root
Ginger-Power
Ginkgo Extract
Ginkgo-Power
Ginseng Extract

Grape Seed-Power 100
Grape Seed-Power 50
Korean Ginseng Power-Herb
Lemon Balm Extract
Milk Thistle Extract
Milk-Thistle Power
Primrose-Power
Saw Palmetto Extract
Saw Palmetto-Power
Saw Palmetto-Power 160
Saw Palmetto-Power 320
Siberian Ginseng
Siberian Ginseng Extract
Siberian Ginseng Power-Herb
St. John's Wort
St. John's Wort Extract
St. John's-Power
St. John's-Power 0.3%
Super Echinacea Extract
Super Echinacea Liquid Extract
Ultra Active Bilberry
Ultra Active Garlic Enteric Coated
Ultra Active Ginkgo Biloba
Ultra Active Milk Thistle
Ultra Active Valerian & Passion Flower
Ultra Active Vitex
Valerian Extract
Valerian-Power
Vitex Extract

**HISTAMINE II RECEPTOR
ANTAGONISTS**
Axid AR
Tagamet HB 200

**INFANTS' AND CHILDREN'S FORMULA
PRODUCTS**
Enfamil
Enfamil Human Milk Fortifier
Enfamil Next Step
Enfamil Next Step Soy
Enfamil Premature Formula
Enfamil Premature Formula with Iron
Enfamil with Iron
Gerber Baby Formula Low Iron
Gerber Baby Formula with Iron
Gerber Soy Baby Formula
Kindercal
Lactofree
Lofenalac
MSUD Diet
Nutramigen
PediaSure with Fiber
Phenyl-Free
Portagen
Pregestimil
ProSobee

**INTERNAL ANALGESIC AND
ANTIPYRETIC PRODUCTS**
Acetaminophen Uniserts
Aleve
Arthriten
Arthritis Pain Formula
Aspergum, Cherry or Orange
Aspirin Free Pain & Fever Relief,
Children's
Aspirin Free Pain Relief
Bayer 8-Hour Aspirin Extended-Release
Bayer Arthritis Pain Regimen Extra
Strength
Bayer Aspirin Extra Strength
Bayer Aspirin Regimen Regular Strength
Bayer Aspirin, Genuine
Bayer Children's Aspirin, Cherry or
Orange

Bayer Plus Extra Strength Buffered
  Aspirin
Doan's Extra Strength
Doan's Regular Strength
Excedrin Extra Strength
Feverall Adult Strength
Feverall Junior Strength
Feverall Sprinkle Caps Powder,
  Children's Strength
Feverall Sprinkle Caps Powder, Junior
  Strength
Feverall, Children's
Feverall, Infants'
Midol IB Cramp Relief Formula
Midol Menstrual Regular Strength
  Multisymptom Formula
Mobigesic
Momentum
Motrin IB
Nuprin
Orudis KT
Percogesic Coated
Prodium
Supac
Tempra 3
Tempra 3, Double Strength
Vanquish
IRON PRODUCTS
Feostat
Fer-In-Sol
Feratab
Fergon
Ferro-Sequels
Ferrous Gluconate
Hytinic
Iron Plus Vitamin C
Nephro-Fer
Slow Fe
Vitron-C
LAXATIVE PRODUCTS
Alophen
Ceo-Two
Colace
Evac-U-Gen
Ex-Lax Extra Gentle
Ex-Lax Gentle Nature Natural
Ex-Lax Maximum Relief Formula
Ex-Lax Original Regular Strength
  Chocolated
Ex-Lax Regular Strength
Fiber Naturale
FiberCon
Fleet Glycerin Adult Size
Fleet Glycerin Child Size
Fleet Laxative
Gentle Laxative
Kellogg's Tasteless Castor Oil
Laxative & Stool Softner
Mag-Ox 400
Metamucil Original Texture, Orange
Metamucil Original Texture, Regular
  Flavor
Metamucil Smooth Texture, Orange
Metamucil Smooth Texture, Sugar Free
  Orange
Metamucil Smooth Texture, Sugar Free
  Regular Flavor
Peri-Colace
Phillips' Milk of Magnesia
Stool Softner
Unilax
Uro-Mag

MENSTRUAL PRODUCTS
Aqua-Ban
Backaid Pills
Diurex Long Acting
Diurex MPR
Diurex PMS
Diurex Water Caplet
Diurex Water Pills
Diurex-2 Water Pills
Lurline PMS
Midol Menstrual Maximum Strength
  Multisymptom Formula
Midol PMS Multisymptom Formula
Midol Teen Multisymptom Formula
MISCELLANEOUS MINERAL PRODUCTS
Chromium Picolinate
Chromium, Organic
Dr. Powers Colloidal Mineral Source
Manganese Chelate
Maxi-Minerals
Selenium, Oceanic
Verazinc
Zinc
ORAL DISCOMFORT PRODUCTS
Dentemp Temporary Filling Mix
Hurricaine, Wild Cherry
Hurricaine, Wild Cherry or Pina Colada
Hurricaine; Wild Cherry, Fina Colada, or
  Watermelon
Lipmagik
Numzit Teething
Peroxyl Hygienic Dental Rinse
Peroxyl Oral Spot Treatment
Probax
Proxigel
Zilactin
Zilactin Baby
Zilactin-B
Zilactin-L
ORAL HYGIENE PRODUCTS
Cepacol Mouthwash/Gargle
Cepacol Mouthwash/Gargle, Mint
Dr. Tichenor's Antiseptic
Tech 2000 Antimicrobial Rinse
ORAL REHYDRATION SOLUTIONS
Infalyte
SLEEP AID PRODUCTS
Arthriten PM
Backaid PM Pills
Doan's P.M. Extra Strength
Dormin
Excedrin PM
Melatonex
Midol PM Night Time Formula
Sleep Rite
Sleep-eze 3
Sleepinal
Tranquil
Tranquil Plus
Unisom Nighttime Sleep Aid
Unisom Pain Relief
SORE THROAT PRODUCTS
Cepacol Sore Throat Maximum Strength,
  Cherry
Cepacol Sore Throat Maximum Strength,
  Cool Menthol
Cepacol Sore Throat Maximum Strength,
  Mint
Cepacol Sore Throat Regular Strength,
  Cherry
Cepacol Sore Throat Regular Strength,
  Original Mint
Entertainer's Secret Throat Relief

Fisherman's Friend, Extra Strong, Sugar
  Free
Fisherman's Friend, Licorice Strong
Fisherman's Friend, Original Extra Strong
Fisherman's Friend, Refreshing Mint,
  Sugar Free
Herbal-Menthol
Ricola Cough Drops, Original Flavor
Ricola Sugar Free Herb Throat Drops,
  Alpine-Mint
Ricola Sugar Free Herb Throat Drops,
  Cherry- or Lemon-Mint
Ricola Sugar Free Herb Throat Drops,
  Mountain Herb
Ricola Throat Drops, Cherry-Mint
Ricola Throat Drops, Honey-Herb
Ricola Throat Drops, Lemon-Mint or
  Orange-Mint
Ricola Throat Drops, Menthol-Eucalyptus
STIMULANT PRODUCTS
Caffedrine
Enerjets
No Doz
No Doz Maximum Strength
Pep-Back
Pep-Back Ultra
Quick-Pep
TOPICAL FLUORIDE PRODUCTS
Fluorigard Anti-Cavity
VITAMIN PRODUCTS
A-D-E with Selenium Tablets
ABC Plus Tablets
Adavite-M Tablets
Adeks Chewable Tablets
Adeks Drops
Akorn Antioxidants Caplets
Antioxidant Formula Softgels
Antioxidant Vitamin & Mineral Formula
  Softgels
B-C-Bid Caplets
Brewers Yeast Tablets
C & E Softgels
C Vitamin Tablets
C Vitamin Timed-Release Tablets
Calcet Plus Tablets
Ceebevim Caplets
Centrum High Potency Liquid
Centrum High Potency Tablets
Centrum Jr. Shamu and His Crew + Extra
  C Chew. Tablets
Centrum Jr. Shamu and His Crew + Extra
  Calcium Chew. Tablets
Centrum Jr. Shamu and His Crew + Iron
  Chew. Tablets
Centrum Silver for Adults 50+
Cevi-Bid Tablets
Chelated Calcium Magnesium Tablets
Chelated Calcium Magnesium Zinc
  Tablets
Chewy Bears Citrus Free Vitamin C
  Chewable Wafers
Children's Chewable Vitamins with Extra
  C Tablets
Clinical Nutrients for Men Tablets
Clinical Nutrients for Women Tablets
Coldvac Lozenges
Compete Tablets
Daily Plus Iron & Calcium Tablets
Daily Vitamins Plus Minerals Tablets
DiabeVite Tablets
Diostate D Tablets
Dolomite Tablets
Eye-Vites Tablets

Fosfree Tablets
Freedavite Tablets
Fruit C Chewable Tablets
Geri-Freeda Tablets
Gevrabon Liquid
Gevral T Tablets
Herpetrol Tablets
Hexavitamin Tablets
Iromin-G Tablets
Jets Chewable Tablets
Kovitonic Liquid
KPN (Key Prenatal) Tablets
LKV (Liquid Kiddie Vitamins) Drops
Mission Prenatal F.A. Tablets
Mission Prenatal H.P. Tablets
Mission Prenatal Tablets
Monocaps Tablets
More Than a Multiple Tablets
Multi-Mineral Tablets
Myadec High-Potency Multivitamin/
    Multimineral Tablets
Natalins Tablets
Nephro-Vite Tablets
Nutri-Mega Softgels
Oncovite Tablets
Os-Cal Fortified Tablets
Oxi-Freeda Tablets
Parvlex Tablets
Peridin-C Tablets
Poly-Vi-Sol Chewable Vitamins
Poly-Vi-Sol Vitamin Drops
Poly-Vi-Sol with Iron Chewable Vitamins
    & Minerals Tablets
Poly-Vi-Sol with Iron Vitamin Drops
Pro-Pep Chewable Tablets
Progen Caplets
Protegra Antioxidant Softgels
Quintabs-M Tablets
Rejuvex for the Mature Woman Caplets
Stress-600 with Zinc Tablets
Stresstabs High Potency Stress Formula +
    Iron Tablets
Stresstabs High Potency Stress Formula
    Plus Zinc Tablets
Stresstabs High Potency Stress Formula
    Tablets
Sunkist Multivitamins Complete Tablets
Sunkist Multivitamins Plus Extra C
    Tablets
Sunkist Multivitamins Plus Iron Tablets
Sunkist Multivitamins Regular Tablets
Super A&D Tablets
Super Dec B-100 Coated Tablets
Super Quints-50 Tablets
Theragran High Potency Multivitamin
    Caplets
Theragran High Potency Multivitamin
    Liquid
Theragran Stress Formula High Potency
    Multivitamin Caplets
Theragran-M High Potency Vitamins
    with Minerals Caplets
Therapeutic B Complex with Vitamin C
    Capsules
Therapeutic Multiple with Minerals
    Tablets
Therapeutic Multivitamin Tablets
Tri-Vi-Sol Vitamins A,D+C Drops
Tri-Vi-Sol With Iron Vitamin A,D+C
    Drops
Ultra-Freeda Tablets
Unilife-A Gelcaps
Variplex-C Tablets

Vi-Daylin Multi-Vitamin Chewable
    Tablets
Vi-Daylin Multi-Vitamin Plus Iron
    Chewable Tablets
Vi-Zac Capsules
Vicon Plus Capsules
Vioday Tablets
Vitalets Chewable Tablets, Flavored or
    Unflavored
Vitalize Liquid

LACTOSE FREE

ANTACID AND ANTIREFLUX PRODUCTS
Almora
Arm & Hammer Pure Baking Soda
Gaviscon
Gaviscon Extra Strength
Gaviscon Extra Strength Liquid
Gaviscon Liquid
Gaviscon-2
Maalox
Maalox Heartburn Relief
Maalox Therapeutic Concentrate
Mag-Ox 400
Phillips' Milk of Magnesia Concentrate,
    Strawberry
Phillips' Milk of Magnesia, Cherry or
    Original Mint
Riopan
Tums E-X Extra Strength, Wintergreen or
    Asst. Fruit Flavors
Tums Ultra, Fruit or Mint Flavors
Tums, Peppermint or Asst. Fruit Flavors
Uro-Mag

ANTHELMINTIC PRODUCTS
Antiminth
Pin-X

ANTIDIARRHEAL PRODUCTS
Diasorb
Kaopectate
Kaopectate, Children's
Pepto-Bismol Maximum Strength
Pepto-Bismol Original Strength
Percy Medicine

ANTIEMETIC PRODUCTS
Dramamine, Children's

APPETITE SUPPRESSANT PRODUCTS
Thinz Back-To-Nature
Thinz-Span

CALCIUM PRODUCTS
Calci-Caps Super
Calci-Mix
Calcium Complex
Calcium Magnesium
Calcium with Vitamins A&D
Caltrate 600 High Potency
Caltrate 600 High Potency+ D
Caltrate Plus
Caltrate Plus Nutrient Enriched,
    Spearmint
Citracal
Citracal + D
Citracal Liquitab
Fem Cal
Mag/Cal Mega
Os-Cal 250 + D
Os-Cal 500
Os-Cal 500 + D

Parvacal 500
Super Cal/Mag
Tums 500; Asst. Fruit or Peppermint
Vita-Cal

COLD, COUGH, AND ALLERGY PRODUCTS
Ambenyl-D Cough
Bromfed
Buckley's DM
Buckley's Mixture
Cepacol Sore Throat Maximum Strength,
    Cherry
Cepacol Sore Throat Maximum Strength,
    Mint
Cepacol Sore Throat Regular Strength,
    Cherry
Cepacol Sore Throat Regular Strength,
    Original Mint
Codimal
Codimal DM
Codimal PH
Comtrex Allergy-Sinus
Comtrex Deep Chest Cold and Conges-
    tion Relief
Comtrex Maximum Strength
Comtrex Maximum Strength Cold and
    Flu Relief
Comtrex Maximum Strength Day & Night
Comtrex Maximum Strength Non-
    Drowsy
Comtrex Maximum Strength Non-
    Drowsy Cold and Flu Releif
Delsym Extended Release
Dorcol Children's Cough
Emagrin Forte
Excedrin Sinus Maximum Strength
Fendol
Fisherman's Friend, Extra Strong, Sugar
    Free
Fisherman's Friend, Licorice Strong
Fisherman's Friend, Original Extra Strong
Fisherman's Friend, Refreshing Mint,
    Sugar Free
GG-Cen
Guaifed
Hayfebrol
Herbal-Menthol
Naldecon DX, Adult
Naldecon DX, Children's
Naldecon DX, Pediatric
Naldecon EX, Children's
Naldecon EX, Pediatric
Naldecon Senior DX
Naldecon Senior EX
Nasal-D
Nolahist
Oranyl
Oranyl Plus
Pertussin CS
Pertussin DM
Ricola Cough Drops, Original Flavor
Ricola Sugar Free Herb Throat Drops,
    Alpine-Mint
Ricola Sugar Free Herb Throat Drops,
    Cherry- or Lemon-Mint
Ricola Sugar Free Herb Throat Drops,
    Mountain Herb
Ricola Throat Drops, Cherry-Mint
Ricola Throat Drops, Honey-Herb
Ricola Throat Drops, Lemon-Mint or
    Orange-Mint
Ricola Throat Drops, Menthol-Eucalyptus
Scot-Tussin Allergy Relief Formula

Scot-Tussin Diabetes CF
Scot-Tussin DM
Scot-Tussin DM Cough Chasers
Scot-Tussin Expectorant
Scot-Tussin Original
Scot-Tussin Senior
Sine-Off Sinus, Cold, and Flu Medicine
   Night Time Formula
Sinulin
Sudafed Children's Cold & Cough
Triaminic DM, Cough Relief
Triaminic Expectorant, Chest & Head
   Congestion
Triaminic Infant, Oral Decongestant
Triaminic Night Time
Triaminic, Cold & Allergy
Triaminicol Multi-Symptom Relief
Vicks 44 Soothing Cough Relief
Vicks 44D Soothing Cough & Head
   Congestion Relief
Vicks 44E Soothing Cough & Chest
   Congestion Relief
Vicks 44m Pediatric Cough & Cold Relief
Vicks 44M Soothing Cough, Cold, & Flu
   Relief
Vicks DayQuil Children's Allergy Relief
Vicks DayQuil Multi-Symptom Cold/Flu
   Relief
Vicks NyQuil Children's Cold/Cough
   Medicine
Vicks NyQuil Multi-Symptom Cold/Flu
   Relief, Cherry
Vicks NyQuil Multi-Symptom Cold/Flu
   Relief, Original

**ENTERAL FOOD SUPPLEMENT
PRODUCTS**
Advera
Boost
Broth Plus
Casec
Choice dm
Citrotein
Compleat Modified Formula
Compleat Pediatric
Comply
Criticare HN
Deliver 2.0
DiabetiSource
Ensure
Ensure High Protein
Ensure Light
Ensure Plus
Ensure Plus HN
Ensure with Fiber
Fibersource
Fibersource HN
Forta Drink
Gelatin Plus
Glucerna
Impact
Impact 1.5
Impact with Fiber
Isocal
Isocal HN
IsoSource
IsoSource 1.5 Cal
IsoSource HN
IsoSource VHN
Isotein HN
Jevity
Lipisorb
Magnacal Renal
MCT Oil

Microlipid
Modical
Nepro
NuBasics
NuBasics Plus
NuBasics VHP
NuBasics with Fiber
Nutren 1.0 Complete
Nutren 1.0 with Fiber Complete
Nutren 1.5 Complete
Nutren 2.0 Complete
Osmolite
Osmolite HN
Peptamen Complete
Peptamen Junior Complete
Peptamen VHP Complete
Perative
Polycose
ProBalance Complete
Promote
Protain XL
Pulmocare
Renalcal Diet
Replete Complete
Replete with Fiber Complete
ReSource
ReSource Crystals
ReSource Diabetic
ReSource Fruit Beverage
ReSource Just for Kids
ReSource Plus
ReSource Yogurt Flavored Beverage
Respalor
SandoSource Peptide
Scandishake Lactose Free
Suplena
Sustacal
Sustacal Basic
Sustacal Plus
Sustacal with Fiber
Tolerex
TraumaCal
Travasorb HN
Travasorb MCT
Travasorb STD
Two Cal HN
Ultracal
Vital High Nitrogen
Vivonex Pediatric
Vivonex T.E.N.

**INFANTS' AND CHILDREN'S FORMULA
PRODUCTS**
Enfamil Next Step Soy
Isomil
Isomil DF
Isomil SF
Kindercal
Lactofree
Lofenalac
MSUD Diet
Nutramigen
Phenyl-Free
Portagen
Pregestimil
ProSobee
RCF (Ross Carbohydrate Free)

**INTERNAL ANALGESIC AND
ANTIPYRETIC PRODUCTS**
Motrin IB

IRON PRODUCTS
Feostat
Fer-In-Sol
Iron Plus Vitamin C

Niferex
Niferex with Vitamin C
Niferex-150

LAXATIVE PRODUCTS
Ceo-Two
Colace
Doxidan
Dr. Caldwell Senna
Ex-Lax Stool Softener
Fiber Naturale
FiberCon
Fleet Babylax
Fleet Glycerin Rectal Applicators
Fleet Mineral Oil Oral Lubricant
Fletcher's Castoria
Fletcher's, Children's Cherry
Haleys M-O, Flavored or Regular
Herb-Lax
Kellogg's Tasteless Castor Oil
Liqui-Doss
Mag-Ox 400
Metamucil Fiber Wafer, Apple Crisp or
   Cinnamon Spice
Metamucil Original Texture, Orange
Metamucil Original Texture, Regular
   Flavor
Metamucil Smooth Texture, Orange
Metamucil Smooth Texture, Sugar Free
   Orange
Metamucil Smooth Texture, Sugar Free
   Regular Flavor
Milkinol
Phillips' Milk of Magnesia Concentrate,
   Strawberry   •
Phillips' Milk of Magnesia; Cherry, Mint,
   or Original
Purge
Therevac Plus
Therevac-SB
Unilax
Uro-Mag

MISCELLANEOUS MINERAL PRODUCTS
Chromium Picolinate
Chromium, Organic
Dr. Powers Colloidal Mineral Source
Manganese Chelate
Maxi-Minerals
Selenium, Oceanic
Zinc

ORAL REHYDRATION SOLUTIONS
Infalyte

SLEEP AID PRODUCTS
Tranquil Plus

SORE THROAT PRODUCTS
Cepacol Sore Throat Maximum Strength,
   Cherry
Cepacol Sore Throat Maximum Strength,
   Cool Menthol
Cepacol Sore Throat Maximum Strength,
   Mint
Cepacol Sore Throat Regular Strength,
   Cherry
Cepacol Sore Throat Regular Strength,
   Original Mint
Fisherman's Friend, Extra Strong, Sugar
   Free
Fisherman's Friend, Licorice Strong
Fisherman's Friend, Original Extra Strong
Fisherman's Friend, Refreshing Mint,
   Sugar Free
Herbal-Menthol
Ricola Cough Drops, Original Flavor
Ricola Sugar Free Herb Throat Drops,
   Alpine-Mint

Ricola Sugar Free Herb Throat Drops,
Cherry- or Lemon-Mint
Ricola Sugar Free Herb Throat Drops,
Mountain Herb
Ricola Throat Drops, Cherry-Mint
Ricola Throat Drops, Honey-Herb
Ricola Throat Drops, Lemon-Mint or
Orange-Mint
Ricola Throat Drops, Menthol-Eucalyptus
VITAMIN PRODUCTS
A-D-E with Selenium Tablets
Adeks Chewable Tablets
Adeks Drops
B-C-Bid Caplets
C Vitamin Tablets
C Vitamin Timed-Release Tablets
Centrum High Potency Liquid
Centrum Silver for Adults 50+
Chewy Bears Citrus Free Vitamin C
Chewable Wafers
Clinical Nutrients for Men Tablets
Clinical Nutrients for Women Tablets
Coldvac Lozenges
Freedavite Tablets
Fruit C Chewable Tablets
Geri-Freeda Tablets
Gevrabon Liquid
Herpetrol Tablets
Jets Chewable Tablets
Kovitonic Liquid
KPN (Key Prenatal) Tablets
LKV (Liquid Kiddie Vitamins) Drops
Monocaps Tablets
More Than a Multiple Tablets
Natalins Tablets
Nutri-Mega Softgels
Oncovite Tablets
Os-Cal Fortified Tablets
Oxi-Freeda Tablets
Parvlex Tablets
Peridin-C Tablets
Poly-Vi-Sol Chewable Vitamins
Poly-Vi-Sol Vitamin Drops
Poly-Vi-Sol with Iron Chewable Vitamins
& Minerals Tablets
Poly-Vi-Sol with Iron Vitamin Drops
Protegra Antioxidant Softgels
Quintabs-M Tablets
Stresstabs High Potency Stress Formula +
Iron Tablets
Stresstabs High Potency Stress Formula
Plus Zinc Tablets
Stresstabs High Potency Stress Formula
Tablets
Super A&D Tablets
Super Dec B-100 Coated Tablets
Super Quints-50 Tablets
Theragran High Potency Multivitamin
Caplets
Theragran High Potency Multivitamin
Liquid
Theragran Stress Formula High Potency
Multivitamin Caplets
Theragran-M High Potency Vitamins
with Minerals Caplets
Tri-Vi-Sol Vitamins A,D+C Drops
Tri-Vi-Sol With Iron Vitamin A,D+C
Drops
Ultra-Freeda Tablets
Unilife-A Gelcaps
Vi-Daylin ADC Vitamins Drops
Vi-Daylin ADC Vitamins Plus Iron Drops
Vi-Daylin Multi-Vitamin Drops

Vi-Daylin Multi-Vitamin Liquid
Vi-Daylin Multi-Vitamin Plus Iron Drops
Vi-Daylin Multi-Vitamin Plus Iron Liquid
Vitalets Chewable Tablets, Flavored or
Unflavored
Vitalize Liquid

PRESERVATIVE FREE

**ANTACID AND ANTIREFLUX
PRODUCTS**
Mylanta
ARTIFICIAL TEAR PRODUCTS
Akwa Tears
Bion Tears
Celluvisc
Hypo Tears
Hypo Tears PF
Lacri-Lube N.P.
Ocucoat PF Lubricating
Refresh
Refresh P.M.
Refresh Plus
Tears Naturale Free
Tears Renewed
ASTHMA INHALANT PRODUCTS
Broncho Saline
Sodium Chloride Inhalation Solution USP
CALCIUM PRODUCTS
Calcium Complex
**COLD, COUGH, AND ALLERGY
PRODUCTS**
Comtrex Maximum Strength Cold and
Flu Relief
Vaporizer in a Bottle Air Wick Inhaler
**INTERNAL ANALGESIC AND
ANTIPYRETIC PRODUCTS**
Aleve
Arthriten
Arthritis Pain Formula
Aspirin Free Pain & Fever Relief,
Children's
Aspirin Free Pain Relief
Aspirin Free, Infants'
Backache from the Makers of Nuprin
BC
BC Arthritis Strength
Bromo-Seltzer
Bufferin Arthritis Strength, Tri-Buffered
Bufferin Extra Strength, Tri-Buffered
Bufferin, Tri-Buffered
Doan's Extra Strength
Doan's Regular Strength
Excedrin Extra Strength
Goody's Extra Strength
Goody's Extra Strength Headache
Momentum
Motrin IB
Nuprin
Percogesic Coated
Prodium [c]
Supac
Tempra 1
Tempra 3
Tempra 3, Double Strength
LAXATIVE PRODUCTS
Fleet Babylax
Fleet Glycerin Rectal Applicators
Fleet Mineral Oil Enema
Fleet Mineral Oil Oral Lubricant

Kellogg's Tasteless Castor Oil
Liqui-Doss
Purge
Therevac Plus
Therevac-SB
MENSTRUAL PRODUCTS
Aqua-Ban
Backaid Pills
Diurex Long Acting
Diurex MPR
Diurex PMS
Diurex Water Caplet
Diurex Water Pills
Diurex-2 Water Pills
Lurline PMS
MISCELLANEOUS NASAL PRODUCTS
Nichols Nasal Douche
**MISCELLANEOUS OPHTHALMIC
PRODUCTS**
AK-NaCl
Lid Wipes-SPF
**OPHTHALMIC DECONGESTANT
PRODUCTS**
Relief
**RIGID GAS-PERMEABLE LENS
PRODUCTS**
Boston Advance Cleaner
Boston Cleaner
SOFT LENS PRODUCTS
Blairex Sterile Saline
Opti-Free SupraClens Daily Protein
Remover
Unisol 4 Saline

PURINE FREE

**ANTACID AND ANTIREFLUX
PRODUCTS**
Alka-Mints
Alka-Seltzer Extra Strength
Alka-Seltzer Gold
Alka-Seltzer Original
Alka-Seltzer, Cherry
Alka-Seltzer, Lemon-Lime
Almora
Arm & Hammer Pure Baking Soda
Dicarbosil
Gaviscon
Gaviscon Extra Strength
Gaviscon-2
Mag-Ox 400
Tums E-X Extra Strength, Wintergreen or
Asst. Fruit Flavors
Tums Ultra, Fruit or Mint Flavors
Tums, Peppermint or Asst. Fruit Flavors
Uro-Mag
ANTIDIARRHEAL PRODUCTS
Diar Aid
Diasorb
Kaopectate
Pepto-Bismol
Pepto-Bismol, Cherry
Rheaban
ANTIEMETIC PRODUCTS
Bonine
Dramamine
Dramamine II Less Drowsy Formula
Dramamine Original
ANTIFLATULENT PRODUCTS
Gas-X

Gas-X Extra Strength
Gelusil
Maalox Antacid Plus Anti-Gas
Maalox Antacid Plus Anti-Gas Extra
 Strength
Maalox Anti-Gas
Maalox Anti-Gas Extra Strength
Riopan Plus
Riopan Plus Double Strength
Tums Anti-Gas/Antacid

APPETITE SUPPRESSANT PRODUCTS

Acutrim 16 Hour Steady Control
Acutrim Late Day Strength
Acutrim Maximum Strength
Amfed T.D.
Dexatrim Caffeine Free Extended
 Duration
Dexatrim Caffeine Free Maximum
 Strength
Dexatrim Caffeine Free with Vitamin C
Dieutrim T.D.
Protrim S.R.

ARTIFICIAL TEAR PRODUCTS

Adsorbotear
Akwa Tears
Bion Tears
Isopto Alkaline
Isopto Tears
Liquifilm Tears
Murine Tears Lubricant
Refresh
Refresh Plus
Tears Naturale
Tears Naturale Free
Tears Naturale II
Tears Plus
Tears Renewed
Ultra Tears

ASTHMA ORAL PRODUCTS

Primatene

CALCIUM PRODUCTS

Calcet
Calci-Caps
Calci-Caps Super
Calci-Caps with Iron
Calci-Chew; Cherry, Lemon, or Orange
Calci-Mix
Calcium Complex
Calcium Magnesium
Caltrate 600 High Potency
Caltrate 600 High Potency+ D
Caltrate Plus
Caltrate Plus Nutrient Enriched,
 Spearmint
Citracal
Citracal + D
Citracal Liquitab
Citron
Fem Cal
Florical
Mag/Cal Mega
Nephro-Calci
Os-Cal 250 + D
Os-Cal 500
Os-Cal 500 + D
Oyster Calcium
Oyster Calcium 500 + D
Oystercal 500
Oystercal-D 250
Parvacal 500
Super Cal/Mag
Tums 500; Asst. Fruit or Peppermint
Vita-Cal

**COLD, COUGH, AND ALLERGY
PRODUCTS**

Alka-Seltzer Plus Cold Medicine
Alka-Seltzer Plus Night-Time Cold
 Medicine
Allerest Maximum Strength
Allerest No Drowsiness
Allergy Relief
Benadryl Allergy
Cepacol Sore Throat Maximum Strength,
 Cherry
Cepacol Sore Throat Maximum Strength,
 Mint
Cepacol Sore Throat Regular Strength,
 Cherry
Cepacol Sore Throat Regular Strength,
 Original Mint
Efidac/24
Hay Fever & Allergy Relief Maximum
 Strength
Herbal-Menthol
Hytuss
Hytuss 2X
Napril
Nasal-D
ND-Gesic
Nolahist
Propagest
Ricola Cough Drops, Original Flavor
Ricola Sugar Free Herb Throat Drops,
 Alpine-Mint
Ricola Sugar Free Herb Throat Drops,
 Cherry- or Lemon-Mint
Ricola Sugar Free Herb Throat Drops,
 Mountain Herb
Ricola Throat Drops, Cherry-Mint
Ricola Throat Drops, Honey-Herb
Ricola Throat Drops, Lemon-Mint or
 Orange-Mint
Ricola Throat Drops, Menthol-Eucalyptus
Scot-Tussin DM Cough Chasers
Sinarest Extra Strength
Sinarest Sinus Medicine
Sine-Off Sinus, Cold, and Flu Medicine
 Night Time Formula
Sinulin
Sinus Relief Extra Strength
Tavist-1 Antihistamine
Tavist-D Antihistamine/Nasal Deconges-
 tant
TheraFlu Flu and Cold Medicine
TheraFlu Flu, Cold, & Cough Medicine
TheraFlu Max. Strength Flu, Cold &
 Cough Medicine NightTime
Triaminicin
Tuss-DM
Vicks 44 Cough, Cold, & Flu Relief
 LiquiCaps
Vicks 44 Non-Drowsy Cough & Cold
 Relief LiquiCaps
Vicks DayQuil Allergy Relief 12-Hour
Vicks DayQuil Multi-Symptom Cold/Flu
 Relief LiquiCaps
Vicks DayQuil Sinus Pressure &
 Congestion Relief
Vicks DayQuil Sinus Pressure & Pain
 Relief with Ibuprofen
Vicks Nyquil Hot Therapy
Vicks NyQuil Multi-Symptom Cold/Flu
 Relief LiquiCaps

**ENTERAL FOOD SUPPLEMENT
PRODUCTS**

Casec

Lipisorb
Moducal
Scandishake
Scandishake (Sweetened with Aspar-
 tame)
Scandishake Lactose Free
Sustacal
Sustacal Plus
TraumaCal
Ultracal

HARD LENS PRODUCTS

Adapettes Sensitive Eyes
Adapt
Blairex Hard Lens Cleaner
Clerz 2
Opti-Clean Daily Cleaner
Opti-Clean II Daily Cleaner for Sensitive
 Eyes
Opti-Free Daily Cleaner
Soaclens

**HISTAMINE II RECEPTOR
ANTAGONISTS**

Tagamet HB 200

**INFANTS' AND CHILDREN'S FORMULA
PRODUCTS**

Enfamil
Enfamil Human Milk Fortifier
Enfamil Next Step
Enfamil Premature Formula
Enfamil Premature Formula with Iron
Enfamil with Iron
Gerber Baby Formula Low Iron
Gerber Baby Formula with Iron
Kindercal
Lactofree
Lofenalac
MSUD Diet
Nutramigen
Phenyl-Free
Portagen
Pregestimil

**INTERNAL ANALGESIC AND
ANTIPYRETIC PRODUCTS**

Acetaminophen Uniserts
Aleve
Aspergum, Cherry or Orange
Aspirin Free Pain & Fever Relief,
 Children's
Aspirin Free Pain Relief
Doan's Extra Strength
Doan's Regular Strength
Feverall Adult Strength
Feverall Junior Strength
Feverall Sprinkle Caps Powder,
 Children's Strength
Feverall Sprinkle Caps Powder, Junior
 Strength
Feverall, Children's
Feverall, Infants'
Motrin IB
Percogesic Coated
Prodium [c]
Supac

IRON PRODUCTS

Feostat
Feratab
Ferro-Sequels
Ferrous Gluconate
Hytinic
Iron Plus Vitamin C
Nephro-Fer
Slow Fe

LAXATIVE PRODUCTS
Alophen
Ceo-Two
Evac-U-Gen
Ex-Lax Extra Gentle
Ex-Lax Gentle Nature Natural
Ex-Lax Maximum Relief Formula
Ex-Lax Original Regular Strength
 Chocolated
Ex-Lax Regular Strength
Ex-Lax Stool Softener
FiberCon
Fleet Glycerin Adult Size
Fleet Glycerin Child Size
Fleet Laxative
Gentle Laxative
Herb-Lax
Laxative & Stool Softner
Mag-Ox 400
Metamucil Fiber Wafer, Apple Crisp or
 Cinnamon Spice
Metamucil Original Texture, Orange
Metamucil Original Texture, Regular
 Flavor
Metamucil Smooth Texture, Orange
Metamucil Smooth Texture, Sugar Free
 Orange
Metamucil Smooth Texture, Sugar Free
 Regular Flavor
Stool Softner
Uro-Mag

MENSTRUAL PRODUCTS
Aqua-Ban
Lurline PMS

MISCELLANEOUS MINERAL PRODUCTS
Chromium, Organic
Manganese Chelate
Maxi-Minerals
Selenium, Oceanic
Zinc

**MISCELLANEOUS OPHTHALMIC
PRODUCTS**
Adsorbonac
Enuclene
Eye-Stream
Lid Wipes-SPF

**OPHTHALMIC DECONGESTANT
PRODUCTS**
AK-Nefrin
Clear eyes ACR Allergy Cold Relief
Clear eyes Lubricating Eye Redness
 Reliever Extra Relief
Estivin II
Isopto-Frin
Murine Tears Plus Lubricant Redness
 Reliever
Naphcon
Naphcon A
Prefrin Liquifilm
Relief
Soothe
Visine Allergy Relief
Visine L.R.
Visine Moisturizing
Visine Original Formula

ORAL HYGIENE PRODUCTS
Scope, Baking Soda

ORAL REHYDRATION SOLUTIONS
Infalyte

**RIGID GAS-PERMEABLE LENS
PRODUCTS**
Opti-Clean II Daily Cleaner for Sensitive
 Eyes

Opti-Free Daily Cleaner

SLEEP AID PRODUCTS
Dormin
Sleep Rite
Sleepinal
Unisom Nighttime Sleep Aid
Unisom Pain Relief

SOFT LENS PRODUCTS
Alcon Enzymatic Cleaner
Clerz 2
Flex-Care for Sensitive Eyes
Mirasept Step 1
Mirasept Step 2
Opti-Clean Daily Cleaner
Opti-Clean II Daily Cleaner for Sensitive
 Eyes
Opti-Free
Opti-Free Daily Cleaner
Opti-Free Enzymatic Cleaner for
 Sensitive Eyes
Opti-Free Express
Opti-Free for Disinfection
Opti-Free SupraClens Daily Protein
 Remover
Opti-One Multi-Purpose
Opti-Soak Conditioning
Opti-Soak Daily Cleaner
Opti-Soak Soothing
Opti-Soft
Opti-Tears Soothing
Pliagel
Preflex for Sensitive Eyes
Unisol 4 Saline

SORE THROAT PRODUCTS
Cepacol Sore Throat Maximum Strength,
 Cherry
Cepacol Sore Throat Maximum Strength,
 Cool Menthol
Cepacol Sore Throat Maximum Strength,
 Mint
Cepacol Sore Throat Regular Strength,
 Cherry
Cepacol Sore Throat Regular Strength,
 Original Mint
Herbal-Menthol
Ricola Cough Drops, Original Flavor
Ricola Sugar Free Herb Throat Drops,
 Alpine-Mint
Ricola Sugar Free Herb Throat Drops,
 Cherry- or Lemon-Mint
Ricola Sugar Free Herb Throat Drops,
 Mountain Herb
Ricola Throat Drops, Cherry-Mint
Ricola Throat Drops, Honey-Herb
Ricola Throat Drops, Lemon-Mint or
 Orange-Mint
Ricola Throat Drops, Menthol-Eucalyptus

STIMULANT PRODUCTS
Caffedrine
Enerjets
Quick-Pep

VITAMIN PRODUCTS
A-D-E with Selenium Tablets
ABC Plus Tablets
Adavite-M Tablets
Adeks Chewable Tablets
Akorn Antioxidants Caplets
Antioxidant Formula Softgels
Antioxidant Vitamin & Mineral Formula
 Softgels
Brewers Yeast Tablets
Bugs Bunny Complete Vitamins Plus
 Minerals Chewable Tablets

Bugs Bunny Plus Iron Chewable Tablets
Bugs Bunny with Extra C Children's
 Chewable Tablets
C & E Softgels
C Vitamin Tablets
C Vitamin Timed-Release Tablets
Calcet Plus Tablets
Ceebevim Caplets
Centrum High Potency Tablets
Centrum Jr. Shamu and His Crew + Extra
 C Chew. Tablets
Centrum Jr. Shamu and His Crew + Extra
 Calcium Chew. Tablets
Centrum Jr. Shamu and His Crew + Iron
 Chew. Tablets
Centrum Silver for Adults 50+
Chelated Calcium Magnesium Tablets
Chelated Calcium Magnesium Zinc
 Tablets
Children's Chewable Vitamins with Extra
 C Tablets
Compete Tablets
Daily Plus Iron & Calcium Tablets
Daily Vitamins Plus Minerals Tablets
DiabeVite Tablets
Dolomite Tablets
Eye-Vites Tablets
Flintstones Children's Chewable Tablets
Flintstones Complete Chewable Tablets
Flintstones Plus Iron Chewable Tablets
Fosfree Tablets
Freedavite Tablets
Fruit C Chewable Tablets
Geri-Freeda Tablets
Gevral T Tablets
Hexavitamin Tablets
Iromin-G Tablets
Jets Chewable Tablets
KPN (Key Prenatal) Tablets
Mission Prenatal F.A. Tablets
Mission Prenatal H.P. Tablets
Mission Prenatal Tablets
Monocaps Tablets
Multi-Mineral Tablets
Natalins Tablets
Nephro-Vite Tablets
Oncovite Tablets
One-A-Day Essential Tablets
One-A-Day Maximum Formula Tablets
Os-Cal Fortified Tablets
Oxi-Freeda Tablets
Parvlex Tablets
Peridin-C Tablets
Poly-Vi-Sol Chewable Vitamins
Poly-Vi-Sol with Iron Chewable Vitamins
 & Minerals Tablets
Progen Caplets
Protegra Antioxidant Softgels
Quintabs-M Tablets
Stress-600 with Zinc Tablets
Stresstabs High Potency Stress Formula +
 Iron Tablets
Stresstabs High Potency Stress Formula
 Plus Zinc Tablets
Stresstabs High Potency Stress Formula
 Tablets
Sunkist Multivitamins Complete Tablets
Sunkist Multivitamins Plus Extra C
 Tablets
Sunkist Multivitamins Plus Iron Tablets
Sunkist Multivitamins Regular Tablets
Super A&D Tablets
Super Dec B-100 Coated Tablets

Super Quints-50 Tablets
Theragran High Potency Multivitamin
  Caplets
Theragran Stress Formula High Potency
  Multivitamin Caplets
Theragran-M High Potency Vitamins
  with Minerals Caplets
Therapeutic B Complex with Vitamin C
  Capsules
Therapeutic Multiple with Minerals
  Tablets
Therapeutic Multivitamin Tablets
Ultra-Freeda Tablets
Unilife-A Gelcaps
Variplex-C Tablets
Vioday Tablets
Vitalets Chewable Tablets, Flavored or
  Unflavored

SODIUM FREE (DIETETICALLY)

ANTACID AND ANTIREFLUX PRODUCTS
Alka-Mints
ALternaGEL
Amitone
Chooz
Dicarbosil
Maalox
Mag-Ox 400
Mylanta Regular Strength
Riopan
Rolaids, Asst. Fruit Flavors or Cherry
Tempo Drops
Tums, Peppermint or Asst. Fruit Flavors
Uro-Mag
XS Hangover Relief

ANTIDIARRHEAL PRODUCTS
Diar Aid
Kaopectate
Lactaid
Percy Medicine

ANTIEMETIC PRODUCTS
Dramamine
Dramamine II Less Drowsy Formula
Dramamine Original
Nauzene

ANTIFLATULENT PRODUCTS
Di-Gel
Gas-X
Gas-X Extra Strength
Gelusil
Kudrox
Little Tummys Infant Gas Relief
Maalox Antacid/Anti-Gas Extra Strength
Mylanta
Mylanta Maximum Strength
Riopan Plus
Riopan Plus Double Strength
Riopan Plus Double Strength, Cherry or
  Mint

APPETITE SUPPRESSANT PRODUCTS
Acutrim 16 Hour Steady Control
Acutrim Late Day Strength
Acutrim Maximum Strength
Amfed T.D.
Dexatrim Caffeine Free Extended
  Duration

Dexatrim Caffeine Free Maximum
  Strength
Dexatrim Caffeine Free with Vitamin C
Dieutrim T.D.
Protrim S.R.
Thinz Back-To-Nature
Thinz-Span

ASTHMA INHALANT PRODUCTS
Bronkaid Mist and Refill

ASTHMA ORAL PRODUCTS
Bronkaid Dual Action Formula
Primatene

CALCIUM PRODUCTS
Calcet
Calci-Caps with Iron
Calci-Chew; Cherry, Lemon, or Orange
Calci-Mix
Caltrate 600 High Potency
Caltrate 600 High Potency+ D
Caltrate Plus
Caltrate Plus Nutrient Enriched,
  Spearmint
Citracal
Citracal + D
Citron
Fem Cal
Mag/Cal Mega
Os-Cal 250 + D
Os-Cal 500
Os-Cal 500 + D
Oyster Calcium
Oyster Calcium 500 + D
Oystercal-D 250
Parvacal 500
Super Cal/Mag
Tums 500; Asst. Fruit or Peppermint

COLD, COUGH, AND ALLERGY PRODUCTS
Advil Cold & Sinus
Allerest No Drowsiness
Benadryl Allergy
Cepacol Sore Throat Maximum Strength,
  Cherry
Cepacol Sore Throat Maximum Strength,
  Mint
Cepacol Sore Throat Regular Strength,
  Cherry
Cepacol Sore Throat Regular Strength,
  Original Mint
Codimal
Coldonyl
Comtrex Deep Chest Cold and Conges-
  tion Relief
Comtrex Maximum Strength
Comtrex Maximum Strength Cold and
  Flu Relief
Comtrex Maximum Strength Non-
  Drowsy
Comtrex Maximum Strength Non-
  Drowsy Cold and Flu Releif
Diabetic Tussin Cough Drops, Cherry
Diabetic Tussin Cough Drops, Menthol-
  Eucalyptus
Diabetic Tussin DM Liqui-Gels
Diabetic Tussin DM Maximum Strength
  Liqui-Gels
Dristan Cold Multi-Symptom
Dristan Sinus
Emagrin Forte
Excedrin Sinus Maximum Strength
Fendol
Herbal-Menthol
Hytuss

Hytuss 2X
Napril
ND-Gesic
Nolahist
Oranyl
Oranyl Plus
Propagest
Ricola Cough Drops, Original Flavor
Ricola Sugar Free Herb Throat Drops,
  Alpine-Mint
Ricola Sugar Free Herb Throat Drops,
  Cherry- or Lemon-Mint
Ricola Sugar Free Herb Throat Drops,
  Mountain Herb
Ricola Throat Drops, Cherry-Mint
Ricola Throat Drops, Honey-Herb
Ricola Throat Drops, Lemon-Mint or
  Orange-Mint
Ricola Throat Drops, Menthol-Eucalyptus
Scot-Tussin DM Cough Chasers
Sinarest Extra Strength
Sinarest Sinus Medicine
Sinulin
Sudafed 12-Hour Extended Release
Sudanyl
Tavist-1 Antihistamine
Tavist-D Antihistamine/Nasal Deconges-
  tant
Tuss-DM
Vicks 44 Cough, Cold, & Flu Relief
  LiquiCaps
Vicks 44 Non-Drowsy Cough & Cold
  Relief LiquiCaps
Vicks DayQuil Multi-Symptom Cold/Flu
  Relief LiquiCaps
Vicks Nyquil Hot Therapy
Vicks NyQuil Multi-Symptom Cold/Flu
  Relief LiquiCaps

ENTERAL FOOD SUPPLEMENT PRODUCTS
MCT Oil
Microlipid

HISTAMINE II RECEPTOR ANTAGONISTS
Tagamet HB 200
Zantac 75

INTERNAL ANALGESIC AND ANTIPYRETIC PRODUCTS
Acetaminophen Uniserts
Actamin Super
Anodynos
Arthriten
Arthritis Pain Formula
Aspercin
Aspercin Extra
Aspermin
Aspermin Extra
Aspirin Free Pain & Fever Relief,
  Children's
Aspirtab
Aspirtab Max
Back-Quell
Backache from the Makers of Nuprin
Bayer 8-Hour Aspirin Extended-Release
Bayer Arthritis Pain Regimen Extra
  Strength
Bayer Aspirin Extra Strength
Bayer Aspirin Regimen Regular Strength
Bayer Aspirin, Genuine
Bayer Children's Aspirin, Cherry or
  Orange
BC
Buffaprin

Buffaprin Extra
Buffasal
Buffasal Max
Bufferin Arthritis Strength, Tri-Buffered
Bufferin Extra Strength, Tri-Buffered
Bufferin, Tri-Buffered
Buffinol
Buffinol Extra
Doan's Extra Strength
Doan's Regular Strength
Dyspel
Emagrin
Excedrin Extra Strength
Feverall Adult Strength
Feverall Junior Strength
Feverall Sprinkle Caps Powder,
   Children's Strength
Feverall Sprinkle Caps Powder, Junior
   Strength
Feverall, Children's
Feverall, Infants'
Midol IB Cramp Relief Formula
Midol Menstrual Regular Strength
   Multisymptom Formula
Mobigesic
Momentum
Motrin IB
Nuprin
Supac
Valorin Super
Vanquish
XS Hangover Relief

IRON PRODUCTS
Feratab
Fergon
Ferrous Gluconate
Nephro-Fer
Slow Fe

LAXATIVE PRODUCTS
Alophen
Doxidan
Dr. Caldwell Senna
Dulcolax
Ex-Lax Original Regular Strength
   Chocolated
Fiber Naturale
FiberCon
Fleet Babylax
Fleet Bisacodyl Enema
Fleet Glycerin Adult Size
Fleet Glycerin Child Size
Fleet Glycerin Rectal Applicators
Fleet Mineral Oil Oral Lubricant
Garfields Tea
Gentle Laxative
Innerclean Herbal
Kellogg's Tasteless Castor Oil
Kondremul
Laxative & Stool Softner
Mag-Ox 400
Metamucil Original Texture, Orange
Metamucil Smooth Texture, Orange
Metamucil Smooth Texture, Sugar Free
   Orange
Metamucil Smooth Texture, Sugar Free
   Regular Flavor
Milkinol
Mitrolan
Stool Softner
Surfak
Therevac Plus
Uro-Mag

MENSTRUAL PRODUCTS
Aqua-Ban
Backaid Pills
Diurex Long Acting
Diurex MPR
Diurex PMS
Diurex Water Caplet
Diurex Water Pills
Diurex-2 Water Pills
Midol Menstrual Maximum Strength
   Multisymptom Formula
Midol PMS Multisymptom Formula
Midol Teen Multisymptom Formula
MISCELLANEOUS MINERAL PRODUCTS
Chromium Picolinate
Chromium, Organic
Manganese Chelate
Maxi-Minerals
Selenium, Oceanic
Zinc
ORAL DISCOMFORT PRODUCTS
Little Teethers Oral Pain Relief
SLEEP AID PRODUCTS
Arthriten PM
Backaid PM Pills
Dormin
Excedrin PM
Melatonex
Midol PM Night Time Formula
Sleep-eze 3
Sleepinal
Tranquil
Tranquil Plus
Unisom Pain Relief
SORE THROAT PRODUCTS
Cepacol Sore Throat Maximum Strength,
   Cherry
Cepacol Sore Throat Maximum Strength,
   Mint
Cepacol Sore Throat Regular Strength,
   Cherry
Cepacol Sore Throat Regular Strength,
   Original Mint
Herbal-Menthol
Ricola Cough Drops, Original Flavor
Ricola Sugar Free Herb Throat Drops,
   Alpine-Mint
Ricola Sugar Free Herb Throat Drops,
   Cherry- or Lemon-Mint
Ricola Sugar Free Herb Throat Drops,
   Mountain Herb
Ricola Throat Drops, Cherry-Mint
Ricola Throat Drops, Honey-Herb
Ricola Throat Drops, Lemon-Mint or
   Orange-Mint
Ricola Throat Drops, Menthol-Eucalyptus
Vicks Chloraseptic Sore Throat, Cherry
   or Menthol
STIMULANT PRODUCTS
Caffedrine
Enerjets
No Doz
No Doz Maximum Strength
Pep-Back
Pep-Back Ultra
Quick-Pep
VITAMIN PRODUCTS
A-D-E with Selenium Tablets
Adeks Chewable Tablets
Antioxidant Formula Softgels
Antioxidant Vitamin & Mineral Formula
   Softgels
B-C-Bid Caplets

Brewers Yeast Tablets
Bugs Bunny Complete Vitamins Plus
   Minerals Chewable Tablets
Bugs Bunny Plus Iron Chewable Tablets
Bugs Bunny with Extra C Children's
   Chewable Tablets
C & E Softgels
C Vitamin Tablets
C Vitamin Timed-Release Tablets
Centrum High Potency Tablets
Centrum Jr. Shamu and His Crew + Extra
   C Chew. Tablets
Centrum Jr. Shamu and His Crew + Extra
   Calcium Chew. Tablets
Centrum Jr. Shamu and His Crew + Iron
   Chew. Tablets
Centrum Silver for Adults 50+
Cevi-Bid Tablets
Chewy Bears Citrus Free Vitamin C
   Chewable Wafers
Children's Chewable Vitamins with Extra
   C Tablets
Clinical Nutrients for Men Tablets
Clinical Nutrients for Women Tablets
Daily Plus Iron & Calcium Tablets
Daily Vitamins Plus Minerals Tablets
Diostate D Tablets
Dolomite Tablets
Eye-Vites Tablets
Flintstones Children's Chewable Tablets
Flintstones Complete Chewable Tablets
Flintstones Plus Iron Chewable Tablets
Freedavite Tablets
Fruit C Chewable Tablets
Geri-Freeda Tablets
Gerimed Tablets
Gevrabon Liquid
Gevral T Tablets
Herpetrol Tablets
Hexavitamin Tablets
Jets Chewable Tablets
Kovitonic Liquid
KPN (Key Prenatal) Tablets
LKV (Liquid Kiddie Vitamins) Drops
Monocaps Tablets
Myadec High-Potency Multivitamin/
   Multimineral Tablets
One-A-Day Essential Tablets
One-A-Day Maximum Formula Tablets
Os-Cal Fortified Tablets
Oxi-Freeda Tablets
Parvlex Tablets
Peridin-C Tablets
Poly-Vi-Sol Vitamin Drops
Poly-Vi-Sol with Iron Vitamin Drops
Pro-Pep Chewable Tablets
Progen Caplets
Protegra Antioxidant Softgels
Quintabs-M Tablets
Stress-600 with Zinc Tablets
Stresstabs High Potency Stress Formula +
   Iron Tablets
Stresstabs High Potency Stress Formula
   Plus Zinc Tablets
Stresstabs High Potency Stress Formula
   Tablets
Sunkist Multivitamins Complete Tablets
Sunkist Multivitamins Plus Extra C
   Tablets
Sunkist Multivitamins Plus Iron Tablets
Sunkist Multivitamins Regular Tablets
Super A&D Tablets
Super Dec B-100 Coated Tablets

Super Quints-50 Tablets
Therapeutic B Complex with Vitamin C
   Capsules
Therapeutic Multiple with Minerals
   Tablets
Therapeutic Multivitamin Tablets
Ultra-Freeda Tablets
Unilife-A Gelcaps
Vitalets Chewable Tablets, Flavored or
   Unflavored
Vitalize Liquid

SUCROSE FREE (DIETETICALLY)

ANTACID AND ANTIREFLUX PRODUCTS
Alka-Seltzer Extra Strength
Alka-Seltzer Gold
Alka-Seltzer Original
Alka-Seltzer, Cherry
Alka-Seltzer, Lemon-Lime
Almora
ALternaGEL
Arm & Hammer Pure Baking Soda
Gaviscon Extra Strength Liquid
Gaviscon Liquid
Maalox
Maalox Heartburn Relief
Maalox Therapeutic Concentrate
Mag-Ox 400
Tums E-X Sugar Free
Uro-Mag

ANTHELMINTIC PRODUCTS
Pin-X

ANTIDIARRHEAL PRODUCTS
Lactaid
Pepto-Bismol Maximum Strength
Pepto-Bismol Original Strength

ANTIEMETIC PRODUCTS
Nauzene

ANTIFLATULENT PRODUCTS
Baby Gasz
CharcoCaps
Gas-X Extra Strength
Little Tummys Infant Gas Relief
Maalox Antacid/Anti-Gas Extra Strength

ASTHMA INHALANT PRODUCTS
Sodium Chloride Inhalation Solution USP

CALCIUM PRODUCTS
Calci-Caps Super
Calci-Mix
Calcium Complex
Calcium Magnesium
Calcium with Vitamins A&D
Caltrate 600 High Potency
Caltrate 600 High Potency+ D
Caltrate Plus
Citracal
Citracal + D
Citracal Liquitab
Fem Cal
Florical
Mag/Cal Mega
Monocal
Nephro-Calci
Os-Cal 250 + D
Os-Cal 500
Oyster Calcium

Oyster Calcium 500 + D
Oystercal 500
Oystercal-D 250
Parvacal 500
Super Cal/Mag

COLD, COUGH, AND ALLERGY PRODUCTS
Benylin Adult Cough Formula
Benylin Multi-Symptom Formula
Buckley's DM
Buckley's Mixture
Clear Cough DM
Clear Cough Night Time
Codimal DM
Coldonyl
Comtrex Deep Chest Cold and Conges-
   tion Relief
Comtrex Maximum Strength Cold and
   Flu Relief
Comtrex Maximum Strength Non-
   Drowsy Cold and Flu Releif
Diabe-tuss DM
Diabetic Tussin Allergy Relief
Diabetic Tussin Cough Drops, Cherry
Diabetic Tussin Cough Drops, Menthol-
   Eucalyptus
Diabetic Tussin DM
Diabetic Tussin DM Liqui-Gels
Diabetic Tussin DM Maximum Strength
Diabetic Tussin DM Maximum Strength
   Liqui-Gels
Diabetic Tussin EX
Diabetic Tussin, Children's
Dimetapp Allergy, Children's
Emagrin Forte
Fendol
Fisherman's Friend, Extra Strong, Sugar
   Free
Fisherman's Friend, Refreshing Mint,
   Sugar Free
Halls Juniors Sugar Free Cough Drops,
   Grape or Orange
Halls Mentho-Lyptus Sugar Free Cough
   Supp. Drops, Bl. Cherry
Halls Mentho-Lyptus Sugar Free Cough
   Supp. Drops, Citrus
Halls Mentho-Lyptus Sugar Free Cough
   Supp. Drops, Menthol
Hayfebrol
Herbal-Menthol
Luden's Maximum Strength Sugar
   Free, Cherry
N'Ice 'N Clear, Cherry Eucalyptus
N'Ice 'N Clear, Menthol Eucalyptus
N'Ice Sore Throat & Cough, Assorted or
   Citrus
N'Ice Sore Throat & Cough, Cherry
N'Ice Sore Throat & Cough, Herbal Mint
   or Honey Lemon
Nasal-D
Oranyl
Oranyl Plus
Propagest
Ricola Sugar Free Herb Throat Drops,
   Alpine-Mint
Ricola Sugar Free Herb Throat Drops,
   Cherry- or Lemon-Mint
Ricola Sugar Free Herb Throat Drops,
   Mountain Herb
Robitussin Sugar Free Cough Drops,
   Cherry or Peppermint
Safe Tussin 30

Scot-Tussin Allergy Relief Formula
Scot-Tussin Diabetes CF
Scot-Tussin DM
Scot-Tussin DM Cough Chasers
Scot-Tussin Expectorant
Scot-Tussin Original
Scot-Tussin Senior
Sine-Off Sinus, Cold, and Flu Medicine
   Night Time Formula
Sinulin
Sudafed Children's Cold & Cough
Sudafed Children's Nasal Decongestant
Sudafed Pediatric Nasal Decongestant
Sudanyl
TheraFlu Max. Strength Flu, Cold &
   Cough Medicine NightTime
Tussar-SF

DENTIFRICE PRODUCTS
Arm & Hammer PeroxiCare
Colgate
Colgate Baking Soda & Peroxide Tartar
   Control
Colgate Baking Soda & Peroxide
   Whitening
Colgate Baking Soda
Colgate Baking Soda Tartar Control
Colgate Junior
Colgate Tartar Control Micro Cleansing
   Formula
Colgate Winterfresh
Natural White
Natural White Baking Soda
Natural White Fights Plaque
Natural White Sensitive
Natural White Tartar Control
Natural White with Peroxide
Pearl Drops Whitening Baking Soda
   Tartar Control
Pearl Drops Whitening Extra Strength
Pearl Drops Whitening Regular Tartar
   Control
Pearl Drops Whitening Toothpolish
Pearl Drops Whitening Toothpolish, Icy
   Cool Mint
Pearl Drops Whitening Toothpolish,
   Spearmint
Slimer
Ultra Brite
Ultra Brite Baking Soda
Ultra Brite Baking Soda & Peroxide

ENTERAL FOOD SUPPLEMENT PRODUCTS
Casec
Criticare HN
Deliver 2.0
DiabetiSource
Impact
Impact 1.5
Impact with Fiber
Isocal
Isocal HN
IsoSource VHN
MCT Oil
Microlipid
Moducal
ReSource Diabetic
SandoSource Peptide
Vivonex Pediatric
Vivonex Plus
Vivonex T.E.N.

GASTRIC DECONTAMINANT PRODUCTS
CharcoAid G

HISTAMINE II RECEPTOR ANTAGONISTS
Axid AR
Tagamet HB 200
Zantac 75

INFANTS' AND CHILDREN'S FORMULA PRODUCTS
Enfamil
Enfamil Human Milk Fortifier
Enfamil Next Step
Enfamil Premature Formula
Enfamil Premature Formula with Iron
Enfamil with Iron
Gerber Baby Formula Low Iron
Gerber Baby Formula with Iron
Lactofree
Lofenalac
MSUD Diet
Nutramigen
Pregestimil
ProSobee

INTERNAL ANALGESIC AND ANTIPYRETIC PRODUCTS
Actamin
Actamin Extra
Actamin Super
Aminofen
Aminofen Max
Anodynos
Arthriten
Aspercin
Aspercin Extra
Aspermin
Aspermin Extra
Aspirin, Enteric Coated
Aspirtab
Aspirtab Max
Back-Quell
Buffaprin
Buffaprin Extra
Buffasal
Buffasal Max
Buffets II
Buffinol
Buffinol Extra
Dyspel
Emagrin
Excedrin Aspirin Free
Mobigesic
Motrin IB
Supac
Tempra Quicklet
Ultraprin
Valorin
Valorin Extra
Valorin Super
Valprin

IRON PRODUCTS
Feostat
Ferro-Sequels
Iron Plus Vitamin C
Irospan
Niferex

LAXATIVE PRODUCTS
Ceo-Two
Citrucel Sugar Free
Evac-Q-Kwik
Ex-Lax Stool Softener
FiberCon
Herb-Lax
Kellogg's Tasteless Castor Oil
Konsyl
Mag-Ox 400

Metamucil Original Texture, Regular Flavor
Metamucil Smooth Texture, Sugar Free Orange
Purge
Unilax
Uro-Mag

MENSTRUAL PRODUCTS
Backaid Pills
Diurex Water Caplet
Lurline PMS

MISCELLANEOUS MINERAL PRODUCTS
Chromium Picolinate
Chromium, Organic
Manganese Chelate
Maxi-Minerals
Selenium, Oceanic
Verazinc
Zinc

ORAL DISCOMFORT PRODUCTS
Baby Gumz
Dentemp Temporary Filling Mix
Little Teethers Oral Pain Relief
Peroxyl Oral Spot Treatment
Probax
Proxigel

ORAL HYGIENE PRODUCTS
Cepacol Mouthwash/Gargle
Cepacol Mouthwash/Gargle, Mint

SORE THROAT PRODUCTS
Cepacol Sore Throat Maximum Strength, Cherry
Cepacol Sore Throat Maximum Strength, Cool Menthol
Cepastat Extra Strength Sore Throat
Cepastat Sore Throat, Cherry
Entertainer's Secret Throat Relief
Fisherman's Friend, Extra Strong, Sugar Free
Fisherman's Friend, Refreshing Mint, Sugar Free
Halls Juniors Sugar Free Cough Drops, Grape or Orange
Halls Mentho-Lyptus Sugar Free Cough Supp. Drops, Bl. Cherry
Halls Mentho-Lyptus Sugar Free Cough Supp. Drops, Citrus
Halls Mentho-Lyptus Sugar Free Cough Supp. Drops, Menthol
Herbal-Menthol
Luden's Maximum Strength Sugar Free, Cherry
N'Ice 'N Clear, Cherry Eucalyptus
N'Ice 'N Clear, Menthol Eucalyptus
N'Ice Sore Throat & Cough, Assorted or Citrus
N'Ice Sore Throat & Cough, Cherry
N'Ice Sore Throat & Cough, Herbal Mint or Honey Lemon
Ricola Sugar Free Herb Throat Drops, Alpine-Mint
Ricola Sugar Free Herb Throat Drops, Cherry- or Lemon-Mint
Ricola Sugar Free Herb Throat Drops, Mountain Herb
Robitussin Sugar Free Cough Drops, Cherry or Peppermint

VITAMIN PRODUCTS
A-D-E with Selenium Tablets
Adeks Chewable Tablets
Akorn Antioxidants Caplets
Antioxidant Formula Softgels
Antioxidant Vitamin & Mineral Formula Softgels

B 50 Complex Capsules or Tablets
B Complex Maxi Tablets
B-C-Bid Caplets
Brewers Yeast Tablets
Buffered C Tablets
C & E Softgels
C Vitamin Tablets
C Vitamin Timed-Release Tablets
Centrum High Potency Tablets
Cevi-Bid Tablets
Chelated Calcium Magnesium Tablets
Chelated Calcium Magnesium Zinc Tablets
Clinical Nutrients for Men Tablets
Clinical Nutrients for Women Tablets
Coldvac Lozenges
Daily Plus Iron & Calcium Tablets
Daily Vitamins Plus Minerals Tablets
DiabeVite Tablets
Diostate D Tablets
Eye-Vites Tablets
Freedavite Tablets
Fruit C Chewable Tablets
Geri-Freeda Tablets
Gerimed Tablets
Herpetrol Tablets
I.L.X. B12 Sugar Free Elixir
Jets Chewable Tablets
Kenwood Therapeutic Liquid
Kovitonic Liquid
KPN (Key Prenatal) Tablets
LKV (Liquid Kiddie Vitamins) Drops
Mature Complete Tablets
Monocaps Tablets
More Than a Multiple Tablets
Multi-Mineral Tablets
Natalins Tablets
Nestabs Tablets
Nutri-Mega Softgels
Os-Cal Fortified Tablets
Oxi-Freeda Tablets
Parvlex Tablets
Peridin-C Tablets
Poly-Vi-Sol Vitamin Drops
Poly-Vi-Sol with Iron Vitamin Drops
Protegra Antioxidant Softgels
Quintabs-M Tablets
Stresstabs High Potency Stress Formula + Iron Tablets
Stresstabs High Potency Stress Formula Plus Zinc Tablets
Stresstabs High Potency Stress Formula Tablets
Super A&D Tablets
Super Dec B-100 Coated Tablets
Super Multiple 42 with Beta Carotene Softgels
Super Quints-50 Tablets
Theragran High Potency Multivitamin Caplets
Theragran Stress Formula High Potency Multivitamin Caplets
Theragran-M High Potency Vitamins with Minerals Caplets
Total Antioxidant Softgels
Tri-Vi-Sol Vitamins A,D+C Drops
Tri-Vi-Sol With Iron Vitamin A,D+C Drops
Ultra-Freeda Tablets
Unilife-A Gelcaps
Vitalets Chewable Tablets, Flavored or Unflavored
Vitalize Liquid

SULFITE FREE

ANTACID AND ANTIREFLUX PRODUCTS
Gaviscon Extra Strength Liquid
Gaviscon Liquid
Maalox
Maalox Heartburn Relief
Maalox Therapeutic Concentrate
Riopan
ANTHELMINTIC PRODUCTS
Antiminth
ANTIDIARRHEAL PRODUCTS
Diasorb
Kaopectate
Kaopectate, Children's
Pepto-Bismol Maximum Strength
Pepto-Bismol Original Strength
Percy Medicine
ANTIEMETIC PRODUCTS
Dramamine, Children's
ANTIFLATULENT PRODUCTS
Maalox Antacid/Anti-Gas Extra Strength
Riopan Plus
Riopan Plus Double Strength, Cherry or Mint
ASTHMA INHALANT PRODUCTS
Broncho Saline
Bronkaid Mist and Refill
Primatene Mist
Sodium Chloride Inhalation Solution USP
COLD, COUGH, AND ALLERGY PRODUCTS
Benadryl Allergy
Benadryl Allergy Decongestant
Buckley's DM
Buckley's Mixture
Dorcol Children's Cough
Hayfebrol
Naldecon DX, Adult
Naldecon DX, Children's
Naldecon EX, Children's
Naldecon EX, Pediatric
Naldecon Senior DX
Naldecon Senior EX
Pertussin CS
Pertussin DM
Scot-Tussin Allergy Relief Formula
Scot-Tussin Diabetes CF
Scot-Tussin DM
Scot-Tussin Expectorant
Scot-Tussin Original
Scot-Tussin Senior
Triaminic DM, Cough Relief
Triaminic Expectorant, Chest & Head Congestion
Triaminic Infant, Oral Decongestant
Triaminic Night Time
Triaminic, Cold & Allergy
Triaminicol Multi-Symptom Relief
Vaporizer in a Bottle Air Wick Inhaler
Vicks 44 Soothing Cough Relief
Vicks 44D Soothing Cough & Head Congestion Relief
Vicks 44e Pediatric Cough & Chest Congestion Relief
Vicks 44E Soothing Cough & Chest Congestion Relief
Vicks 44m Pediatric Cough & Cold Relief
Vicks 44M Soothing Cough, Cold, & Flu Relief
Vicks DayQuil Children's Allergy Relief
Vicks DayQuil Multi-Symptom Cold/Flu Relief
Vicks NyQuil Children's Cold/Cough Medicine
Vicks NyQuil Multi-Symptom Cold/Flu Relief, Cherry
Vicks NyQuil Multi-Symptom Cold/Flu Relief, Original
INTERNAL ANALGESIC AND ANTIPYRETIC PRODUCTS
Aspirin Free, Infants'
Tempra 1
Tempra 2
IRON PRODUCTS
Feostat
Fer-In-Sol
Ircon FA
LAXATIVE PRODUCTS
Agoral, Marshmallow or Raspberry
Colace
Dr. Caldwell Senna
Fleet Babylax
Fleet Mineral Oil Oral Lubricant
Fleet Prep Kit 2
Fletcher's Castoria
Fletcher's, Children's Cherry
Kellogg's Tasteless Castor Oil
Liqui-Doss
Purge
Therevac Plus
Therevac-SB

MISCELLANEOUS NASAL PRODUCTS
Breathe Free
HuMIST Saline
Nasal Moist
Ocean
Pretz
ORAL DISCOMFORT PRODUCTS
Dentemp Temporary Filling Mix
Hurricaine, Wild Cherry
Hurricaine, Wild Cherry or Pina Colada
Hurricaine; Wild Cherry, Pina Colada, or Watermelon
Lipmagik
Oragesic
Peroxyl Hygienic Dental Rinse
TOPICAL DECONGESTANT PRODUCTS
Dristan
Dristan 12-Hour
Otrivin
Otrivin Pediatric
Pretz-D
Privine
Rhinall
Vicks Sinex 12-Hour Ultra Fine Mist
Vicks Sinex Ultra Fine Mist
Vicks Vapor Inhaler
VITAMIN PRODUCTS
Adeks Drops
Centrum High Potency Liquid
Gevrabon Liquid
Kovitonic Liquid
LKV (Liquid Kiddie Vitamins) Drops
Poly-Vi-Sol Vitamin Drops
Poly-Vi-Sol with Iron Vitamin Drops
Theragran High Potency Multivitamin Liquid
Tri-Vi-Sol Vitamins A,D+C Drops
Tri-Vi-Sol With Iron Vitamin A,D+C Drops
Vitalize Liquid

GERIATRIC FORMULATION

COLD, COUGH, AND ALLERGY PRODUCTS
Naldecon Senior DX
Naldecon Senior EX
ENTERAL FOOD SUPPLEMENT PRODUCTS
ProBalance Complete
LAXATIVE PRODUCTS
Evac-U-Gen
VITAMIN PRODUCTS
B-C-Bid Caplets
Centrum Silver for Adults 50+
Cevi-Bid Tablets
Geri-Freeda Tablets
Gerimed Tablets
Gevrabon Liquid
Mature Complete Tablets
Unicap Senior Tablets

PEDIATRIC FORMULATION

ANTACID AND ANTIREFLUX PRODUCTS
Mylanta Children's Upset Stomach Relief
Mylanta Children's Upset Stomach Relief, Bubble Gum or Fruit
ANTHELMINTIC PRODUCTS
Pin-X
ANTIDIARRHEAL PRODUCTS
Kaopectate, Children's
ANTIEMETIC PRODUCTS
Dramamine, Children's
ANTIFLATULENT PRODUCTS
Baby Gasz
Little Tummys Infant Gas Relief
Mylicon, Infant's
Phazyme Gas Relief
ASTHMA AUXILIARY DEVICES
Assess Low Range
Mini-Wright AFS Low Range
CALCIUM PRODUCTS
Chewy Bears Chewable Calcium
CALLUS, CORN, WART, & INGROWN TOENAIL PRODUCTS
Duofilm Wart Remover Patch for Kids
COLD, COUGH, AND ALLERGY PRODUCTS
Benadryl Allergy
Benylin Pediatric Cough Formula
Diabetic Tussin, Children's
Dimetapp Allergy, Children's
Dimetapp Cold & Allergy Quick Dissolve
Dimetapp Cold & Fever, Children's
Dimetapp Decongestant, Pediatric
Dorcol Children's Cough
Halls Juniors Sugar Free Cough Drops, Grape or Orange
Mentholatum Cherry Chest Rub for Kids
Naldecon DX, Children's
Naldecon DX, Pediatric
Naldecon EX, Children's
Naldecon EX, Pediatric
Pedia Care Cold-Allergy
Pedia Care Cough-Cold Formula
Pedia Care Infants' Decongestant

Pedia Care Infants' Decongestant Plus
  Cough
Pedia Care Night Rest Cough-Cold
  Formula
Pertussin CS
Redacon DX
Robitussin Pediatric
Robitussin Pediatric Cough
Robitussin Pediatric Cough & Cold
Robitussin Pediatric Night Relief
St. Joseph Cough Suppressant for
  Children
Sudafed Children's Cold & Cough
Sudafed Children's Nasal Decongestant
Sudafed Pediatric Nasal Decongestant
Triaminic AM, Non-Drowsy Cough &
  Decongestant Formula
Triaminic AM, Non-Drowsy Deconges-
  tant Formula
Triaminic DM, Cough Relief
Triaminic Expectorant, Chest & Head
  Congestion
Triaminic Infant, Oral Decongestant
Triaminic Night Time
Triaminic Sore Throat, Throat Pain &
  Cough
Triaminic, Cold & Allergy
Triaminicol Multi-Symptom Relief
Tylenol Children's Cold Multi-Symptom
Tylenol Children's Cold Plus Cough
Tylenol Children's Flu
Tylenol Infants' Cold Decongestant and
  Fever Reducer
Vicks 44e Pediatric Cough & Chest
  Congestion Relief
Vicks 44m Pediatric Cough & Cold Relief
Vicks DayQuil Children's Allergy Relief
Vicks NyQuil Children's Cold/Cough
  Medicine

DENTIFRICE PRODUCTS
Colgate Junior
Crest for Kids, Sparkle Fun
First Teeth Baby Toothpaste
Orajel Baby Tooth & Gum Cleanser
Pete & Pam Toothpaste Pre-measured
  Strips
Slimer
Tom's Natural for Children, with Calcium
  & Fluoride

**DIAPER RASH AND PRICKLY HEAT
PRODUCTS**
A + D Ointment with Zinc Oxide
Balmex
Caldesene Medicated
Desitin
Desitin Cornstarch Baby Powder
Desitin Daily Care
Diapa-Kare
Diaparene Cornstarch Baby Powder
Diaparene Diaper Rash
Diaper Guard
Dyprotex
Flanders Buttocks Ointment
Gold Bond Baby Powder
Gold Bond Cornstarch Plus Medicated
  Baby Powder
Johnson's Baby Cream
Johnson's Baby Powder
Johnson's Baby Powder Cornstarch
Johnson's Baby, Medicated
Johnson's Diaper Rash Ointment
Little Bottoms
Resinol Diaper Rash
ZBT Baby Powder

DRY SKIN PRODUCTS
Johnson's Baby Lotion
Johnson's Ultra Sensitive Baby Cream
Johnson's Ultra Sensitive Baby Lotion
Little Noses Saline Moisturizing
Stevens Baby

**ENTERAL FOOD SUPPLEMENT
PRODUCTS**
Compleat Pediatric
Peptamen Junior Complete
ReSource Just for Kids
Vivonex Pediatric

**INFANTS' AND CHILDREN'S FORMULA
PRODUCTS**
Carnation Alsoy
Carnation Follow-Up
Carnation Follow-Up Soy
Carnation Good Start
Enfamil
Enfamil Human Milk Fortifier
Enfamil Next Step
Enfamil Next Step Soy
Enfamil Premature Formula
Enfamil Premature Formula with Iron
Enfamil with Iron
Gerber Baby Formula Low Iron
Gerber Baby Formula with Iron
Gerber Soy Baby Formula
Isomil
Isomil DF
Isomil SF
Kindercal
Lactofree
Lofenalac
MSUD Diet
Nutramigen
PediaSure
PediaSure with Fiber
Phenyl-Free
Portagen
Pregestimil
ProSobee
RCF (Ross Carbohydrate Free)
Similac
Similac PM 60/40
Similac Special Care 24 with Iron
Similac Toddler's Best; Berry, Chocolate,
  or Vanilla
Similac with Iron

INSECT REPELLENT PRODUCTS
Camp Lotion for Kids
Coppertone Bug & Sun Kids Formula
  SPF 30
Off! Skintastic for Kids
Skedaddle! for Children
Skedaddle! for Children SPF 15

**INTERNAL ANALGESIC AND
ANTIPYRETIC PRODUCTS**
Acetaminophen Suspension, Children's
  Flavored
Advil, Children's
Aspirin Free Pain & Fever Relief,
  Children's
Aspirin Free, Infants'
Bayer Children's Aspirin, Cherry or
  Orange
Feverall Sprinkle Caps Powder,
  Children's Strength
Feverall Sprinkle Caps Powder, Junior
  Strength
Feverall, Children's
Feverall, Infants'

Liquiprin for Children
Motrin, Children's
Motrin, Junior Strength
Tempra 1
Tempra 2
Tempra 3
Tempra 3, Double Strength
Tempra Quicklet
Tylenol Junior Strength Swallowable
Tylenol Junior Strength, Fruit Burst
Tylenol Junior Strength, Fruit Flavor
Tylenol Junior Strength, Grape
Tylenol, Children's Bubble Gum Flavor
Tylenol, Children's Cherry
Tylenol, Children's Cherry or Grape
Tylenol, Children's Fruit Burst
Tylenol, Children's Fruit Flavor
Tylenol, Children's Grape
Tylenol; Infants' Suspension, Cherry or
  Grape

IRON PRODUCTS
Fer-In-Sol

LAXATIVE PRODUCTS
Fleet Babylax
Fleet Glycerin Child Size
Fleet Ready-to-Use Enema for Children
Fletcher's Castoria
Fletcher's, Children's Cherry
Senokot Children's

**MISCELLANEOUS DIABETES
PRODUCTS**
Cleanlet Kids
tenderfoot

MISCELLANEOUS NASAL PRODUCTS
Little Noses Saline

ORAL DISCOMFORT PRODUCTS
Anbesol Baby, Grape
Anbesol Baby, Original
Baby Gumz
Dr. Hand's Teething
Little Teethers Oral Pain Relief
Orabase Baby
Orajel Baby
Orajel Baby Nighttime Formula
Zilactin Baby

ORAL REHYDRATION SOLUTIONS
Kao Lectrolyte Individual Packets,
  Flavored or Unflavored
Naturalyte, Bubblegum or Unflavored
Naturalyte, Fruit Flavored or Grape
Pedialyte
Pedialyte Freezer Pops
Revital Ice Freezer Pops

OSTOMY APPLIANCES
Little Ones Active Life Drainable
  Pouches
Little Ones Sur-Fit Drainable Pouches

**POISON IVY, OAK, AND SUMAC
PRODUCTS**
Benadryl Itch Stopping Children's
  Formula
Cortizone-5 for Kids

SORE THROAT PRODUCTS
Halls Juniors Sugar Free Cough Drops,
  Grape or Orange
Sucrets Children's Sore Throat, Cherry

SUNSCREEN AND SUNTAN PRODUCTS
Bain de Soleil All Day for Kids Water-
  proof Sunblock
Bio Sun Children
Bull Frog for Kids
Coppertone Kids Colorblock Disappear-
  ing Purple Sunblock

Coppertone Kids Sunblock
Coppertone Little Licks Sunblock Lip
  Balm
Hawaiian Tropic Baby Faces Sunblock
Hawaiian Tropic Just for Kids Sunblock
Neutrogena Kids Sunblock
Nivea Sun Kids
PreSun for Kids
Snoopy Sunblock
TI-Baby Natural Sunblock
Water Babies UVA/UVB Sunblock

TOPICAL DECONGESTANT PRODUCTS
Little Noses Decongestant
Otrivin Pediatric

TOPICAL FLUORIDE PRODUCTS
Fluoride Foam
Reach Act for Kids

VITAMIN PRODUCTS
A Kid's Companion Wafers
Adeks Drops
Bugs Bunny Complete Vitamins Plus
  Minerals Chewable Tablets
Bugs Bunny Plus Iron Chewable Tablets
Bugs Bunny with Extra C Children's
  Chewable Tablets
Centrum Jr. Shamu and His Crew + Extra
  C Chew. Tablets
Centrum Jr. Shamu and His Crew + Extra
  Calcium Chew. Tablets
Centrum Jr. Shamu and His Crew + Iron
  Chew. Tablets
Chewy Bears Citrus Free Vitamin C
  Chewable Wafers

Chewy Bears Complete Chewable
  Tablets
Children's Chewable Vitamins with Extra
  C Tablets
Children's Multi-Vitamin Liquid
Circus Chews Complete Chewable
  Tablets
Circus Chews with Beta Carotene
  Chewable Tablets
Circus Chews with Calcium Chewable
  Tablets
Circus Chews with Extra Vitamin C
  Tablets
Circus Chews with Iron
Flintstones Children's Chewable Tablets
Flintstones Complete Chewable Tablets
Flintstones Plus Extra C Children's
  Chewable Tablets
Flintstones Plus Iron Chewable Tablets
Garfield Complete Vitamins with
  Minerals Chewable Tablets
Garfield Regular Vitamins Chewable
  Tablets
Garfield Vitamins Plus Extra C Chewable
  Tablets
Garfield Vitamins Plus Iron Chewable
  Tablets
Jets Chewable Tablets
Kovitonic Liquid
LKV (Liquid Kiddie Vitamins) Drops
Poly-Vi-Sol Chewable Vitamins

Poly-Vi-Sol Vitamin Drops
Poly-Vi-Sol with Iron Chewable Vitamins
  & Minerals Tablets
Poly-Vi-Sol with Iron Vitamin Drops
Sesame Street Complete Vitamins &
  Minerals Chewable Tablets
Sesame Street Vitamins Plus Extra C
  Chewable Tablets
Sesame Street Vitamins Plus Iron
  Chewable Tablets
Sunkist Multivitamins Complete Tablets
Sunkist Multivitamins Plus Extra C
  Tablets
Sunkist Multivitamins Plus Iron Tablets
Sunkist Multivitamins Regular Tablets
Tri-Vi-Sol Vitamins A,D+C Drops
Tri-Vi-Sol With Iron Vitamin A,D+C
  Drops
Unicap Jr. Chewable Tablets
Vi-Daylin ADC Vitamins Drops
Vi-Daylin ADC Vitamins Plus Iron Drops
Vi-Daylin Multi-Vitamin Chewable
  Tablets
Vi-Daylin Multi-Vitamin Drops
Vi-Daylin Multi-Vitamin Plus Iron
  Chewable Tablets
Vi-Daylin Multi-Vitamin Plus Iron Drops
Vita-Lea for Children Tablets
Vita-Lea for Infants & Toddlers Powder
Vitalets Chewable Tablets, Flavored or
  Unflavored

New Product Tables

HIV TEST KITS

Product Manufacturer/Supplier	No. of Tests	Reaction Time (business days)	Comments
** **Confide HIV Testing Service** Direct Access Diagnostics	1	7, after laboratory's receipt	to order test, dial 1-800-THE-TEST · read the pre-counseling booklet about HIV and AIDS · prick fingertip with lancet provided · apply three drops of blood to precoded test card · tear identification code tab from test card and mail in postage-paid envelope to certified laboratory for HIV-1 antibody testing · to obtain test result, call the Confide Test Result Center seven days later and enter the kit's personal identification number · all callers have the opportunity to speak directly with a counselor (anonymously and in confidence) · referrals for further testing are provided when necessary
** **Home Access** Home Access Health	1	7, after laboratory's receipt	to order test, dial 1-800-HIV-TEST · register anonymously via telephone with identification code number and receive professional pre-test telephone counseling · prick fingertip with lancet provided, then apply blood sample to test card · seal card in protective barrier pouch and mail to central processing laboratory for HIV-1 antibody testing · call seven days later to obtain test result · pre- and post-test counseling available any time
** **Home Access Express** Home Access Health	1	3, after laboratory's reciept	test procedure is identical to Home Access, except that the test card is sent to laboratory via FedEx and result is available in three days

** New listing

These products became available after publication of Handbook of Nonprescription Drugs, 11th Edition.

URINE TEST KITS

	Product Manufacturer/Supplier	No. of Tests	Reaction Time (min)	Comments
**	**EZ-Detect Urine Blood Test** Biomerica	6	1	one step procedure to detect the presence of blood · collect urine sample in cup provided · dip test strip · after one minute, match test strip pad color to color chart on test strip vial label · strip's control area indicates any presence of vitamin C · strip is highly sensitive
**	**HealthCheck Uri-Test Nitrite** Health-Mark Diagnostics	3	1	collect urine sample in cup provided · dip test strip · after one minute, match test strip pad color to results chart · a positive result is indicated by appearance of any shade of pink color
**	**UTI Home Screening** Consumers Choice	6	1	test urine which has remained in the bladder a minimum of 4-6 hours · either collect in a clean, dry container and dip test strip, or pass test strip directly through urine stream · after one minute, match test strip pad color to color chart on test strip vial label · a positive result is indicated by appearance of any shade of pink color

** New listing

DRUGS OF ABUSE TEST KITS

	Product Manufacturer/Supplier	No. of Tests	Reaction Time (business days)	Comments
**	**Dr. Brown's Home Drug Testing System** Personal Health & Hygiene	1	1-3, after laboratory's receipt	approved by the Food and Drug Administration · collect urine sample in cup provided · transfer sample into the two sealable plastic tubes, enclose in the plastic pouch and postage-paid bubble mailer, and mail to certified testing laboratory for analysis · obtain result by calling toll-free telephone number and giving the kit's identification number · referrals for counseling and medical help will be offered
**	**Parent's Alert** ChemTrak	1	3, after laboratory's receipt	collect urine sample in cup provided · enclose in the specimen bag and overnight shipping pouch, and send via Airborne Express to certified laboratory for analysis · obtain result by calling toll-free telephone number and giving the kit's code number · counseling is available before, during, and after testing, and referrals for additional counseling may be offered · test indicates the presence of LSD and Ecstasy in addition to the standardly indicated drugs
**	**PDT-90 Personal Drug Testing Service** Psychemedics	1	5, after laboratory's receipt	can detect drugs of abuse for the previous approximate 90-day period · collect a small snip of hair (60-80 strands, 1.5" in length, from back crown of the head) and mail to testing laboratory for analysis · obtain results by calling toll-free telephone number and giving the kit's code number · referrals for counseling may be offered

** New listing

HORMONAL SUPPLEMENTS

Product Manufacturer/Supplier	Dosage Form	Hormone	Other Ingredients
** **DHEA** Natrol	tablet	dehydroepiandrosterone, 5mg; 10mg; 25mg	
** **DHEA** Natrol	capsule	dehydroepiandrosterone, 25mg	
** **DHEA** Breckenridge Ph'cal	tablet	dehydroepiandrosterone, 25mg	
** **DHEA** American Health	tablet	dehydroepiandrosterone, 25mg	
** **DHEA** Young Again Products	cream	dehydroepiandrosterone, 1%	
** **DHEA** Young Again Products	tablet	dehydroepiandrosterone, 25mg	
** **DHEA for Men** Celestial Seasonings	timed-release caplet	vitamin A, 2500 IU · vitamin C, 60mg · vitamin E, 15 IU · dehydroepiandrosterone, 25mg	
** **DHEA for Women** Celestial Seasonings	timed-release caplet	vitamin A, 2500 IU · vitamin C, 60mg · vitamin E, 15 IU · dehydroepiandrosterone, 5mg	
** **DHEA Therapeutic** Breckenridge Ph'cal	cream	dehydroepiandrosterone, 1%	
** **Preferred DHEA** Reese Chemical	capsule	dehydroepiandrosterone, 50mg · ascorbyl palmitate, 15mg	
** **Preferred DHEA Therapeutic** Reese Chemical	cream	dehydroepiandrosterone, 1%	water · propylene glycol · sorbitol · glyceryl stearate · stearic acid · dimethicone · vitamin E · benzoin gum salt
** **Pregnenolone** Young Again Products	cream	pregnenolone, 2%	
** **Pregnenolone** Young Again Products	tablet	pregnenolone, 25mg	
** **Triple Hormone** Young Again Products	tablet	dehydroepiandrosterone, 25mg · pregnenolone, 25mg · melatonin, 2mg	

** New listing

In-Home Testing and Monitoring Product Tables

FECAL OCCULT BLOOD TEST KITS

Product [a] Manufacturer/Supplier	No. of Tests	Comments
ColoCARE ChemTrak	3	use for three consecutive bowel movements · flush toilet twice before each bowel movement · pad is floated in toilet bowl with specimen · observe for 30 seconds · pad check area on left will turn blue and/or green, the other will not · positive result is appearance of a blue color on the test pad · flush pad away when test is complete
EZ-Detect Stool Blood Test Biomerica	5	one step procedure · use for three consecutive bowel movements · flush toilet twice before each bowel movement · test pad is floated in toilet bowl with specimen · observe for up to 2 minutes · positive result appears as a blue-green color on test pad · no diet restrictions (vitamin C and rare meat are okay) · avoid anti-inflammatory medications and those that cause internal bleeding

[a] Other nonprescription test kits for fecal occult blood may be obtained from physicians.

See Chapter 3, "In-Home Testing and Monitoring Products," for more information about these products.

OVULATION PREDICTION TEST KITS

Product Manufacturer/Supplier	No. of Tests	Reaction Time (min)	Indication of Positive Result	Comments
Answer 1-Step Ovulation Test Carter Products	5	5	test line color similar to or darker than reference line color	test any time of day · reduce liquid intake 2 hrs before testing · positive result indicates ovulation should occur within 24-36 hrs
Clearplan Easy Unipath Diagnostics	5	5	test line color in large window is similar to or darker than line color in small window	test any time of day, but test at same time each day · use concentrated (at least 4 hrs) urine specimen · positive result indicates ovulation should occur within 24-36 hrs · blue line in small window indicates test is complete and performed correctly
Conceive Ovulation Test Quidel	5	3	pink-to-purple test line color is darker than reference line color	test any time of day, but collect at same time each day · positive result indicates ovulation should occur within 24-40 hrs
** **early Ovulation predictor** Selfcare	5	3	test line color is darker than control line color	positive result indicates ovulation should occur within 24-72 hrs
EZ-LH Biomerica	6 & 10	1-5	comparison of test band to control band · pink band appears	one step procedure
First Response 1-Step Ovulation Predictor Test Carter Products	5	5	test line color similar to or darker than reference line color	test any time of day · reduce liquid intake 2 hrs before testing · positive result indicates ovulation should occur within 24-36 hrs
OvuKIT Quidel	6 & 9	60	blue test stick color is darker than the surge guide test	use urine collected between 10am and 8pm · do not use first morning urine · collect at same time each day · positive result indicates ovulation should occur within 24-40 hrs
OvuQUICK Quidel	6 & 9	4	color of test result area on test pad matches or is darker than the reference spot	use urine collected between 10am and 8pm · do not use first morning urine · collect at same time each day · positive result indicates ovulation should occur within 24-40 hrs
Q Test for Ovulation Prediction Quidel	5	35	result pad on test strip changes color from pale blue to dark blue	test any time of day · predicts ovulation within 20-44 hrs · error control pad on test strip indicates if test is performed correctly

** New listing

See Chapter 3, "In-Home Testing and Monitoring Products," for more information about these products.

PREGNANCY TEST KITS

Product Manufacturer/Supplier	No. of Tests	Reaction Time (min)	Indication of Positive Result	Control	Comments
Answer Pregnancy Test Carter Products	1	3	2 pink lines appear in result window		test any time of day · use as soon as first day of missed pleriod
Answer Quick & Simple 1-Step Stick Pregnancy Test Carter Products	1 & 2	2	2 pink lines appear in result window		test any time of day · use as soon as first day of missed period · one step procedure · hold test stick in urine stream
Clearblue Easy Unipath Diagnostics	1 & 2	1	blue line appears in large window	blue line in small window indicates test is complete and performed correctly	use any time after missed period · one step procedure · hold test stick in stream of concentrated (at least 6 hrs.) urine · hold stick downward during testing
Conceive Pregnancy Test Quidel	1 & 2	1-3	pink-to-purple test line appears	blue control line appears	use any time after missed period
Confirm Durex Consumer	1 & 2	3	appearance of blue line in both the test and control windows		use any time after missed period · one step procedure · hold test stick in urine stream
e.p.t. Warner-Lambert Consumer	1 & 2	3	pink line appears in round results window	square control window always shows a pink line	use first day of missed period · one step procedure · hold test stick in urine stream
early Pregnancy test Selfcare	1	1	pink line appears in square test window	pink line appears in round reference window	use any time after missed period · one step · choice of test methods: either hold test stick in urine stream or dip test stick in a cup of collected urine
First Response 1-Step Pregnancy Test Carter Products	1 & 2	2	2 pink lines appear in result window		test any time of day · use as soon as first day of missed period · one step procedure · hold test stick in urine stream
Fortel Midstream Biomerica	1 & 2	1-5	pink band appears in large test window		use as soon as first day of missed period · one step procedure
Fortel Plus Biomerica	1 & 2	1	pink band appears in test window		use as soon as first day of missed period · one step
Nimbus Quick Strip Biomerica	25	1-5	pink band appears in test window		one step procedure
Precise § Becton Dickinson Consumer	1 & 2	1	end-of-test window turns pink, blue check mark appears in result window	error control bar in result window indicates test is working correctly	use any time after missed period · one step procedure
Q-Test For Pregnancy Quidel	1	positive results as early as 9	test strip result pad turns blue	error control pad on test strip indicates if test is performed correctly	use any time after missed period · negative results can be verified in 16 minutes
RapidVue Quidel	1	1	pink-to-purple test line appears	blue control line appears	use any time after missed period · one step procedure · add 3 drops from urine collection to test well of test cassette

See Chapter 3, "In-Home Testing and Monitoring Products," for more information about these products.

CHOLESTEROL TEST KITS

Product [a] Manufacturer/Supplier	No. of Tests	Reaction Time (min)	Comments
CholesTrak ChemTrak	1 & 2	12-15	can test at any time; but do not test within 4 hrs of taking 500mg or more of vitamin C, or a standard dose of acetaminophen (may cause falsely low result) · prick fingertip, according to package instructions/supplies, to obtain blood sample · apply one or more drops of blood into the blood well, to fill · wait two to four minutes, then pull tab of test device · test is complete 12 minutes later after the "OK" indicator has turned purple, and "END" indicator turns green · read test device like a thermometer, and check the result chart for cholesterol level
** **HealthCheck** Health-Mark Diagnostics	1	3	apply one drop of blood onto test strip · read result color and compare with result chart · result indicates one of three groups: desirable, borderline, or high risk for heart disease

** New listing

[a] These products measure total cholesterol only. If a result of 200mg/dL or greater is obtained, the patient should see a physician for further evaluation.

See Chapter 3, "In-Home Testing and Monitoring Products," for more information about these products.

ELECTRONIC OSCILLOMETRIC BLOOD PRESSURE MONITOR PRODUCTS

Product Manufacturer/Supplier	Comments
** **A&D UA-702 Manual Inflation Digital B.P. Monitor** A&D Medical	inflates and deflates manually · low-battery indicator · automatic shut off
** **A&D UA-751 Auto-Inflation with Printer Digital B.P. Monitor** A&D Medical	inflates and deflates automatically · jumbo display · memory recall of 14 readings with date and time · prints in list or graph format
** **A&D UA-767 One-Step Auto-Inflation Digital B.P. Monitor** A&D Medical	inflates and deflates automatically · jumbo display · single-button operation · low-battery indicator · automatic shut off
** **A&D UA-777 One-Step Auto-Inflation Digital B.P. Monitor** A&D Medical	fuzzy logic operation · deflates automatically · single-button operation
** **A&D UB-211 Finger Digital B.P. Monitor** A&D Medical	compact, portable · inflates automatically · adjustable finger cuff · ergonomic design fits in either hand · low-battery indicator · automatic shut off
** **A&D UB-302 Compact Wrist Digital B.P. Monitor** A&D Medical	one-step single-button operation · inflates automatically
** **A&D UB-325 Wrist Digital B.P. Monitor** A&D Medical	inflates and deflates automatically · jumbo display · low-battery indicator · automatic shut off · 2-person memory recall (14 readings per person)
Labtron 02-707 Digital B.P./Pulse Monitor Graham-Field	compact, palm-sized · inflates manually, deflates automatically · self adjusting D-bar cuff · pressure release valve · lcd display · automatic shut off · comes with zippered vinyl carrying case · several cuff sizes available
Labtron 02-847 Automatic Digital B.P./Pulse Monitor Graham-Field	fully automatic, portable · inflates automatically · self adjusting D-bar cuff · automatic pressure release valve · lcd display · low-battery indicator · automatic shut off · comes with zippered vinyl carrying case · several cuff sizes available
Labtron 02-857 Auto. B.P. Kit w/Memory & Extra-Large Display Graham-Field	memory recall of last reading · inflates automatically with nine preset settings · easy three-step procedure · self adjusting D-bar cuff · extra-large lcd display · 2.5-minute automatic shut off · comes with zippered vinyl carrying case, four "AA" batteries
Labtron 02-947 Automatic Digital B.P./Pulse with Printer Graham-Field	fully automatic, portable · permanent record of time, date, systolic, diastolic, and pulse measurements · self adjusting D-bar cuff · built-in automatic pump · large lcd display · comes with one extra roll of chart paper, zippered vinyl carrying case, four "AA" batteries · several cuff sizes available
Labtron 02-949 Finger B.P./Pulse Monitor Graham-Field	compact, lightweight, portable · adjustable finger cuff · inflates and deflates automatically · digital display · low-battery indicator · comes with four "AAA" batteries
** **Labtron 02-959 Automatic Wrist B.P. Monitor** Graham-Field	large lcd display of blood pressure, pulse rate, graphic symbols, time, and date · automatic shut off · portable, self-contained in carrying case with storage compartment for cuff · comes with four "AA" batteries · two-person memory recall · 1.5 lbs.
Lumiscope 1060 Digital Blood Pressure Monitor Lumiscope	memory recall of last reading · D-bar cuff · inflates manually · preset automatic deflation valve · automatic shut off
Lumiscope 1083N Finger Blood Pressure Monitor Lumiscope	adjustable finger cuff · inflates automatically · digital display · preset automatic deflation · automatic shut off · memory recall of last reading

See Chapter 3, "In-Home Testing and Monitoring Products," for more information about these products.

ELECTRONIC OSCILLOMETRIC BLOOD PRESSURE MONITOR PRODUCTS - continued

Product Manufacturer/Supplier	Comments
Lumiscope 1085M Auto Inflation Blood Pressure Monitor Lumiscope	jumbo lcd display · memory recall of last reading · D-bar cuff · inflates automatically · preset automatic deflation rate · automatic shut off
** **Lumiscope 1090 Wrist Blood Pressure Monitor** Lumiscope	inflates automatically · fuzzy logic operation · large lcd display of blood pressure, pulse, time, and date · storage compartment for cuff inside the unit's carrying case · two-person memory recall (14 readings per person)
Marshall 82 Manual Inflation Blood Pressure Monitor Omron Healthcare	contoured D-ring cuff inflates manually and deflates automatically · large digital display
Marshall 92 Manual Inflation Blood Pressure Monitor Omron Healthcare	contoured D-ring cuff inflates and deflates automatically · large digital display · memory recall
Marshall 97 Measurement Print-out Blood Pressure Monitor Omron Healthcare	prints systolic, diastolic, and pulse measurements · contoured D-ring cuff inflates and deflates automatically · digital display
Marshall F-89 Finger Blood Pressure Monitor Omron Healthcare	adjustable finger cuff inflates and deflates automatically · digital display
Omron HEM-412C Manual Inflation B.P. Monitor Omron Healthcare	contoured D-ring cuff inflates manually and deflates automatically · digital display
Omron HEM-601 Wrist B.P. Monitor Omron Healthcare	inflates and deflates automatically · jumbo digital display · built-in cuff storage feature
Omron HEM-602 Wrist B.P. Monitor with Memory Omron Healthcare	displays up to seven readings in digital and bar-graph form · cuff inflates and deflates automatically · jumbo digital display · built-in cuff storage feature · includes four "AA" batteries
Omron HEM-605 Compact Wrist B.P. Monitor Omron Healthcare	convenient watch-style design · measures blood pressure and pulse directly from the wrist · small, pre-formed wrist cuff · inflates and deflates automatically · easy-to-read display panel folds down when not in use · comes with storage case and two "AA" batteries
Omron HEM-703CP Measurement Print-out B.P. Monitor Omron Healthcare	contoured D-ring cuff inflates and deflates automatically · digital display
Omron HEM-704C Self-Storing B.P. Monitor Omron Healthcare	curved contour D-ring cuff inflates and deflates automatically · jumbo digital display · folds into its own carrying case
Omron HEM-705CP Memory, Print-out, and Graph B.P. Monitor Omron Healthcare	prints in numerical and bar-graph form · curved contour D-ring cuff inflates and deflates automatically · large digital display · memory of 14 readings
Omron HEM-706 Fuzzy Logic B.P. Monitor Omron Healthcare	automatically determines ideal cuff inflation level · curved contour D-ring cuff · large digital display · built-in cuff storage
Omron HEM-711 Smart-Inflate Fuzzy Logic B.P. Monitor Omron Healthcare	automatically determines ideal cuff inflation level · curved contour D-ring cuff with "How To Apply" label · large digital display

See Chapter 3, "In-Home Testing and Monitoring Products," for more information about these products.

ELECTRONIC OSCILLOMETRIC BLOOD PRESSURE MONITOR PRODUCTS - continued

Product Manufacturer/Supplier	Comments
Omron HEM-712C Automatic Inflation B.P. Monitor Omron Healthcare	contoured D-ring cuff inflates and deflates automatically · digital display · memory recall
Omron HEM-806F Deluxe Finger B.P. Monitor Omron Healthcare	finger cuff adjusts automatically · digital display · comes with carrying case and two "AA" batteries
Omron HEM-808F Travel Finger B.P. Monitor Omron Healthcare	compact, self-store design · inflates and deflates automatically · large digital display · includes two "AAA" batteries
Omron HEM-815F Finger B.P. Monitor Omron Healthcare	adjustable finger cuff inflates and deflates automatically · digital display
** **Sunbeam 7624 Manual Digital B.P. Monitor** Sunbeam Consumer	inflates manually · one-touch operation · jumbo display · memory recall of last reading
** **Sunbeam 7654 Digital B.P. Monitor** Sunbeam Consumer	inflates automatically · jumbo display · fuzzy logic operation · memory recall of last reading
Sunbeam 7655-10 Digital Finger B.P. Monitor Sunbeam Consumer	inflates automatically · adjustable finger cuff · over- or under-inflation indicator
Sunbeam 7684 Digital Wrist Unit B.P. Monitor Sunbeam Consumer	inflates automatically · jumbo display · fuzzy logic operation · two-person memory recall (14 readings per person) · 2.5 lbs.
** **Sunbeam 7685 Digital Wrist Unit B.P. Monitor** Sunbeam Consumer	inflates automatically · jumbo display · memory recall of last reading · 2.5 lbs.

** New listing

See Chapter 3, "In-Home Testing and Monitoring Products," for more information about these products.

Internal Analgesic and Antipyretic Product Table

INTERNAL ANALGESIC AND ANTIPYRETIC PRODUCTS

Product [a] Manufacturer/Supplier	Dosage Form	Acetamin-ophen	Aspirin	Ibuprofen	Other Analgesics	Other Ingredients [b]
ACETAMINOPHEN						
AL AF PE **Acetaminophen Suspension, Children's Flavored** Multisource	drops	80mg/0.8ml				
AF CA GL PU SO **Acetaminophen Uniserts** Upsher-Smith Labs	suppository	120mg; 325mg; 650mg				
AF CA SU **Actamin** Buffington	tablet	325mg				
AF CA SU **Actamin Extra** Buffington	tablet	500mg				
AF SO SU **Actamin Super** Buffington	tablet	500mg				caffeine, 65mg
AF **Alka-Seltzer** Bayer Consumer	caplet	500mg				calcium carbonate, 380mg · crospovidone · docusate sodium · hydroxypropyl methylcellulose · lecithin · magnesium stearate · polyvinylpyrrolidone · sodium benzoate · sodium hexametaphosphate · sodium starch glycolate · starch · stearic acid
AF CA SU **Aminofen** Dover Ph'cal	tablet	324mg				
AF CA SU **Aminofen Max** Dover Ph'cal	tablet	500mg				
AF **Anacin Aspirin Free Maximum Strength** Whitehall-Robins Healthcare	tablet	500mg				calcium stearate · croscarmellose sodium · D&C red#7 lake · FD&C blue#1 lake · hydroxypropyl methylcellulose · polyethylene glycol · povidone · propylene glycol · starch · stearic acid · titanium dioxide
AF CA GL PR PU SO PE **Aspirin Free Pain & Fever Relief, Children's** Hudson	chewable tablet	80mg				
AF CA GL PR PU **Aspirin Free Pain Relief** Hudson	tablet	325mg				

See Chapter 4, "Internal Analgesic and Antipyretic Products," for more information about these products.

INTERNAL ANALGESIC AND ANTIPYRETIC PRODUCTS - continued

	Product [a] Manufacturer/Supplier	Dosage Form	Acetamin- ophen	Aspirin	Ibuprofen	Other Analgesics	Other Ingredients [b]
AF CA GL PR PU	**Aspirin Free Pain Relief** Hudson	caplet · tablet	500mg				
AL AF CA PR SL PE	**Aspirin Free, Infants'** Hudson	drops	80mg/0.8ml				
AF CA PR	**Bromo-Seltzer** Warner-Lambert Consumer	granular effervescent	325mg/capful				sodium bicarbonate, 2.78g/capful · citric acid, 2.22g/capful
**	**Dynafed EX.** BDI Ph'cals	tablet	500mg				
AF CA SO SU	**Dyspel** Dover Ph'cal	tablet	325mg				ephedrine sulfate, 8mg · atropine sulfate, 0.06mg
AF	**Excedrin Aspirin Free** Bristol-Myers Products	caplet	500mg				caffeine, 65mg · benzoic acid · carnauba wax · corn starch · D&C red#27 lake · D&C yellow#10 lake · FD&C blue#1 lake · hydroxypropyl methylcellulose · magnesium stearate · methylparaben · microcrystalline cellulose · mineral oil · polysorbate 20 · povidone · propylene glycol · propylparaben · simethicone emulsion · sorbitan monolaurate · stearic acid · titanium dioxide · may also contain: croscarmellose sodium · FD&C red#40 · saccharin sodium · sodium starch glycolate
AF GL SU	**Excedrin Aspirin Free** Bristol-Myers Products	geltab	500mg				caffeine, 65mg · benzoic acid · corn starch · FD&C blue#1 · FD&C red#40 · FD&C yellow#6 · gelatin · glycerin · hydroxypropyl methylcellulose · magnesium stearate · methylparaben · microcrystalline cellulose · mineral oil · polysorbate 20 · povidone · propylene glycol · propylparaben · simethicone emulsion · sorbitan monolaurate · stearic acid · titanium dioxide · may also contain: croscarmellose sodium · sodium starch glycolate

See Chapter 4, "Internal Analgesic and Antipyretic Products," for more information about these products.

INTERNAL ANALGESIC AND ANTIPYRETIC PRODUCTS - continued

	Product [a] Manufacturer/Supplier	Dosage Form	Acetamin- ophen	Aspirin	Ibuprofen	Other Analgesics	Other Ingredients [b]
PR SO	**Excedrin Extra Strength** Bristol-Myers Products	caplet · tablet	250mg	250mg			caffeine, 65mg · benzoic acid · hydroxypropyl cellulose · hydroxypropyl methylcellulose · microcrystalline cellulose · mineral oil · polysorbate 20 · povidone · propylene glycol · simethicone emulsion · sorbitan monolaurate · stearic acid · may also contain: carnauba wax · FD&C blue#1 · saccharin sodium · titanium dioxide
GL	**Excedrin Extra Strength** Bristol-Myers Products	geltab	250mg	250mg			caffeine, 65mg · benzoic acid · D&C yellow#10 lake · disodium EDTA · FD&C blue#1 lake · FD&C red#40 lake · ferric oxide · gelatin · glycerin · hydroxypropyl cellulose · hydroxypropyl methylcellulose · maltitol solution · microcrystalline cellulose · mineral oil · pepsin · polysorbate 20 · povidone · propylene glycol · propyl gallate · simethicone emulsion · sorbitan monolaurate · stearic acid · titanium dioxide
AF CA GL PU SO	**Feverall Adult Strength** Upsher-Smith Labs	suppository	650mg				
AF CA GL PU SO	**Feverall Junior Strength** Upsher-Smith Labs	suppository	325mg				
AF CA GL PU SO PE	**Feverall Sprinkle Caps Powder, Children's Strength** Upsher-Smith Labs	capsule	80mg				
AF CA GL PU SO PE	**Feverall Sprinkle Caps Powder, Junior Strength** Upsher-Smith Labs	capsule	160mg				
AF CA GL PU SO PE	**Feverall, Children's** Upsher-Smith Labs	suppository	120mg				
AF CA GL PU SO PE	**Feverall, Infants'** Upsher-Smith Labs	suppository	80mg				

See Chapter 4, "Internal Analgesic and Antipyretic Products," for more information about these products.

INTERNAL ANALGESIC AND ANTIPYRETIC PRODUCTS - continued

	Product [a] Manufacturer/Supplier	Dosage Form	Acetamin-ophen	Aspirin	Ibuprofen	Other Analgesics	Other Ingredients [b]
AL AF CA PE	**Liquiprin for Children** Menley & James Labs	drops	48mg/ml				dextrose · fructose · sucrose · fruit flavor · D&C red#33 · FD&C red#40 · propylparaben · methylparaben · glycerin · citric acid · polyethylene glycol · sodium citrate · sodium gluconate · sweetener
AF CA GL SO	**Midol Menstrual Regular Strength Multisymptom Formula** Bayer Consumer	caplet	325mg				pyrilamine maleate, 12.5mg
AF CA GL PR PU	**Percogesic Coated** Medtech	tablet	325mg				phenyltoloxamine citrate, 30mg · cellulose · flavor · FD&C yellow#6 hydroxypropyl methylcellulose · magnesium stearate · polyethylene glycol · povidone · purified water · silica gel · starch · stearic acid · sucrose
AF CA	**Stanback AF Extra-Strength** Stanback	powder	950mg				
AF	**Tapanol Extra Strength** Republic Drug	caplet · tablet	500mg				
AL AF CA PR SL PE	**Tempra 1** Bristol-Myers Products	drops	80mg/0.8ml				citric acid · D&C red#33 · FD&C blue#1 · FD&C red#40 · glycerin · grape flavor · propylene glycol · sodium benzoate · sodium citrate · saccharin sodium · water
AL AF CA SL PE	**Tempra 2** Bristol-Myers Products	syrup	160mg/5ml				BHA · citric acid · D&C red#33 · FD&C blue#1 · FD&C red#40 flavors · polyethylene glycol · propylene glycol · sodium benzoate · sodium citrate · saccharin sodium · sorbitol · water
AF CA GL PR PE	**Tempra 3** Bristol-Myers Products	chewable tablet	80mg				aspartame · croscarmellulose sodium · D&C red#27 aluminum lake · FD&C blue#1 aluminum lake · glycine · grape flavor · magnesium stearate · mannitol · microcrystalline cellulose · sodium citrate
AF CA GL PR PE	**Tempra 3, Double Strength** Bristol-Myers Products	chewable tablet	160mg				aspartame · croscarmellulose sodium · D&C red#27 aluminum lake · FD&C blue#1 aluminum lake · glycine · grape flavor · magnesium stearate · mannitol · microcrystalline cellulose · sodium citrate
** AF CA SU PE	**Tempra Quicklet** Bristol-Myers Products	tablet	80mg; 160mg				aspartame · citric acid · D&C red#27 lake · FD&C blue#1 lake · flavor · magnesium stearate · mannitol · potassium carbonate · silicon dioxide · sodium bicarbonate

See Chapter 4, "Internal Analgesic and Antipyretic Products," for more information about these products.

INTERNAL ANALGESIC AND ANTIPYRETIC PRODUCTS - continued

Product [a] Manufacturer/Supplier	Dosage Form	Acetamin- ophen	Aspirin	Ibuprofen	Other Analgesics	Other Ingredients [b]
AF CA **Tylenol Extended Relief** McNeil Consumer	timed-release caplet	650mg (immediate release, 325mg · slow, continuous release, 325mg)				corn starch · hydroxyethyl cellulose · hydroxypropyl methylcellulose · magnesium stearate · microcrystalline cellulose · povidone · powdered cellulose · pregelatinized starch · sodium starch glycolate · titanium dioxide · triacetin
AF CA **Tylenol Extra Strength** McNeil Consumer	caplet	500mg				cellulose · corn starch · hydroxypropyl methylcellulose · magnesium stearate · polyethylene glycol · sodium starch glycolate · red#40
AF CA **Tylenol Extra Strength** McNeil Consumer	gelcap · geltab	500mg				benzyl alcohol · butylparaben · castor oil · cellulose · corn starch · edetate calcium disodium · gelatin · hydroxypropyl methylcellulose · magnesium stearate · methylparaben · propylparaben · sodium lauryl sulfate · sodium propionate · sodium starch glycolate · titanium dioxide · blue#1 · blue#2 · red#40 · yellow#10
AF CA **Tylenol Extra Strength** McNeil Consumer	tablet	500mg				magnesium stearate · cellulose · sodium starch glycolate · corn starch
AF CA **Tylenol Extra Strength Adult** McNeil Consumer	liquid	166.7mg/5ml				alcohol, 7% · citric acid · flavors · glycerin · polyethylene glycol · purified water · sodium benzoate · sorbitol · sucrose · blue#1 · yellow#6 · yellow#10
AF CA PE **Tylenol Junior Strength Swallowable** McNeil Consumer	caplet	160mg				cellulose · corn starch · ethylcellulose · magnesium stearate · sodium lauryl sulfate · sodium starch glycolate
** AF PE **Tylenol Junior Strength, Fruit Burst** McNeil Consumer	chewable tablet	160mg				aspartame · cellulose · citric acid · corn starch · flavors · magnesium stearate · mannitol · red#7 · may contain: ethylcellulose or cellulose acetate · povidone
AF CA PE **Tylenol Junior Strength, Fruit Flavor** McNeil Consumer	chewable tablet	160mg				aspartame · cellulose · citric acid · corn starch · ethylcellulose · flavors · magnesium stearate · mannitol · red#7
AF CA PE **Tylenol Junior Strength, Grape** McNeil Consumer	chewable tablet	160mg				aspartame · cellulose · cellulose acetate · citric acid · corn starch · flavors · magnesium stearate · mannitol · povidone · blue#1 · red#7 · red#30

See Chapter 4, "Internal Analgesic and Antipyretic Products," for more information about these products.

INTERNAL ANALGESIC AND ANTIPYRETIC PRODUCTS - continued

	Product [a] Manufacturer/Supplier	Dosage Form	Acetamin-ophen	Aspirin	Ibuprofen	Other Analgesics	Other Ingredients [b]
AF CA	**Tylenol Regular Strength** McNeil Consumer	caplet	325mg				cellulose · hydroxypropyl methylcellulose · magnesium stearate · polyethylene glycol · sodium starch glycolate · corn starch · red#40
AF CA	**Tylenol Regular Strength** McNeil Consumer	tablet	325mg				cellulose · corn starch · magnesium stearate · sodium starch glycolate
AF CA PE	**Tylenol, Children's Bubble Gum Flavor** McNeil Consumer	chewable tablet	80mg				aspartame · cellulose · flavors · magnesium stearate · mannitol · povidone · red#7 · may contain: ethylcellulose or cellulose acetate · gum arabic · maltodextrin
AL AF CA PE	**Tylenol, Children's Bubble Gum Flavor** McNeil Consumer	suspension	80mg/2.5ml				butylparaben · cellulose · citric acid · corn syrup · flavors · glycerin · propylene glycol · purified water · sodium benzoate · sorbitol · xanthan gum · D&C red#33 · FD&C red#40
AL AF CA PE	**Tylenol, Children's Cherry** McNeil Consumer	elixir	80mg/2.5ml				benzoic acid · citric acid · flavors · glycerin · polyethylene glycol · propylene glycol · sodium benzoate · sorbitol · sucrose · purified water · red#33 (Cherry) · red#40
AL AF CA PE	**Tylenol, Children's Cherry or Grape** McNeil Consumer	suspension	80mg/2.5ml				butylparaben · cellulose · citric acid · corn syrup · flavors · glycerin · propylene glycol · purified water · sodium benzoate · sorbitol · xanthan gum · FD&C red#40 · FD&C blue#1 (Grape) · D&C red#33 (Grape)
** AF PE	**Tylenol, Children's Fruit Burst** McNeil Consumer	chewable tablet	80mg				aspartame · cellulose · citric acid · corn starch · flavors · magnesium stearate · mannitol · red#7 · may contain: ethylcellulose or cellulose acetate · povidone
AF CA PE	**Tylenol, Children's Fruit Flavor** McNeil Consumer	chewable tablet	80mg				aspartame · cellulose · citric acid · corn starch · ethylcellulose · flavors · magnesium stearate · mannitol · red#7
AF CA PE	**Tylenol, Children's Grape** McNeil Consumer	chewable tablet	80mg				aspartame · cellulose · citric acid · corn starch · flavors · magnesium stearate · mannitol · povidone · blue#1 · red#7 · red#30 · may contain: ethylcellulose or cellulose acetate

See Chapter 4, "Internal Analgesic and Antipyretic Products," for more information about these products.

INTERNAL ANALGESIC AND ANTIPYRETIC PRODUCTS - continued

	Product [a] Manufacturer/Supplier	Dosage Form	Acetamin-ophen	Aspirin	Ibuprofen	Other Analgesics	Other Ingredients [b]
AL AF CA PE	**Tylenol; Infants' Suspension, Cherry or Grape** McNeil Consumer	drops	80mg/0.8ml				butylparaben · cellulose · citric acid · corn syrup · flavors · glycerin · propylene glycol · purified water · sodium benzoate · sorbitol · xanthan gum · FD&C red#40 (Cherry) · D&C red#33 · FD&C blue#1
AF CA SU	**Valorin** Otis Clapp & Son	tablet	325mg				
AF CA SU	**Valorin Extra** Otis Clapp & Son	tablet	500mg				
AF SO SU	**Valorin Super** Otis Clapp & Son	tablet	500mg				caffeine, 65mg
** AF SO	**XS Hangover Relief** Lee Consumer	liquid	1000mg/15ml				calcium citrate, 1250mg/15ml · magnesium trisilicate, 750mg/15ml · calcium carbonate, 350mg/15ml · caffeine, 125mg/15ml · glucose · purified water · methylparaben · xanthan gum · glycerin · propylparaben · peppermint oil · FD&C yellow#5 · FD&C blue#1
	ASPIRIN						
	Anacin Whitehall-Robins Healthcare	caplet		400mg			caffeine, 32mg · hydroxypropyl methylcellulose · iron oxide · microcrystalline cellulose · polyethylene glycol · starch · surfactant · lecithin · simethicone
	Anacin Whitehall-Robins Healthcare	tablet		400mg			caffeine, 32mg · hydroxypropyl methylcellulose · microcrystalline cellulose · polyethylene glycol · surfactant · starch
	Anacin Maximum Strength Whitehall-Robins Healthcare	tablet		500mg			caffeine, 32mg · hydroxypropyl methylcellulose · microcrystalline cellulose · polyethylene glycol · starch · surfactant
SO SU	**Anodynos** Buffington	tablet		410mg		salicylamide, 30mg	caffeine, 60mg
CA GL PR SO	**Arthritis Pain Formula** Medtech	caplet		500mg			magnesium hydroxide, 100mg · aluminum hydroxide, 27mg · hydrogenated vegetable oil · microcrystalline cellulose · starch · surfactant
CA	**Ascriptin Arthritis Pain** Novartis Consumer	caplet		325mg			magnesium hydroxide, 75mg · aluminum hydroxide, 75mg · calcium carbonate · carnauba wax · hydroxypropyl methylcellulose · magnesium stearate · microcrystalline cellulose · propylene glycol · starch · talc · titanium dioxide

See Chapter 4, "Internal Analgesic and Antipyretic Products," for more information about these products.

INTERNAL ANALGESIC AND ANTIPYRETIC PRODUCTS - continued

Product [a] Manufacturer/Supplier	Dosage Form	Acetamin-ophen	Aspirin	Ibuprofen	Other Analgesics	Other Ingredients [b]
** **Ascriptin Enteric Adult Low Strength** Novartis Consumer	tablet		81mg			hydroxypropyl methylcellulose · methacrylic acid copolymer · microcrystalline cellulose · polyethylene glycol · polysorbate 80 · pregelatinized starch · sodium lauryl sulfate · talc · titanium dioxide · triacetin
** **Ascriptin Enteric Regular Strength** Novartis Consumer	tablet		325mg			carnauba wax · hydroxypropyl methylcellulose · methacrylic acid copolymer · microcrystalline cellulose · polyethylene glycol · polysorbate 80 · pregelatinized starch · sodium lauryl sulfate · talc · titanium dioxide · triacetin
CA **Ascriptin Maximum Strength** Novartis Consumer	caplet		500mg			magnesium hydroxide, 80mg · dried aluminum hydroxide gel, 80mg · calcium carbonate · carnauba wax · hydroxypropyl methylcellulose · magnesium stearate · microcrystalline cellulose · propylene glycol · starch · talc · titanium dioxide
CA **Ascriptin Regular Strength** Novartis Consumer	tablet		325mg			magnesium hydroxide, 50mg · dried aluminum hydroxide gel, 50mg · calcium carbonate · carnauba wax · hydroxypropyl methylcellulose · magnesium stearate · microcrystalline cellulose · propylene glycol · starch · talc · titanium dioxide
CA SO SU **Aspercin** Otis Clapp & Son	tablet		324mg			
CA SO SU **Aspercin Extra** Otis Clapp & Son	tablet		500mg			
CA GL PU **Aspergum, Cherry or Orange** Schering-Plough Healthcare	gum		227mg			flavor
CA SO SU **Aspermin** Buffington	tablet		324mg			
CA SO SU **Aspermin Extra** Buffington	tablet		500mg			
Aspirin Multisource	suppository		125mg; 300mg; 600mg			
SU **Aspirin, Enteric Coated** Paddock Labs	tablet		650mg			
CA SO SU **Aspirtab** Dover Ph'cal	tablet		324mg			

See Chapter 4, "Internal Analgesic and Antipyretic Products," for more information about these products.

INTERNAL ANALGESIC AND ANTIPYRETIC PRODUCTS - continued

	Product [a] / Manufacturer/Supplier	Dosage Form	Acetamin-ophen	Aspirin	Ibuprofen	Other Analgesics	Other Ingredients [b]
CA SO SU	**Aspirtab Max** / Dover Ph'cal	tablet		500mg			
CA SO SU	**Back-Quell** / Otis Clapp & Son	tablet		425mg			ephedrine sulfate · atropine sulfate
CA GL SO	**Bayer 8-Hour Aspirin Extended-Release** / Bayer Consumer	timed-release caplet		650mg			guar gum · micorcrystalline · cellulose · starch · other ingredients
CA GL SO	**Bayer Arthritis Pain Regimen Extra Strength** / Bayer Consumer	caplet		500mg			D&C yellow#10 · FD&C yellow#6 · hydroxypropyl methylcellulose · iron oxide · methacrylic acid · copolymer · starch · titanium dioxide · triacetin
CA GL SO	**Bayer Aspirin Extra Strength** / Bayer Consumer	caplet · tablet		500mg			starch · triacetin
**	**Bayer Aspirin Regimen Adult Low Strength with Calcium** / Bayer Consumer	caplet		81mg			calcium carbonate, 250mg · colloidal silicon dioxide · FD&C blue#2 lake · hydroxypropyl methylcellulose · microcrystalline cellulose · propylene glycol · sodium starch glycolate · titanium dioxide · zinc stearate
CA GL SO	**Bayer Aspirin Regimen Regular Strength** / Bayer Consumer	caplet		325mg			D&C yellow#10 · FD&C yellow#6 · hydroxypropyl methylcellulose · methacrylic acid copolymer · starch · titanium dioxide · triacetin
CA GL SO	**Bayer Aspirin, Genuine** / Bayer Consumer	caplet · tablet		325mg			starch · triacetin
CA GL SO PE	**Bayer Children's Aspirin, Cherry or Orange** / Bayer Consumer	chewable tablet		81mg			dextrose · FD&C yellow#6 · flavor · saccharin sodium · starch
CA GL	**Bayer Plus Extra Strength Buffered Aspirin** / Bayer Consumer	caplet		500mg			calcium carbonate · magnesium carbonate · magnesium oxide
DY PR SO	**BC** / Block Drug	tablet		325mg			salicylamide, 95mg · caffeine, 16mg
DY PR	**BC** / Block Drug	powder		650mg			salicylamide, 195mg · caffeine, 32mg
DY PR	**BC Arthritis Strength** / Block Drug	powder		742mg			salicylamide, 222mg · caffeine, 36mg
CA SO SU	**Buffaprin** / Buffington	tablet		325mg			magnesium oxide

See Chapter 4, "Internal Analgesic and Antipyretic Products," for more information about these products.

INTERNAL ANALGESIC AND ANTIPYRETIC PRODUCTS - continued

	Product [a] Manufacturer/Supplier	Dosage Form	Acetamin- ophen	Aspirin	Ibuprofen	Other Analgesics	Other Ingredients [b]
CA SO SU	**Buffaprin Extra** Buffington	tablet		500mg			magnesium oxide
CA SO SU	**Buffasal** Dover Ph'cal	tablet		324mg			magnesium oxide
CA SO SU	**Buffasal Max** Dover Ph'cal	tablet		500mg			magnesium oxide
CA PR SO	**Bufferin Arthritis Strength, Tri-Buffered** Bristol-Myers Products	caplet		500mg			calcium carbonate, 222.3mg · magnesium oxide, 88.9mg · magnesium carbonate, 55.6mg · benzoic acid · citric acid · corn starch · FD&C blue#1 · hydroxypropyl methylcellulose · magnesium stearate · mineral oil · polysorbate 20 · povidone · propylene glycol · simethicone emulsion · sodium phosphate · sorbitan monolaurate · titanium dioxide · may also contain: carnauba wax · zinc stearate
**	**Bufferin Enteric** Bristol-Myers Products	tablet		81mg			FD&C yellow#6 aluminum lake · hydroxypropyl methylcellulose · methacrylic acid copolymer · microcrystalline cellulose · polyethylene glycol · polysorbate 80 · pregelatinized starch · sodium lauryl sulfate · talc · titanium dioxide · triacetin
CA PR SO	**Bufferin Extra Strength, Tri-Buffered** Bristol-Myers Products	tablet		500mg			calcium carbonate, 222.3mg · magnesium oxide, 88.9mg · magnesium carbonate, 55.6mg · benzoic acid · citric acid · corn starch · FD&C blue#1 · hydroxypropyl methylcellulose · magnesium stearate · mineral oil · polysorbate 20 · povidone · propylene glycol · simethicone emulsion · sodium phosphate · sorbitan monolaurate · titanium dioxide · may also contain: carnauba wax · zinc stearate
CA PR SO	**Bufferin, Tri-Buffered** Bristol-Myers Products	tablet		325mg			calcium carbonate, 158mg · magnesium oxide, 63mg · magnesium carbonate, 39mg · benzoic acid · citric acid · corn starch · FD&C blue#1 · hydroxypropyl methylcellulose · magnesium stearate · mineral oil · polysorbate 20 · povidone · propylene glycol · simethicone emulsion · sodium phosphate · sorbitan monolaurate · titanium dioxide · may also contain: carnauba wax · zinc stearate

See Chapter 4, "Internal Analgesic and Antipyretic Products," for more information about these products.

INTERNAL ANALGESIC AND ANTIPYRETIC PRODUCTS - continued

	Product [a] Manufacturer/Supplier	Dosage Form	Acetamin-ophen	Aspirin	Ibuprofen	Other Analgesics	Other Ingredients [b]
SU	**Buffets II** Jones Medical	tablet	162mg	226.8mg			aluminum hydroxide, 50mg · caffeine, 32.4mg
CA SO SU	**Buffinol** Otis Clapp & Son	tablet		325mg			magnesium oxide
CA SO SU	**Buffinol Extra** Otis Clapp & Son	tablet		500mg			magnesium oxide
	Cope Mentholatum	tablet		421mg			caffeine, 32mg · magnesium hydroxide · dried aluminum hydroxide gel · corn starch · hydrogenated vegetable oil · microcrystalline cellulose · sodium lauryl sulfate · talc · colloidal silicon dioxide · polyvinylpyrrolidone
	Ecotrin Adult Low Strength SmithKline Beecham	tablet		81mg			carnauba wax · D&C yellow#10 · FD&C yellow#6 · hydroxypropyl methylcellulose · methacrylic acid copolymer · microcrystalline cellulose · polyethylene glycol · polysorbate 80 · propylene glycol · silicon dioxide · starch · stearic acid · talc · titanium dioxide · triethyl citrate
	Ecotrin Maximum Strength SmithKline Beecham	caplet · tablet		500mg			carnauba wax · colloidal silicon dioxide · FD&C yellow#6 · hydroxypropyl methylcellulose · maltodextrin · methacrylic acid copolymer · microcrystalline cellulose · pregelatinized starch · propylene glycol · simethicone · sodium hydroxide · sodium starch glycolate · stearic acid · talc · titanium dioxide · triethyl citrate
	Ecotrin Regular Strength SmithKline Beecham	tablet		325mg			carnauba wax · colloidal silicon dioxide · FD&C yellow#6 · hydroxypropyl methylcellulose · maltodextrin · methacrylic acid copolymer · microcrystalline cellulose · pregelatinized starch · propylene glycol · simethicone · sodium hydroxide · sodium starch glycolate · stearic acid · talc · titanium dioxide · triethyl citrate
SO SU	**Emagrin** Otis Clapp & Son	tablet		410mg		salicylamide, 60mg	caffeine, 30mg
DY PR	**Goody's Extra Strength** Goody's Ph'cals	tablet	130mg	260mg			caffeine, 16.25mg
DY PR	**Goody's Extra Strength Headache** Goody's Ph'cals	powder	260mg	520mg			caffeine, 32.5mg · lactose · potassium chloride
	Halfprin Low Strength Enteric Coated Kramer Labs	tablet		81mg; 162mg			

See Chapter 4, "Internal Analgesic and Antipyretic Products," for more information about these products.

INTERNAL ANALGESIC AND ANTIPYRETIC PRODUCTS - continued

	Product [a] Manufacturer/Supplier	Dosage Form	Acetamin- ophen	Aspirin	Ibuprofen	Other Analgesics	Other Ingredients [b]
	Heartline BDI Ph'cals	tablet		81mg			
CA	**Norwich Aspirin** Chattem	caplet · tablet		325mg; 500mg			starch · hydroxypropyl methylcellulose · polyethylene glycol
	P-A-C Lee Consumer	tablet		400mg			anhydrous caffeine, 32mg · cellulose · corn starch · croscarmellose sodium · sucrose · FD&C blue #2 · FD&C yellow #5 (tartrazine)
	Regiprin Enteric Coated Republic Drug	tablet		81mg			
	St. Joseph Low Dose Adult Aspirin Schering-Plough Healthcare	caplet · chewable tablet		81mg			fruit flavor
	Stanback, Original Formula Stanback	powder		650mg		salicylamide, 200mg	caffeine, 32mg
DY GL PR PU SO SU	**Supac** Mission Pharmacal	tablet	160mg	230mg			calcium gluconate, 60mg · caffeine, 33mg
GL SO	**Vanquish** Bayer Consumer	caplet	194mg	227mg			magnesium hydroxide, 50mg · caffeine, 33mg · dried aluminum hydroxide gel, 25mg
	IBUPROFEN						
AF	**Advil** Whitehall-Robins Healthcare	gel caplet			200mg		croscarmellose sodium · FD&C red#40 · FD&C yellow#6 · gelatin · glycerin · hydroxypropyl methylcellulose · iron oxides · lecithin · pharmaceutical glaze · propyl gallate · silicon dioxide · simethicone · sodium lauryl sulfate · starch · stearic acid · titanium dioxide · triacetin
** AF PE	**Advil, Children's** Whitehall-Robins Healthcare	suspension			100mg/5ml		sucrose · glycerin · sorbitol solution · microcrystalline cellulose · polysorbate 80 · sodium benzoate · citric acid · xanthan gum · carboxy methylcellulose sodium · artificial guarana flavor · artificial sweetner · disodium edetate · FD&C red#40 · purified water

See Chapter 4, "Internal Analgesic and Antipyretic Products," for more information about these products.

INTERNAL ANALGESIC AND ANTIPYRETIC PRODUCTS - continued

Product [a] Manufacturer/Supplier	Dosage Form	Acetamin-ophen	Aspirin	Ibuprofen	Other Analgesics	Other Ingredients [b]
** AF	**Advil, Junior Strength** Whitehall-Robins Healthcare	tablet			100mg		acetylated monoglycerides · carnauba wax · colloidal silicon dioxide · croscarmellose sodium · iron oxides · methylparaben · microcrystalline cellulose · povidone · pregelatinized starch · propylene glycol · propylparaben · shellac · sodium benzoate · starch · stearic acid · sucrose · titanium dioxide
**	**Dynafed IB** BDI Ph'cals	tablet			200mg		
AF	**Haltran** Lee Consumer	tablet			200mg		carnauba wax · corn starch · hydroxypropyl methylcellulose · propylene glycol · silicon dioxide · pregelatinized starch · stearic acid · titanium dioxide
AF CA GL SO	**Midol IB Cramp Relief Formula** Bayer Consumer	tablet			200mg		
AF CA DY GL LA PR PU SO SU	**Motrin IB** McNeil Consumer	caplet · tablet			200mg		carnauba wax · corn starch · hydroxypropyl methylcellulose · propylene glycol · silicon dioxide · pregelatinized starch · stearic acid · titanium dioxide
AF CA GL PU SU	**Motrin IB** McNeil Consumer	gelcap			200mg		benzyl alcohol · butylparaben · butyl alcohol · castor oil · colloidal silicon dioxide · edetate calcium disodium · FD&C yellow #6 · gelatin · hydroxypropyl methylcellulose · iron oxide black · magnesium stearate · methylparaben · microcrystalline cellulose · povidone · pregelatinized starch · propylene glycol · propylparaben · SDA 3 A alcohol · sodium lauryl sulfate · sodium propionate · sodium starch glycolate · starch · titanium dioxide
AL PE	**Motrin, Children's** McNeil Consumer	suspension			100mg/5ml		citric acid · corn starch · artificial flavors · glycerin · polysorbate 80 · purified water · sodium benzoate · sucrose · xanthan gum · FD&C red#40 · D&C yellow#10

See Chapter 4, "Internal Analgesic and Antipyretic Products," for more information about these products.

INTERNAL ANALGESIC AND ANTIPYRETIC PRODUCTS - continued

	Product [a] Manufacturer/Supplier	Dosage Form	Acetamin- ophen	Aspirin	Ibuprofen	Other Analgesics	Other Ingredients [b]
** AF PE	**Motrin, Children's** McNeil Consumer	chewable tablet			50mg		aspartame · citric acid · flavors · hydroxyethyl cellulose · hydroxypropyl methylcellulose · magnesium stearate · mannitol · microcrystalline cellulose · povidone · sodium lauryl sulfate · sodium starch glycolate · FD&C yellow#6
** AF PE	**Motrin, Children's** McNeil Consumer	drops			50mg/1.25ml		citric acid · corn starch · artificial flavors · glycerin · polysorbate 80 · purified water · sodium benzoate · sorbitol · sucrose · xanthan gum · FD&C red#40
** AF PE	**Motrin, Junior Strength** McNeil Consumer	chewable tablet			100mg		aspartame · citric acid · flavors · hydroxyethyl cellulose · hydroxypropyl methylcellulose · magnesium stearate · mannitol · microcrystalline cellulose · povidone · sodium lauryl · sulfate · sodium starch glycolate · FD&C yellow#6
** AF PE	**Motrin, Junior Strength** McNeil Consumer	caplet			100mg		carnauba wax · colloidal silicon dioxide · corn starch · hydroxypropyl methylcellulose · microcrystalline cellulose · polydextrose · polyethylene glycol · propylene glycol · sodium starch glycolate · titanium dioxide · triacetin · D&C yellow#10 · FD&C yellow#6
AF CA GL PR SO	**Nuprin** Bristol-Myers Products	caplet · tablet			200mg		carnauba wax · corn starch · D&C yellow#10 · FD&C yellow#6 · hydroxypropyl methylcellulose · propylene glycol · silicon dioxide · stearic acid · titanium dioxide
AF CA SU	**Ultraprin** Otis Clapp & Son	tablet			200mg		
AF CA SU	**Valprin** Buffington	tablet			200mg		
	OTHER ANALGESICS						
AF	**Actron** Bayer Consumer	caplet · tablet				ketoprofen, 12.5mg	corn starch · croscarmellose sodium · hydroxypropyl methylcellulose · lactose · magnesium stearate · microcrystalline cellulose · polyethylene glycol · titanium dioxide
AF CA GL PR PU	**Aleve** Bayer Consumer	caplet · tablet				naproxen sodium, 220mg (naproxen, 200mg · sodium, 20mg)	magnesium stearate · microcrystalline cellulose · povidone · purified water · talc · Opadry YS-1-4215

See Chapter 4, "Internal Analgesic and Antipyretic Products," for more information about these products.

INTERNAL ANALGESIC AND ANTIPYRETIC PRODUCTS - continued

	Product [a] Manufacturer/Supplier	Dosage Form	Acetamin-ophen	Aspirin	Ibuprofen	Other Analgesics	Other Ingredients [b]
AF DY GL PR SO SU	**Arthriten** Alva-Amco Pharmacal	tablet	250mg			magnesium salicylate tetrahydrate, 377mg	magnesium carbonate · magnesium oxide · calcium carbonate
	Arthropan Purdue Frederick	liquid				choline salicylate, 174mg/ml (equivalent to aspirin, 130mg)	
AF	**Azo-Dine [c]** Republic Drug	tablet				phenazopyridine HCl, 97.2mg	
AF	**Azo-Standard [c]** PolyMedica Ph'cals	tablet				phenazopyridine HCl, 95mg	
AF CA PR SO	**Backache from the Makers of Nuprin** Bristol-Myers Products	caplet				magnesium salicylate tetrahydrate, 580mg (equivalent to anhydrous magnesium salicylate, 467mg)	carnauba wax · hydrogenated vegetable oil · hydroxypropyl methylcellulose · magnesium stearate · microcrystalline cellulose · polyethylene glycol · polysorbate 80 · titanium dioxide
	Cystex Numark Labs	tablet				sodium salicylate, 162.5mg	methenamine, 162mg · benzoic acid, 32mg
AF CA GL PR PU SO	**Doan's Extra Strength** Novartis Consumer	caplet				magnesium salicylate tetrahydrate, 580mg	magnesium stearate · microcrystalline cellulose · Opadry white · polyethylene glycol · stearic acid
AF CA GL PR PU SO	**Doan's Regular Strength** Novartis Consumer	caplet				magnesium salicylate tetrahydrate, 377mg	FD&C yellow#6 · magnesium stearate · microcrystalline cellulose · Opadry light green · polyethylene glycol · stearic acid
	Magnesium Salicylate Multisource	caplet				magnesium salicylate, 467mg	
AF DY GL SO SU	**Mobigesic** B. F. Ascher	tablet				magnesium salicylate, 325mg	phenyltoloxamine citrate, 30mg
AF CA GL PR SO	**Momentum** Medtech	caplet				magnesium salicylate tetrahydrate 580mg (equivalent to magnesium salicylate anhydrous, 467mg)	hydrogenated vegetable oil · hydroxypropyl methylcellulose · microcrystalline cellulose · polyethylene glycol · polysorbate 80 · titanium dioxide

See Chapter 4, "Internal Analgesic and Antipyretic Products," for more information about these products.

INTERNAL ANALGESIC AND ANTIPYRETIC PRODUCTS - continued

	Product [a] Manufacturer/Supplier	Dosage Form	Acetamin- ophen	Aspirin	Ibuprofen	Other Analgesics	Other Ingredients [b]
AF CA GL	**Orudis KT** Whitehall-Robins Healthcare	caplet · tablet				ketoprofen, 12.5mg	cellulose · D&C yellow#10 lake · FD&C blue#1 lake · iron oxide · pharmaceutical glaze · povidone · silica · sodium benzoate · sodium lauryl sulfate · starch · stearic acid · sugar · titanium dioxide · wax · FD&C yellow#5 lake (tartrazine)
AF CA GL PR PU	**Prodium [c]** Breckenridge Ph'cal	tablet				phenazopyridine HCl, 95mg	dextrose · FD&C red#40 aluminum lake · FD&C blue#2 aluminum lake · hydroxypropyl cellulose · polysorbate · povidone · sodium starch glycolate · starch · titanium dioxide · carnauba wax · ethylcellulose · Opaspray maroon
AF	**Re-Azo [c]** Reese Chemical	tablet				phenazopyridine HCl, 97.5mg	
**	**Uristat [c]** Advanced Care Products	tablet				phenazopyridine HCl, 95mg	lactose monohydrate · sodium starch glycolate · corn starch · hydrogenated vegetable oil · colloidal silicon dioxide · magnesium stearate
**	**UroFemme [c]** Kramer Labs	tablet				phenazopyridine HCl, 95mg	

** New listing

[a] For products that contain an analgesic and a sleep aid, see the Sleep Aid Products table. For products that are indicated for diuresis but may also contain an analgesic, see the Menstrual Products table.

[b] Caffeine may be effective as an adjuvant analgesic.

[c] Urinary tract analgesic

See Chapter 4, "Internal Analgesic and Antipyretic Products," for more information about these products.

External Analgesic Product Table

EXTERNAL ANALGESIC PRODUCTS

Product Manufacturer/Supplier	Dosage Form	Counterirritant	Other Ingredients
** **Absorbine Arthritis Strength** W. F. Young	liquid	menthol, 4% · capsaicin, 0.025% (from capsicum oleoresin)	plant extracts of calendula, echinacea, wormwood · chloroxylenol · iodine · potassium iodide · thymol · water
Absorbine Jr. W. F. Young	liquid	menthol, 1.27%	plant extracts of calendula, echinacea, wormwood · acetone · chloroxylenol · FD&C blue#1 · FD&C yellow#5 · iodine · potassium iodide · thymol · wormwood oil · water
Absorbine Jr. Extra Strength W. F. Young	liquid	menthol, 4%	plant extracts of calendula, echinacea, wormwood · acetone · chloroxylenol · FD&C blue#1 · iodine · potassium iodide · thymol · wormwood oil · water
Absorbine Jr. Power Gel W. F. Young	gel	menthol, 4%	hydroalcoholic gel base
** **Arctic** Systems Design	pump spray	menthol, 8%	isopropyl alcohol · deionized water · eucalyptus oil · oil of origanum · peppermint oil
Arthricare Double Ice Pain Relieving Rub Del Ph'cals	gel	menthol, 4% · camphor, 3.1%	
Arthricare Pain Relieving Rub Del Ph'cals	cream	menthol, 1.25% · methyl nicotinate, 0.25% · capsicum oleoresin, 0.025%	
Arthricare Triple Medicated Pain Relieving Rub Del Ph'cals	cream	methyl salicylate, 30% · menthol, 1.25% · methyl nicotinate, 0.25%	
** **ArthriCare Ultra** Del Ph'cals	gel	menthol, 2% · capsaicin, 0.075%	aloe vera gel · carbomer · cetyl alcohol · DMDM hydantoin
Arthritis Hot Thompson Medical	cream	methyl salicylate, 15% · menthol, 10%	methylparaben · glyceryl monostearate · lanolin · trolamine · citric acid · propylene glycol · stearic acid · water
** **Arthur Itis** Stellar Health Products	cream · liquid	capsaicin, 0.025%	trolamine salicylate, 10%
Aspercreme Thompson Medical	lotion		trolamine salicylate, 10% · glyceryl monostearate · stearic acid · lanolin · cetyl alcohol · isopropyl palmitate · propylparaben · methylparaben · propylene glycol · sodium lauryl sulfate · potassium phosphate · water · aloe
Aspercreme Thompson Medical	cream		trolamine salicylate, 10% · cetyl alcohol · stearic acid · mineral oil · propylparaben · water · methylparaben · glycerin · potassium phosphate monobasic · aloe
** **Aspergel** Thompson Medical	gel		trolamine salicylate, 10% · aloe vera gel · hydroxyethyl cellulose · PEG-8 · polyglycerylmethacrylate · propylene glycol · purified water · SD alcohol 40
Banalg Muscle Pain Reliever Forest Ph'cals	lotion	methyl salicylate, 4.9% · camphor, 2% · menthol, 1%	greaseless base
Ben Gay Arthritis Formula Non-Greasy Pain Relieving Pfizer Consumer	cream	methyl salicylate, 30% · menthol, 8%	greaseless nonstaining emulsion base

See Chapter 5, "External Analgesic Products," for more information about these products.

EXTERNAL ANALGESIC PRODUCTS - continued

Product Manufacturer/Supplier	Dosage Form	Counterirritant	Other Ingredients
Ben Gay Greaseless Formula Pain Relieving Pfizer Consumer	cream	methyl salicylate, 15% · menthol, 10%	greaseless nonstaining emulsion base
Ben Gay Original Formula Pain Relieving Pfizer Consumer	ointment	methyl salicylate, 18.3% · menthol, 16%	oleaginous base
Ben Gay Ultra Strength Pain Relieving Pfizer Consumer	cream	methyl salicylate, 30% · menthol, 10% · camphor, 4%	greaseless nonstaining emulsion base
Ben Gay Vanishing Scent Non-Greasy Pain Relieving Pfizer Consumer	gel	menthol, 2.5%	hydroalcoholic gel base
Betuline Ferndale Labs	lotion	methyl salicylate · camphor · menthol	peppermint oil · water soluble base
** **Buckley's White Rub** W. K. Buckley	ointment	menthol, 3.6% · methyl salicylate, 1.2%	camphor · thymol · oil of turpentine · oil of hemlock · capsicum oleoresin · white beeswax · paraffin wax · mineral oil sodium borate
Campho-phenique Pain Relieving Antiseptic Bayer Consumer	gel · liquid	camphor, 10.8% · phenol, 4.7%	eucalyptus oil
** **Capzasin-HP** Thompson Medical	cream	capsaicin, 0.075%	benzyl alcohol · cetyl alcohol · glyceryl monostearate · isopropyl myristate · PEG-100 stearate · purified water · sorbitol solution · white petrolatum
** **Capzasin-HP** Thompson Medical	lotion	capsaicin, 0.075%	dimethicone copolyol · DMDM hydantoin· hydroxyethyl cellulose · propylene glycol · purified water · SD alcohol 40
** **Capzasin-P** Thompson Medical	lotion	capsaicin, 0.025%	dimethicone copolyol · DMDM hydantoin· hydroxyethyl cellulose · propylene glycol · purified water · SD alcohol 40
Capzasin-P Thompson Medical	cream	capsaicin, 0.025%	benzyl alcohol · cetyl alcohol · glyceryl monostearate · isopropyl myristate · polyoxyl 40 stearate · water · sorbitol · white petrolatum
Cool Heat Republic Drug	gel	menthol, 2%	
Deep-Down BIRA	cream	methyl salicylate, 15% · menthol, 5% · camphor, 0.5%	SD alcohol, 40.5%
Dencorub Alvin Last	cream	methyl salicylate, 15% · camphor, 3.1% · menthol, 1.25%	water · stearic acid · beeswax · paraffin · glycol stearate · petrolatum · glycerin · mineral oil · triethanolamine · lanolin · eucalyptus oil · isobornyl acetate
Dencorub Alvin Last	liquid	capsaicin, 0.025% (from capsicum oleoresin)	water · quince seed · benzoic acid · disodium EDTA · algin · mullein extract · myrrh extract · valerian
** **Dolorac** GenDerm	cream	capsaicin, 0.25%	benzyl alcohol · cetyl alcohol · glyceryl monostearate · isopropyl myristate · polyoxyethylene stearate blend · sorbitol solution · petrolatum · water
** **Double Cap** Breckenridge Ph'cal	cream	capsaicin, 0.5%	sorbitol, 70% · purified water · glyceryl monostearate · cetyl alcohol · isopropyl myristate · benzyl alcohol · white petrolatum · polyoxyl 40 stearate
** **Epso-Pine Bath Salts** Majestic Drug	granule	methyl salicylate · eucalyptus oil	magnesium sulfate · balsam peru · pine needle oil · FD&C blue#1 · FD&C yellow#5

See Chapter 5, "External Analgesic Products," for more information about these products.

EXTERNAL ANALGESIC PRODUCTS - continued

Product Manufacturer/Supplier	Dosage Form	Counterirritant	Other Ingredients
Eucalyptamint Arthritis Pain Reliever Novartis Consumer	ointment	menthol, 16%	lanolin · eucalyptus oil
Eucalyptamint Muscle Pain Relief Novartis Consumer	cream	menthol, 8%	carbomer 980 · eucalyptus oil · fragrance · propylene glycol · SD alcohol 3A · triethanolamine · Tween 80 · water
Exocaine Medicated Rub Del Ph'cals	cream	methyl salicylate, 25%	
Exocaine Odor Free Del Ph'cals	cream		trolamine salicylate, 10%
Exocaine Plus Rub Del Ph'cals	cream	methyl salicylate, 30%	
Flexall Chattem	gel	menthol, 7% · methyl salicylate	allantoin · aloe vera gel · carbomer 940 · eucalyptus oil · glycerin · peppermint oil · SD aldohol 38-B · steareth-2 · steareth-21 · thyme oil · tocopheryl acetate · triethanolamine · water
Flexall 454 Maximum Strength Chattem	gel	menthol, 16% · methyl salicylate	allantoin · aloe vera gel · carbomer 940 · diisopropyl adipate · eucalyptus oil · glycerin · peppermint oil · SD alcohol 38-B · steareth-2 · steareth-21 · triethanolamine · tocopheryl acetate · thyme oil · water
** **Flexall Ultra Plus** Chattem	gel	menthol, 16% · methyl salicylate, 10% · camphor, 3.1%	allantoin · aloe vera gel · carbomer 940 · diisopropyl adipate · eucalyptus oil · glycerin · peppermint oil · SD alcohol 38-B · steareth-2 · steareth-21 · thyme oil · tocopheryl acetate · triethanolamine · water
** **Flexcin** Breckenridge Ph'cal	cream	capsaicin	purified water · glyceryl monostearate · cetyl alcohol · isopropyl myristate · benzyl alchohol · white petrolatum · polyoxyl 40 stearate · sorbitol ·
Gold Bond Medicated Anti-Itch Chattem	cream	menthol, 1% · methyl salicylate, 1%	lidocaine, 4% · cetearyl alcohol · DMDM hydantoin · eucalyptol · glyceryl stearate · methylparaben · petrolatum · propylene glycol · simethicone · sorbic acid · sorbitol · thymol · tocopherol · water · zinc oxide
Gold Bond Medicated, Extra Strength Chattem	powder	menthol, 0.8% · methyl salicylate	zinc oxide, 5% · eucalyptol · salicylic acid · talc · thymol · zinc stearate
Gold Bond Medicated, Regular Strength Chattem	powder	menthol, 0.15% · methyl salicylate	zinc oxide, 1% · eucalyptol · salicylic acid · talc · thymol · zinc stearate
Gordogesic Gordon Labs	cream	methyl salicylate, 10%	propylene glycol · cetyl alcohol · mineral oil · stearic acid · white wax · triethanolamine · sodium lauryl sulfate · methylparaben · propylparaben
Heet Medtech	liniment	methyl salicylate, 15% · camphor, 3.6% · capsaicin, 0.025% (as capsicum oleoresin)	alcohol, 70% · acetone
Icy Hot Chattem	cream	methyl salicylate, 30% · menthol, 10%	water · emulsifying wax · stearic acid · triethanolamine · cetyl esters · carbomer

See Chapter 5, "External Analgesic Products," for more information about these products.

EXTERNAL ANALGESIC PRODUCTS - continued

	Product Manufacturer/Supplier	Dosage Form	Counterirritant	Other Ingredients
**	**Icy Hot Arthritis Therapy** Chattem	gel	capsaicin, 0.025%	allantoin · aloe vera gel · benzyl alcohol · copolymer 940 · diazolidinyl urea · diisopropyl adipate · emulsyfying wax · FD&C blue#1 · glycerin · isopropyl myristrate · maleated soybean oil · methylparaben · oleth-3 phosphate · propylene glycol · propylparaben · steareth-2 · steareth-21 · tocopheryl acetate · tridecyl neopentanoate · triethanolamine · water
	Icy Hot Chill Stick Chattem	stick	methyl salicylate, 30% · menthol, 10%	ceresin · cyclomethcone · hydrogenated castror oil · microcrystalline wax · paraffin · PEG-150 distearate · propylene glycol · stearic acid · stearyl alcohol
	Icy Hot Extra Strength Long-Lasting Balm Pain Reliever Chattem	ointment	methyl salicylate, 29% · menthol, 7.6%	paraffin · white petrolatum
**	**Iodex with Methyl Salicylate** Lee Consumer	ointment	methyl salicylate, 4.8%	iodine, 4.7% · oleic acid · petrolatum
	Menthacin Mentholatum	cream	menthol, 4% · capsaicin, 0.025% ·	caprylic/capric triglyceride · carbomer 1342 · carbomer 940 · cetyl alcohol · diazolidinyl urea · glyceryl stearate · sodium lauryl sulfate · maleated soybean oil · methylparaben · polysorbate 60 · propylene glycol · propylparaben · sorbitan stearate · trolamine · water
	Mentholatum Mentholatum	ointment	camphor, 9% · natural menthol, 1.3%	fragrance · petrolatum · titanium dioxide
	Mentholatum Deep Heating Mentholatum	lotion	methyl salicylate, 20% · menthol, 6%	carbomer 941 · lanolin oil · mineral oil · polysorbate 60 · sorbitan stearate · trolamine · water
	Mentholatum Deep Heating Arthritis Formula Mentholatum	cream	methyl salicylate, 30% · menthol, 8%	glyceryl stearate · sodium lauryl sulfate · isoceteth-20 · poloxamer 407 · quaternium-15 · sorbitan stearate · water
	Mentholatum Deep Heating Rub Mentholatum	cream	methyl salicylate, 12.7% · menthol, 5.8%	chloroxylenol · fragrance · glyceryl stearate · sodium lauryl sulfate · lanolin · water
	Methagual Gordon Labs	ointment	methyl salicylate, 8% · guaiacol, 2%	petrolatum · white wax · methylparaben · propylparaben
	Minit-Rub Bristol-Myers Products	cream	methyl salicylate, 15% · menthol, 3.5% · camphor, 2.3%	calcium benzoate · lanolin · polysorbate 20 · sodium alginate · sorbitol · water · may also contain: methylchloroisothiazoline/methylisothiazoline · DMDM hydantoin
	Mobisyl B. F. Ascher	cream		trolamine salicylate, 10%
	Myoflex Novartis Consumer	cream		trolamine salicylate, 10% · cetyl alcohol · disodium EDTA · fragrance · propylene glycol · sodium lauryl sulfate · stearyl alcohol · water · white wax
	Noxzema Original Procter & Gamble	cream	camphor · menthol · phenol	water · stearic acid · linseed oil · soybean oil · fragrance · ammonium hydroxide · gelatin · clove oil · eucalyptus oil · calcium hydroxide

See Chapter 5, "External Analgesic Products," for more information about these products.

EXTERNAL ANALGESIC PRODUCTS - continued

Product Manufacturer/Supplier	Dosage Form	Counterirritant	Other Ingredients
Noxzema Original Procter & Gamble	lotion	camphor · menthol · phenol	water · stearic acid · soybean oil · propylene glycol · fragrance · linseed oil · gelatin · calcium hydroxide · cetyl alcohol · clove oil · eucalyptus oil · carbomer · triethanolamine
Pain Gel Plus Mentholatum	lotion	menthol, 4%	aloe vera gel · carbomer 934 · dye · fragrance · isopropyl alcohol · methylparaben · propylparaben · squalane · triethanolamine · vitamin E acetate · water
Pain Patch Mentholatum	pad	menthol, 154mg	
** **Pain-X** B. F. Ascher	gel	menthol, 5% · camphor, 4% · purified capsaicin, 0.05%	aloe vera gel
PainBreak Stevens Skin Softener	cream	menthol, 5% · methyl salicylate, 5%	deionized water · glyceryl stearate · stearic acid · jojoba oil · glycerin · cetyl alcohol · apricot kernel oil · sweet almond oil · castor oil · cetyl palmitate · cetearyl octanoate · panthenol · diazolidinyl urea · methylparaben · propylparaben · magnesium aluminum silicate · squalene · methyl gluceth 20 · tocopherol acetate · avocado oil · aloe vera gel · TEA salicylate
** **Pharmacist's Creme** Reese Chemical	cream	methyl salicylate, 15% · menthol, 10% · capsaicin, 0.025%	water · stearic acid · glyceryl strearate SE · PEG-40 stearate · steareth-2 · triethanolamine · carbomer · propylene glycol · diazolidinyl urea · methylparaben · propylparaben
Sarna Stiefel Labs	lotion	camphor, 0.5% · menthol, 0.5%	
Sloan's C. B. Fleet	liniment	turpentine oil, 47% · capsaicin, 0.025% (from capsicum oleoresin)	
Soltice Quick Rub Oakhurst	cream	camphor, 5.1% · menthol, 5.1%	greaseless base
Sportscreme Thompson Medical	cream		trolamine salicylate, 10% · cetyl alcohol · FD&C blue#1 · FD&C yellow#5 · fragrance · glycerin · methylparaben · mineral oil · potassium phosphate monobasic · propylparaben · stearic acid · water
Sportscreme Thompson Medical	lotion		trolamine salicylate, 10% · cetyl alcohol · fragrance · glyceryl monostearate · isopropyl palmitate · lanolin anhydrous · methylparaben · potassium phosphate monobasic · propylene glycol · propylparaben · sodium lauryl sulfate · stearic acid · water
Thera-Gesic Mission Pharmacal	cream	methyl salicylate, 15% · menthol, 1%	water · dimethylpolysiloxane · glycerin · carbopol · triethanolamine · sodium lauryl sulfate · methylparaben · propylparaben
** **TheraPatch** CNS	transdermal patch	methyl salicylate, 11% · camphor, 3.5% · menthol, 2%	karaya gum vehicle · fragrances · quaternium-15 · plant extracts
Therapeutic Mineral Ice Bristol-Myers Products	gel	menthol, 2%	ammonium hydroxide · carbomer 934 · cupric sulfate · FD&C blue#1 · isopropyl alcohol · magnesium sulfate · sodium hydroxide · thymol · water
Therapeutic Mineral Ice Exercise Formula Bristol-Myers Products	gel	menthol, 4%	ammonium hydroxide · carbomer · cupric sulfate · FD&C blue#1 · fragrance · isopropyl alcohol · magnesium sulfate · sodium hydroxide · thymol · water
Unguentine Mentholatum	ointment	phenol, 1%	eucalyptus oil · oleostearine · petrolatum · thyme oil · zinc oxide

See Chapter 5, "External Analgesic Products," for more information about these products.

EXTERNAL ANALGESIC PRODUCTS - continued

Product Manufacturer/Supplier	Dosage Form	Counterirritant	Other Ingredients
Unguentine Plus Mentholatum	cream	phenol, 0.5%	lidocaine HCl, 2% · fragrance · glyceryl stearate · isoceteth-20 · isopropyl palmitate · methylparaben · mineral oil · poloxamer 407 · propylparaben · quaternium-15 · sorbitan stearate · tetrasodium EDTA · water
Vicks VapoRub Procter & Gamble	cream	camphor, 5.2% · menthol, 2.8% · eucalyptus oil, 1.2% · spirits of turpentine	carbomer 954 · cedarleaf oil · cetyl alcohol · cetyl palmitate · cyclomethicone copolyol · dimethicone copolyol · dimethicone · EDTA · glycerin · imidazolidinyl urea · isopropyl palmitate · methylparaben · nutmeg oil · PEG-100 stearate · propylparaben · purified water · sodium hydroxide · stearic acid · stearyl alcohol · thymol · titanium dioxide
Vicks VapoRub Procter & Gamble	ointment	camphor, 4.8% · menthol, 2.6% · eucaplyptus oil, 1.2% · spirits of turpentine	cedarleaf oil · nutmeg oil · special petrolatum · thymol
Vicks VapoSteam Procter & Gamble	liquid	camphor, 6.2% · menthol, 3.2% · eucalyptus oil, 1.5%	alcohol, 78% · cedarleaf oil · nutmeg oil · poloxamer 124 · silicone · laureth-7
Wonder Ice Pedinol Pharmacal	gel	menthol	water · SD alcohol 40, 8% · mineral oil · petrolatum · propylene glycol · hydrogenated vegetable oil · beeswax · carbomer · triethanolamine · phenylcarbinol · glycerin · potassuim sorbate · sodium benzoate · diazolidinyl urea · phenoxyethanol · EDTA · paraffin wax · sorbitan stearate · cetyl alcohol · cetyl esters · polysorbate 20 · sulfonated castor oil · sodium borate · methylparaben · propylparaben · fragrance · FD&C blue#1
Zostrix GenDerm	cream	capsaicin, 0.025%	benzyl alcohol · cetyl alcohol · glyceryl monostearate · isopropyl myristate · polyoxyethylene stearate blend · sorbitol solution · petrolatum · water
Zostrix Sports GenDerm	cream	capsaicin, 0.075%	benzyl alcohol · cetyl alcohol · glyceryl monostearate · isopropyl myristate · PEG-100 stearate · purified water · sorbitol solution · white petrolatum
Zostrix-HP GenDerm	cream	capsaicin, 0.075%	benzyl alcohol · cetyl alcohol · glyceryl monostearate · isopropyl myristate · polyoxyethylene stearate blend · sorbitol solution · petrolatum · water

** New listing

§ Manufacturer/supplier did not confirm information for this edition. Product listing is reprinted from the '96-97 edition.

See Chapter 5, "External Analgesic Products," for more information about these products.

Vaginal and Menstrual Product Tables

VAGINAL ANTIFUNGAL PRODUCTS

	Product Manufacturer/Supplier	Dosage Form	Antifungal	Antiseptic	Other Ingredients
	Femizol-7 Lake Consumer	cream	clotrimazole, 1%		benzyl alcohol · cetearyl alcohol · cetyl esters wax · 2-octyldodecanol · polysorbate 60 · purified water · sodium phosphate monobasic · sorbitan monostearate
**	**Femizol-M** Lake Consumer	cream	miconazole nitrate, 2%	benzoic acid	BHA · mineral oil · peglicol 5 oleate · pegoxyol 7 stearate · purified water
	Femstat 3 Bayer Consumer	cream	butoconazole nitrate, 2%		cetyl alcohol · glyceryl stearate · PEG-100 stearate · methylparaben · propylparaben · mineral oil · polysorbate 60 · propylene glycol · sorbitan monostearate · stearyl alcohol · purified water
	Gyne-Lotrimin Schering-Plough Healthcare	cream	clotrimazole, 1%		cetyl esters wax · octyl dodecanol · polysorbate 60 · water · sorbitan monostearate · benzyl alcohol · cetearyl alcohol
**	**Gyne-Lotrimin 3 Combination Pack** Schering-Plough Healthcare	cream; suppository	cream: clotrimazole, 1% · suppository: clotrimazole, 200mg		
**	**Gyne-Lotrimin 3 Inserts** Schering-Plough Healthcare	suppository	clotrimazole, 200mg		
	Gyne-Lotrimin Inserts Schering-Plough Healthcare	suppository	clotrimazole, 100mg	povidone	corn starch · lactose · magnesium stearate
**	**Monistat 3 Combination Pack** Advanced Care Products	cream; suppository	cream: miconazole nitrate, 2% suppository: miconazole nitrate, 200mg		cream: BHA mineral oil · peglicol 5 oleate · pegoxyol 7 stearate · purified water · benzoic acid suppository: hydrogenated vegetable oil base
	Monistat 7 Advanced Care Products	suppository	miconazole nitrate, 100mg		hydrogenated vegetable oil base
	Monistat 7 Advanced Care Products	cream	miconazole nitrate, 2%		BHA · mineral oil · peglicol 5 oleate · pegoxyol 7 stearate · purified water · benzoic acid
**	**Mycelex-3** Bayer Consumer	cream	butoconazole nitrate, 2%		cetyl alcohol · glyceryl stearate · PEG-100 stearate · methylparaben · propylparaben · mineral oil · polysorbate 60 · propylene glycol · sorbitan · monostearate · stearyl alcohol · purified water
	Mycelex-7 Bayer Consumer	cream	clotrimazole, 1%		cetyl esters wax · octyldodecanol · polysorbate 60 · water · sorbitan monostearate · benzyl alcohol · cetostearyl alcohol
	Mycelex-7 Inserts Bayer Consumer	suppository	clotrimazole, 100mg	povidone	corn starch · lactose · magnesium stearate
**	**Vagistat-1** Bristol-Myers Products	ointment	tioconazole, 6.5%		butylated hydroxyanisole · magnesium aluminum silicate · white petrolatum

See Chapter 6, "Vaginal and Menstrual Products," for more information about these products.

FEMININE HYGIENE PRODUCTS

Product Manufacturer/Supplier	Dosage Form	Antimicrobial	Antipruritic/ Anesthetic/ Counterirritant	Hydrocortisone	Other Ingredients
Betadine Medicated Douche Purdue Frederick	liquid	povidone-iodine, 10%			
Betadine Premixed Medicated Disposable Douche Purdue Frederick	liquid	povidone-iodine, 0.3%			
Feminique Douche, Baby Powder or Spring Fresh Scent § Quality Health Products	liquid	octoxynol-9			deionized water · lactic acid · sodium lactate · diazolidinyl urea · methylparaben · disodium EDTA · fragrance
Feminique Douche, Extra Cleansing § Quality Health Products	liquid	octoxynol-9			deionized water · vinegar
Feminique Douche, Natural Vinegar & Water § Quality Health Products	liquid				water · vinegar · sorbic acid
Feminique Feminine Cloth Towelettes § Quality Health Products	wipe	octoxynol-9			water · propylene glycol · sodium benzoate · sodium lactate · fragrance · lactic acid · quaternium-15 · sodium lauryl sulfate
Gyne-cort Combe	cream			0.5%	
Gyne-cort Extra Strength 10 Combe	cream			1%	
Lanacane Creme Combe	cream	benzethonium chloride, 0.1% · chlorothymol	benzocaine, 6%		aloe · dioctyl sodium sulfosuccinate · ethoxydiglycol fragrance · glycerin · glyceryl stearate SE · isopropyl alcohol · methylparaben · propylparaben · sodium borate · stearic acid · sulfated castor oil · triethanolamine · water · zinc oxide · pyrithione zinc
** **Lanacane Maximum Strength** Combe	cream	benzethonium chloride, 0.2%	benzocaine, 20%		acetylated lanolin alcohol · aloe · cetyl acetate · cetyl alcohol · dimethicone · fragrance · glycerin · glyceryl stearate · isopropyl myristate · methylparaben · mineral oil · PEG-100 stearate · propylparaben · sorbitan stearate · stearamidopropyl PG-dimonium chloride phosphate · water · pyrithione zinc

See Chapter 6, "Vaginal and Menstrual Products," for more information about these products.

FEMININE HYGIENE PRODUCTS - continued

	Product Manufacturer/Supplier	Dosage Form	Antimicrobial	Antipruritic/ Anesthetic/ Counterirritant	Hydrocortisone	Other Ingredients
	Massengill Disp. Douche, Fresh Mtn. Breeze or Spring Rain SmithKline Beecham	liquid	cetylpyridinium chloride · octoxynol-9			purified water · SD alcohol 40 · lactic acid · sodium lactate · propylene glycol · diazolidinyl urea · methylparaben · propylparaben · disodium EDTA · fragrance · D&C yellow#10 (Mtn. Breeze) · FD&C blue#1 (Mtn Breeze)
	Massengill Disp. Douche, Vinegar & Water Extra Cleansing SmithKline Beecham	liquid	cetylpyridinium chloride · octoxynol-9			purified water · sodium citrate · citric acid · vinegar · diazolidinyl urea · edetate disodium
	Massengill Disposable Douche, Baking Soda SmithKline Beecham	liquid	sodium bicarbonate			sanitized water
	Massengill Disposable Douche, Vinegar & Water Extra Mild SmithKline Beecham	liquid				purified water · sodium citrate · citric acid · vinegar
	Massengill Douche, Country Flowers or Fresh Baby Pwdr. Scent SmithKline Beecham	liquid	cetylpyridinium chloride · octoxynol-9			purified water · sodium citrate · citric acid · SD alcohol 40 · diazolidinyl urea · fragrance · disodium edetate · FD&C blue#1 · FD&C red#28 (Country Flowers)
	Massengill Douche, Unscented SmithKline Beecham	powder		methyl salicylate · phenol · thymol · menthol		eucalyptus oil · ammonium alum · sodium chloride · PEG-8 · D&C yellow#10 · FD&C yellow#6
FR	**Massengill Medicated Disposable Douche** SmithKline Beecham	liquid	povidone-iodine, 0.3%			purified water
	Massengill Medicated Towelette SmithKline Beecham	wipe			0.5%	diazolidinyl urea · DMDM hydantoin · isopropyl myristate · methylparaben · propylparaben · polysorbate 60 · propylene glycol · sorbitan stearate · steareth-2 · steareth-21 · water
	Massengill Towelette, Baby Powder or Unscented SmithKline Beecham	wipe	cetylpyridinium chloride · octoxynol-9			water · lactic acid · sodium lactate · potassium sorbate · disodium EDTA · fragrance

See Chapter 6, "Vaginal and Menstrual Products," for more information about these products.

FEMININE HYGIENE PRODUCTS - continued

	Product Manufacturer/Supplier	Dosage Form	Antimicrobial	Antipruritic/ Anesthetic/ Counterirritant	Hydrocortisone	Other Ingredients
	Norforms, Fresh Flowers Scent C. B. Fleet	suppository	benzethonium chloride			PEG-18 · PEG-32 · PEG-20 stearate · fragrance · methylparaben · lactic acid
FR	**Norforms, Unscented** C. B. Fleet	suppository	benzethonium chloride			PEG-18 · PEG-32 · PEG-20 stearate · methylparaben · lactic acid
	PMC Disposable Douche Thomas & Thompson	liquid	boric acid, 82%	thymol, 0.3% · phenol, 0.2% · menthol		ammonium aluminum sulfate, 16% · eucalyptus oil · peppermint oil
	PMC Douche Thomas & Thompson	powder	boric acid, 82%	thymol, 0.3% · phenol, 0.2% · menthol		ammonium aluminum sulfate, 16% · eucalyptus oil · peppermint oil
**	**Summer's Eve Disposable Douche, Ultra** C. B. Fleet	liquid	octoxynol-9			sodium chloride · decyl glucoside · citric acid · sodium benzoate · disodium EDTA · fragrance · water
	Summer's Eve Disposable Douche, Vinegar & Water C. B. Fleet	liquid	benzoic acid			vinegar · water
	Summer's Eve Douche C. B. Fleet	liquid	povidone-iodine, 0.3%			water · citric acid
	Summer's Eve Douche, Extra-Cleansing Vinegar & Water C. B. Fleet	liquid	benzoic acid			purified water · sodium chloride · vinegar
	Summer's Eve Douche; Musk, Touch of Spring, or White Flowers C. B. Fleet	liquid	octoxynol-9			citric acid · sodium benzoate · disodium EDTA · fragrance · water
	Summer's Eve Feminine Powder C. B. Fleet	powder	octoxynol-9 · benzethonium chloride			corn starch · tricalcium phosphate · fragrance
	Summer's Eve Feminine Wash Cleansing Cloths C. B. Fleet	wipe	octoxynol-9			purified water · sodium benzoate · fragrance · citric acid · disodium EDTA
	Trimo-San Milex Products	jelly	oxyquinoline sulfate, 0.025%			glycerin · carbomer · sodium citrate · citric acid · methylparaben · simethicone · lilac perfume · sodium lauryl sulfate · triethanolamine
	Vaginex Douche § Quality Health Products	liquid	povidone-iodine, 30%			
	Vaginex Medicated § Quality Health Products	powder	8-hydroxyquinoline · 8-hydroxyquinoline sulfate			zinc oxide · corn starch · fragrance · isostearic acid · PPG-20 methyl glucose ether · talc

See Chapter 6, "Vaginal and Menstrual Products," for more information about these products.

FEMININE HYGIENE PRODUCTS - continued

Product Manufacturer/Supplier	Dosage Form	Antimicrobial	Antipruritic/ Anesthetic/ Counterirritant	Hydrocortisone	Other Ingredients
Vaginex, Scented or Unscented § Quality Health Products	cream			1%	
Vagisil Combe	cream	resorcinol, 2%	benzocaine, 5%		
Yeast-X C. B. Fleet	cream			1%	
Yeast-Gard Advanced, Sensitive Formula Lake Consumer	cream	benzalkonium chloride, 0.13%	benzocaine, 5%		deionized water · glyceryl stearate · mineral oil · cetyl alcohol · PEG-100 stearate · aloe vera gel · isopropyl palmitate · isopropyl myristate · isopropyl stearate · lanolin alcohol · triethanolamine · methylparaben · propylparaben · carbomer 940 · vitamin E · fragrance · trisodium HEDTA
Yeast-Gard Disposable Douche Lake Consumer	solution	povidone-iodine, 0.3%			purified water
Yeast-Gard Disposable Douche Premix Lake Consumer	liquid	octoxynol-9			purified water · lactic acid · sodium lactate · sodium benzoate · aloe vera
Yeast-Gard Douche Concentrate Lake Consumer	liquid	povidone-iodine, 10%			
Yeast-Gard Maximum Strength Lake Consumer	cream	benzalkonium chloride, 0.13%	benzocaine, 20%		deionized water · propylene glycol · cetyl alcohol · isopropyl palmitate · glyceryl stearate · sodium lauryl sulfate · aloe vera gel · methylparaben · propylparaben · vitamin E · fragrance · tetrasodium HEDTA

** New listing
§ Manufacturer/supplier did not confirm information for this edition. Product listing is reprinted from the '96-97 edition.

See Chapter 6, "Vaginal and Menstrual Products," for more information about these products.

MENSTRUAL PRODUCTS

Product [a] Manufacturer/Supplier	Dosage Form	Analgesic	Diuretic	Other Ingredients
Aqua-Ban Thompson Medical AF CA GL PR PU SO	tablet		pamabrom, 50mg	FD&C blue#1 aluminum lake · titanium dioxide · hydroxypropyl methylcellulose · microcrystalline cellulose · propylene glycol · croscarmellose sodium · carnauba wax · lactose · magnesium stearate · polyethylene glycol · polysorbate 80 · starch
Backaid Pills Alva-Amco Pharmacal AF CA GL PR SO SU	caplet	acetaminophen, 500mg	pamabrom, 25mg	
Diurex Long Acting Alva-Amco Pharmacal GL PR SO	timed-release capsule	potassium salicylate · acetaminophen	caffeine, 195mg	
Diurex MPR Alva-Amco Pharmacal AF CA GL PR SO	caplet	acetaminophen, 500mg	pamabrom, 25mg	
Diurex PMS Alva-Amco Pharmacal AF CA GL PR SO	caplet	acetaminophen, 500mg	pamabrom, 25mg	pyrilamine maleate, 15mg
Diurex Water Caplet Alva-Amco Pharmacal AF CA GL PR SO SU	caplet		pamabrom, 50mg	
Diurex Water Pills Alva-Amco Pharmacal GL PR SO	tablet	potassium salicylate · salicylamide	caffeine	
Diurex-2 Water Pills Alva-Amco Pharmacal AF CA GL PR SO	tablet	magnesium salicylate tetrahydrate, 202mg	pamabrom, 25mg	iron · calcium
Fem-1 BDI Ph'cals	tablet	acetaminophen, 500mg	pamabrom, 25mg	
Lurline PMS Fielding AF CA GL PR PU SU	tablet	acetaminophen, 500mg	pamabrom, 25mg	pyridoxine HCl, 50mg
Midol Menstrual Maximum Strength Multisymptom Formula Bayer Consumer AF GL SO	caplet	acetaminophen, 500mg	caffeine, 60mg	pyrilamine maleate, 15mg
Midol Menstrual Maximum Strength Multisymptom Formula Bayer Consumer AF	gelcap	acetaminophen, 500mg	caffeine, 60mg	pyrilamine maleate, 15mg

See Chapter 6, "Vaginal and Menstrual Products," for more information about these products.

MENSTRUAL PRODUCTS - continued

Product [a] Manufacturer/Supplier	Dosage Form	Analgesic	Diuretic	Other Ingredients
AF CA	**Midol PMS Maximum Strength Multisymptom Formula** Bayer Consumer	gelcap	acetaminophen, 500mg	pamabrom, 25mg	pyrilamine maleate, 15mg · croscarmellose sodium · D&C red#27 lake · disodium EDTA · FD&C blue#1 · FD&C red#40 lake · gelatin · glycerin · hydroxypropyl methylcellulose · iron oxide · magnesium stearate · microcrystalline cellulose · starch · stearic acid · titanium dioxide · triacetin
AF CA GL SO	**Midol PMS Multisymptom Formula** Bayer Consumer	caplet	acetaminophen, 500mg	pamabrom, 25mg	pyrilamine maleate, 15mg
AF CA GL SO	**Midol Teen Multisymptom Formula** Bayer Consumer	caplet	acetaminophen, 400mg	pamabrom, 25mg	
AF CA	**Odrinil Water Pills** Fox Pharmacal	tablet		pamabrom, 25mg	dicalcium phosphate · cellulose · stearic acid · silica · coating materials · yellow#10 · yellow#6
**	**Pamprin** Chattem	gelcap	acetaminophen, 500mg	pamabrom, 25mg	pyrilamine maleate, 15mg
CA	**Pamprin Maximum Pain Relief** Chattem	caplet	acetaminophen, 250mg · magnesium salicylate, 250mg	pamabrom, 25mg	
AF CA	**Pamprin Multisymptom Formula** Chattem	caplet · tablet	acetaminophen, 500mg	pamabrom, 25mg	pyrilamine maleate, 15mg
AF CA	**Premsyn PMS** Chattem	caplet	acetaminophen, 500mg	pamabrom, 25mg	pyrilamine maleate, 15mg
**	**Premsyn PMS** Chattem	gelcap	acetaminophen, 500mg	pamabrom, 25mg	pyrilamine maleate, 15mg
**	**Repose PMS** GumTech	gum			magnesium oxide, 25mg · pyridoxine, 2mg · sorbitol powder · gum base · maltitol syrup · mannitol powder · mint and other natural flavors · resinous glaze · dong quai · dandelion leaf · carnauba wax · titanium dioxide coating

** New listing

[a] This table lists only products that contain a diuretic; some may contain an analgesic and a diuretic. For other products used in the management of dysmenorrhea, see the Internal Analgesic and Antipyretic Products table.

See Chapter 6, "Vaginal and Menstrual Products," for more information about these products.

VAGINAL LUBRICANT PRODUCTS

	Product Manufacturer/Supplier	Dosage Form	Lubricant/Humectant	Preservative	Other Ingredients
	Astroglide Biofilm	gel	glycerin · propylene glycol	polyquaternium #5 · methylparaben · propylparaben	purified water
** **FR**	**Born Again Vaginal Moisturizing** Alvin Last	gel	glycerin	methylparaben	water · wild yam extract · sodium alginate · tocopheryl acetate · citric acid
	Feminease Parnell Ph'cals	cream	mineral oil · stearic acid · glycerin · propylene glycol · lecithin	benzoic acid · BHT	purified water · yerba santa · cetyl alcohol · glyceryl stearate · isopropyl myristate · PEG- 40 stearate · squalene · dimethicone · diazolidinyl urea · PEG-12 oleate · sulfated castor oil
	Gyne-Moistrin Schering-Plough Healthcare	gel	propylene glycol	methylparaben · propylparaben	polyglyceryl methacrylate · water
	H-R Lubricating Carter Products	jelly	propylene glycol	propylparaben · methylparaben	hydroxypropyl methylcellulose · carbomer 934P · sodium hydroxide
	K-Y Jelly Advanced Care Products	jelly	glycerin	chlorhexidine gluconate · methylparaben	glucono delta lactone · sodium hydroxide · hydroxyethyl cellulose · purified water · sodium hydroxide
**	**K-Y Liquid** Advanced Care Products	liquid	glycerin · propylene glycol	methylparaben · benzoic acid	sorbitol · Natrosol 250H · sodium hydroxide · purified water
** **FR**	**K-Y Long Lasting** Advanced Care Products	gel	glycerin · mineral oil · hydrogenated palm glyceride	methylparaben · sorbic acid	purified water · PVM/MA decadiene crosspolymer · calcium-sodium salt of MVE/MA copolymer · vitamin E · sodium hydroxide
	Lubrin Inserts Kenwood Labs	suppository	glycerin		PEG-6-32 · PEG-20 · caprylic/capric triglyceride · PEG-40 stearate · polysorbate 80
FR	**Maxilube** Mission Pharmacal	jelly	silicone oil · sodium lauryl sulfate · glycerin	methylparaben · propylparaben	water · triethanolamine · carbomer 934
	Moist Again Vaginal Moisturizing Lake Consumer	gel	glycerin	chlorhexidine gluconate · sodium benzoate · potassium sorbate · diazolidinyl urea · sorbic acid	water · carbomer · triethanolamine · aloe vera · citric acid
	Replens Warner-Lambert Consumer	gel	mineral oil · hydrogenated palm oil glyceride · glycerin	sorbic acid	carbomer 934P · polycarbophil
	Surgel Ulmer Pharmacal	gel	propylene glycol · glycerin		carboxymethylcellulose sodium · phenyl mercuric nitrate
	Women's Health Formula Lubricating Lake Consumer	gel	glycerin	chlorhexidine gluconate · methylparaben	glucono delta lactone · hydroxyethyl cellulose · sodium hydroxide · water
**	**Wondergel Personal Liquid** Lake Consumer	gel	glycerin · propylene glycol	methylparaben · potassium sorbate · sodium benzoate	water · hydroxyethyl cellulose · DMDM · hydantoin · ginseng · aloe vera

See Chapter 6, "Vaginal and Menstrual Products," for more information about these products.

Contraceptive Product Tables

CONDOM PRODUCTS

Product Manufacturer/Supplier	Material [a]	Spermicide	Comments
Avanti Durex Consumer	polyurethane	No	lubricated
Avanti Super Thin Durex Consumer	polyurethane	No	lubricated
** **CarePlus** Selfcare	latex	nonoxynol-9, 100mg (suppository)	condoms packaged with separate spermicide inserts (suppositories) · reservoir end · lubricated
Class Act Ribbed and Sensitive Carter Products	latex	No	reservoir end · lubricated · ribbed
Class Act Ribbed and Sensitive with Spermicide Carter Products	latex	Yes	reservoir end · spermicidal lubricant · ribbed
** **Class Act Smooth Sensation** Carter Products	latex	No	reservoir end · lubricated
** **Class Act Smooth Sensation with Spermicide** Carter Products	latex	Yes	reservoir end · spermicidal lubricant
Class Act Ultra Thin and Sensitive Carter Products	latex	No	reservoir end · lubricated · ultra thin
Class Act Ultra Thin and Sensitive with Spermicide Carter Products	latex	Yes	reservoir end · spermicidal lubricant · ultra thin
Fourex [a] Durex Consumer	animal membrane [a]	No	pre-moistened capsule or pre-moistened foil
Fourex with Spermicide [a] Durex Consumer	animal membrane [a]	nonoxynol-9, 7%	spermicidally lubricated foil
Gold Circle Coin Durex Consumer	latex	No	reservoir end
Gold Circle Rainbow Coin Durex Consumer	latex	No	reservoir end · contoured shape · colored
** **LifeStyles Extra Strength with Spermicide** Ansell	latex	nonoxynol-9	
** **LifeStyles Lubricated** Ansell	latex	No	lubricated
** **LifeStyles Spermicidally Lubricated** Ansell	latex	nonoxynol-9	spermicidal lubricant
** **LifeStyles Ultra Sensitive** Ansell	latex	No	ultra thin
** **LifeStyles Ultra Sensitive with Spermicide** Ansell	latex	nonoxynol-9	ultra thin

See Chapter 7, "Contraceptive Methods and Products," for more information about these products.

CONDOM PRODUCTS - continued

Product Manufacturer/Supplier	Material [a]	Spermicide	Comments
** **LifeStyles Vibra-Ribbed** Ansell	latex	No	ribbed
** **LifeStyles Vibra-Ribbed with Spermicide** Ansell	latex	nonoxynol-9	ribbed
** **LifeStyles; Assorted Colors, Form Fitting, or Studded** Ansell	latex	No	colored, contoured shape, or rubber studs
Naturalamb [a] Carter Products	lamb cecum [a]	No	lubricated
Naturalamb with Spermicide [a] Carter Products	lamb cecum [a]	Yes	spermicidal lubricant
Ramses Extra Strength with Spermicide Durex Consumer	latex	nonoxynol-9, 8%	reservoir end · spermicidal lubricant
Ramses Extra with Spermicide Durex Consumer	latex	nonoxynol-9, 5%	reservoir end · spermicidal lubricant · regular or ribbed
Ramses Sensitol Durex Consumer	latex	No	reservoir end · lubricated
Ramses Ultra Thin Durex Consumer	latex	No	reservoir end · lubricated · regular or ribbed
Ramses Ultra Thin with Spermicide Durex Consumer	latex	nonoxynol-9, 5%	reservoir end · spermicidal lubricant · regular or ribbed
Reality Female Condom § Female Health	polyurethane	No	thin, soft, loose-fitting sheath with two flexible rings · inner ring aids in insertion and holds device in place over the cervix · outer ring remains outside the vagina after insertion · may be inserted hours before intercourse · prelubricated with silicone · packaged with extra water-based lubricant · disposable, for one-time use only
Saxon Gold Rainbow Durex Consumer	latex	No	reservoir end · contoured shape · colored · lubricated
Saxon Gold Ultra with Spermicide, Clear or Rainbow Durex Consumer	latex	nonoxynol-9, 6.6%	reservoir end · contoured shape · clear or colored · spermicidal lubricant
Saxon Gold Ultra Lube Durex Consumer	latex	No	reservoir end · contoured shape · water-based lubricant
Saxon Gold Ultra Ribbed Durex Consumer	latex	No	reservoir end · contoured shape · lubricated
Saxon Gold Ultra Sensitive Durex Consumer	latex	No	reservoir end · contoured shape · lubricated

See Chapter 7, "Contraceptive Methods and Products," for more information about these products.

CONDOM PRODUCTS - continued

Product Manufacturer/Supplier	Material [a]	Spermicide	Comments
Sheik Classic Durex Consumer	latex	No	reservoir end · regular or lubricated
Sheik Classic with Spermicide Durex Consumer	latex	nonoxynol-9, 8%	reservoir end · spermicidal lubricant
Sheik Excita Extra with Spermicide Durex Consumer	latex	nonoxynol-9, 8%	reservoir end · spermicidal lubricant · ribbed
Sheik Fiesta Durex Consumer	latex	No	reservoir end · assorted colors · lubricated
Sheik Super Thin Durex Consumer	latex	No	reservoir end · lubricated · regular or ribbed
Sheik Super Thin with Spermicide Durex Consumer	latex	nonoxynol-9, 8%	reservoir end · spermicidal lubricant · regular or ribbed
Touch Durex Consumer	latex	No	reservoir end · available styles are regular, ribbed, sunrise colors, and thin ultra sensitive
Touch Lubricated Durex Consumer	latex	No	reservoir end · lubricated
Touch with Spermicide Durex Consumer	latex	nonoxynol-9, 8%	reservoir end · spermicidal lubricant
Trojan Carter Products	latex	No	non-lubricated · rounded end
Trojan Extra Strength Carter Products	latex	No	reservoir end · golden color · lubricated
Trojan Extra Strength with Spermicide Carter Products	latex	Yes	reservoir end · spermicidal lubricant
Trojan Magnum Carter Products	latex	No	reservoir end · larger size · lubricated
Trojan Magnum with Spermicide Carter Products	latex	Yes	reservoir end · larger size · spermicidal lubricant
Trojan Naturalube Carter Products	latex	No	reservoir end · contoured shape · lubricated · ribbed/textured
Trojan Plus Carter Products	latex	No	reservoir end · contoured shape · golden color · lubricated
Trojan Plus 2 with Spermicide Carter Products	latex	Yes	reservoir end · contoured shape · spermicidal lubricant
Trojan Ribbed Carter Products	latex	No	reservoir end · golden color · lubricated · ribbed/textured
Trojan Ribbed with Spermicide Carter Products	latex	Yes	reservoir end · spermicidal lubricant · ribbed/textured

See Chapter 7, "Contraceptive Methods and Products," for more information about these products.

CONDOM PRODUCTS - continued

Product Manufacturer/Supplier	Material [a]	Spermicide	Comments
** **Trojan Ultra Pleasure** Carter Products	latex	No	bulbous shaped reservoir end · lubricated
** **Trojan Ultra Pleasure with Spermicide** Carter Products	latex	Yes	bulbous shaped reservoir end · spermicidal lubricant
Trojan Ultra Texture Carter Products	latex	No	reservoir end · lubricated · textured
Trojan Ultra Texture with Spermicide Carter Products	latex	Yes	reservoir end · spermicidal lubricant · textured
Trojan Ultra Thin Carter Products	latex	No	receptacle end · lubricated
Trojan Ultra Thin with Spermicide Carter Products	latex	Yes	receptacle end · spermicidal lubricant
Trojan Very Sensitive Carter Products	latex	No	reservoir end · contoured shape · lubricated
Trojan Very Sensitive with Spermicide Carter Products	latex	Yes	reservoir end · contoured shape · spermicidal lubricant
Trojan-Enz Carter Products	latex	No	reservoir end · lubricated or non-lubricated
Trojan-Enz Large Carter Products	latex	No	reservoir end · larger size · lubricated
Trojan-Enz Large with Spermicide Carter Products	latex	Yes	reservoir end · larger size · spermicidal lubricant
Trojan-Enz with Spermicide Carter Products	latex	Yes	reservoir end · spermicidal lubricant

** New listing

[a] Animal membrane condoms are more porous than latex ones and may allow transmission of the AIDS virus. Animal membrane condoms are not to be used for the prevention of sexually transmitted diseases.

See Chapter 7, "Contraceptive Methods and Products," for more information about these products.

SPERMICIDE PRODUCTS

Product Manufacturer/Supplier	Dosage Form	Spermicide	Other Ingredients
Advantage 24 [a] Lake Consumer	gel	nonoxynol-9, 3.5%	purified water · glycerin · mineral oil · polycarbophil · hydrogenated palm oil glyceride · carbomer 934P · methylparaben · sorbic acid · sodium hydroxide
** **CarePlus** Selfcare	condom; spermicide insert (suppository)	nonoxynol-9, 100mg (suppository)	packaged with condoms
Conceptrol Advanced Care Products	gel	nonoxynol-9, 4%	cellulose gum · lactic acid · methylparaben · povidone · propylene glycol · purified water · sorbic acid · sorbitol solution
Conceptrol Inserts Advanced Care Products	suppository	nonoxynol-9, 5.56%	polyethylene glycol 1000 · polyethylene glycol 1450 · povidone · sodium bicarbonate · citric acid · compound TL-LDK
Delfen Advanced Care Products	foam	nonoxynol-9, 12.5%	benzoic acid · cetyl alcohol · diethylaminoethyl stearamide · glacial acetic acid · methylparaben · perfume · polyvinyl alcohol · propylene glycol · purified water · carboxymethylcellulose sodium · sorbic acid · stearic acid
Emko Schering-Plough Healthcare	foam	nonoxynol-9, 12%	benzethonium chloride · propellants · glyceryl stearate
Encare Thompson Medical	suppository	nonoxynol-9, 100mg	polyethylene glycol · tartaric acid · sodium citrate · sodium bicarbonate
Gynol II [a] Advanced Care Products	jelly	nonoxynol-9, 2%	lactic acid · methylparaben · povidone · propylene glycol · purified water · carboxymethylcellulose sodium · sorbic acid · sorbitol solution
Gynol II ES [a] Advanced Care Products	jelly	nonoxynol-9, 3%	lactic acid · methylparaben · povidone · propylene glycol · purified water · carboxymethylcellulose sodium · sorbic acid · sorbitol solution
K-Y Plus [a] Advanced Care Products	jelly	nonoxynol-9, 2.2%	cremophor · hydroxyethyl cellulose · methylparaben · propylene glycol · purified water · sorbic acid
Koromex [a] § Quality Health Products	jelly	nonoxynol-9, 3%	
Koromex § Quality Health Products	foam	nonoxynol-9, 12.5%	acetic acid · cetyl alcohol · fragrance · isobutane · isopropyl alcohol · laureth-4 · PEG-50 stearate · propylene glycol · sodium acetate water
Koromex Crystal Clear [a] § Quality Health Products	gel	nonoxynol-9, 3%	
Koromex Inserts § Quality Health Products	suppository	nonoxynol-9, 125mg (5%)	lactic acid · polyethylene glycol
Ortho-Gynol [a] Advanced Care Products	jelly	octoxynol-9, 1%	benzoic acid · castor oil · fragrance · glacial acetic acid · methylparaben · potassium hydroxide · propylene glycol · purified water · sorbic acid · carboxymethylcellulose sodium
Semicid Inserts Whitehall-Robins Healthcare	suppository	nonoxynol-9, 100mg	benzethonium chloride · citric acid · D&C red#21 lake · D&C red#33 lake · methylparaben · polyethylene glycol · water
Shur-Seal [a] Milex Products	jelly	nonoxynol-9, 2%	water · propylene glycol · methylcellulose · methylparaben · simethicone · boric acid · citric acid

See Chapter 7, "Contraceptive Methods and Products," for more information about these products.

SPERMICIDE PRODUCTS - continued

Product Manufacturer/Supplier	Dosage Form	Spermicide	Other Ingredients
VCF [a] Apothecus Ph'cal	gel	nonoxynol-9, 3%	propylene glycol · cellulose gum · sorbitol · polyvinylpyrrolidone · lactic acid · methylparaben · EDTA · water
VCF Vaginal Contraceptive Film Apothecus Ph'cal	film square	nonoxynol-9, 28%	glycerin · polyvinyl alcohol

** New listing

[a] For use with a diaphragm

§ Manufacturer/supplier did not confirm information for this edition. Product listing is reprinted from the '96-97 edition.

See Chapter 7, "Contraceptive Methods and Products," for more information about these products.

Cold, Cough, and Allergy
Product Tables

MISCELLANEOUS NASAL PRODUCTS

	Product Manufacturer/Supplier	Dosage Form	Primary Ingredients	Preservative	Other Ingredients
	4-Way Saline Moisturizing Mist Bristol-Myers Products	spray	sodium chloride	benzalkonium chloride	water · boric acid · sodium borate · eucalyptol · menthol · polysorbate 80 · glycerin
	Ayr B. F. Ascher	gel	sodium chloride, 0.5%	propylene glycol · methylparaben · propylparaben	diazolidinyl urea · carbomer · tocopherol acetate · glyceryl polymethacrylate · aloe vera gel · glycerin
	Ayr B. F. Ascher	drops · spray	sodium chloride, 0.65%	benzalkonium chloride · thimerosal	
SL	**Breathe Free** Thompson Medical	spray	sodium chloride, 0.65%	benzalkonium chloride	monobasic sodium · dibasic sodium
SL	**HuMIST Saline** Scherer Labs	spray	sodium chloride, 0.65%	chlorobutanol, 0.35%	sodium phosphate dibasic anhydrous · sodium phosphate monobasic · disodium EDTA
PE	**Little Noses Saline** Vetco	drops · spray	sodium chloride, 0.65%	benzalkonium chloride · thimerosal	disodium phosphate · sodium phosphate
**	**Nasal Moist** Blairex Labs	gel		methylparaben · propylparaben	aloe vera · sodiun chloride · allantoin · purified water · propylene glycol · hydroxyethyl cellulose
SL	**Nasal Moist** Blairex Labs	pump spray · solution	sodium chloride, 0.65%	benzyl alcohol	
	NaSal Saline Moisturizer Bayer Consumer	drops · spray	sodium chloride, 0.65%	thimerosal, 0.001% · benzalkonium chloride	
PR	**Nichols Nasal Douche** Alvin Last	powder	sodium chloride		sodium bicarbonate · sodium borate · menthol · eucalyptol
	Nose Better Natural Mist Lee Consumer	spray	glycerin, 1% · sodium chloride, 0.35%	benzalkonium chloride	water · potassium phosphate · fragrance · disodium EDTA · hydroxypropyl methylcellulose · sodium hydroxide
SL	**Ocean** Fleming	spray	sodium chloride, 0.65%	benzyl alcohol · benzalkonium chloride	
SL	**Pretz** Parnell Ph'cals	solution · spray	glycerin, 3%	phenylmercuric nitrate	citric acid · sodium citrate · sodium chloride · water · yerba santa
	Salinex Muro Ph'cal	drops · spray	sodium chloride, 0.4%	benzalkonium chloride, 0.01% · propylene glycol	disodium edetate · hydroxypropyl methylcellulose · polyethylene glycol · purified water · sodium phosphate

** New listing

See Chapter 8, "Cold, Cough and Allergy Products," for more information about these products.

COLD, COUGH, AND ALLERGY PRODUCTS

	Product Manufacturer/Supplier	Dosage Form	Decongestant	Antihistamine
AF	**A.R.M. Caplet** Menley & James Labs	caplet	phenylpropanolamine HCl, 25mg	chlorpheniramine maleate, 4mg
AF GL	**Actifed** Warner-Lambert Consumer	tablet	pseudoephedrine HCl, 60mg	triprolidine HCl, 2.5mg
AF	**Actifed Allergy Daytime/Nighttime** Warner-Lambert Consumer	Daytime, caplet; Nighttime, caplet	Daytime: pseudoephedrine HCl, 30mg Nighttime: pseudoephedrine HCl, 30mg	Nighttime: diphenhydramine HCl, 25mg
AF	**Actifed Sinus Daytime/Nighttime** Warner-Lambert Consumer	Daytime, caplet; Nighttime, caplet	Daytime: pseudoephedrine HCl, 30mg Nighttime: pseudoephedrine HCl, 30mg	Nighttime: diphenhydramine HCl, 25mg
AF GL SO	**Advil Cold & Sinus** Whitehall-Robins Healthcare	caplet · tablet	pseudoephedrine HCl, 30mg	
**	**Aler-Dryl** Reese Chemical	caplet		diphenhydramine HCl, 50mg
**	**Aler-Releaf** Reese Chemical	timed-release capsule	phenylpropanolamine HCl, 75mg	chloropheniramine maleate, 4mg
	Alka-Seltzer Plus Cold & Cough Medicine Bayer Consumer	effervescent tablet	phenylpropanolamine bitartrate, 20mg	chlorpheniramine maleate, 2mg
AF	**Alka-Seltzer Plus Cold & Cough Medicine Liqui-Gels** Bayer Consumer	softgel	pseudoephedrine HCl, 30mg	chlorpheniramine maleate, 2mg
PU	**Alka-Seltzer Plus Cold Medicine** Bayer Consumer	effervescent tablet	phenylpropanolamine bitartrate, 20mg	chlorpheniramine maleate, 2mg
AF	**Alka-Seltzer Plus Cold Medicine Liqui-Gels** Bayer Consumer	softgel	pseudoephedrine HCl, 30mg	chlorpheniramine maleate, 2mg
	Alka-Seltzer Plus Flu & Body Aches Bayer Consumer	effervescent tablet	phenylpropanolamine bitartrate, 20mg	chlorpheniramine maleate, 2mg
AF	**Alka-Seltzer Plus Flu & Body Aches Liqui-Gels** Bayer Consumer	softgel	pseudoephedrine HCl, 30mg	
PU	**Alka-Seltzer Plus Night-Time Cold Medicine** Bayer Consumer	effervescent tablet	phenylpropanolamine bitartrate, 20mg	doxylamine succinate, 6.25mg
	Alka-Seltzer Plus Night-Time Cold Medicine Liqui-Gels Bayer Consumer	softgel	pseudoephedrine HCl, 30mg	doxylamine succinate, 6.25mg
	Alka-Seltzer Plus Sinus Medicine Bayer Consumer	effervescent tablet	phenylpropanolamine bitartrate, 20mg	
	Aller-med Republic Drug	caplet		diphenhydramine HCl, 25mg
AF GL PU	**Allerest Maximum Strength** Novartis Consumer	tablet	pseudoephedrine HCl, 30mg	chlorpheniramine maleate, 2mg
AF GL PU SO	**Allerest No Drowsiness** Novartis Consumer	tablet	pseudoephedrine HCl, 30mg	

See Chapter 8, "Cold, Cough and Allergy Products," for more information about these products.

Analgesic	Expectorant	Antitussive	Other Ingredients
			D&C yellow#10 · FD&C yellow#6 · lactose · starch · magnesium stearate · gelatin · carnauba wax · hydroxypropyl methylcellulose · polyethylene glycol · sodium starch glycolate
			lactose · sucrose · magnesium stearate · potato starch · titanium dioxide · flavor · hydroxypropyl methylcellulose · polyethylene glycol · povidone · corn starch
			carnauba wax · lactose · polyethylene glycol · titanium dioxide · magnesium stearate · microcrystalline cellulose · crospovidone · hydroxypropyl methylcellulose · Nighttime only: FD&C blue#1 aluminum lake · polysorbate 80
Daytime: acetaminophen, 500mg Nighttime: acetaminophen, 500mg			carnauba wax · crospovidone · hydroxypropyl methylcellulose · magnesium stearate · microcrystalline cellulose · polyethylene glycol · povidone · pregelatinized corn starch · stearic acid · titanium dioxide · Nighttime only: FD&C blue#1 aluminum lake · polysorbate 80 · sodium starch glycolate
ibuprofen, 200mg			carnauba or equivalent wax · croscarmellose sodium · iron oxides · methylparaben · microcrystalline cellulose · propylparaben · silicon dioxide · sodium benzoate · sodium lauryl sulfate · starch · stearic acid · sucrose · titanium dioxide
			D&C yellow#10 · di-pac compressed sugar · microcrystalline cellulose · sodium starch glycolate · stearic acid · pregelatinized starch
			sucrose · starch · talc · diacalcium phosphate · D&C yellow#10 · FD&C red#3 · FD&C yellow#6 · gelatin · pharmaceutical glaze
aspirin, 500mg		dextromethorphan hydrobromide, 10mg	aspartame · citric acid · flavor · sodium bicarbonate (sodium, 506mg) · tableting aids
acetaminophen, 325mg		dextromethorphan hydrobromide, 10mg	D&C red#33 · FD&C blue#1 · gelatin · glycerin · polyethylene glycol · potssium acetate · povidone · purified water · sorbitol · titanium dioxide
aspirin, 325mg			citric acid · flavors · sodiun bicarbonate
acetaminophen, 325mg			FD&C blue#1 · FD&C red#40 · gelatin · glycerin · polyethylene glycol · potassium acetate · povidone · purified water · sorbitol · titanium dioxide
acetaminophen, 325mg		dextromethorphan hydrobromide, 10mg	aspartame · calcium carbonate · citric acid · croscarmellose sodium · D&C yellow#10 · flavor · maltodextrin · mannitol · polyvinylpyrrolidone · sodium bicarbonate · saccharin sodium · sorbitol · starch · stearic acid · tableting aids
acetaminophen, 325mg		dextromethorphan hydrobromide, 10mg	FD&C red#40 · gelatin · glycerin · polyethylene glycol · povidone · propylene glycol · purified water · sorbitol · titanium dioxide
aspirin, 500mg		dextromethorphan hydrobromide, 15mg	aspartame · citric acid · flavors · sodium bicarbonate · tableting aids
acetaminophen, 325mg		dextromethorphan hydrobromide, 10mg	D&C yellow#10 · FD&C blue#1 · gleatin · glycerin · polyethylene glycol · potassium acetate · povidone · purified water · sorbitol · titanium dioxide
aspirin, 325mg			aspartame · citric acid · flavor · sodium bicarbonate · tableting aids
			corn starch · blue#1 · hydroxypropyl methylcellulose · lactose · microcrystalline cellulose · polyethylene glycol · polysorbate 80 · stearic acid · titanium dioxide
acetaminophen, 325mg			corn starch · hydroxypropyl methylcellulose · microcrystalline cellulose · polyethylene glycol · polysorbate 80 · stearic acid · titanium dioxide

COLD, COUGH, AND ALLERGY PRODUCTS - continued

	Product Manufacturer/Supplier	Dosage Form	Decongestant	Antihistamine
AF GL PU	**Allergy Relief** Hudson	tablet		chlorpheniramine maleate, 2mg
** LA	**Ambenyl-D Cough** Forest Ph'cals	syrup	pseudoephedrine HCl, 30mg/5ml	
DY	**BC Allergy·Sinus·Cold** Block Drug	powder	phenylpropanolamine HCl, 25mg	chlorpheniramine maleate, 4mg
DY	**BC Sinus·Cold** Block Drug	powder	phenylpropanolamine HCl, 25mg	
AF PU SO	**Benadryl Allergy** Warner-Lambert Consumer	capsule		diphenhydramine HCl, 25mg
AF PU	**Benadryl Allergy** Warner-Lambert Consumer	tablet		diphenhydramine HCl, 25mg
AL SL	**Benadryl Allergy** Warner-Lambert Consumer	liquid		diphenhydramine HCl, 12.5mg/5ml
PE	**Benadryl Allergy** Warner-Lambert Consumer	chewable tablet		diphenhydramine HCl, 12.5mg
AL SL	**Benadryl Allergy Decongestant** Warner-Lambert Consumer	liquid	pseudoephedrine HCl, 30mg/5ml	diphenhydramine HCl, 12.5mg/5ml
AF	**Benadryl Allergy Decongestant** Warner-Lambert Consumer	tablet	pseudoephedrine HCl, 60mg	diphenhydramine HCl, 25mg
AL DY	**Benadryl Allergy Dye-Free** Warner-Lambert Consumer	liquid		diphenhydramine HCl, 12.5mg/5ml
DY	**Benadryl Allergy Dye-Free Liqui-gels** Warner-Lambert Consumer	softgel		diphenhydramine HCl, 25mg
AF	**Benadryl Allergy/Cold** Warner-Lambert Consumer	tablet	pseudoephedrine HCl, 30mg	diphenhydramine HCl, 12.5mg
AF	**Benadryl Allergy/Sinus/Headache Formula** Warner-Lambert Consumer	caplet	pseudoephedrine HCl, 30mg	diphenhydramine HCl, 12.5mg
AL SU	**Benylin Adult Cough Formula** Warner-Lambert Consumer	liquid		
AL	**Benylin Cough Suppressant Expectorant** Warner-Lambert Consumer	liquid		
AL SU	**Benylin Multi-Symptom Formula** Warner-Lambert Consumer	liquid	pseudoephedrine HCl, 15mg/5ml	

See Chapter 8, "Cold, Cough and Allergy Products," for more information about these products.

Analgesic	Expectorant	Antitussive	Other Ingredients
	guaifenesin, 100mg/5ml	dextromethorphan hydrobromide, 15mg/5ml	sucrose · sodium chloride · ethyl alcohol · menthol · citric acid · saccharin sodium · sorbitol · flavors
aspirin, 650mg			
aspirin, 650mg			
			lactose · magnesium stearate · D&C red#28 · FD&C red#3 · FD&C red#40 · FD&C blue#1 · gelatin · glyceryl monooleate · titanium dioxide
			candellila wax · croscarmellose sodium · dibasic calcium phosphate dihydrate · D&C red#27 aluminum lake · hydroxypropyl methylcellulose · microcrystalline cellulose · polyethylene glycol · polysorbate 80 · stearic acid · titanium dioxide · zinc stearate · pregelatinized starch
			FD&C red#40 · D&C red#33 · glycerin · sodium citrate · flavors · sodium benzoate · citric acid · poloxamer 407 · sugar · water · sodium chloride
			aspartame · dextrates · D&C red#27 aluminum lake · FD&C blue#1 aluminum lake · flavors · magnesium stearate · magnesium trisilicate · tartaric acid
			saccharin sodium · sodium citrate · sodium benzoate · sorbitol · glycerin · flavors · FD&C red #40 · FD&C blue #1 · citric acid · poloxamer 407 · polysorbate 20 · sodium chloride · purified water
			croscarmellose sodium · dibasic calcium phosphate dihydrate · FD&C blue#1 aluminum lake · hydroxypropyl methylcellulose · microcrystalline cellulose · polyethylene glycol · polysorbate 80 · pregelatinized starch · stearic acid · titanium dioxide · zinc stearate
			glycerin · sodium citrate · saccharin sodium · sodium benzoate · flavor · citric acid · sodium carboxymethyl cellulose · sorbitol solution · water
			gelatin · glycerin · polyethylene glycol 400 · sorbitol
acetaminophen, 500mg			candellila wax · croscarmellose sodium · hydroxypropyl cellulose · hydroxypropyl methylcellulose · magnesium stearate · microcrystalline cellulose · polyethylene glycol · pregelatinized starch · propylene glycol · sodium starch glycolate · starch · stearic acid · titanium dioxide · zinc stearate · edible ink
acetaminophen, 500mg			candellila wax · starch · croscarmellose sodium · D&C yellow#10 aluminum lake · FD&C yellow#6 aluminum lake · hydroxypropyl cellulose · hydroxypropyl methylcellulose · microcrystalline cellulose · polyethylene glycol · polysorbate 80 · stearic acid · titanium dioxide · zinc stearate · FD&C blue#1 aluminum lake · pregelatinized starch · sodium starch glycolate · edible red ink
		dextromethorphan hydrobromide, 15mg/5ml	glycerin · saccharin sodium · sodium benzoate · sodium citrate · citric acid · D&C red#33 · FD&C red#40 · flavors · poloxamer 407 · polysorbate 20 · sodium carboxymethyl cellulose · sorbitol solution · caramel · purified water
	guaifenesin, 100mg/5ml	dextromethorphan hydrobromide, 5mg/5ml	sodium benzoate · sodium citrate · saccharin sodium · caramel · citric acid · D&C red#33 · disodium edetate · FD&C red#40 · flavor · poloxamer 407 · polyethylene glycol · propyl gallate · propylene glycol · sodium chloride · sorbitol solution · purified water
	guaifenesin, 100mg/5ml	dextromethorphan hydrobromide, 5mg/5ml	saccharin sodium · sodium benzoate · sodium citrate · caramel · citric acid · D&C red#33 · edetate disodium · FD&C red#40 · flavor · poloxamer 407 · polyethylene glycol 1450 · propyl gallate · propylene glycol · sodium chloride · sorbitol solution · purified water

COLD, COUGH, AND ALLERGY PRODUCTS - continued

	Product Manufacturer/Supplier	Dosage Form	Decongestant	Antihistamine
AL PE	**Benylin Pediatric Cough Formula** Warner-Lambert Consumer	liquid		
AL LA	**Bromfed** Muro Ph'cal	syrup	pseudoephedrine HCl, 30mg/5ml	brompheniramine maleate, 2mg/5ml
** AL DY GL LA SU SL	**Buckley's DM** W. K. Buckley	syrup	pseudoephedrine HCl, 30mg/5ml	
** AL DY GL LA SU SL	**Buckley's Mixture** W. K. Buckley	syrup		
** AF GL LA PU SO	**Cepacol Sore Throat Maximum Strength, Cherry** J. B. Williams	lozenge		
AF GL LA PU SO	**Cepacol Sore Throat Maximum Strength, Mint** J. B. Williams	lozenge		
AF GL LA PU SO	**Cepacol Sore Throat Regular Strength, Cherry** J. B. Williams	lozenge		
AF GL LA PU SO	**Cepacol Sore Throat Regular Strength,** **Original Mint** J. B. Williams	lozenge		
	Cerose-DM Wyeth-Ayerst Labs	liquid	phenylephrine HCl, 10mg/5ml	chlorpheniramine maleate, 4mg/5ml
	Cheracol D Roberts Ph'cal	liquid		
	Cheracol Plus Roberts Ph'cal	syrup	phenylpropanolamine HCl, 25mg	chlorpheniramine, 4mg
	Chlor-Trimeton 12-Hour Allergy Schering-Plough Healthcare	tablet		chlorpheniramine maleate, 12mg
	Chlor-Trimeton 12-Hour Allergy Decongestant Schering-Plough Healthcare	tablet	pseudoephedrine sulfate, 120mg	chlorpheniramine maleate, 8mg
AL	**Chlor-Trimeton 4-hour Allergy** Schering-Plough Healthcare	syrup		chlorpheniramine maleate, 2mg/5ml

See Chapter 8, "Cold, Cough and Allergy Products," for more information about these products.

Analgesic	Expectorant	Antitussive	Other Ingredients
		dextromethorphan hydrobromide, 7.5mg/5ml	glycerin · flavors · saccharin sodium · sodium benzoate · sodium citrate · citric acid · FD&C blue#1 · FD&C red#40 · poloxamer 407 · polysorbate 20 · sodium carboxymethyl cellulose · sorbitol solution · purified water
			citric acid · FD&C yellow#6 · flavor · glycerin · methylparaben · sodium benzoate · sodium citrate · saccharin sodium · sorbitol · sucrose · purified water
		dextromethorphan hydrobromide, 12.5mg/5ml	glycerin · ammonium carbonate · carrageenan · menthol · canada balsam · pine needle oil · camphor · butylparaben · propylparaben · saccharin sodium · tincture of capsicum
		dextromethorphan hydrobromide, 12.5mg/5ml	glycerin · ammonium carbonate · carrageenan · menthol · canada balsam · pine needle oil · camphor · butylparaben · propylparaben · saccharin sodium · tincture of capsicum
		menthol, 3.6mg	benzocaine, 10mg · cetylpyridinium chloride · D&C red#33 · FD&C red#40 · flavor · glucose · sucrose
		menthol, 2mg	benzocaine, 10mg · cetylpyridinium chloride · D&C yellow#10 · FD&C yellow#6 · flavor · glucose · sucrose
		menthol, 3.6mg	cetylpyridinium chloride · D&C red#33 · FD&C red#40 · flavor · glucose · sucrose
		menthol, 2mg	cetylpyridinium chloride · D&C yellow#10 · FD&C yellow#6 · flavor · glucose · sucrose
		dextromethorphan hydrobromide, 15mg/5ml	alcohol, 2.4% · flavors · citric acid · disodium edetate · FD&C yellow#6 · glycerin · saccharin sodium · sodium benzoate · sodium citrate · sodium propionate · water
	guaifenesin, 100mg	dextromethorphan hydrobromide, 10mg	alcohol, 4.75% · benzoic acid · fructose · glycerin · propylene glycol · sodium chloride · sucrose
		dextromethorphan hydrobromide, 20mg	alcohol, 8% · glycerin · methylparaben · propylene glycol · propylparaben · sodium chloride · sorbitol solution

COLD, COUGH, AND ALLERGY PRODUCTS - continued

	Product Manufacturer/Supplier	Dosage Form	Decongestant	Antihistamine
	Chlor-Trimeton 4-Hour Allergy Schering-Plough Healthcare	tablet		chlorpheniramine maleate, 4mg
	Chlor-Trimeton 4-Hour Allergy Decongestant Schering-Plough Healthcare	tablet	pseudoephedrine sulfate, 60mg	chlorpheniramine maleate, 4mg
AF	**Chlor-Trimeton 6-Hour Allergy, Sinus, Headache** Schering-Plough Healthcare	caplet	phenylpropanolamine HCl, 12.5mg	chlorpheniramine maleate, 2mg
	Chlor-Trimeton 8-Hour Allergy Schering-Plough Healthcare	tablet		chlorpheniramine maleate, 8mg
	Chlor-Trimeton Non-Drowsy 4-Hour Schering-Plough Healthcare	tablet	pseudoephedrine sulfate, 60mg	
AL DY SU	**Clear Cough DM** Vetco	liquid		
AL DY SU	**Clear Cough Night Time** Vetco	liquid		doxylamine succinate, 2.08mg/5ml
AL SO	**Codimal** Schwarz Pharma	capsule	pseudoephedrine HCl, 30mg	chlorpheniramine maleate, 2mg
AF LA SO	**Codimal** Schwarz Pharma	tablet	pseudoephedrine HCl, 30mg	chlorpheniramine maleate, 2mg
AL DY LA SU	**Codimal DM** Schwarz Pharma	syrup	phenylephrine HCl, 5mg/5ml	pyrilamine maleate, 8.3mg/5ml
AL LA	**Codimal PH** Schwarz Pharma	syrup	phenylephrine HCl, 5mg/5ml	pyrilamine maleate, 8.3mg/5ml
**	**Cold Control** Reese Chemical	caplet	pseudoedphedrine HCl, 60mg	diphenhydramine HCl, 25mg
**	**Coldmax** Reese Chemical	timed-release capsule	phenylpropanolamine HCl, 75mg	chlorpheniramine maleate, 4mg
AF SO SU	**Coldonyl** Dover Ph'cal	tablet	phenylephrine HCl, 5mg	
AF GL LA	**Comtrex Allergy-Sinus** Bristol-Myers Products	caplet · tablet	pseudoephedrine HCl, 30mg	chlorpheniramine maleate, 2mg
**	**Comtrex Allergy-Sinus Daytime** Bristol-Myers Products	caplet	pseudoephedrine HCl, 30mg	

See Chapter 8, "Cold, Cough and Allergy Products," for more information about these products.

Analgesic	Expectorant	Antitussive	Other Ingredients
acetaminophen, 500mg			
	guaifenesin, 100mg/5ml	dextromethorphan hydrobromide, 15mg/5ml	purified water · benzoic acid · citric acid · glycerin · sorbitol · flavor
acetaminophen, 166.67mg/5ml		dextromethorphan hydrobromide, 5mg/5ml	ascorbic acid · benzoic acid · citric acid · gelatin · glycerin · potassium citrate · propylene glycol · purified water · sorbitol · polysorbate 80 · berry flavor
acetaminophen, 325mg			
acetaminophen, 325mg			
		dextromethorphan hydrobromide, 10mg/5ml	
		codeine phosphate, 10mg/5ml[a]	
acetaminophen, 500mg			corn starch · D&C red#27 lake · FD&C blue#1 lake · FD&C red#40 lake · lactose anhydrous · magnesium stearate · pregelatinized starch · sodium alginate · stearic acid · talc
			sucrose · starch · talc · dicalcium phosphate · D&C yellow #10 · FD&C red#3 · FD&C yellow#6 · gelatin · pharmaceutical glaze
acetaminophen, 325mg			
acetaminophen, 500mg			benzoic acid · carnauba wax · corn starch · D&C yellow#10 lake · FD&C blue#1 lake · FD&C red#40 lake · hydroxypropyl methylcellulose · mineral oil · polysorbate 20 · povidone · propylene glycol · simethicone emulsion · sodium citrate · sorbitan monolaurate · stearic acid · titanium dioxide · may also contain: crospovidone · D&C yellow#10 · erythorbic acid · FD&C blue#1 · magnesium stearate · methylparaben · microcrystalline cellulose · polysorbate 80 · propylparaben · silicon dioxide · wood cellulose
acetaminophen, 500mg			benzoic acid · corn starch · D&C yellow#10 lake · FD&C red#40 · hydroxypropyl methylcellulose · mineral oil · polysorbate 20 · povidone · propylene glycol · simethicone emulsion · sorbitan monolaurate · stearic acid · titanium dioxide · may also contain: carnauba wax · D&C yellow#10 · FD&C red#40

COLD, COUGH, AND ALLERGY PRODUCTS - continued

Product Manufacturer/Supplier	Dosage Form	Decongestant	Antihistamine
** AF GL LA SO SU **Comtrex Deep Chest Cold and Congestion Relief** Bristol-Myers Products	liqui-gel	phenylpropanolamine HCl, 12.5mg	
AF GL LA SO **Comtrex Maximum Strength** Bristol-Myers Products	liqui-gel	phenylpropanolamine HCl, 12.5mg	chlorpheniramine maleate, 2mg
LA PR **Comtrex Maximum Strength Cold and Flu Relief** Bristol-Myers Products	liquid	pseudoephedrine HCl, 60mg/30ml	chlorpheniramine maleate, 4mg/30ml
AF GL LA SO SU **Comtrex Maximum Strength Cold and Flu Relief** Bristol-Myers Products	caplet · tablet	pseudoephedrine HCl, 30mg	chlorpheniramine maleate, 2mg
AF LA **Comtrex Maximum Strength Day & Night** Bristol-Myers Products	Day, caplet; Night, liquid	Day: pseudoephedrine HCl, 30mg Night: pseudoephedrine HCl, 60mg/30ml	Night: chlorpheniramine maleate, 4mg/30ml
AF GL LA **Comtrex Maximum Strength Day & Night** Bristol-Myers Products	Day, caplet; Night, tablet	Day: pseudoephedrine HCl, 30mg Night: pseudoephedrine HCl, 30mg	Night: chlorpheniramine maleate, 2mg
AF GL LA SO **Comtrex Maximum Strength Non-Drowsy** Bristol-Myers Products	liqui-gel	phenylpropanolamine HCl, 12.5mg	
AF GL LA SO SU **Comtrex Maximum Strength Non-Drowsy Cold and Flu Relief** Bristol-Myers Products	caplet	pseudoephedrine HCl, 30mg	
AF **Congestac** Menley & James Labs	caplet	pseudoephedrine HCl, 60mg	
Contac 12-Hour Allergy SmithKline Beecham	tablet		clemastine fumarate, 1.34mg (equivalent to clemastine, 1mg)
Contac 12-Hour Cold SmithKline Beecham	timed-release capsule	phenylpropanolamine HCl, 75mg	chlorpheniramine maleate, 8mg
Contac 12-Hour Cold Maximum Strength SmithKline Beecham	caplet	phenylpropanolamine HCl, 75mg	chlorpheniramine maleate, 12mg
Contac Day & Night Allergy/Sinus SmithKline Beecham	Day, caplet; Night, caplet	Day: pseudoephedrine HCl, 60mg Night: pseudoephedrine HCl, 60mg	Night: diphenhydramine HCl, 50mg

See Chapter 8, "Cold, Cough and Allergy Products," for more information about these products.

Analgesic	Expectorant	Antitussive	Other Ingredients
acetaminophen, 325mg	guaifenesin, 200mg	dextromethorphan hydrobromide, 10mg	FD&C red#40 · gelatin · glycerin · polyethylene glycol · povidone · propylene glycol · silicon dioxide · sorbitol · titanium dioxide · water
acetaminophen, 500mg		dextromethorphan hydrobromide, 15mg	D&C yellow#10 · FD&C red#40 · gelatin · glycerin · polyethylene glycol · povidone · propylene glycol · silicon dioxide · sorbitol · titanium dioxide · water
acetaminophen, 1000mg/30ml		dextromethorphan hydrobromide, 30mg/30ml	alcohol, 10% · benzoic acid · D&C yellow#10 · FD&C blue#1 · FD&C red#40 · flavors · glycerin · polyethylene glycol · povidone · saccharin sodium · sodium citrate · sucrose water
acetaminophen, 500mg		dextromethorphan hydrobromide, 15mg	benzoic acid · corn starch · D&C yellow#10 aluminum lake · FD&C red#40 aluminum lake · hydroxypropyl methylcellulose · magnesium stearate · methylparaben · mineral oil · polysorbate 20 · povidone · propylene glycol · propylparaben · simethicone emulsion · sorbitan monolaurate · stearic acid · titanium dioxide · may also contain: carnauba wax · D&C yellow#10 · FD&C red#40
Day: acetaminophen, 500mg Night: acetaminophen, 1000mg/30ml		Day: dextromethorphan hydrobromide, 15mg Night: dextromethorphan hydrobromide, 30mg/30ml	Day: benzoic acid · corn starch · D&C yellow#10 lake · D&C red#40 lake · hydroxypropyl methylcellulose · magnesium stearate · methylparaben · mineral oil · polysorbate 20 · povidone · propylene glycol · propylparaben · simethicone emulsion · sorbitan monolaurate · stearic acid · titanium dioxide · may also contain: carnauba wax · D&C yellow#10 · FD&C red#40 Night: alcohol, 10% · sucrose · benzoic acid · D&C yellow#10 · FD&C blue#1 · FD&C red#40 · flavors · glycerin · polyethylene glycol · povidone · saccharin sodium · sodium citrate · sucrose water
Day: acetaminophen, 500mg Night: acetaminophen, 500mg		Day: dextromethorphan hydrobromide, 15mg Night: dextromethorphan hydrobromide, 15mg	benzoic acid · corn starch · D&C yellow#10 lake · D&C red#40 lake · FD&C blue#1 lake (Night) · hydroxypropyl methylcellulose · magnesium stearate · methylparaben · mineral oil · polysorbate 20 · povidone · propylene glycol · propylparaben · simethicone emulsion · sorbitan monolaurate · stearic acid · titanium dioxide · may also contain: carnauba wax · sodium citrate · D&C yellow#10 · FD&C red#40
acetaminophen, 500mg		dextromethorphan hydrobromide, 15mg	FD&C yellow#6 · gelatin · glycerin · polyethylene glycol · povidone · propylene glycol · silicon dioxide · sorbitol · titanium dioxide · water
acetaminophen, 500mg		dextromethorphan hydrobromide, 15mg	benzoic acid · corn starch · D&C yellow#10 lake · FD&C red#40 lake · hydroxypropyl methylcellulose · magnesium stearate · methylparaben · mineral oil · polysorbate 20 · povidone · propylene glycol · propylparaben · simethicone emulsion · sorbitan monolaurate · stearic acid · titanium dioxide · may also contain: carnauba wax · D&C yellow#10 · FD&C red#40
	guaifenesin, 400mg		microcrystalline cellulose · croscarmellose sodium · starch · povidone · hydroxypropyl methylcellulose · magnesium stearate · polyethylene glycol · silicon dioxide
			colloidal silicon dioxide · corn starch · lactose · povidone · pregelatinized starch · stearic acid
			benzyl alcohol · butylparaben · colors · edetate calcium disodium · gelatin · methylparaben · pharmaceutical glaze · polysorbate 80 · propylparaben · sodium lauryl sulfate · sodium propionate · starch · sucrose
			acetylated monoglycerides · carnauba wax · colloidal silicon dioxide · ethylcellulose · hydroxypropyl methylcellulose · lactose · stearic acid · titanium dioxide
Day: acetaminophen, 650mg Night: acetaminophen, 650mg			colors · hydroxypropyl methylcellulose · magnesium stearate · microcrystalline cellulose · polyethylene glycol · polysorbate 80 · silicon dioxide · starch · stearic acid · titanium dioxide

COLD, COUGH, AND ALLERGY PRODUCTS - continued

	Product Manufacturer/Supplier	Dosage Form	Decongestant	Antihistamine
	Contac Day & Night Cold/Flu SmithKline Beecham	Day, caplet; Night, caplet	Day: pseudoephedrine HCl, 60mg Night: pseudoephedrine HCl, 60mg	Night: diphenhydramine HCl, 50mg
	Contac Non-Drowsy SmithKline Beecham	caplet	pseudoephedrine HCl, 30mg	
	Contac Severe Cold & Flu Maximum Strength SmithKline Beecham	caplet	phenylpropanolamine HCl, 12.5mg	chlorpheniramine maleate, 2mg
AF	**Coricidin Cold & Flu** Schering-Plough Healthcare	tablet		chlorpheniramine maleate, 2mg
	Coricidin Cough & Cold Schering-Plough Healthcare	tablet		chlorpheniramine maleate, 4mg
AF	**Coricidin D** Schering-Plough Healthcare	tablet	phenylpropanolamine HCl, 12.5mg	chlorpheniramine maleate, 2mg
DY	**Cough-X** B. F. Ascher	lozenge		
**	**Creo-Terpin** Lee Consumer	liquid		
	DayGel Republic Drug	liquid-cap	pseudoephedrine HCl, 30mg	
AL LA	**Delsym Extended Release** Medeva Ph'cals	suspension		
AL	**Demazin** Schering-Plough Healthcare	syrup	phenylpropanolamine HCl, 12.5mg/5ml	chlorpheniramine maleate, 2mg/5ml
	Demazin Schering-Plough Healthcare	timed-release tablet	phenylpropanolamine HCl, 25mg	chlorpheniramine maleate, 4mg
AL DY SU	**Diabe-tuss DM** Paddock Labs	syrup		
AL DY SU	**Diabetic Tussin Allergy Relief** Health Care Products	syrup		chlorpheniramine maleate, 2mg
DY SO SU	**Diabetic Tussin Cough Drops, Cherry** Health Care Products	tablet		
DY SO SU	**Diabetic Tussin Cough Drops, Menthol-Eucalyptus** Health Care Products	tablet		
AL DY SU	**Diabetic Tussin DM** Health Care Products	syrup		

See Chapter 8, "Cold, Cough and Allergy Products," for more information about these products.

Analgesic	Expectorant	Antitussive	Other Ingredients
Day: acetaminophen, 650mg Night: acetaminophen, 650mg		Day: dextromethorphan hydrobromide, 30mg	color · hydroxypropyl methylcellulose · magnesium stearate · microcrystalline cellulose · polyethylene glycol · polysorbate 80 · silicon dioxide · starch · stearic acid · titanium dioxide
acetaminophen, 325mg		dextromethorphan hydrobromide, 15mg	carnauba wax · colloidal silicon dioxide · hydroxypropyl methylcellulose · magnesium stearate · microcrystalline cellulose · polyethylene glycol · polysorbate 80 · starch · stearic acid · titanium dioxide
acetaminophen, 500mg		dextromethorphan hydrobromide, 15mg	FD&C blue#1 · cellulose · hydroxypropyl methylcellulose · polyethylene glycol · polysorbate 80 · povidone · sodium starch glycolate · starch · stearic acid · titanium dioxide
acetaminophen, 325mg			
		dextromethorphan hydrobromide, 30mg	
acetaminophen, 325mg			
		dextromethorphan hydrobromide, 5mg	benzocaine, 2mg
		dextromethorphan hydrobromide, 10mg/15ml	water · corn syrup · alcohol, 25% · sodium glycerophosphate · saccharin sodium · sodium EDTA · hydrochloric acid · orange oil · FD&C blue#1 · FD&C yellow#5
acetaminophen, 250mg	guaifenesin, 100mg	dextromethorphan hydrobromide, 10mg	
		dextromethorphan polistirex (equivalent to 30mg/5ml dextromethorphan hydrobromide)	citric acid · ethylcellulose · FD&C yellow#6 · flavor · high fructose corn syrup · methylparaben · polyethylene glycol 3350 · polysorbate 80 · propylene glycol · propylparaben · purified water · sucrose · tragacanth · vegetable oil · xanthan gum
		dextromethorphan, 15mg/5ml	sorbitol
			hydroxypropyl methylcellulose · calcium saccharin · methylparaben · artificial flavors · purified water · may contain citric acid
		menthol, 5mg · eucalyptus oil	acesulfame potassium · flavor · isomalt
		menthol, 6mg · eucalyptus oil	acesulfame potassium · flavor · isomalt
	guaifenesin, 100mg/5ml	dextromethorphan hydrobromide, 10mg/5ml	hydroxypropyl methylcellulose · calcium saccharin · methylparaben · potassium sorbate · povidone · artificial flavors · menthol · purified water · may contain citric acid

COLD, COUGH, AND ALLERGY PRODUCTS - continued

	Product Manufacturer/Supplier	Dosage Form	Decongestant	Antihistamine
** DY SO SU	**Diabetic Tussin DM Liqui-Gels** Health Care Products	gelcap		
AL DY SU	**Diabetic Tussin DM Maximum Strength** Health Care Products	syrup		
** DY SO SU	**Diabetic Tussin DM Maximum Strength Liqui-Gels** Health Care Products	gelcap		
AL DY SU	**Diabetic Tussin EX** Health Care Products	syrup		
AL DY SU PE	**Diabetic Tussin, Children's** Health Care Products	syrup		
	Dimetane Allergy Extentabs Whitehall-Robins Healthcare	timed-release tablet		brompheniramine maleate, 12mg
AL	**Dimetapp** Whitehall-Robins Healthcare	elixir	phenylpropanolamine HCl, 12.5mg/5ml	brompheniramine maleate, 2mg/5ml
	Dimetapp 12-Hour Maximum Strength Extentabs Whitehall-Robins Healthcare	timed-release tablet	phenylpropanolamine HCl, 75mg	brompheniramine maleate, 12mg
	Dimetapp 4-Hour Maximum Strength Whitehall-Robins Healthcare	tablet	phenylpropanolamine HCl, 25mg	brompheniramine maleate, 4mg
	Dimetapp 4-Hour Maximum Strength Liqui-Gels Whitehall-Robins Healthcare	softgel	phenylpropanolamine HCl, 25mg	brompheniramine maleate, 4mg
	Dimetapp Allergy Whitehall-Robins Healthcare	tablet		brompheniramine maleate, 4mg
	Dimetapp Allergy Liqui-Gels Whitehall-Robins Healthcare	softgel		brompheniramine maleate, 4mg
	Dimetapp Allergy Sinus Whitehall-Robins Healthcare	caplet	phenylpropanolamine HCl, 12.5mg	brompheniramine maleate, 2mg
AL DY SU PE	**Dimetapp Allergy, Children's** Whitehall-Robins Healthcare	elixir		brompheniramine maleate, 2mg/5ml
	Dimetapp Cold & Allergy Whitehall-Robins Healthcare	chewable tablet	phenylpropanolamine HCl, 6.25mg	brompheniramine maleate, 1mg

See Chapter 8, "Cold, Cough and Allergy Products," for more information about these products.

Analgesic	Expectorant	Antitussive	Other Ingredients
	guaifenesin, 100mg	dextromethorphan hydrobromide, 10mg	propylene glycol · polyethylene glycol 400 · povidone · gelatin · glycerin · purified water
	guaifenesin, 200mg/5ml	dextromethorphan hydrobromide, 10mg/5ml	acesulfame K · hydroxypropyl methylcellulose · aspartame · methylparaben · potassium sorbate · artificial flavors · menthol · purified water · may contain citric acid
	guaifenesin, 200mg	dextromethorphan hydrobromide, 10mg	polyethylene glycol 400 · povidone · propylene glycol
	guaifenesin, 100mg/5ml	menthol	hydroxypropyl methylcellulose · calcium saccharin · methylparaben · potassium sorbate · povidone · artificial flavors · purified water · may contain citric acid
	guaifenesin, 100mg/5ml	dextromethorphan hydrobromide, 10mg/5ml · menthol	hydroxypropyl methylcellulose · calcium saccharin · methylparaben · potassium sorbate · povidone · artificial flavors · purified water · may contain citric acid
			acacia · acetylated monoglycerides · calcium carbonate · calcium sulfate · carnauba wax · cellulose acetate phthalate · corn starch · diethyl phthalate · edible ink · FD&C blue#2 aluminum lake · FD&C red#3 · gelatin · guar gum · magnesium stearate · pharmaceutical glaze · polysorbates · stearic acid · sucrose · titanium dioxide · wheat flour · white wax · may contain: FD&C red#40 aluminum lake · FD&C yellow#6 aluminum lake · acetone
			citric acid · FD&C blue#1 · FD&C red#40 · grape flavor · glycerin · saccharin sodium · sodium benzoate · sorbitol · water
			acacia · acetylated monoglycerides · calcium sulfate · carnauba wax · castor wax or oil · citric acid · edible inks · FD&C blue#1 · FD&C blue#2 aluminum lake · gelatin · magnesium stearate · magnesium trisilicate · pharmaceutical glaze · polysorbates · povidone · silicon dioxide · stearyl alcohol · sucrose · titanium dioxide · wheat flour · white wax · may contain: FD&C red#40 aluminum lake · FD&C yellow#6 aluminum lake · acetone
			corn starch · FD&C blue#1 aluminum lake · magnesium stearate · microcrystalline cellulose
			D&C red#33 · FD&C blue#1 · gelatin · glycerin · mannitol · pharmaceutical glaze · polyethylene glycol · povidone · propylene glycol · sorbitan · sorbitol · titanium dioxide · water
			corn starch · D&C yellow#10 lake · dibasic calcium phosphate · FD&C yellow#6 lake · lactose · magnesium stearate · polyethylene glycol
			FD&C green#3 · gelatin · glycerin · mannitol · pharmaceutical glaze · polyethylene glycol · povidone · propylene glycol · sorbitan · sorbitol · titanium dioxide · water
acetaminophen, 500mg			corn starch · hydroxypropyl cellulose · hydroxypropyl methylcellulose · magnesium stearate · methylparaben · microcrystalline cellulose · polysorbate 20 · povidone · propylparaben · propylene glycol · stearic acid · titanium dioxide · water
			citric acid · grape flavor · glycerin · sodium benzoate · sorbitol · water · maltol
			aspartame · citric acid · crospovidone · D&C red#30 aluminum lake · D&C red#7 calcium lake · FD&C blue#1 aluminum lake · grape flavor · glycine · magnesium stearate · mannitol · microcrystalline cellulose · pregelatinized starch · silicon dioxide · sorbitol · stearic acid

COLD, COUGH, AND ALLERGY PRODUCTS - continued

	Product Manufacturer/Supplier	Dosage Form	Decongestant	Antihistamine
** PE	**Dimetapp Cold & Allergy Quick Dissolve** Whitehall-Robins Healthcare	tablet	phenylpropanolamine HCl, 6.25mg	brompheniramine maleate, 1mg
	Dimetapp Cold & Cough Maximum Strength Liqui-Gels Whitehall-Robins Healthcare	softgel	phenylpropanolamine HCl, 25mg	brompheniramine maleate, 4mg
AL PE	**Dimetapp Cold & Fever, Children's** Whitehall-Robins Healthcare	suspension	pseudoephedrine HCl, 15mg/5ml	brompheniramine maleate, 1mg/5ml
	Dimetapp Decongestant Non-Drowsy Liqui-Gels Whitehall-Robins Healthcare	softgel	pseudoephedrine HCl, 30mg	
AL PE	**Dimetapp Decongestant, Pediatric** Whitehall-Robins Healthcare	drops	pseudoephedrine HCl, 7.5mg/0.8ml	
AL	**Dimetapp DM** Whitehall-Robins Healthcare	elixir	phenylpropanolamine HCl, 12.5mg/5ml	brompheniramine maleate, 2mg/5ml
	Disophrol Chronotabs Sustained Action Schering-Plough Healthcare	timed-release tablet	pseudoephedrine sulfate, 120mg	dexbrompheniramine maleate, 6mg
AL LA SL PE	**Dorcol Children's Cough** Novartis Consumer	syrup	pseudoephedrine HCl, 15mg/5ml	
** AL	**Double Tussin DM** Reese Chemical	liquid		
	Dristan Cold & Cough Liqui-Gels Whitehall-Robins Healthcare	softgel	pseudoephedrine HCl, 30mg	
AF GL	**Dristan Cold Maximum Strength No Drowsiness** Whitehall-Robins Healthcare	caplet	pseudoephedrine HCl, 30mg	
	Dristan Cold Maximum Strength No Drowsiness Whitehall-Robins Healthcare	gel caplet	pseudoephedrine HCl, 30mg	
AF GL SO	**Dristan Cold Multi-Symptom** Whitehall-Robins Healthcare	tablet	phenylephrine HCl, 5mg	chlorpheniramine maleate, 2mg
AF GL	**Dristan Cold Multi-Symptom Maximum Strength** Whitehall-Robins Healthcare	gel caplet	pseudoephedrine HCl, 30mg	brompheniramine maleate, 2mg
AF GL SO	**Dristan Sinus** Whitehall-Robins Healthcare	caplet	pseudoephedrine HCl, 30mg	
AF	**Drixoral Allergy Sinus** Schering-Plough Healthcare	timed-release tablet	pseudoephedrine sulfate, 60mg	dexbrompheniramine maleate, 3mg

See Chapter 8, "Cold, Cough and Allergy Products," for more information about these products.

Analgesic	Expectorant	Antitussive	Other Ingredients
			aspartame · FD&C blue#2 · FD&C red#40 · cherry flavor 51.849 · grape flavor 5-118-15 · gelatin · glycerin · mannitol · purified water
		dextromethorphan hydrobromide, 20mg	FD&C red #40 · gelatin · glycerin · mannitol · pharmaceutical glaze · polyethylene glycol · povidone · propylene glycol · sorbitan · sorbitol · titanium dioxide · water
acetaminophen, 160mg/5ml			carboxymethylcellulose sodium · citric acid · D&C red#33 · disodium edetate · FD&C blue#1 · flavors · glycerin · high fructose corn syrup · maltol · methylparaben · microcrystalline cellulose · polysorbate 80 · potassium sorbate · propylene glycol · propylparaben · sorbitol · sucrose · water · xanthan gum · caramel
			FD&C blue#1 · gelatin · glycerin · mannitol · pharmaceutical glaze · polyethylene glycol · povidone · propylene glycol · sorbitan · sorbitol · titanium dioxide · water
			caramel · citric acid · FD&C blue#1 · D&C red #33 · grape flavor · glycerin · high fructose corn syrup · maltol · menthol · polyethylene glycol · propylene glycol · sodium benzoate · sorbitol · sucrose · water
		dextromethorphan hydrobromide, 10mg/5ml	citric acid · FD&C blue#1 · FD&C red#40 · red grape flavor · glycerin · propylene glycol · saccharin sodium · sodium benzoate · sorbitol · water
	guaifenesin, 50mg/5ml	dextromethorphan hydrobromide, 5mg/5ml	benzoic acid · flavors · purified water · sodium hydroxide · sucrose · red#40 · tartaric acid · blue#1 · edetate disodium · glycerin · propylene glycol
	guaifenesin, 200mg/5ml	dextromethorphan hydrobromide, 30mg/5ml	caramel color · citric acid · FD&C red#40 · flavors · menthol · propylene glycol · purified water · sodium benzoate · sodium citrate · sorbitol solution
acetaminophen, 250mg	guaifenesin, 100mg	dextromethorphan hydrobromide, 10mg	D&C yellow#10 · FD&C red#40 · gelatin · glycerin · mannitol · polyethylene glycol · povidone · propylene glycol · sorbitan · sorbitol · water
acetaminophen, 500mg			calcium stearate · croscarmellose sodium · D&C red#7 lake · D&C yellow#10 lake · FD&C yellow#6 lake · hydrogenated vegetable oil · hydroxypropyl methylcellulose · microcrystalline cellulose · pharmaceutical glaze · polyethylene glycol · povidone · starch · stearic acid · titanium dioxide · alcohol · n-butyl alcohol
acetaminophen, 500mg			calcium stearate · croscarmellose sodium · D&C red#27 lake · D&C yellow#10 lake · EDTA · FD&C blue#1 lake · FD&C red#40 lake · gelatin · glycerin · hydrogenated vegetable oil · hydroxypropyl methylcellulose · iron oxide · lecithin · microcrystalline cellulose · pharmaceutical glaze · polyethylene glycol · povidone · simethicone · starch · stearic acid · titanium dioxide
acetaminophen, 325mg			calcium stearate · croscarmellose sodium · D&C yellow#10 lake · FD&C yellow#10 lake · hydroxypropyl methylcellulose · microcrystalline cellulose · polyethylene glycol · povidone · starch · stearic acid · may also contain: D&C red#7 lake · pharmaceutical glaze · titanium dioxide
acetaminophen, 500mg			calcium stearate · croscarmellose sodium · D&C red#30 · EDTA D&C red#40 lake · gelatin · glycerin · hydrogenated vegetable oil · hydroxypropyl methylcellulose · iron oxide · lecithin · microcrystalline cellulose · pharmaceutical glaze · polyethylene glycol · povidone · simethicone · starch · stearic acid · titanium dioxide · triacetin
ibuprofen, 200mg			carnauba or equivalent wax · croscarmellose sodium · iron oxide · methylparaben · microcrystalline cellulose · propylparaben · silicon dioxide · sodium benzoate · sodium lauryl sulfate · starch · stearic acid · sucrose · titanium dioxide · mineral spirits · black ink
acetaminophen, 500mg			

COLD, COUGH, AND ALLERGY PRODUCTS - continued

	Product Manufacturer/Supplier	Dosage Form	Decongestant	Antihistamine
	Drixoral Cold & Allergy Schering-Plough Healthcare	timed-release tablet	pseudoephedrine sulfate, 120mg	dexbrompheniramine maleate, 6mg
AF	**Drixoral Cold & Flu** Schering-Plough Healthcare	timed-release tablet	pseudoephedrine sulfate, 60mg	dexbrompheniramine maleate, 3mg
	Drixoral Nasal Decongestant Non-Drowsy Formula Schering-Plough Healthcare	timed-release tablet	pseudoephedrine sulfate, 120mg	
	Duadacin Kenwood Labs	capsule	phenylpropanolamine HCl, 12.5mg	chlorpheniramine maleate, 2mg
	Dynafed Jr. BDI Ph'cals	tablet	pseudoephedrine HCl, 30mg	
	Dynafed Plus BDI Ph'cals	tablet	pseudoephedrine HCl, 30mg	
	Dynafed Pseudo BDI Ph'cals	tablet	pseudoephedrine HCl, 60mg	
	Efidac 24 Chlorpheniramine Novartis Consumer	timed-release tablet		chlorpheniramine maleate, 16mg
AF GL PU	**Efidac/24** Novartis Consumer	timed-release tablet	pseudoephedrine HCl, 240mg	
AF LA SO SU	**Emagrin Forte** Otis Clapp & Son	tablet	phenylephrine HCl, 5mg	
AF GL LA SO	**Excedrin Sinus Maximum Strength** Bristol-Myers Products	caplet	pseudoephedrine HCl, 30mg	
	Fedahist Schwarz Pharma	tablet	pseudoephedrine HCl, 60mg	chlorpheniramine maleate, 4mg
LA SO SU	**Fendol** Buffington	tablet	phenylephrine HCl, 5mg	
GL LA SU	**Fisherman's Friend, Extra Strong, Sugar Free** Bristol-Myers Products	lozenge		
GL LA	**Fisherman's Friend, Licorice Strong** Bristol-Myers Products	lozenge		
GL LA	**Fisherman's Friend, Original Extra Strong** Bristol-Myers Products	lozenge		
GL LA SU	**Fisherman's Friend, Refreshing Mint, Sugar Free** Bristol-Myers Products	lozenge		
LA	**GG-Cen** Schwarz Pharma	capsule		
AL LA	**Guaifed** Muro Ph'cal	syrup	pseudoephedrine HCl, 30mg/5ml	

See Chapter 8, "Cold, Cough and Allergy Products," for more information about these products.

Analgesic	Expectorant	Antitussive	Other Ingredients
acetaminophen, 500mg			
acetaminophen, 325mg			
acetaminophen, 325mg			
acetaminophen, 500mg			
			cellulose · cellulose acetate · FD&C blue#1 · hydroxypropyl methylcellulose · hydroxypropyl cellulose · polysorbate 80 · povidone · sodium chloride · titanium dioxide · magnesium stearate · polyethylene glycol
acetaminophen, 260mg	guaifenesin, 101mg		caffeine, 32mg
acetaminophen, 500mg			benzoic acid · corn starch · D&C yellow#10 lake · FD&C red#40 lake · hydroxypropyl methylcellulose · mineral oil · polysorbate 20 · povidone · propylene glycol · simethicone emulsion · sorbitan monolaurate · stearic acid · titanium dioxide · may also contain: carnauba wax · D&C yellow#10 · FD&C red#40
			lactose · colloidal silicon dioxide · magnesium stearate · microcrystalline cellulose · stearic acid · talc
acetaminophen, 354mg · salicylamide, 65mg	guaifenesin, 101mg		caffeine, 32mg
		menthol, 10mg · eucalyptus oil	sorbitol · natural licorice · magnesium stearate · capsicum
		menthol, 6mg	sugar · licorice · edible gums · anise oil
		menthol, 10mg · eucalyptus oil	sugar · licorice · edible gums · capsicum
		menthol, 3mg · peppermint oil	sorbitol · magnesium stearate · aspartame · phenylalanine
	guaifenesin, 200mg		
	guaifenesin, 200mg/5ml	menthol	benzoic acid · cherry flavor · citric acid · edetate disodium · FD&C red#40 · FD&C blue#1 · glycerin · polyethylene glycol · povidone · purified water · saccharin sodium · sodium citrate · sorbitol · sucrose · vanillin

COLD, COUGH, AND ALLERGY PRODUCTS - continued

	Product Manufacturer/Supplier	Dosage Form	Decongestant	Antihistamine
SU PE	**Halls Juniors Sugar Free Cough Drops, Grape or Orange** Warner-Lambert Consumer	lozenge		
	Halls Mentho-Lyptus Cough Supp. Drops, Cherry Warner-Lambert Consumer	lozenge		
	Halls Mentho-Lyptus Cough Supp. Drops, Honey-Lemon Warner-Lambert Consumer	lozenge		
	Halls Mentho-Lyptus Cough Supp. Drops, Mentho-Lyptus Warner-Lambert Consumer	lozenge		
	Halls Mentho-Lyptus Cough Supp. Drops, Spearmint Warner-Lambert Consumer	lozenge		
	Halls Mentho-Lyptus Ex. Strength Cough Supp. Drops, Ice Blue Warner-Lambert Consumer	lozenge		
SU	**Halls Mentho-Lyptus Sugar Free Cough Supp. Drops, Bl. Cherry** Warner-Lambert Consumer	lozenge		
SU	**Halls Mentho-Lyptus Sugar Free Cough Supp. Drops, Citrus** Warner-Lambert Consumer	lozenge		
SU	**Halls Mentho-Lyptus Sugar Free Cough Supp. Drops, Menthol** Warner-Lambert Consumer	lozenge		
	Halls Plus Max. Strength; Cherry, Honey-Lemon, Mentho-Lyptus Warner-Lambert Consumer	lozenge		
** AF GL PU	**Hay Fever & Allergy Relief Maximum Strength** Hudson	tablet	pseudoephedrine HCl, 30mg	chlorpheniramine maleate, 2mg
AL DY GL LA SU SL	**Hayfebrol** Scot-Tussin Pharmacal	liquid	pseudoephedrine HCl, 30mg/5ml	chlorpheniramine maleate, 2mg/5ml
DY GL LA PU SO SU	**Herbal-Menthol** Shaklee	lozenge		
	Hold Menley & James Labs	lozenge		
**	**Humibid GC** Menley & James Labs	caplet	pseudoephedrine HCl, 30mg	

See Chapter 8, "Cold, Cough and Allergy Products," for more information about these products.

Analgesic	Expectorant	Antitussive	Other Ingredients
		menthol, 2.5 mg	acesulfame · potassium · isomalt · natural flavor · red#40 (Grape) · blue#1 (Grape) · yellow#6 (Orange)
		menthol, 7.6mg	corn syrup · flavor · sucrose · eucalyptus oil · blue#2 · red#40
		menthol, 8.6mg	flavor · corn syrup · sucrose · eucalyptus oil · beta carotene
		menthol, 7mg	corn syrup · flavor · sucrose · eucalyptus oil
		menthol, 6mg	flavor · blue#1 · corn syrup · sucrose · beta carotene · eucalyptus oil
		menthol, 12mg	flavor · blue#1 · corn syrup · sucrose · eucalyptus oil
		menthol, 5mg	acesulfame potassium · blue#1 · flavor · isomalt · red#40 · eucalyptus oil · citric acid
		menthol, 5mg	acesulfame potassium · flavor · isomalt · yellow#5 · citric acid · eucalyptus oil
		menthol, 6mg	acesulfame potassium · flavor · isomalt · eucalyptus oil
		menthol, 10mg	eucalyptus oil · corn syrup · acesulfame potassium · flavoring · glycerin · high fructose corn syrup · sucrose · Cherry: blue#2 · red#40 · Honey-Lemon: honey · yellow#6 · yellow#10 · Mentho-Lyptus: citric acid
		menthol	methylparaben · propylparaben · cherry-mint flavor · glycerin · hydroxymethylcellulose · potassium benzoate · citric acid · propylene glycol · sorbitol
		menthol, 6mg (from peppermint)	brown rice syrup · corn syrup · honey · horehound extract · marshmallow root extract · peppermint oil · thyme extract · eucalyptus oil
		dextromethorphan hydrobromide, 5mg	corn syrup · sucrose · vegetable oil · flavors · FD&C blue#1 · FD&C red#40 · FD&C yellow#5 · FD&C yellow#10
	guaifenesin, 200mg	dextromethorphan hydrobromide, 10mg	

COLD, COUGH, AND ALLERGY PRODUCTS - continued

	Product Manufacturer/Supplier	Dosage Form	Decongestant	Antihistamine
AF GL PU SO	**Hytuss** Hyrex Ph'cals	tablet		
AF GL PU SO	**Hytuss 2X** Hyrex Ph'cals	capsule		
AL	**Ipsatol** Kenwood Labs	syrup	phenylpropanolamine HCl, 9mg/5ml	
	Isodettes Block Drug	lozenge		
SU	**Luden's Maximum Strength Sugar Free, Cherry §** Hershey Foods	lozenge		
	Luden's Maximum Strength, Cherry § Hershey Foods	lozenge		
	Luden's Maximum Strength, Menthol Eucalyptus § Hershey Foods	lozenge		
	Mentholatum Mentholatum	ointment		
PE	**Mentholatum Cherry Chest Rub for Kids** Mentholatum	ointment		
	Mini Pseudo BDI Ph'cals	tablet	pseudoephedrine HCl, 60mg	
AF	**Motrin IB Sinus** McNeil Consumer	caplet · tablet	pseudoephedrine HCl,30mg	
SU	**N'Ice 'N Clear, Cherry Eucalyptus** SmithKline Beecham	lozenge		
SU	**N'Ice 'N Clear, Menthol Eucalyptus** SmithKline Beecham	lozenge		
SU	**N'Ice Sore Throat & Cough, Assorted or Citrus** SmithKline Beecham	lozenge		
** SU	**N'Ice Sore Throat & Cough, Cherry** SmithKline Beecham	lozenge		
** SU	**N'Ice Sore Throat & Cough, Herbal Mint or Honey Lemon** SmithKline Beecham	lozenge		
AL LA SL	**Naldecon DX, Adult** Apothecon	liquid	phenylpropanolamine HCl, 12.5mg/5ml	
AL LA SL PE	**Naldecon DX, Children's** Apothecon	syrup	phenylpropanolamine HCl, 6.25mg/5ml	

See Chapter 8, "Cold, Cough and Allergy Products," for more information about these products.

Analgesic	Expectorant	Antitussive	Other Ingredients
	guaifenesin, 100mg		
	guaifenesin, 200mg		
	guaifenesin, 100mg/5ml	dextromethorphan hydrobromide, 10mg/5ml	
		menthol, 10mg	benzocaine, 6mg · corn syrup · flavor · FD&C red#40 · FD&C blue#1 · sucrose · propylene glycol · sodium bicarbonate · water
		menthol, 10mg · eucalyptus oil	isomalt · hydrogenated starch hydrolysate · citric acid · malic acid · flavoring · acesulfame potassium · artificial color
		menthol, 10mg · eucalyptus oil	sugar · corn syrup · citric acid · malic acid · flavoring · artificial color
		menthol, 10mg · eucalyptus oil	sugar · corn syrup
		camphor, 9% · natural menthol, 1.3%	fragrance · petrolatum · titanium dioxide
		camphor, 4.7% · natural menthol, 2.6% · eucalyptus oil, 1.2%	fragrance · petrolatum · steareth-2 · titanium dioxide
ibuprofen, 200mg			cellulose · corn starch · glyceryl triacetate · hydroxpropyl methylcellulose · silicon dioxide · sodium lauryl sulfate · sodium starch glycolate · stearic acid · titanium dioxide · red#40 aluminum lake
		menthol, 7mg	flavors · D&C red#33 · sorbitol · tartaric acid · FD&C yellow#6
		menthol, 5mg	citric acid · flavors · sorbitol
		menthol, 5mg	ascorbic acid (Asst.) · citric acid · flavors · natural colors · sodium citrate · sorbitol · tartaric acid (Asst.)
		menthol 5mg	colors · sorbitol · flavors · tartaric acid
		menthol 5mg	citric acid · colors · flavor · sodium citrate · sorbitol · ascorbic acid (Lemon)
	guaifenesin, 200mg/5ml	dextromethorphan hydrobromide, 10mg/5ml	
	guaifenesin, 100mg/5ml	dextromethorphan hydrobromide, 5mg/5ml	

COLD, COUGH, AND ALLERGY PRODUCTS - continued

	Product Manufacturer/Supplier	Dosage Form	Decongestant	Antihistamine
AL LA PE	**Naldecon DX, Pediatric** Apothecon	drops	phenylpropanolamine HCl, 6.25mg/ml	
AL LA SL PE	**Naldecon EX, Children's** Apothecon	syrup	phenylpropanolamine HCl, 6.25mg/5ml	
AL LA SL PE	**Naldecon EX, Pediatric** Apothecon	drops	phenylpropanolamine HCl, 6.25mg/ml	
AL LA SL GE	**Naldecon Senior DX** Apothecon	liquid		
AL LA SL GE	**Naldecon Senior EX** Apothecon	liquid		
AF GL PU SO	**Napril** Randob Labs	tablet	pseudoephedrine HCl, 60mg	chlorpheniramine maleate, 4mg
AF CA DY GL LA PU SU	**Nasal-D** Shaklee	tablet	pseudoephedrine HCl, 60mg (from ephedra)	
**	**Nasalcrom** Pharmacia & Upjohn	nasal spray		cromolyn sodium, 40mg/1ml
AF GL PU SO	**ND-Gesic** Hyrex Ph'cals	tablet	phenylephrine HCl, 5mg	pyrilamine maleate, 12.5mg · chlorpheniramine maleate, 2mg
	NiteGel Republic Drug	liquid-cap	pseudoephedrine HCl, 30mg	doxylamine succinate, 6.25mg
AF DY GL LA PU SO	**Nolahist** Carnrick Labs	tablet		phenindamine tartrate, 25mg
	Novahistine SmithKline Beecham	elixir	phenylephrine HCl, 5mg/5ml	chlorpheniramine maleate, 2mg/5ml
	Novahistine DH SmithKline Beecham	liquid	pseudoephedrine HCl, 30mg/5ml	chlorpheniramine maleate, 2mg/5ml
	Novahistine DMX SmithKline Beecham	syrup	pseudoephedrine HCl, 30mg/5ml	
	Novahistine Expectorant SmithKline Beecham	liquid	pseudoephedrine HCl, 30mg/5ml	

See Chapter 8, "Cold, Cough and Allergy Products," for more information about these products.

Analgesic	Expectorant	Antitussive	Other Ingredients
	guaifenesin, 50mg/ml	dextromethorphan hydrobromide, 5mg/ml	
	guaifenesin, 100mg/5ml		
	guaifenesin, 50mg/ml		
	guaifenesin, 200mg/5ml	dextromethorphan hydrobromide, 10mg/5ml	citric acid · D&C yellow#10 · FD&C yellow#6 · natural and artificial flavors · propylene glycol · Prosweet MM24 · saccharin sodium · sodium benzoate · sodium citrate · sorbitol solution · purified water
	guaifenesin, 200mg/5ml		citric acid · FD&C blue#1 · FD&C red#40 · natural and artificial flavors · polyethylene glycol · saccharin sodium · sodium benzoate · sodium citrate · sorbitol solution · purified water
			lactose · corn starch · stearic acid · magnesium stearate
			calcium stearate · croscarmellose sodium · dicalcium phosphate · eucalyptus leaf extract · eucalyptus oil · glycerin · hydroxypropyl methylcellulose · maltodextrin · microcrystalline cellulose · peppermint leaf extract · peppermint oil · thyme extract
			purified water · benzalkonium chloride, 0.01% · disodium edetate, 0.01%
acetaminophen, 300mg			
acetaminophen, 250mg		dextromethorphan hydrobromide, 10mg	
			alcohol, 5% · sorbitol · D&C yellow#10 · FC&C blue#1 · flavors · glycerin · sodium chloride · water
		codeine phosphate, 10mg/5ml[a]	alcohol, 5% · invert sugar · saccharin sodium · sorbitol · FD&C blue#1 · FD&C red#40 · flavors · glycerin · hydrochloric acid · sodium chloride · water
	guaifenesin, 100mg/5ml	dextromethorphan hydrobromide, 10mg/5ml	alcohol, 10% · saccharin sodium · sorbitol · FD&C red#40 · FD&C yellow#6 · flavors · glycerin · hydrochloric acid · invert sugar · sodium chloride · water
	guaifenesin, 100mg/5ml	codeine phosphate, 10mg/5ml[a]	alcohol, 7.5% · saccharin sodium · sorbitol · invert sugar · D&C yellow#10 · FD&C blue#1 · FD&C red#40 · flavors · glycerin · hydrochloric acid · sodium chloride · sodium gluconate · water

COLD, COUGH, AND ALLERGY PRODUCTS - continued

	Product Manufacturer/Supplier	Dosage Form	Decongestant	Antihistamine
AF LA SO SU	**Oranyl** Otis Clapp & Son	tablet	pseudoephedrine HCl, 30mg	
AF LA SO SU	**Oranyl Plus** Otis Clapp & Son	tablet	pseudoephedrine HCl, 30mg	
	Ornex Maximum Strength Menley & James Labs	caplet	pseudoephedrine HCl, 30mg	
	Ornex Regular Strength Menley & James Labs	caplet	pseudoephedrine HCl, 30mg	
	P.C. Nasal Decongestant Republic Drug	tablet	pseudoephedrine, 30mg	
** PE	**Pedia Care Cold-Allergy** Pharmacia & Upjohn	chewable tablet	pseudoephedrine HCl, 15mg	chlorpheniramine maleate, 1mg
AF PE	**Pedia Care Cough-Cold Formula** Pharmacia & Upjohn	chewable tablet	pseudoephedrine HCl, 15mg	chlorpheniramine maleate, 1mg
AL PE	**Pedia Care Cough-Cold Formula** Pharmacia & Upjohn	liquid	pseudoephedrine HCl, 15mg/5ml	chlorpheniramine maleate, 1mg/5ml
AL PE	**Pedia Care Infants' Decongestant** Pharmacia & Upjohn	drops	pseudoephedrine HCl, 7.5mg/0.8ml	
AL PE	**Pedia Care Infants' Decongestant Plus Cough** Pharmacia & Upjohn	drops	pseudoephedrine HCl, 7.5mg/0.8ml	
AL PE	**Pedia Care Night Rest Cough-Cold Formula** Pharmacia & Upjohn	liquid	pseudoephedrine HCl, 15mg/5ml	chlorpheniramine maleate, 1mg/5ml
AL LA SL PE	**Pertussin CS** Blairex Labs	liquid		
LA SL	**Pertussin DM** Blairex Labs	liquid		
DY	**Pinex Concentrate** Alvin Last	syrup		
	Prominicol Cough Republic Drug	syrup	phenylpropanolamine HCl, 12.5mg	chlorpheniramine maleate, 2mg
AF DY GL PU SO SU	**Propagest** Carnrick Labs	tablet	phenylpropanolamine HCl, 25mg	
	Protac DM Republic Drug	liquid		

See Chapter 8, "Cold, Cough and Allergy Products," for more information about these products.

Analgesic	Expectorant	Antitussive	Other Ingredients
acetaminophen, 500mg			
acetaminophen, 500mg			crospovidone · hydroxypropyl methylcellulose · magnesium stearate · microcrystalline cellulose · polyethylene glycol · polysorbate 80 · povidone · starch · titanium dioxide
acetaminophen, 325mg			crospovidone · FD&C blue#1 · hydroxypropyl methylcellulose · magnesium stearate · microcrystalline cellulose · polyethylene glycol · polysorbate 80 · povidone · starch · titanium dioxide
			aspartame · cellulose · citric acid · corn starch · flavors · mannitol · colloidal silicon dioxide · stearic acid · D&C red#7
		dextromethorphan hydrobromide, 5mg	aspartame · cellulose · citric acid · flavors · magnesium stearate · magnesium trisilicate · mannitol · corn starch · D&C red#7
		dextromethorphan hydrobromide, 5mg/5ml	citric acid · corn syrup · flavors · glycerin · propylene glycol · sodium benzoate · carboxymethylcellulose sodium · sorbitol · purified water · red#40
			benzoic acid · citric acid · flavors · glycerin · polyethylene glycol · propylene glycol · purified water · sodium benzoate · sorbitol · sucrose · red#40
		dextromethorphan hydrobromide, 2.5mg/0.8ml	citric acid · flavors · glycerin · purified water · sodium benzoate · sorbitol
		dextromethorphan hydrobromide, 7.5mg/5ml	citric acid · corn syrup · flavors · glycerin · propylene glycol · sodium benzoate · carboxymethylcellulose sodium · sorbitol · purified water · red#40
		dextromethorphan hydrobromide, 7mg/10ml	citric acid · colors · flavor · sorbic acid · sorbitol · sucrose · water
		dextromethorphan hydrobromide, 30mg/10ml	caramel · carboxymethylcellulose sodium · citric acid · D&C red#33 · flavor · sorbic acid · sorbitol · sugar · water
		dextromethorphan hydrobromide, 7.5mg/5ml (when diluted to 16fl.oz.)	alcohol, 16% (3% when diluted) · purified water · sucrose · glycerin · honey · flavor · caramel · sodium hydroxide
		dextromethorphan hydrobromide, 10mg	
	guaifenesin, 100mg	dextromethorphan hydrobromide, 10mg	

COLD, COUGH, AND ALLERGY PRODUCTS - continued

	Product Manufacturer/Supplier	Dosage Form	Decongestant	Antihistamine
AL	**Protac SF** Republic Drug	liquid		chlorpheniramine maleate, 2mg
**	**Protac Troches** Republic Drug	lozenge		
AF	**Pyrroxate** Lee Consumer	caplet	phenylpropanolamine HCl, 25mg	chlorpheniramine maleate, 4mg
**	**Recofen** Reese Chemical	caplet		
** AL PE	**Redacon DX** Reese Chemical	drops	phenylpropanolamine HCl, 6.25 mg/ml	
AL DY	**REM Liquid** Alvin Last	liquid		
**	**Rephenyl** Reese Chemical	caplet	phenylpropanolamine HCl, 37.5mg	
AF DY GL LA PU SO	**Ricola Cough Drops, Original Flavor** Ricola	lozenge		
AF DY GL LA PU SO SU	**Ricola Sugar Free Herb Throat Drops, Alpine-Mint** Ricola	lozenge		
AF DY GL LA PU SO SU	**Ricola Sugar Free Herb Throat Drops, Cherry- or Lemon-Mint** Ricola	lozenge		
AF DY GL LA PU SO SU	**Ricola Sugar Free Herb Throat Drops, Mountain Herb** Ricola	lozenge		
AF DY GL LA PU SO	**Ricola Throat Drops, Cherry-Mint** Ricola	lozenge		

See Chapter 8, "Cold, Cough and Allergy Products," for more information about these products.

Analgesic	Expectorant	Antitussive	Other Ingredients
		dextromethorphan hydrobromide, 15mg	
		menthol, 10mg	benzocaine, 6mg
acetaminophen, 500mg			benzyl alcohol · butylparaben · erythrosine sodium · gelatin · glycerin · magnesium stearate · methylparaben · propylparaben · sodium lauryl sulfate · sodium propionate · starch · talc
	guaifenesin, 200mg	dextromethorphan hydrobromide, 15mg	corn starch · lactose · pregelatinized starch · D&C yellow#10 · magnesium stearate · sodium starch · glycolate
	guaifenesin, 50mg/ml	dextromethorphan hydrobromide, 5mg/ml	
		dextromethorphan hydrobromide, 5mg/5ml · eucalyptol	corn syrup · sucrose · glycerin · purified water · caramel · sodium chloride · sodium benzoate · licorice · anise oil · disodium EDTA · citric acid · sodium citrate
	guaifenesin, 200mg		corn starch · D&C yellow#10 · FD&C yellow#6 · lactose · magnesium stearate · pregelatinized corn starch · sodium starch glycolate · microcrystalline cellulose
		menthol, 3mg	sugar · glucose syrup · caramelized sugar · extracts of peppermint, lemon balm, thyme, sage, hyssop, elder, linden flowers, wild thyme, horehound, angelica root, and peppermint oil
		menthol, 4.8mg	extracts of peppermint, lemon balm, lady's mantle, linden flowers, and elder · natural flavorings · citric acid · aspartame · chlorophyll · isomalt
		menthol, 1mg	extracts of peppermint, lemon balm, lady's mantle, linden flowers, and elder · citric acid · lemon and peppermint oils (Lemon-Mint) · cherry and peppermint flavorings (Cherry-Mint) · cherry and elderberry concentrates (Cherry-Mint) · ascorbic acid · aspartame · flavorings (Lemon-Mint) · isomalt
		menthol, 1.5mg	extracts of peppermint, lemon balm, thyme, sage, hyssop, elder, linden flowers, wild thyme, horehound, and angelica root · caramel coloring · aspartame · peppermint oil · isomalt
		menthol, 1.5mg	sugar · glucose syrup · citric acid · extracts of peppermint, lemon balm, thyme, sage, hyssop, elder, linden flowers, wild thyme, horehound, and angelica root · cherry concentrate · elder concentrate · cherry flavorings · peppermint oil

COLD, COUGH, AND ALLERGY PRODUCTS - continued

	Product Manufacturer/Supplier	Dosage Form	Decongestant	Antihistamine
AF DY GL LA PU SO	**Ricola Throat Drops, Honey-Herb** Ricola	lozenge		
AF DY GL LA PU SO	**Ricola Throat Drops, Lemon-Mint or Orange-Mint** Ricola	lozenge		
AF DY GL LA PU SO	**Ricola Throat Drops, Menthol-Eucalyptus** Ricola	lozenge		
AL	**Robitussin** Whitehall-Robins Healthcare	syrup		
AL	**Robitussin CF** Whitehall-Robins Healthcare	syrup	phenylpropanolamine HCl, 12.5mg/5ml	
	Robitussin Cold & Cough Liqui-Gels Whitehall-Robins Healthcare	softgel	pseudoephedrine HCl, 30mg	
	Robitussin Cold, Cough, & Flu Liqui-Gels Whitehall-Robins Healthcare	softgel	pseudoephedrine HCl, 30mg	
	Robitussin Cough Calmers Whitehall-Robins Healthcare	lozenge		
	Robitussin Cough Drops, Cherry or Menthol Eucalyptus Whitehall-Robins Healthcare	lozenge		
	Robitussin Cough Drops, Honey-Lemon Whitehall-Robins Healthcare	lozenge		
	Robitussin DM Whitehall-Robins Healthcare	syrup		
	Robitussin Liquid Center Cough Drops, Cherry w/ Honey-Lemon Whitehall-Robins Healthcare	lozenge		
	Robitussin Liquid Center Cough Drops, Honey-Lemon w/ Cherry Whitehall-Robins Healthcare	lozenge		
	Robitussin Liquid Center Cough Drops, Menthol Euc. w/Cherry Whitehall-Robins Healthcare	lozenge		
	Robitussin Maximum Strength Cough Whitehall-Robins Healthcare	liquid		

See Chapter 8, "Cold, Cough and Allergy Products," for more information about these products.

Analgesic	Expectorant	Antitussive	Other Ingredients
		menthol, 2.4mg	honey · sugar · corn syrup · extracts of peppermint, lemon balm, thyme, sage, hyssop, elder, linden flowers, wild thyme, horehound, angelica root, and peppermint oil
		menthol, 1.25mg	sugar · glucose syrup · citric acid · extracts of lemon balm, orange-mint (Orange-Mint), peppermint, thyme, sage, hyssop, elder, linden flowers, wild thyme, horehound, and angelica root · lemon oil (Lemon-Mint) · peppermint oil · orange flavoring (Orange-Mint) · natural coloring (Lemon-Mint) · paprika extract (Orange-Mint)
		menthol, 4.5mg	sugar · glucose syrup · extracts of peppermint, lemon balm, thyme, sage, hyssop, elder, linden flowers, wild thyme, horehound, angelica root, peppermint oil, and eucalyptus oil · chlorophyll
	guaifenesin, 100mg/5ml		caramel · citric acid · FD&C red#40 · flavors · glucose · glycerin · high fructose corn syrup · saccharin sodium · sodium benzoate · water
	guaifenesin, 100mg/5ml	dextromethorphan hydrobromide, 10mg/5ml	citric acid · FD&C red#40 · flavors · glycerin · propylene glycol · saccharin sodium · sodium benzoate · sorbitol · water
	guaifenesin, 200mg	dextromethorphan hydrobromide, 10mg	FD&C blue#1 · FD&C red#40 · gelatin · glycerin · polyethylene glycol · povidone · propylene glycol · sorbitan · sorbitol · water
acetaminophen, 250mg	guaifenesin, 100mg	dextromethorphan hydrobromide, 10mg	D&C yellow#10 · FD&C red#40 · gelatin · glycerin · polyethylene glycol · povidone · propylene glycol 400 · sorbitol · water
		dextromethorphan hydrobromide, 5mg	corn syrup · FD&C red #40 · cherry flavor · sucrose · menthol flavor
		menthol, 7.4mg · eucalyptus oil	corn syrup · FD&C red#40 (Cherry) · flavors (Cherry) · sucrose
		menthol, 10mg · eucalyptus oil	corn syrup · D&C yellow#10 · FD&C yellow#6 · flavors · sucrose · lemon oil · honey · may contain starch
	guaifenesin, 100mg/5ml	dextromethorphan hydrobromide, 10mg/5ml	citric acid · FD&C red#40 · flavors · glucose · glycerin · high fructose corn syrup · saccharin sodium · sodium benzoate · water
		menthol, 8mg · eucalyptus oil	corn syrup · FD&C red#40 · flavors · glycerin · high fructose corn syrup · honey · lemon oil · sorbitol · sucrose · water
		menthol, 10mg · eucalyptus oil	corn syrup · D&C yellow #10 aluminum lake · FD&C yellow #6 aluminum lake · flavors · glycerin · high fructose corn syrup · honey · lemon oil · sorbitol · sucrose · water
		menthol, 8mg · eucalyptus oil	corn syrup · flavors · glycerin · high fructose corn syrup · sorbitol · sucrose · water
		dextromethorphan hydrobromide, 15mg/5ml	alcohol, 1.4% · citric acid · FD&C red#40 · flavors · glycerin · glucose · high fructose corn syrup · saccharin sodium · sodium benzoate · water

COLD, COUGH, AND ALLERGY PRODUCTS - continued

	Product Manufacturer/Supplier	Dosage Form	Decongestant	Antihistamine
	Robitussin Maximum Strength Cough & Cold Whitehall-Robins Healthcare	liquid	pseudoephedrine HCl, 30mg/5ml	
AL	**Robitussin Night Relief** Whitehall-Robins Healthcare	liquid	pseudoephedrine HCl, 10mg/5ml	pyrilamine maleate, 8.33mg/5ml
	Robitussin Night-Time Cold Formula Whitehall-Robins Healthcare	softgel	pseudoephedrine HCl, 30mg	doxylamine succinate, 6.25mg
AL	**Robitussin PE** Whitehall-Robins Healthcare	syrup	pseudoephedrine HCl, 30mg/5ml	
AL PE	**Robitussin Pediatric** Whitehall-Robins Healthcare	drops	pseudoephedrine HCl, 15mg/2.5ml	
AL PE	**Robitussin Pediatric Cough** Whitehall-Robins Healthcare	liquid		
AL PE	**Robitussin Pediatric Cough & Cold** Whitehall-Robins Healthcare	liquid	pseudoephedrine HCl, 15mg/5ml	
AL PE	**Robitussin Pediatric Night Relief** Whitehall-Robins Healthcare	liquid	pseudoephedrine HCl, 15mg/5ml	chlorpheniramine maleate, 1mg/5ml
	Robitussin Severe Congestion Liqui-Gels Whitehall-Robins Healthcare	softgel	pseudoephedrine HCl, 30mg	
SU	**Robitussin Sugar Free Cough Drops, Cherry or Peppermint** Whitehall-Robins Healthcare	lozenge		
AL DY SU	**Safe Tussin 30** Kramer Labs	liquid		
AL DY GL LA SU SL	**Scot-Tussin Allergy Relief Formula** Scot-Tussin Pharmacal	liquid		diphenhydramine HCl, 12.5mg/5ml
** AL DY GL LA SU SL	**Scot-Tussin Diabetes CF** Scot-Tussin Pharmacal	liquid		
AL DY GL LA SU SL	**Scot-Tussin DM** Scot-Tussin Pharmacal	liquid		chlorpheniramine maleate, 2mg/5ml

See Chapter 8, "Cold, Cough and Allergy Products," for more information about these products.

Analgesic	Expectorant	Antitussive	Other Ingredients
		dextromethorphan hydrobromide, 15mg/5ml	alcohol, 1.4% · citric acid · FD&C red#40 · flavors · glycerin · glucose · high fructose corn syrup · saccharin sodium · sodium benzoate · water
acetaminophen, 108.33mg/5ml		dextromethorphan hydrobromide, 5mg/5ml	citric acid · FD&C blue#1 · FD&C red#40 · cherry flavor · glycerin · propylene glycol · saccharin sodium · sodium benzoate · sorbitol · water
acetaminophen, 325mg		dextromethorphan hydrobromide, 15mg	D&C green#5 · D&C yellow#10 · FD&C green#3 · FD&C yellow#6 · gelatin · glycerin · polyethylene glycol · povidone · propylene glycol · sodium acetate · sorbitan · sorbitol · water
	guaifenesin, 100mg/5ml		citric acid · FD&C red#40 · flavors · glucose · glycerin · high fructose corn syrup · maltol · propylene glycol · saccharin sodium · sodium benzoate · water · maltol
	guaifenesin, 100mg/2.5ml	dextromethorphan hydrobromide, 5mg/2.5ml	citric acid · FD&C red#40 · flavors · glycerin · high fructose corn syrup · menthol · polyethylene glycol · propylene glycol · saccharin sodium · sodium benzoate · carboxymethylcellulose sodium · sorbitol · water
		dextromethorphan hydrobromide, 7.5mg/5ml	citric acid · FD&C red#40 · cherry flavor · glycerin · propylene glycol · saccharin sodium · sodium benzoate · sorbitol · water
		dextromethorphan hydrobromide, 7.5mg/5ml	citric acid · FD&C red#40 · cherry flavor · glycerin · propylene glycol · saccharin sodium · sodium benzoate · sorbitol · water
		dextromethorphan hydrobromide, 7.5mg/5ml	citric acid · FD&C blue#1 · FD&C red#40 · flavors · glycerin · high fructose corn syrup · propylene glycol · saccharin sodium · sodium benzoate · sorbitol · water
	guaifenesin, 200mg		FD&C green#3 · gelatin · glycerin · polyethylene glycol · povidone · propylene glycol · sorbitol
		menthol, 10mg · eucalyptus oil	aspartame · canola oil · FD&C blue#1 aluminum lake · FD&C red#40 aluminum lake (Cherry) · flavors · lycasin · isomalt · water
	guaifenesin, 200mg/5ml	dextromethorphan hydrobromide, 30mg/5ml	citric acid · benzoic acid · glycerin · sorbitol · peppermint · menthol · water
		menthol	methylparaben · propylparaben · propylene glycol · glycerin · cherry-strawberry flavor · benzoic acid · citric acid · hydroxymethylcellulose · Magnasweet-110
		dextromethorphan hydrobromide, 10mg/5ml · menthol	hydroxymethylcellulose · methylparaben · propylparaben · potassium benzoate · citric acid · glycerin · propylene glycol · cherry-strawberry flavor · Magnasweet-110
		dextromethorphan hydrobromide, 15mg/5ml · menthol	glycerin · propylene glycol · citric acid · potassium benzoate · hydroxymethylcellulose · methylparaben · propylparaben · cherry-strawberry flavor · Magnasweet-110

COLD, COUGH, AND ALLERGY PRODUCTS - continued

	Product Manufacturer/Supplier	Dosage Form	Decongestant	Antihistamine
AF DY GL LA PU SO SU	**Scot-Tussin DM Cough Chasers** Scot-Tussin Pharmacal	lozenge		
AL DY GL LA SU SL	**Scot-Tussin Expectorant** Scot-Tussin Pharmacal	liquid		
AL DY GL LA SU SL	**Scot-Tussin Original** Scot-Tussin Pharmacal	liquid	phenylephrine HCl, 4.2mg/5ml	pheniramine maleate, 13.33mg/5ml
AL DY GL LA SU SL	**Scot-Tussin Senior** Scot-Tussin Pharmacal	liquid		
**	**Sinadrin Plus** Reese Chemical	tablet	pseudoephedrine HCl, 60mg	dexbrompheniramine maleate, 2mg
**	**Sinadrin Super** Reese Chemical	tablet	phenylpropanolamine HCl, 25mg	chlorpheniramine maleate, 4mg
AF GL PU SO	**Sinarest Extra Strength** Novartis Consumer	tablet	pseudoephedrine HCl, 30mg	chlorpheniramine maleate, 2mg
AF GL PU SO	**Sinarest Sinus Medicine** Novartis Consumer	tablet	pseudoephedrine HCl, 30mg	chlorpheniramine maleate, 2mg
AF	**Sine-Aid IB** McNeil Consumer	caplet	pseudoephedrine HCl, 30mg	
AF	**Sine-Aid Maximum Strength** McNeil Consumer	tablet	pseudoephedrine HCl, 30mg	
AF	**Sine-Aid Maximum Strength** McNeil Consumer	caplet	pseudoephedrine HCl, 30mg	
AF	**Sine-Aid Maximum Strength** McNeil Consumer	gelcap	pseudoephedrine HCl, 30mg	
	Sine-Off Maximum Strength No Drowsiness Formula Hogil Ph'cal	caplet	pseudoephedrine HCl, 30mg	
	Sine-Off Sinus Medicine Hogil Ph'cal	caplet	pseudoephedrine HCl, 30mg	chlorpheniramine maleate, 2mg

See Chapter 8, "Cold, Cough and Allergy Products," for more information about these products.

Analgesic	Expectorant	Antitussive	Other Ingredients
		dextromethorphan hydrobromide, 2.5mg · peppermint oil	sorbitol
	guaifenesin, 100mg/5ml	menthol	glycerin · propylene glycol · citric acid · benzoic acid · methylparaben · propylparaben · hydroxypropyl methylcellulose · aspartame · grape flavor
sodium salicylate, 83.3mg/5ml			sodium citrate, 83.3mg/5ml · caffeine citrate, 25mg/5ml · glycerin · potassium benzoate · saccharin sodium · methylparaben · propylparaben · hydroxymethylcellulose · cherry-strawberry flavor · Magnasweet-110
	guaifenesin, 200mg/5ml	dextromethorphan hydrobromide, 15mg/5ml · menthol	aspartame · citric acid · hydroxypropyl methylcellulose · benzoic acid · methylparaben · propylparaben · glycerin · propylene glycol · peppermint-stick flavor
acetominophen, 500mg			lactose · corn starch · D&C yellow#10 · FD&C blue#1 · povidone · stearic acid · magnesium stearate
acetaminophen, 500mg			pregelatinized corn starch · stearic acid · sodium starch glycolate · D&C yellow#10
acetaminophen, 500mg			corn starch · hydroxypropyl methylcellulose · microcrystalline cellulose · polyethylene glycol · polysorbate 80 · polyvinylpyrrolidone · stearic acid · titanium dioxide
acetaminophen, 325mg			corn starch · yellow#10 · yellow#6 · hydroxypropyl methylcellulose · microcrystalline cellulose · polyethylene glycol · polysorbate 80 · polyvinylpyrrolidone · stearic acid · titanium dioxide
ibuprofen, 200mg			cellulose · corn starch · glyceryl triacetate · hydroxypropyl methylcellulose · silicon dioxide · sodium lauryl sulfate · sodium starch glycolate · stearic acid · titanium dioxide · red#40 aluminum lake · yellow#10 aluminum lake
acetaminophen, 500mg			cellulose · corn starch · magnesium stearate · sodium starch glycolate
acetaminophen, 500mg			cellulose · corn starch · hydroxypropyl methylcellulose · magnesium stearate · polyethylene glycol · sodium starch glycolate · titanium dioxide · blue#1 · red#40
acetaminophen, 500mg			benzyl alcohol · butylparaben · castor oil · cellulose · corn starch · edetate calcium disodium · gelatin · hydroxypropyl methylcellulose · iron oxide black · magnesium stearate · methylparaben · propylparaben · sodium lauryl sulfate · sodium propionate · sodium starch glycolate · titanium dioxide · FD&C red#40
acetaminophen, 500mg			crospovidone · FD&C red#40 · hydroxypropyl methylcellulose · magnesium stearate · microcrystalline cellulose · polyethylene glycol · polysorbate 80 · povidone · starch · titanium dioxide
acetaminophen, 500mg			carnauba wax · hydroxypropyl methylcellulose · magnesium stearate · microcrystalline cellulose · polydextrose · polyethylene glycol · povidone · sodium starch · glycolate · starch · stearic acid · titanium dioxide · triacetin · FD&C yellow#6 · D&C yellow#10

COLD, COUGH, AND ALLERGY PRODUCTS - continued

	Product Manufacturer/Supplier	Dosage Form	Decongestant	Antihistamine
** AF GL LA PU SU	**Sine-Off Sinus, Cold, and Flu Medicine Night Time Formula** Hogil Ph'cal	gel caplet	pseudoephedrine HCl, 30mg	diphenhydramine HCl, 25mg
	Singlet SmithKline Beecham	caplet	pseudoephedrine HCl, 60mg	chlorpheniramine maleate, 4mg
AF LA PU SO SU	**Sinulin** Carnrick Labs	tablet	phenylpropanolamine HCl, 25mg	chlorpheniramine maleate, 4mg
AF GL PU	**Sinus Relief Extra Strength** Hudson	tablet	pseudoephedrine HCl, 30mg	chlorpheniramine maleate, 2mg
AF	**Sinutab Non-Drying** Warner-Lambert Consumer	liquid-cap	pseudoephedrine HCl, 30mg	
AF	**Sinutab Sinus Allergy Medication Maximum Strength** Warner-Lambert Consumer	caplet · tablet	pseudoephedrine HCl, 30mg	chlorpheniramine maleate, 2mg
AF	**Sinutab Sinus without Drowsiness Maximum Strength** Warner-Lambert Consumer	caplet · tablet	pseudoephedrine HCl, 30mg	
	Sinutol Maximum Strength Republic Drug	tablet	pseudoephedrine HCl, 30mg	
	Spec-T Sore Throat Cough Suppressant Apothecon	lozenge		
	Spec-T Sore Throat Decongestant Apothecon	lozenge	phenylpropanolamine HCl, 10.5mg · phenylephrine HCl, 5mg	
AL PE	**St. Joseph Cough Suppressant for Children** Schering-Plough Healthcare	syrup		
	Sucrets 4-Hour Cough Suppressant, Cherry or Menthol SmithKline Beecham	lozenge		
AF	**Sudafed** Warner-Lambert Consumer	tablet	pseudoephedrine HCl, 60mg	
AF	**Sudafed** Warner-Lambert Consumer	tablet	pseudoephedrine HCl, 30mg	
AF SO	**Sudafed 12-Hour Extended Release** Warner-Lambert Consumer	timed-release caplet	pseudoephedrine HCl, 120mg	

See Chapter 8, "Cold, Cough and Allergy Products," for more information about these products.

Analgesic	Expectorant	Antitussive	Other Ingredients
acetaminophen, 500mg			croscarmellose sodium · D&C red#28 · FD&C blue#1 · yellow#6 · gelatin · hydroxypropyl methylcellulose · polysorbate 80 · silicon dioxide · sodium lauryl sulfate · stearic acid · titanium dioxide
acetaminophen, 650mg			D&C red#27 · D&C yellow#10 · FD&C blue#1 · hydroxypropyl cellulose · hydroxypropyl methylcellulose · magnesium stearate · microcrystalline cellulose · polyethylene glycol 8000 · pregelatinized starch · sodium starch glycolate · sucrose · titanium dioxide
acetaminophen, 650mg			
acetaminophen, 500mg			
	guaifenesin, 200mg		gelatin · sorbitol · FD&C blue#1 · povidone · polyethylene glycol · propylene glycol
acetaminophen, 500mg			pregelatinized starch · FD&C yellow#6 aluminum lake · D&C yellow#10 aluminum lake · croscarmellose sodium · crospovidone · microcrystalline cellulose · povidone · stearic acid · zinc stearate · caplet only: carnauba wax · hydroxypropyl cellulose · hydroxypropyl methylcellulose · polyethylene glycol · titanium dioxide
acetaminophen, 500mg			pregelatinized starch · D&C yellow#10 aluminum lake · FD&C yellow#6 aluminum lake · croscarmellose sodium · crospovidone · microcrystalline cellulose · povidone · stearic acid · zinc stearate · caplet only: carnauba wax · hydroxypropyl methylcellulose · polyethylene glycol · titanium dioxide
acetaminophen, 500mg			
		dextromethorphan hydrobromide, 10mg	benzocaine, 10mg · FD&C yellow#5 (tartrazine) · FD&C yellow#6 · dextrose · flavor · glucose · glycerin · propylene glycol · sucrose
			benzocaine, 10mg · FD&C blue#1 · yellow#5 (tartrazine) · dextrose · flavor · glucose · glycerin · propylene glycol · sucrose
		dextromethorphan hydrobromide, 7.5mg/5ml	
		dextromethorphan hydrobromide, 15mg	corn syrup · FD&C blue #1 · D&C yellow #10 (Menthol) · FD&C red#40 (Cherry) · Cherry or menthol-eucalyptus flavor · magnesium trisilicate · menthol · mineral oil · sucrose
			corn starch · dibasic calcium phosphate · sucrose · talc · sodium starch glycolate · acacia · carnauba wax · hydroxypropyl methylcellulose · magnesium stearate · pharmaceutical glaze · polysorbate 60 · stearic acid · titanium dioxide · pregelatinized corn starch · edible ink
			dibasic calcium phosphate · FD&C red#40 aluminum lake · yellow#6 aluminum lake · potato starch · sodium benzoate · acacia · carnauba wax · magnesium stearate · pharmaceutical glaze · polysorbate 60 · povidone · stearic acid · talc · titanium dioxide · corn starch · sucrose · edible ink
			hydroxypropyl methylcellulose · magnesium stearate · microcrystalline cellulose · polyethylene glycol · povidone · titanium dioxide · edible ink

COLD, COUGH, AND ALLERGY PRODUCTS - continued

	Product Manufacturer/Supplier	Dosage Form	Decongestant	Antihistamine
AL LA SU PE	**Sudafed Children's Cold & Cough** Warner-Lambert Consumer	liquid	pseudoephedrine HCl, 15mg/5ml	
AL SU PE	**Sudafed Children's Nasal Decongestant** Warner-Lambert Consumer	liquid	pseudoephedrine HCl, 15mg/5ml	
** AF SU PE	**Sudafed Children's Nasal Decongestant** Warner-Lambert Consumer	chewable tablet	pseudoephedrine HCl, 15mg	
AF	**Sudafed Cold & Cough** Warner-Lambert Consumer	liquid-cap	pseudoephedrine HCl, 30mg	
** AF	**Sudafed Cold & Sinus** Warner-Lambert Consumer	liquid-cap	pseudoephedrine HCl, 30mg	
AL DY SU PE	**Sudafed Pediatric Nasal Decongestant** Warner-Lambert Consumer	drops	pseudoephedrine HCl, 7.5mg/0.8ml	
AF	**Sudafed Severe Cold Formula** Warner-Lambert Consumer	caplet · tablet	pseudoephedrine HCl, 30mg	
AF	**Sudafed Sinus Non-Drowsy Maximum Strength** Warner-Lambert Consumer	caplet · tablet	pseudoephedrine HCl, 30mg	
AF	**Sudafed Sinus Non-Drying Non-Drowsy Maximum Strength** Warner-Lambert Consumer	liquid-cap	pseudoephedrine HCl, 30mg	
SO SU	**Sudanyl** Dover Ph'cal	tablet	pseudoephedrine HCl, 30mg	
AF GL PU SO	**Tavist-1 Antihistamine** Novartis Consumer	tablet		clemastine fumarate, 1.34mg
AF GL PU SO	**Tavist-D Antihistamine/Nasal Decongestant** Novartis Consumer	tablet	phenylpropanolamine HCl, 75mg	clemastine fumarate, 1.34mg
	Teldrin Hogil Ph'cal	timed-release capsule	phenylpropanolamine HCl, 75mg	chlorpheniramine maleate, 8mg
**	**Tetra-Formula** Reese Chemical	lozenge		
	Tetrahist Republic Drug	tablet	pseudoephedrine HCl, 30mg	chlorpheniramine maleate, 2mg
**	**Theracaps** Reese Chemical	caplet	phenylpropanolamine HCl, 37.5mg	pyrilamine maleate, 50mg
** AL	**Theracof** Reese Chemical	liquid	phenylpropanolamine HCl 8.3mg/5ml	pyrilamine maleate, 8.3/5ml

See Chapter 8, "Cold, Cough and Allergy Products," for more information about these products.

Analgesic	Expectorant	Antitussive	Other Ingredients
	guaifenesin, 100mg/5ml	dextromethorphan hydrobromide, 5mg/5ml	caramel · citric acid · D&C red#33 · edetate disodium · FD&C red#40 · flavors · poloxamer 407 · polyethylene glycol 1450 · propyl gallate · propylene glycol · saccharin sodium · sodium benzoate · sodium chloride · sodium citrate · sorbitol solution · purified water
			citric acid · edetate disodium · FD&C red#40 · FD&C blue#1 · flavors · glycerin · poloxamer 407 · polyethylene glycol 1450 · povidone k-90 · saccharin sodium · sodium benzoate · sodium citrate · sorbitol solution · purified water
			ascorbic acid · aspartame · carnauba wax · citric acid · crospovidone · FD&C yellow#6 aluminum lake · flavors · hydroxypropyl methylcellulose · magnesium stearate · mannitol · microcrystalline cellulose · sodium chloride · tartaric acid
acetaminophen, 250mg	guaifenesin, 100mg	dextromethorphan hydrobromide, 10mg	D&C yellow#10 · FD&C red#40 · gelatin · glycerin · polyethylene glycol · povidone · propylene glycol · purified water · sorbitol · edible white ink
acetaminophen, 325mg			FD&C blue#1 · FD&C red#40 · gelatin · glycerin · pharmaceutical glaze · polyethylene glycol · povidone · purified water · sodium acetate · sorbitol special · titanium dioxide
			carboxymethyl cellulose sodium · citric acid · flavors · glycerin · poloxamer 407 · saccharin sodium · sodium benzoate · sodium chloride · sodium citrate · sorbitol solution · purified water
acetaminophen, 500mg		dextromethorphan hydrobromide, 15mg	pregelatinized corn starch · microcrystalline cellulose · carnauba wax · crospovidone · hydroxypropyl methylcellulose · polyethylene glycol · povidone · stearic acid · titanium dioxide · magnesium stearate
acetaminophen, 500mg			povidone · pregelatinized corn starch · carnauba wax · crospovidone · FD&C yellow#6 aluminum lake · hydroxymethyl cellulose · magnesium stearate · microcrystalline cellulose · polyethylene glycol · polysorbate 80 · stearic acid · titanium dioxide
	guaifenesin, 200mg		FD&C blue#1 · gelatin · glycerin · polyethylene glycol · povidone · propylene glycol · sorbitol · edible ink
			lactose · povidone · starch · talc · stearic acid
			colloidal silicon dioxide · yellow#10 · dibasic calcium phosphate dihydrate · lactose · magnesium stearate · methylcellulose · polyethylene glycol · povidone · starch · synthetic polymers · titanium dioxide
			benzyl alcohol · butylparaben · D&C red#33 · edetate calcium disodium · FD&C red#3 · FD&C yellow#6 · gelatin · methylparaben · pharmaceutical glaze · propylparaben · sodium lauryl sulfate · sodium propionate · starch · sucrose · other ingredients · may also contain polysorbate 80
		dextromethorphan hydrobromide, 7.5mg	benzocaine, 15mg · sucrose · corn sugar solids · glycerin · propylene glycol · dextrose · vanillin · FD&C blue#1 · FD&C red#40 · artificial cherry flavor
acetaminophen, 325mg		dextromethorphan hydrobromide, 15mg	
acetaminophen, 500 mg		dextromethorphan hydrobromide, 30mg	starch · stearic acid · lactose · microcrystalline cellulose
acetaminophen, 108.3mg/5ml		dextromethorphan hydrobromide, 5mg/5ml	cerellose dextrose · glycerine · grape wine flavor · honey flavor · menthol crystals · methylparaben · phosphoric acid · propylene glycol · propylparaben · sodium chloride · saccharin sodium · sorbitol · sugar · water · artificial marshmallow flavor

COLD, COUGH, AND ALLERGY PRODUCTS - continued

	Product Manufacturer/Supplier	Dosage Form	Decongestant	Antihistamine
AF GL PU	**TheraFlu Flu and Cold Medicine** Novartis Consumer	individual packet	pseudoephedrine HCl, 60mg	chlorpheniramine maleate, 4mg
AF GL PU	**TheraFlu Flu, Cold, & Cough Medicine** Novartis Consumer	individual packet	pseudoephedrine HCl, 60mg	chlorpheniramine maleate, 4mg
AF	**TheraFlu Max. Strength Flu & Cold Medicine For Sore Throat** Novartis Consumer	individual packet	pseudoephedrine HCl, 60mg	chlorpheniramine maleate, 4mg
AF GL PU	**TheraFlu Max. Strength Flu, Cold & Cough Medicine NightTime** Novartis Consumer	individual packet	pseudoephedrine HCl, 60mg	chlorpheniramine maleate, 4mg
** AF PU SU	**TheraFlu Max. Strength Flu, Cold & Cough Medicine NightTime** Novartis Consumer	caplet	pseudoephendrine · HCl, 30mg	chlorpheniramine maleate, 2mg
AF	**Theraflu Maximum Strength Non-Drowsy** Novartis Consumer	caplet	pseudoephedrine HCl, 30mg	
AF DY	**TheraFlu Maximum Strength Sinus Non-Drowsy** Novartis Consumer	caplet	pseudoephedrine HCl, 30mg	
	Tolu-Sed DM Scherer Labs	liquid		
	Tri-Fed Republic Drug	tablet	pseudoephedrine HCl, 60mg	triprolidine HCl, 2.5mg
AL DY PE	**Triaminic AM, Non-Drowsy Cough & Decongestant Formula** Novartis Consumer	syrup	pseudoephedrine HCl, 15mg/5ml	
AL DY PE	**Triaminic AM, Non-Drowsy Decongestant Formula** Novartis Consumer	syrup	pseudoephedrine HCl, 15mg/5ml	
AL LA SL PE	**Triaminic DM, Cough Relief** Novartis Consumer	syrup	phenylpropanolamine HCl, 6.25mg/5ml	
AL LA SL PE	**Triaminic Expectorant, Chest & Head Congestion** Novartis Consumer	liquid	phenylpropanolamine HCl, 6.25mg/5ml	
AL DY LA SL PE	**Triaminic Infant, Oral Decongestant** Novartis Consumer	drops	pseudoephedrine HCl, 7.5mg/0.8ml	

See Chapter 8, "Cold, Cough and Allergy Products," for more information about these products.

Analgesic	Expectorant	Antitussive	Other Ingredients
acetaminophen, 650mg			natural lemon flavors · sucrose · ascorbic acid · citric acid · sodium citrate · titanium dioxide · tribasic calcium phosphate · pregelatinized starch · yellow#6 · yellow#10
acetaminophen, 650mg		dextromethorphan hydrobromide, 20mg	natural lemon flavors · sucrose · ascorbic acid · citric acid · sodium citrate · titanium dioxide · tribasic calcium phosphate · pregelatinized starch · yellow#6 · yellow#10
acetaminophen, 1000mg			acesulfame · natural apple and cinnamon flavors · ascorbic acid · aspartame · blue#1 · citric acid · maltodextrin · red#40 · silicon dioxide · sodium citrate · sucrose · tribasic calcium phosphate · yellow#10
acetaminophen, 1000mg		dextromethorphan hydrobromide, 30mg	ascorbic acid · citric acid · natural lemon flavors · maltol · pregelatinized starch · silicon dioxide · sodium citrate · sucrose · titanium dioxide · tribasic calcium phosphate · yellow#6 · yellow#10
acetaminophen, 500mg		dextromethorphan hydrobromide, 15mg	blue #1 · colloidal silicon dioxide · croscarmellose · sodium · gelatin · hydroxypropyl cellulose · hydroxypropyl methylcellulose · lactose · magnesium stearate · methylparaben · polydextrose · polyethylene glycol · pregelatinized starch · titanium dioxide · triacetin · yellow #6 · yellow #10 ·
acetaminophen, 500mg		dextromethorphan hydrobromide, 15mg	colloidal silicon dioxide · croscarmellose sodium · gelatin · hydroxypropyl cellulose · hydroxypropyl methylcellulose · lactose · magnesium stearate · methylparaben · polydextrose · polyethylene glycol · pregelatinized starch · red#40 · titanium dioxide · triacetin · yellow#6 · yellow#10
acetaminophen, 500mg			colloidal silicon dioxide · croscarmellose sodium · hydroxypropyl methylcellulose · lactose · magnesium stearate · methylcellulose · methylparaben · polyethylene glycol · povidone · pregelatinized starch · titanium dioxide
	guaifenesin, 100mg/5ml	dextromethorphan hydrobromide, 10mg/5ml	alcohol, 10%
		dextromethorphan hydrobromide, 7.5mg/5ml	benzoic acid · citric acid · dibasic sodium phosphate · edetate disodium · flavors · propylene glycol · purified water · sorbitol · sucrose
			benzoic acid · edetate disodium · flavors · purified water · sodium hydroxide · sorbitol · sucrose
		dextromethorphan hydrobromide, 5mg/5ml	sorbitol · sucrose · benzoic acid · blue#1 · flavors · propylene glycol · purified water · red#40 · sodium chloride
	guaifenesin, 50mg/5ml		saccharin · sorbitol · sucrose · benzoic acid · edetate disodium · flavors · purified water · saccharin sodium · sodium hydroxide · yellow#6 · yellow#10
			benzoic acid · edetate disodium · flavors · purified water · sodium chloride · sorbitol solution · sucrose

COLD, COUGH, AND ALLERGY PRODUCTS - continued

	Product Manufacturer/Supplier	Dosage Form	Decongestant	Antihistamine
AL LA SL PE	**Triaminic Night Time** Novartis Consumer	liquid	pseudoephedrine HCl, 15mg/5ml	chlorpheniramine maleate, 1mg/5ml
AL PE	**Triaminic Sore Throat, Throat Pain & Cough** Novartis Consumer	liquid	pseudoephedrine HCl, 15mg/5ml	
AL LA SL PE	**Triaminic, Cold & Allergy** Novartis Consumer	syrup	phenylpropanolamine HCl, 6.25mg/5ml	chlorpheniramine maleate, 1mg/5ml
AF GL PU	**Triaminicin** Novartis Consumer	tablet	phenylpropanolamine HCl, 25mg	chlorpheniramine maleate, 4mg
AL LA SL PE	**Triaminicol Multi-Symptom Relief** Novartis Consumer	liquid	phenylpropanolamine HCl, 6.25mg/5ml	chlorpheniramine maleate, 1mg/5ml
AF GL PU SO	**Tuss-DM** Hyrex Ph'cals	tablet		
	Tussar-2 Rhône-Poulenc Rorer Ph'cals	syrup	pseudoephedrine HCl, 30mg/5ml	
AL	**Tussar-DM** Rhône-Poulenc Rorer Ph'cals	syrup	pseudoephedrine HCl, 30mg/5ml	chlorpheniramine maleate, 2mg/5ml
SU	**Tussar-SF** Rhône-Poulenc Rorer Ph'cals	syrup	pseudoephedrine HCl, 30mg/5ml	
AF	**Tylenol Allergy Sinus Maximum Strength** McNeil Consumer	gelcap · geltab	pseudoephedrine HCl, 30mg	chlorpheniramine maleate, 2mg
AF	**Tylenol Allergy Sinus Maximum Strength** McNeil Consumer	caplet	pseudoephedrine HCl, 30mg	chlorpheniramine maleate, 2mg
AF	**Tylenol Allergy Sinus NightTime Maximum Strength** McNeil Consumer	caplet	pseudoephedrine HCl, 30mg	diphenhydramine HCl, 25mg
AF PE	**Tylenol Children's Cold Multi-Symptom** McNeil Consumer	chewable tablet	pseudoephedrine HCl, 7.5mg	chlorpheniramine maleate, 0.5mg
AL AF PE	**Tylenol Children's Cold Multi-Symptom** McNeil Consumer	liquid	pseudoephedrine HCl, 15mg/5ml	chlorpheniramine maleate, 1mg/5ml
AL AF PE	**Tylenol Children's Cold Plus Cough** McNeil Consumer	liquid	pseudoephedrine HCl, 15mg/5ml	chlorpheniramine maleate, 1mg/5ml
AF PE	**Tylenol Children's Cold Plus Cough** McNeil Consumer	chewable tablet	pseudoephedrine HCl, 7.5mg	chlorpheniramine maleate, 0.5mg

See Chapter 8, "Cold, Cough and Allergy Products," for more information about these products.

Analgesic	Expectorant	Antitussive	Other Ingredients
		dextromethorphan hydrobromide, 7.5mg/5ml	sorbitol · sucrose · benzoic acid · blue#1 · citric acid · flavors · propylene glycol · purified water · red#33 · dibasic sodium phosphate
acetaminophen, 160mg/5ml		dextromethorphan hydrobromide, 7.5mg/5ml	benzoic acid · blue#1 · dibasic sodium phosphate · edetate disodium · flavors · glycerin · polyethylene glycol · propylene glycol · purified water · red#33 · red#40 · sucrose · tartaric acid
			sorbitol · sucrose · benzoic acid · edetate disodium · flavors · purified water · sodium hydroxide · yellow#6
acetaminophen, 650mg			colloidal silicon dioxide · croscarmellose sodium · hydroxypropyl cellulose · lactose · magnesium stearate · methylcellulose · methylparaben · polyethylene glycol · povidone · pregelatinized starch · red#40 · titanium dioxide · yellow#10
		dextromethorphan hydrobromide, 5mg/5ml	benzoic acid · flavor · propylene glycol · purified water · red#40 · sodium chloride · sorbitol · sucrose
	guaifenesin, 200mg	dextromethorphan hydrobromide, 10mg	
	guaifenesin, 100mg/5ml	codeine phosphate, 10mg/5ml[a]	alcohol, 2.5% · artificial flavors · citric acid · D&C yellow#10 · FD&C blue#1 · glycerin · methylparaben · methyl salicylate · propylene glycol · saccharin sodium · sodium citrate · sorbitol · sucrose · water
		dextromethorphan hydrobromide, 15mg/5ml	artificial flavors · citric acid · FD&C red#40 · glucose · glycerin · methylparaben · sodium citrate · sucrose · water
	guaifenesin, 100mg/5ml	codeine phosphate, 10mg/5ml[a]	citric acid · FD&C red#40 · glycerin · methylparaben · methyl salicylate · propylene glycol · saccharin sodium · sodium citrate · sorbitol · water
acetaminophen, 500mg			benzyl alcohol · butylparaben · castor oil · corn starch · cellulose · edetate calcium disodium · gelatin · hydroxypropyl methylcellulose · magnesium stearate · methylparaben · propylparaben · sodium lauryl sulfate · sodium propionate · sodium starch glycolate · titanium dioxide · blue#1 · blue#2 · yellow#10
acetaminophen, 500mg			carnauba wax · cellulose · corn starch · hydroxypropyl cellulose · hydroxypropyl methylcellulose · iron oxide black · magnesium stearate · polyethylene glycol · sodium starch glycolate · titanium dioxide · blue#1 · yellow#6 · yellow#10
acetaminophen, 500mg			cellulose · corn starch · hydroxypropyl methylcellulose · iron oxide black · magnesium stearate · polyethylene glycol · polysorbate 80 · sodium citrate · sodium starch glycolate · titanium dioxide · blue#1 · yellow#10
acetaminophen, 80mg			aspartame · basic polymethacrylate · cellulose acetate · citric acid · flavors · hydroxypropyl methylcellulose · magnesium stearate · mannitol · microcrystalline cellulose · blue#1 · red#7
acetaminophen, 160mg/5ml			benzoic acid · citric acid · flavors · glycerin · malic acid · polyethylene glycol · propylene glycol · sodium benzoate · sorbitol · sucrose · purified water · blue#1 · red#40
acetaminophen, 160mg/5ml		dextromethorphan hydrobromide, 5mg/5ml	citric acid · corn syrup · flavors · polyethylene glycol · propylene glycol · sodium benzoate · carboxymethylcellulose sodium · sorbitol · purified water · red#33 · red#40
acetaminophen, 80mg		dextromethorphan hydrobromide, 2.5mg	aspartame · basic polymethacrylate · cellulose acetate · colloidal silicon dioxide · flavors · hydroxypropyl methylcellulose · mannitol · microcrystalline cellulose · stearic acid · red #7

COLD, COUGH, AND ALLERGY PRODUCTS - continued

	Product Manufacturer/Supplier	Dosage Form	Decongestant	Antihistamine
** AF PE	**Tylenol Children's Flu** McNeil Consumer	liquid	pseudoephedrine HCl, 15mg/5ml	chlorpheniramine maleate, 1mg/5ml
AF	**Tylenol Cold Medication Multi-Symptom Formula** McNeil Consumer	caplet · tablet	pseudoephedrine HCl, 30mg	chlorpheniramine maleate, 2mg
AF	**Tylenol Cold Multi-Symptom** McNeil Consumer	individual packet	pseudoephedrine HCl, 60mg/packet	chlorpheniramine maleate, 4mg/packet
AF	**Tylenol Cold No Drowsiness Formula** McNeil Consumer	caplet	pseudoephedrine HCl, 30mg	
AF	**Tylenol Cold No Drowsiness Formula** McNeil Consumer	gelcap	pseudoephedrine HCl, 30mg	
** AF	**Tylenol Cold Severe Congestion Multi-Symptom** McNeil Consumer	caplet	pseudoephedrine HCl, 30mg	
AF	**Tylenol Cough Multi-Symptom** McNeil Consumer	liquid		
AF	**Tylenol Cough with Decongestant Multi-Symptom** McNeil Consumer	liquid	pseudoephedrine, HCl, 60mg/15ml	
AF	**Tylenol Flu Maximum Strength** McNeil Consumer	gelcap	pseudoephedrine HCl, 30mg	
AF	**Tylenol Flu NightTime Maximum Strength** McNeil Consumer	gelcap	pseudoephedrine HCl, 30mg	diphenhydramine HCl, 25mg
AF	**Tylenol Flu NightTime Maximum Strength Hot Medication** McNeil Consumer	individual packet	pseudoephedrine HCl, 60mg	diphenhydramine HCl, 50mg
AL AF PE	**Tylenol Infants' Cold Decongestant and Fever Reducer** McNeil Consumer	drops	pseudoephedrine HCl, 7.5mg/0.8ml	
AF	**Tylenol Severe Allergy Maximum Strength** McNeil Consumer	caplet		diphenhydramine HCl, 12.5mg
AF	**Tylenol Sinus Maximum Strength** McNeil Consumer	caplet · tablet	pseudoephedrine HCl, 30mg	

See Chapter 8, "Cold, Cough and Allergy Products," for more information about these products.

Analgesic	Expectorant	Antitussive	Other Ingredients
acetaminophen, 160mg/5ml		dextromethorphan hydrobromide, 7.5mg/5ml	citric acid · corn syrup · flavors · polyethylene glycol · propylene glycol · sodium benzoate · sodium carboxymethycellulose · sorbitol · purified water · red#33 · red#40
acetaminophen, 325mg		dextromethorphan hydrobromide, 15mg	cellulose · corn starch · glyceryl triacetate (caplet) · hydroxypropyl methylcellulose (caplet) · iron oxide black (caplet) · magnesium stearate · sodium starch glycolate · titanium dioxide (caplet) · blue#1 (caplet) · yellow#6 · yellow#10
acetaminophen, 650mg/packet		dextromethorphan hydrobromide, 30mg/packet	aspartame · citric acid · corn starch · flavors · sodium citrate · sucrose · red#40 · yellow#10
acetaminophen, 325mg		dextromethorphan hydrobromide, 15mg	cellulose · corn starch · glyceryl triacetate · hydroxypropyl methylcellulose · iron oxide black · magnesium stearate · sodium starch glycolate · titanium dioxide · blue#1 · yellow#10
acetaminophen, 325mg		dextromethorphan hydrobromide, 15mg	benzyl alcohol · butylparaben · castor oil · cellulose · corn starch · edetate calcium disodium · gelatin · hydroxypropyl methylcellulose · magnesium stearate · methylparaben · propylparaben · sodium propionate · sodium lauryl sulfate · sodium starch glycolate · titanium dioxide · red #40 · yellow #10
acetaminophen, 325mg	guaifenesin, 200mg	dextromethorphan hydrobromide, 15mg	carnauba wax · cellulose · colloidal silicon dioxide · corn starch · hydroxypropyl methylcellulose · iron oxide · povidone · pregelatinized starch · propylene glycol · sodium starch glycolate · stearic acid · titanium dioxide · triacetin · blue#1 · yellow#6 · yellow#10
acetaminophen, 650mg/15ml		dextromethorphan hydrobromide, 30mg/15ml	alcohol, 5% · citric acid · flavors · high fructose corn syrup · polyethylene glycol · propylene glycol · purified water · sodium benzoate · carboxymethylcellulose sodium · saccharin sodium · sorbitol · red #40
acetaminophen, 650mg/15ml		dextromethorphan hydrobromide, 30mg/15ml	alcohol, 5% · citric acid · flavors · high fructose corn syrup · polyethylene glycol · propylene glycol · purified water · sodium benzoate · carboxymethylcellulose sodium · saccharin sodium · sorbitol · blue#1 · red #40
acetaminophen, 500mg		dextromethorphan hydrobromide, 15mg	benzyl alcohol · butylparaben · castor oil · cellulose · corn starch · edetate calcium disodium · gelatin · hydroxypropyl methylcellulose · iron oxide black · magnesium stearate · methylparaben · propylparaben · sodium lauryl sulfate · sodium propionate · sodium starch glycolate · titanium dioxide · red#40 · blue#1
acetaminophen, 500mg			benzyl alcohol · butylparaben · castor oil · cellulose · corn starch · edetate calcium disodium · gelatin · hydroxypropyl methylcellulose · iron oxide black · magnesium stearate · methylparaben · propylparaben · sodium citrate · sodium lauryl sulfate · sodium propionate · sodium starch glycolate · titanium dioxide · D&C red#28 · FD&C blue#1
acetaminophen, 1000mg			ascorbic acid · aspartame · citric acid · flavors · sodium citrate · sucrose · yellow#10 · blue#1 · red#40 · yellow#6 · may also contain silicon dioxide
acetaminophen, 80mg/0.8ml			citric acid · corn syrup · flavors · polyethylene glycol · propylene glycol · purified water · sodium benzoate · saccharin · FD&C red#40
acetaminophen, 500mg			cellulose · corn starch · hydroxypropyl cellulose · hydroxypropyl methylcellulose · iron oxide black · magnesium stearate · polyethylene glycol · sodium citrate · sodium starch glycolate · titanium dioxide · yellow#6 · yellow#10
acetaminophen, 500mg			carnauba wax (caplet) · cellulose · corn starch · hydroxypropyl methylcellulose (caplet) · magnesium stearate · polyethylene glycol (caplet) · polysorbate 80 (caplet) · sodium starch glycolate · titanium dioxide (caplet) · blue#1 · yellow#6 (tablet) · red#40 (caplet) · yellow#10

COLD, COUGH, AND ALLERGY PRODUCTS - continued

	Product Manufacturer/Supplier	Dosage Form	Decongestant	Antihistamine
AF	**Tylenol Sinus Maximum Strength** McNeil Consumer	gelcap · geltab	pseudoephedrine HCl, 30mg	
PR SL	**Vaporizer in a Bottle Air Wick Inhaler** Columbia Labs	nasal inhaler		
AF PU SO	**Vicks 44 Cough, Cold, & Flu Relief LiquiCaps** Procter & Gamble	softgel	pseudoephedrine HCl, 30mg	chlorpheniramine maleate, 2mg
AF PU SO	**Vicks 44 Non-Drowsy Cough & Cold Relief LiquiCaps** Procter & Gamble	softgel	pseudoephedrine HCl, 60mg	
LA SL	**Vicks 44 Soothing Cough Relief** Procter & Gamble	liquid		
LA SL	**Vicks 44D Soothing Cough & Head Congestion Relief** Procter & Gamble	liquid	pseudoephedrine HCl, 12mg/5ml	
AL SL PE	**Vicks 44e Pediatric Cough & Chest Congestion Relief** Procter & Gamble	liquid		
LA SL	**Vicks 44E Soothing Cough & Chest Congestion Relief** Procter & Gamble	liquid		
AL LA SL PE	**Vicks 44m Pediatric Cough & Cold Relief** Procter & Gamble	liquid	pseudoephedrine HCl, 30mg/15ml	chlorpheniramine maleate, 2mg/15ml
LA SL	**Vicks 44M Soothing Cough, Cold, & Flu Relief** Procter & Gamble	liquid	pseudoephedrine HCl, 15mg/5ml	chlorpheniramine maleate, 1mg/5ml
**	**Vicks Chloraseptic Cough and Throat Drops, Cherry or Lemon** Procter & Gamble	lozenge		
**	**Vicks Chloraseptic Cough and Throat Drops, Menthol** Procter & Gamble	lozenge		
	Vicks Cough Drops, Cherry Procter & Gamble	lozenge		
	Vicks Cough Drops, Menthol Procter & Gamble	lozenge		
AF GL PU	**Vicks DayQuil Allergy Relief 12-Hour** Procter & Gamble	tablet	phenylpropanolamine HCl, 75mg	brompheniramine maleate, 12mg

See Chapter 8, "Cold, Cough and Allergy Products," for more information about these products.

Analgesic	Expectorant	Antitussive	Other Ingredients
acetaminophen, 500mg			benzyl alcohol · butylparaben · castor oil · cellulose · corn starch · edetate calcium disodium · gelatin · hydroxypropyl methylcellulose · iron oxide black · magnesium stearate · methylparaben · propylparaben · sodium lauryl sulfate · sodium propionate · sodium starch glycolate · titanium dioxide · FD&C blue#1 · D&C yellow #10
		camphor, 3.6% · menthol, 0.55% · eucalyptus oil · oil of peppermint	isopropyl alcohol, 71.4% · methyl salicylate · oil of white camphor · isobornyl acetate · oil of spike lavender · propylene glycol · isoamyl acetate · resin fixative-D
acetaminophen, 250mg		dextromethorphan hydrobromide, 10mg	D&C red#33 lake · FD&C blue#1 · gelatin · glycerin · polyethylene glycol · povidone · propylene glycol · purified water
		dextromethorphan hydrobromide, 30mg	D&C red#33 · FD&C blue#1 · FD&C red#40 · gelatin · glycerin · polyethylene glycol · povidone · purified water · sorbitol
		dextromethorphan hydrobromide, 10mg/5ml	alcohol, 5% · carboxymethylcellulose sodium · citric acid · FD&C blue#1 · FD&C red#40 · flavor · high fructose corn syrup · polyethylene oxide · polyoxyl 40 stearate · propylene glycol · purified water · sodium benzoate · sodium citrate · saccharin sodium
		dextromethorphan hydrobromide, 10mg/5ml	alcohol, 5% · citric acid · FD&C blue#1 · FD&C red#40 · flavor · high fructose corn syrup · polyethylene oxide · polyoxyl 40 stearate · propylene glycol · purified water · saccharin sodium · sodium benzoate · sodium citrate · sucrose · carboxymethylcellulose sodium
	guaifenesin, 100mg/15ml	dextromethorphan hydrobromide, 10mg/15ml	carboxymethylcellulose sodium · citric acid · FD&C red#40 · flavor · high fructose corn syrup · polyethylene oxide · polyoxyl 40 stearate · propylene glycol · purified water · saccharin sodium · sodium benzoate · sodium citrate
	guaifenesin, 200mg/15ml	dextromethorphan hydrobromide, 20mg/15ml	alcohol, 5% · carboxymethylcellulose sodium · citric acid · FD&C blue#1 · FD&C red#40 · flavor · high fructose corn syrup · polyethylene oxide · polyoxyl 40 stearate · propylene glycol · purified water · saccharin sodium · sodium benzoate · sodium citrate · sucrose
		dextromethorphan hydrobromide, 15mg/15ml	carboxymethylcellulose sodium · citric acid · FD&C red#40 · flavor · high fructose corn syrup · polyethylene oxide · polyoxyl 40 stearate · propylene glycol · purified water · saccharin sodium · sodium benzoate · sodium citrate
acetaminophen, 162.5mg/5ml		dextromethorphan hydrobromide, 7.5mg/5ml	alcohol, 10% · carboxymethylcellulose sodium · citric acid · FD&C blue#1 · FD&C red#40 · flavor · high fructose corn syrup · polyethylene glycol · polyethylene oxide · propylene glycol · purified water · saccharin sodium · sodium citrate
		menthol, 8.4mg	corn syrup · FD&C blue#2 (Cherry) · FD&C red#40 (Cherry) · D&C yellow#10 (Lemon) · FD&C yellow#6 (Lemon) · flavors · sucrose
		menthol, 8.4mg	corn syrup · FD&C blue#1 · flavors · sucrose
		menthol, 1.7mg	ascorbic acid · citric acid · corn syrup · FD&C blue#1 · FD&C red #40 · sucrose · eucalyptus oil
		menthol, 3.3mg	ascorbic acid · caramel · corn syrup · sucrose · eucalyptus oil
			dimethyl polysiloxane oil · FD&C blue#1 aluminum lake · hydroxypropyl methylcellulose · lactose · magnesium stearate · polyethylene glycol · talc · titanium dioxide

COLD, COUGH, AND ALLERGY PRODUCTS - continued

	Product Manufacturer/Supplier	Dosage Form	Decongestant	Antihistamine
AL LA SL PE	**Vicks DayQuil Children's Allergy Relief** Procter & Gamble	liquid	pseudoephedrine HCl, 30mg/15ml	chlorpheniramine maleate, 2mg/15ml
AL LA SL	**Vicks DayQuil Multi-Symptom Cold/Flu Relief** Procter & Gamble	liquid	pseudoephedrine HCl, 60mg/30ml	
AF GL PU SO	**Vicks DayQuil Multi-Symptom Cold/Flu Relief LiquiCaps** Procter & Gamble	softgel	pseudoephedrine HCl, 30mg	
AF GL PU	**Vicks DayQuil Sinus Pressure & Congestion Relief** Procter & Gamble	caplet	phenylpropanolamine HCl, 25mg	
AF PU	**Vicks DayQuil Sinus Pressure & Pain Relief with Ibuprofen** Procter & Gamble	caplet	pseudoephedrine HCl, 30mg	
AL LA SL PE	**Vicks NyQuil Children's Cold/Cough Medicine** Procter & Gamble	liquid	pseudoephedrine HCl, 30mg/15ml	chlorpheniramine maleate, 2mg/15ml
AF GL PU SO	**Vicks Nyquil Hot Therapy** Procter & Gamble	individual packet	pseudoephedrine HCl, 60mg	doxylamine succinate, 12.5mg
AF GL PU SO	**Vicks NyQuil Multi-Symptom Cold/Flu Relief LiquiCaps** Procter & Gamble	softgel	pseudoephedrine HCl, 30mg	doxylamine succinate, 6.25mg
LA SL	**Vicks NyQuil Multi-Symptom Cold/Flu Relief, Cherry** Procter & Gamble	liquid	pseudoephedrine HCl, 60mg/30ml	doxylamine succinate, 12.5mg/30ml
LA SL	**Vicks NyQuil Multi-Symptom Cold/Flu Relief, Original** Procter & Gamble	liquid	pseudoephedrine HCl, 60mg/30ml	doxylamine succinate, 12.5mg/30ml
	Vicks Original Cough Drops, Cherry Procter & Gamble	lozenge		
	Vicks Original Cough Drops, Menthol Procter & Gamble	lozenge		
	Vicks VapoRub Procter & Gamble	cream		
	Vicks VapoRub Procter & Gamble	ointment		
	Vicks VapoSteam Procter & Gamble	liquid		

See Chapter 8, "Cold, Cough and Allergy Products," for more information about these products.

Analgesic	Expectorant	Antitussive	Other Ingredients
			citric acid · D&C red#33 · FD&C green#3 · flavor · methylparaben · potassium sorbate · propylene glycol · purified water · sodium citrate · sorbitol · sucrose
acetaminophen, 650mg/30ml		dextromethorphan hydrobromide, 20mg/30ml	citric acid · FD&C yellow#6 · flavor · glycerin · polyethylene glycol · propylene glycol · purified water · saccharin sodium · sodium citrate · sucrose
acetaminophen, 250mg		dextromethorphan hydrobromide, 10mg	FD&C red#40 · FD&C yellow#6 · gelatin · polyethylene glycol · povidone · propylene glycol · purified water · sorbitol special
	guaifenesin, 200mg		colloidal silicon dioxide · crospovidone · FD&C yellow#6 aluminum lake · hydroxypropyl methylcellulose · microcrystalline cellulose · polyethylene glycol · polysorbate 80 · povidone · stearic acid · titanium dioxide
ibuprofen, 200mg			carnauba or equivalent wax · croscarmellose sodium · iron oxide · methylparaben · microcrystalline cellulose · propylparaben · silicon dioxide · sodium benzoate · sodium lauryl sulfate · starch · stearic acid · sucrose · titanium dioxide
		dextromethorphan hydrobromide, 15mg/15ml	citric acid · FD&C red#40 · flavor · potassium sorbate · propylene glycol · purified water · sodium citrate · sucrose
acetaminophen, 1000mg		dextromethorphan hydrobromide, 30mg	citric acid · flavor · sucrose
acetaminophen, 250mg		dextromethorphan hydrobromide, 10mg	D&C yellow#10 · FD&C blue#1 · gelatin · glycerin · polyethylene glycol · povidone · propylene glycol · purified water · sorbitol special
acetaminophen, 1000mg/30ml		dextromethorphan hydrobromide, 30mg/30ml	alcohol, 10% · citric acid · FD&C blue#1 · FD&C red#40 · flavor · high fructose corn syrup · polyethylene glycol · propylene glycol · purified water · saccharin sodium · sodium citrate
acetaminophen, 1000mg/30ml		dextromethorphan hydrobromide, 30mg/30ml	alcohol, 10% · citric acid · D&C yellow#10 · FD&C green#3 · FD&C yellow#6 · flavor · high fructose corn syrup · polyethylene glycol · propylene glycol · purified water · saccharin sodium · sodium citrate
		menthol, 3.1mg	citric acid · corn syrup · FD&C blue#1 · FD&C red#40 · flavor · sucrose
		menthol, 6.6mg	caramel · corn syrup · flavor · sucrose · tolu balsam · benzyl alcohol · camphor · eucalyptus oil · thymol
		camphor, 5.2% · menthol, 2.8% · eucalyptus oil, 1.2%	carbomer 954 · cedarleaf oil · cetyl alcohol · cetyl palmitate · cyclomethicone copolyol · dimethicone · EDTA · glycerin · imidazolidinyl urea · isopropyl palmitate · methylparaben · nutmeg oil · PEG-100 stearate · propylparaben · spirits of turperntine · thymol · purified water · sodium hydroxide · stearic acid · stearyl alcohol · titanium dioxide
		camphor, 4.8% · menthol, 2.6% · eucalyptus oil, 1.2%	cedarleaf oil · nutmeg oil · special petrolatum · spirits of turpentine · thymol
		camphor, 6.2%	alcohol, 78% · cedarleaf oil · nutmeg oil · poloxamer 124 · silicone · menthol · eucalyptus oil · laureth-7

TOPICAL DECONGESTANT PRODUCTS

	Product Manufacturer/Supplier	Dosage Form	Sympathomimetic	Preservative	Other Ingredients
	4-Way Fast Acting Bristol-Myers Products	nasal spray	phenylephrine HCl, 0.5% · naphazoline HCl, 0.05%	benzalkonium chloride	pyrilamine maleate, 0.2% · water · boric acid/sodium borate
	4-Way Long Lasting Bristol-Myers Products	nasal spray	oxymetazoline HCl, 0.05%	phenylmercuric acetate, 0.002% · benzalkonium chloride	glycine · sorbitol · water
	4-Way Mentholated Bristol-Myers Products	nasal spray	phenylephrine HCl, 0.5% · naphazoline HCl, 0.05%	benzalkonium chloride	pyrilamine maleate, 0.2% · camphor · eucalyptol · menthol · poloxamer 188 · polysorbate 80 · water · boric acid/sodium borate
	Afrin 12-Hour Schering-Plough Healthcare	nasal drops · nasal pump spray · nasal spray	oxymetazoline HCl, 0.05%	benzalkonium chloride · propylene glycol	disodium edetate · polyethylene glycol 1450 · povidone · sodium phosphate dibasic · sodium phosphate monobasic · water
	Afrin 12-Hour, Cherry Schering-Plough Healthcare	nasal spray	oxymetazoline HCl, 0.05%	benzalkonium chloride · benzyl alcohol · propylene glycol	disodium edetate · flavor · polyethylene glycol 1450 · sodium phosphate dibasic · sodium phosphate monobasic · water
	Afrin 12-Hour, Menthol Schering-Plough Healthcare	nasal spray	oxymetazoline HCl, 0.05%	benzalkonium chloride	camphor · eucalyptol · menthol · polysorbate 80
**	**Afrin 4-Hour Extra Moisturizing** Schering-Plough Healthcare	nasal spray	phenylephrine HCl, 0.5%	benzalkonium chloride, 0.14%	
	Afrin Extra Moisturizing Formula Schering-Plough Healthcare	nasal spray	oxymetazoline HCl, 0.05%	benzalkonium chloride · propylene glycol	polyethylene glycol 1450 · povidone · glycerin
	Afrin Sinus Schering-Plough Healthcare	nasal spray	oxymetazoline HCl, 0.05%	benzalkonium chloride · benzyl alcohol · propylene glycol	camphor · eucalyptol · menthol · polysorbate 80
	Benzedrex Menley & James Labs	nasal inhaler	propylhexedrine, 250mg		menthol · lavender oil
	Cheracol Roberts Ph'cal	nasal pump spray	oxymetazoline HCl, 0.05%	phenylmercuric acetate, 0.002% in an aqueous solution of benzalkonium chloride	glycine · sodium hydroxide · sorbitol · artificial cherry flavor · purified water
SL	**Dristan** Whitehall-Robins Healthcare	nasal spray	phenylephrine HCl, 0.5%	benzalkonium chloride, 0.02% · benzyl alcohol · disodium EDTA	pheniramine maleate, 0.2% · disodium phosphate · hydroxypropyl methylcellulose · phosphoric acid · sodium chloride · water
SL	**Dristan 12-Hour** Whitehall-Robins Healthcare	nasal spray	oxymetazoline HCl, 0.05%	benzalkonium chloride, 0.02% · thimerosal, 0.002%	hydroxypropyl methylcellulose · potassium phosphate · sodium chloride · sodium phosphate · water
	Duration Schering-Plough Healthcare	nasal spray	oxymetazoline HCl, 0.05%	benzalkonium chloride · propylene glycol	disodium edetate, polyethylene glycol 1450, povidone
PE	**Little Noses Decongestant** Vetco	nasal drops	phenylephrine HCl, 0.125%	thimerosal, 0.001% · benzalkonium chloride	citric acid · purified water · sodium chloride · sodium citrate
	Neo-Synephrine 12-Hour Bayer Consumer	nasal spray	oxymetazoline HCl, 0.05%	phenylmercuric acetate, 0.002% · benzalkonium chloride	
	Neo-Synephrine Extra Bayer Consumer	nasal drops · nasal spray	phenylephrine HCl, 1%	thimerosal, 0.001% · benzalkonium chloride	
	Neo-Synephrine Extra Moisturizing 12-Hour Bayer Consumer	nasal spray	oxymetazoline HCl, 0.05%	phenylmercuric acetate, 0.002% · benzalkonium chloride	glycine · purified water · sorbitol · may contain sodium chloride · glycerin
	Neo-Synephrine Mild Bayer Consumer	nasal drops · nasal spray	phenylephrine HCl, 0.25%	benzalkonium chloride · thimerosal, 0.001%	

See Chapter 8, "Cold, Cough and Allergy Products," for more information about these products.

TOPICAL DECONGESTANT PRODUCTS - continued

	Product Manufacturer/Supplier	Dosage Form	Sympathomimetic	Preservative	Other Ingredients
	Neo-Synephrine Regular Bayer Consumer	nasal drops · nasal spray	phenylephrine HCl, 0.5%	thimerosal, 0.001% · benzalkonium chloride	
SL	**Otrivin** Novartis Consumer	nasal drops · nasal spray	xylometazoline HCl, 0.1%	benzalkonium chloride, 0.02%	disodium edetate · sodium phosphate monobasic · sodium chloride · sodium phosphate dibasic · purified water
SL PE	**Otrivin Pediatric** Novartis Consumer	nasal drops	xylometazoline HCl, 0.05%	benzalkonium chloride, 0.02%	disodium edetate · sodium phosphate monobasic · sodium chloride · sodium phosphate dibasic · purified water
SL	**Pretz-D** Parnell Ph'cals	nasal spray	ephedrine, 0.25%	phenylmercuric acetate	glycerin, 3% · citric acid · sodium citrate · sodium chloride · yerba santa
SL	**Privine** Novartis Consumer	nasal drops · nasal spray	naphazoline HCl, 0.05%	benzalkonium chloride, 0.02%	disodium edetate · sodium chloride · dibasic sodium phosphate · monobasic sodium phosphate · purified water
SL	**Privine** Novartis Consumer	nasal solution	naphazoline HCl, 0.05%	benzalkonium chloride	disodium edetate dihydrate · hydrochloric acid · purified water · sodium chloride · trolamine
SL	**Rhinall** Scherer Labs	nasal drops · nasal spray	phenylephrine HCl, 0.25%	chlorobutanol · benzalkonium chloride	sodium bisulfite · sodium chloride · sorbitol · Tween 80 · disodium EDTA
SL	**Vicks Sinex 12-Hour Ultra Fine Mist** Procter & Gamble	nasal spray	oxymetazoline HCl, 0.05%	benzalkonium chloride · chlorhexidine gluconate	camphor · menthol · eucalyptol · disodium EDTA · potassium phosphate · purified water · sodium chloride · sodium phosphate · tyloxapol
SL	**Vicks Sinex Ultra Fine Mist** Procter & Gamble	nasal spray	phenylephrine HCl, 0.5%	benzalkonium chloride · chlorhexidine gluconate	camphor · eucalyptol · menthol · citric acid · purified · disodium EDTA · water · tyloxapol
SL	**Vicks Vapor Inhaler** Procter & Gamble	nasal inhaler	levodesoxyephedrine, 50mg/inhaler		bornyl acetate · camphor · lavender oil · menthol

** New listing

See Chapter 8, "Cold, Cough and Allergy Products," for more information about these products.

SORE THROAT PRODUCTS

	Product Manufacturer/Supplier	Dosage Form	Anesthetic [a]	Antibacterial [a]	Other Ingredients
**	**Bi-Zets** Reese Chemical	lozenge	benzocaine, 15mg		sucrose · corn sugar solids · glycerin · orange juice flavor · FD&C yellow#6
	Celestial Seasonings Soothers Herbal Throat Drops, Asst. Warner-Lambert Consumer	lozenge	menthol		corn syrup · pectin · natural flavors · oils of: angelica root, anise star, ginger, lemon grass, sage, white thyme · sucrose · Cherry: cherry · elderberry · pineapple juice · Golden: extracts of: chicory root, ginseng root, horehound, peppermint · Honey-Lemon Chamomile: chamomile flower extract · citric acid · honey · lemon juice · tea extract · Orange: beta carotene · citric acid · orange juice
** AF GL LA PU SO	**Cepacol Sore Throat Maximum Strength, Cherry** J. B. Williams	lozenge	benzocaine, 10mg · menthol, 3.6mg	cetylpyridinium chloride	D&C red#33 · FD&C red#40 · flavor · glucose · sucrose
** AF GL LA PU SU	**Cepacol Sore Throat Maximum Strength, Cherry** J. B. Williams	pump spray	dyclonine HCl, 0.1%	cetylpyridinium chloride	colors · flavors · dibasic sodium phosphate · glycerin · phosphoric acid · poloxamer · potassium sorbate · sorbitol · water
** AF GL LA PU SU	**Cepacol Sore Throat Maximum Strength, Cool Menthol** J. B. Williams	pump spray	dyclonine HCl, 0.1%	cetylpyridinium chloride	dibasic sodium phosphate · colors · flavors · glycerin · phosphoric acid · poloxamer · potassium sorbate · polysorbate 20 · saccharin sodium · sorbitol · water
AF GL LA PU SO	**Cepacol Sore Throat Maximum Strength, Mint** J. B. Williams	lozenge	benzocaine, 10mg · menthol, 2mg	cetylpyridinium chloride	D&C yellow#10 · FD&C yellow#6 · flavor · glucose · sucrose
AF GL LA PU SO	**Cepacol Sore Throat Regular Strength, Cherry** J. B. Williams	lozenge	menthol, 3.6mg	cetylpyridinium chloride	D&C red#33 · FD&C red#40 · flavor · glucose · sucrose
AF GL LA PU SO	**Cepacol Sore Throat Regular Strength, Original Mint** J. B. Williams	lozenge	menthol, 2mg	cetylpyridinium chloride	D&C yellow#10 · FD&C yellow#6 · flavor · glucose · sucrose
SU	**Cepastat Extra Strength Sore Throat** SmithKline Beecham	lozenge	phenol, 29mg · eucalyptus oil · menthol		antifoam emulsion · caramel · gum crystal · sorbitol

See Chapter 8, "Cold, Cough and Allergy Products," for more information about these products.

SORE THROAT PRODUCTS - continued

	Product Manufacturer/Supplier	Dosage Form	Anesthetic [a]	Antibacterial [a]	Other Ingredients
SU	**Cepastat Sore Throat, Cherry** SmithKline Beecham	lozenge	phenol, 14.5mg · menthol		antifoam emulsion · D&C red#33 · FD&C yellow#6 · flavor · gum crystal · saccharin sodium · sorbitol
	Cheracol Sore Throat Roberts Ph'cal	spray	phenol, 1.4%	alcohol, 12.5%	glycerin · propylene glycol · sodium citrate · saccharin sodium · citric acid · sorbitol
DY GL SU	**Entertainer's Secret Throat Relief** KLI Corp.	pump spray			water · glycerin · carboxymethylcellulose sodium · aloe vera gel · potassium chloride · dibasic sodium phosphate · flavor · methylparaben · propylparaben
GL LA SU	**Fisherman's Friend, Extra Strong, Sugar Free** Bristol-Myers Products	lozenge	menthol, 10mg · eucalyptus oil		sorbitol · natural licorice · magnesium stearate · capsicum
GL LA	**Fisherman's Friend, Licorice Strong** Bristol-Myers Products	lozenge	menthol, 6mg		sugar · licorice · edible gums · anise oil
GL LA	**Fisherman's Friend, Original Extra Strong** Bristol-Myers Products	lozenge	menthol, 10mg · eucalyptus oil		sugar · licorice · edible gums · capsicum
GL LA SU	**Fisherman's Friend, Refreshing Mint, Sugar Free** Bristol-Myers Products	lozenge	menthol, 3mg		sorbitol · peppermint oil · magnesium stearate · aspartame · phenylalanine
SU PE	**Halls Juniors Sugar Free Cough Drops, Grape or Orange** Warner-Lambert Consumer	lozenge	menthol, 2.5mg		acesulfame potassium · isomalt · natural flavor · eucalyptus oil · red#40 (Grape) · blue#1 (Grape) · yellow#6 (Orange)
	Halls Mentho-Lyptus Cough Supp. Drops, Cherry Warner-Lambert Consumer	lozenge	menthol, 7.6mg		corn syrup · flavor · sucrose · eucalyptus oil · blue#2 · red#40
	Halls Mentho-Lyptus Cough Supp. Drops, Honey-Lemon Warner-Lambert Consumer	lozenge	menthol, 8.6mg		flavor · corn syrup · sucrose · eucalyptus oil · beta carotene
	Halls Mentho-Lyptus Cough Supp. Drops, Mentho-Lyptus Warner-Lambert Consumer	lozenge	menthol, 7mg		corn syrup · flavor · sucrose · eucalyptus oil
	Halls Mentho-Lyptus Cough Supp. Drops, Spearmint Warner-Lambert Consumer	lozenge	menthol, 6mg		flavor · blue#1 · corn syrup · sucrose · eucalyptus oil

See Chapter 8, "Cold, Cough and Allergy Products," for more information about these products.

SORE THROAT PRODUCTS - continued

	Product Manufacturer/Supplier	Dosage Form	Anesthetic [a]	Antibacterial [a]	Other Ingredients
	Halls Mentho-Lyptus Ex. Strength Cough Supp. Drops, Ice Blue Warner-Lambert Consumer	lozenge	menthol, 12mg		flavor · blue#1 · corn syrup · sucrose · eucalyptus oil
SU	**Halls Mentho-Lyptus Sugar Free Cough Supp. Drops, Bl. Cherry** Warner-Lambert Consumer	lozenge	menthol, 5mg		acesulfame potassium · blue#1 · flavor · isomalt · red#40 · eucalyptus oil · citric acid
SU	**Halls Mentho-Lyptus Sugar Free Cough Supp. Drops, Citrus** Warner-Lambert Consumer	lozenge	menthol, 5mg		acesulfame potassium · flavor · isomalt · yellow#5 · citric acid · eucalyptus oil
SU	**Halls Mentho-Lyptus Sugar Free Cough Supp. Drops, Menthol** Warner-Lambert Consumer	lozenge	menthol, 6mg		acesulfame potassium · flavor · isomalt · eucalyptus oil
	Halls Plus Max. Strength; Cherry, Honey-Lemon, Mentho-Lyptus Warner-Lambert Consumer	lozenge	menthol, 10mg		eucalyptus oil · corn syrup · acesulfame potassium · flavoring · glycerin · high fructose corn syrup · sucrose · Cherry: blue#2 · red#40 · Honey-Lemon: honey · yellow#6 · yellow#10 · Mentho-Lyptus: citric acid
DY GL LA PU SO SU	**Herbal-Menthol** Shaklee	lozenge	menthol, 6mg (from peppermint)		brown rice syrup · corn syrup · honey · horehound extract · marshmallow root extract · peppermint oil · thyme extract · eucalyptus oil
	Isodettes Block Drug	lozenge	menthol, 10mg · benzocaine, 6mg		corn syrup · flavor · FD&C red#40 · FD&C blue#1 · sucrose · propylene glycol · sodium bicarbonate · water
	Isodettes, Cherry Block Drug	spray	phenol, 1.4%		propylene glycol · flavor · FD&C red#40 · water · sodium hydroxide
	Isodettes, Menthol Block Drug	spray	phenol, 1.4%		glycerin · flavor · menthol · sodium saccharin · D&C green#5 · D&C yellow#10 · FD&C green#3 · water
SU	**Luden's Maximum Strength Sugar Free, Cherry §** Hershey Foods	lozenge	menthol, 10mg · eucalyptus oil		isomalt · hydrogenated starch hydrolysate · citric acid · malic acid · flavoring · acesulfame potassium · artificial color
	Luden's Maximum Strength, Cherry § Hershey Foods	lozenge	menthol, 10mg · eucalyptus oil		sugar · corn syrup · citric acid · malic acid · flavoring · artificial color
	Luden's Maximum Strength, Menthol Eucalyptus § Hershey Foods	lozenge	menthol, 10mg · eucalyptus oil		sugar · corn syrup

See Chapter 8, "Cold, Cough and Allergy Products," for more information about these products.

SORE THROAT PRODUCTS - continued

	Product Manufacturer/Supplier	Dosage Form	Anesthetic [a]	Antibacterial [a]	Other Ingredients
	Luden's Original Menthol § Hershey Foods	lozenge	menthol		sugar · corn syrup · flavoring · caramel color
SU	**N'Ice 'N Clear, Cherry Eucalyptus** SmithKline Beecham	lozenge	menthol, 7mg		flavors · D&C red#33 · sorbitol · tartaric acid · FD&C yellow #6
SU	**N'Ice 'N Clear, Menthol Eucalyptus** SmithKline Beecham	lozenge	menthol, 5mg		citric acid · flavors · sorbitol
SU	**N'Ice Sore Throat & Cough, Assorted or Citrus** SmithKline Beecham	lozenge	menthol, 5mg		ascorbic acid (Asst.) · citric acid · natural colors · flavors · sodium citrate · sorbitol · tartaric acid (Asst.)
** SU	**N'Ice Sore Throat & Cough, Cherry** SmithKline Beecham	lozenge	menthol, 5mg		colors · sorbitol · flavors · tartaric acid
** SU	**N'Ice Sore Throat & Cough, Herbal Mint or Honey Lemon** SmithKline Beecham	lozenge	menthol, 5mg		citric acid · colors · flavor · sodium citrate · sorbitol · ascorbic acid (Lemon)
	Painalay Sore Throat Gargle Medtech	spray	phenol, 1.4%		
**	**Protac Troches** Republic Drug	lozenge	menthol, 10mg · benzocaine, 6mg		
AF DY GL LA PU SO	**Ricola Cough Drops, Original Flavor** Ricola	lozenge	menthol, 3mg		sugar · glucose syrup · caramelized sugar · extracts of: peppermint, lemon balm, thyme, sage, hyssop, elder, linden flowers, wild thyme, horehound, angelica root, peppermint oil
AF DY GL LA PU SO SU	**Ricola Sugar Free Herb Throat Drops, Alpine-Mint** Ricola	lozenge	menthol, 4.8mg		extracts of: peppermint, lemon balm, lady's mantle, linden flowers, elder · natural flavorings · citric acid · aspartame · chlorophyll · isomalt
AF DY GL LA PU SO SU	**Ricola Sugar Free Herb Throat Drops, Cherry- or Lemon-Mint** Ricola	lozenge	menthol, 1mg		extracts of: peppermint, lemon balm, lady's mantle, linden flowers, elder · citric acid · lemon and peppermint oils (Lemon-Mint) · cherry and peppermint flavorings (Cherry-Mint) · cherry and elderberry concentrates (Cherry-Mint) · ascorbic acid · aspartame · flavorings (Lemon-Mint) · isomalt

See Chapter 8, "Cold, Cough and Allergy Products," for more information about these products.

SORE THROAT PRODUCTS - continued

	Product Manufacturer/Supplier	Dosage Form	Anesthetic [a]	Antibacterial [a]	Other Ingredients
AF DY GL LA PU SO SU	**Ricola Sugar Free Herb Throat Drops, Mountain Herb** Ricola	lozenge	menthol, 1.5mg		extracts of: peppermint, lemon balm, thyme, sage, hyssop, elder, linden flowers, wild thyme, horehound, angelica root · caramel coloring · aspartame · peppermint oil · isomalt
AF DY GL LA PU SO	**Ricola Throat Drops, Cherry-Mint** Ricola	lozenge	menthol, 1.5mg		sugar · glucose syrup · citric acid · extracts of: peppermint, lemon balm, thyme, sage, hyssop, elder, linden flowers, wild thyme, horehound, angelica root · cherry concentrate · elder concentrate · cherry flavorings · peppermint oil
AF DY GL LA PU SO	**Ricola Throat Drops, Honey-Herb** Ricola	lozenge	menthol, 2.4mg		honey · sugar · corn syrup · extracts of: peppermint, lemon balm, thyme, sage, hyssop, elder, linden flowers, wild thyme, horehound, angelica root, peppermint oil
AF DY GL LA PU SO	**Ricola Throat Drops, Lemon-Mint or Orange-Mint** Ricola	lozenge	menthol, 1.25mg		sugar · glucose syrup · citric acid · extracts of: lemon balm, orange-mint (Orange-Mint), peppermint, thyme, sage, hyssop, elder, linden flowers, wild thyme, horehound, angelica root · lemon oil (Lemon-Mint) · peppermint oil · orange flavoring (Orange-Mint) · natural coloring (Lemon-Mint) · paprika extract (Orange-Mint)
AF DY GL LA PU SO	**Ricola Throat Drops, Menthol-Eucalyptus** Ricola	lozenge	menthol, 4.5mg		sugar · glucose syrup · extracts of: peppermint, lemon balm, thyme, sage, hyssop, elder, linden flowers, wild thyme, horehound, angelica root, peppermint oil, eucalyptus oil · chlorophyll
	Robitussin Cough Drops, Cherry or Menthol Eucalyptus Whitehall-Robins Healthcare	lozenge	menthol, 7.4mg · eucalyptus oil		corn syrup · FD&C red#40 (Cherry) · flavors (Cherry) · sucrose
	Robitussin Cough Drops, Honey-Lemon Whitehall-Robins Healthcare	lozenge	menthol, 10mg · eucalyptus oil		corn syrup · D&C yellow#10 · FD&C yellow#6 · flavors · sucrose · lemon oil · candy base · honey
	Robitussin Liquid Center Cough Drops, Cherry w/ Honey-Lemon Whitehall-Robins Healthcare	lozenge	menthol, 8mg · eucalyptus oil		corn syrup · FD&C red#40 · flavors · glycerin · high fructose corn syrup · honey · lemon oil · methylparaben · propylparaben · sodium benzoate · sorbitol · sucrose · candy base · water

See Chapter 8, "Cold, Cough and Allergy Products," for more information about these products.

SORE THROAT PRODUCTS - continued

	Product Manufacturer/Supplier	Dosage Form	Anesthetic [a]	Antibacterial [a]	Other Ingredients
	Robitussin Liquid Center Cough Drops, Honey-Lemon w/ Cherry Whitehall-Robins Healthcare	lozenge	menthol, 10mg · eucalyptus oil		D&C yellow#10 aluminum lake · FD&C yellow#6 aluminum lake · flavors · glycerin · high fructose corn syrup · honey · lemon oil · sorbitol · sucrose · titanium dioxide · water · candy base · glycerin · water
	Robitussin Liquid Center Cough Drops, Menthol Euc. w/Cherry Whitehall-Robins Healthcare	lozenge	menthol, 8mg · eucalyptus oil		corn syrup · flavors · glycerin · high fructose corn syrup · sorbitol · sucrose · water · candy base
SU	**Robitussin Sugar Free Cough Drops, Cherry or Peppermint** Whitehall-Robins Healthcare	lozenge	menthol, 10mg		aspartame · canola oil · FD&C blue#1 aluminum lake · FD&C red#40 aluminum lake (Cherry) · flavors · eucalyptus oil · lycasin · isomalt · water · candy base
	Spec-T Sore Throat Anesthetic Apothecon	lozenge	benzocaine, 10mg		agar FD&C red#40 · glucose · glycerin · sucrose · flavor
	Spec-T Sore Throat Cough Suppressant Apothecon	lozenge	benzocaine, 10mg		dextromethorphan hydrobromide, 10mg · FD&C yellow#5 (tartrazine) · FD&C yellow#6 · dextrose · flavor · glucose · glycerin · propylene glycol · sucrose
	Spec-T Sore Throat Decongestant Apothecon	lozenge	benzocaine, 10mg		phenylpropanolamine HC1, 10.5mg · phenylephrine HCl, 5mg · FD&C blue#1 · yellow#5 (tartrazine) · dextrose · flavor · glucose · glycerin · propylene glycol · sucrose
PE	**Sucrets Children's Sore Throat, Cherry** SmithKline Beecham	lozenge	dyclonine HCl, 1.2mg		citric acid · corn syrup · FD&C blue#1 · FD&C red#40 · flavor · mineral oil · silicon dioxide · sucrose
	Sucrets Maximum Strength Sore Throat, Vapor Black Cherry SmithKline Beecham	lozenge	dyclonine HCl, 3mg		corn syrup · FD&C blue#1 · FD&C red#40 · flavors · menthol · mineral oil · silicon dioxide · sucrose · tartaric acid
	Sucrets Maximum Strength Sore Throat, Wintergreen SmithKline Beecham	lozenge	dyclonine HCl, 3mg		citric acid · corn syrup · D&C yellow#10 · flavors · mineral oil · silicon dioxide · sucrose
	Sucrets Sore Throat, Assorted Flavors SmithKline Beecham	lozenge	dyclonine HCl, 2mg		citric acid · corn syrup · D&C yellow#10 · FD&C blue#1 · FD&C red#40 · flavors · mineral oil · silicon dioxide · sucrose · tartaric acid
	Sucrets Sore Throat, Original Mint SmithKline Beecham	lozenge		hexylresorcinol, 2.4mg	corn syrup · D&C yellow#10 · FD&C blue#1 · flavors · mineral oil · silicon dioxide · sucrose

See Chapter 8, "Cold, Cough and Allergy Products," for more information about these products.

SORE THROAT PRODUCTS - continued

	Product Manufacturer/Supplier	Dosage Form	Anesthetic [a]	Antibacterial [a]	Other Ingredients
**	**Tetra-Formula** Reese Chemical	lozenge	benzocaine, 15mg		dextromethorphan hydrobromide, 7.5mg · sucrose · corn sugar solids · glycerin · propylene glycol · dextrose · vanillin · FD&C blue#1 · FD&C red#40 · artificial cherry flavor
AL AF SO	**Vicks Chloraseptic Sore Throat, Cherry or Menthol** Procter & Gamble	spray	phenol, 1.4%		colors · flavors · glycerin · purified water · saccharin sodium · FD&C red#40 (Cherry) · D&C green#5 (Menthol) · D&C yellow#10 (Menthol)
	Vicks Chloraseptic Sore Throat, Cherry or Menthol Procter & Gamble	lozenge	menthol, 10mg · benzocaine, 6mg		corn syrup · FD&C yellow#10 (Menthol) · FD&C blue#1 · FD&C red#40 · FD&C yellow#6 (Menthol) · flavor · sucrose
	Vicks Cough Drops, Cherry Procter & Gamble	lozenge	menthol, 1.7mg		ascorbic acid · citric acid · corn syrup · FD&C blue#1 · FD&C red#40 · sucrose · eucalyptus oil · flavor
	Vicks Cough Drops, Menthol Procter & Gamble	lozenge	menthol, 3.3mg		ascorbic acid · caramel · corn syrup · sucrose · eucalyptus oil
	Vicks Original Cough Drops, Cherry Procter & Gamble	lozenge	menthol, 3.1mg		citric acid · corn syrup · FD&C blue#1 · FD&C red#40 · flavor · sucrose
	Vicks Original Cough Drops, Menthol Procter & Gamble	lozenge	menthol, 6.6mg		camphor · caramel · corn syrup · flavor · sucrose · tolu balsam · thymol · benzyl alcohol · eucalyptus oil

** New listing

§ Manufacturer/supplier did not confirm information for this edition. Product listing is reprinted from the '96-97 edition.

[a] Phenol is both an anesthetic and an antibacterial agent.

See Chapter 8, "Cold, Cough and Allergy Products," for more information about these products.

Asthma Product Tables

ASTHMA AUXILIARY DEVICES

Product Manufacturer/Supplier	Comments
PEAK FLOW METERS	
PE **Assess Low Range** HealthScan Products	measures within range of 30-390 Liters/min · accurate to ±5% · made from impact resistant polycarbonate plastic · transparent, to encourage regular cleaning · one-year warranty · disposable cardboard pediatric-sized mouthpiece available · main body dimensions: 8" x 1.5" x 1.3", weight: 2.6 oz.
Assess Standard Range HealthScan Products	measures within range of 60-880 Liters/min · accurate to ±5% · made from impact resistant polycarbonate plastic · transparent, to encourage regular cleaning · one-year warranty · disposable cardboard mouthpiece available · main body dimensions: 8" x 1.5" x 1.3", weight: 2.6 oz.
PE **Mini-Wright AFS Low Range** Clement Clarke	measures within range of 30-400 Liters/min · accurate to better than ±5% · individually custom calibrated for accuracy · disposable cardboard pediatric-sized mouthpiece available
Mini-Wright Standard Range Clement Clarke	measures within range of 60-850 Liters/min · accurate to better than ±5% · individually custom calibrated for accuracy · disposable cardboard mouthpiece available · can be disassembled for easy maintenance

See Chapter 9, "Asthma Products," for more information about these products.

ASTHMA INHALANT PRODUCTS

	Product Manufacturer/Supplier	Dosage Form [a]	Epinephrine	Other Ingredients
AL	**Asthma Haler** Menley & James Labs	oral inhaler	0.16mg base/spray (epinephrine bitartrate, 0.3mg/spray)	cetylpyridinium chloride · propellants · sorbitan trioleate
AL	**Asthma Nefrin** Menley & James Labs	solution for nebulization	2.25% base (as racemic epinephrine HCl)	chlorobutanol, 0.5% · benzoic acid · potassium metabisulfite · sodium metabisulfate · sodium chloride · propylene glycol · purified water
	Breatheasy Pascal	oral inhaler	2.2% (as epinephrine HCl)	benzyl alcohol, 1% · isotonic salts, 0.5%
AL PR SL	**Broncho Saline** Blairex Labs	solution		sodium chloride, 0.9%
SO SL	**Bronkaid Mist and Refill** Bayer Consumer	oral inhaler	0.25mg base/spray (as nitrate and HCl salts)	alcohol, 33%
	Bronkaid Mist Suspension Bayer Consumer	oral inhaler	epinephrine bitartrate, 7mg/ml	
	Micro NEFRIN Bird Products	solution for nebulization	2.25% base (as racemic epinephrine HCl)	chlorobutanol, 0.5g
SL	**Primatene Mist** Whitehall-Robins Healthcare	oral inhaler	5.5mg/ml	alcohol, 34% · ascorbic acid · fluorocarbons (propellant) · water · hydrochloric acid · nitric acid
AL PR SU SL	**Sodium Chloride Inhalation Solution USP** Dey Labs	solution		sodium chloride, 0.45%; 0.9%

See Chapter 9, "Asthma Products," for more information about these products.

ASTHMA ORAL PRODUCTS

	Product Manufacturer/Supplier	Dosage Form	Ephedrine [a]	Other Ingredients
GL SO	**Bronkaid Dual Action Formula** Bayer Consumer	caplet	25mg (as sulfate)	guaifenesin, 400mg
	Dynafed Two-Way BDI Ph'cals	tablet	25mg (as HCl)	guaifenesin, 200mg · magnesium stearate · ditab
	Mini Two-Way Action BDI Ph'cals	tablet	25mg (as HCl)	guaifenesin, 200mg · magnesium stearate · ditab
GL PU SO	**Primatene** Whitehall-Robins Healthcare	tablet	12.5mg (as HCl)	guaifenesin, 200mg · crospovidone · FD&C yellow#6 lake · magnesium stearate · microcrystalline cellulose · povidone · silicon dioxide · purified water

[a] Several states have placed restrictions on the nonprescription status of ephedrine due to its abuse potential.

See Chapter 9, "Asthma Products," for more information about these products.

Sleep Aid and Stimulant Product Tables

SLEEP AID PRODUCTS

	Product Manufacturer/Supplier	Dosage Form	Antihistamine	Other Ingredients
**	**Alka-Seltzer PM** Bayer Consumer	effervescent tablet	diphenhydramine citrate, 38mg	aspirin, 325mg · acesulfame potassium · aspartame · citric acid · flavors · sodium bicarbonate · tableting aids
AF	**Anacin P.M. Aspirin Free** Whitehall-Robins Healthcare	caplet	diphenhydramine HCl, 25mg	acetaminophen, 500mg · calcium stearate · FD&C blue#1 lake · hydroxypropyl methylcellulose · magnesium stearate · microcrystalline cellulose · polyethylene glycol · povidone · starch · stearic acid · titanium dioxide
DY GL SO	**Arthriten PM** Alva-Amco Pharmacal	caplet	diphenhydramine HCl, 25mg	acetaminophen, 250mg · magnesium salicylate, 250mg · magnesium carbonate · magnesium oxide · calcium carbonate
AF GL SO	**Backaid PM Pills** Alva-Amco Pharmacal	caplet	diphenhydramine HCl, 25mg	acetaminophen, 500mg
	Bayer PM Extra Strength Bayer Consumer	caplet	diphenhydramine HCl, 25mg	aspirin, 500mg · colloidal silicon dioxide · dibasic calcium phosphate · dibutyl sebacate · ethylcellulose · FD&C blue#1 lake · FD&C blue#2 lake · hydroxypropyl methylcellulose · microcrystalline cellulose · oleic acid · propylene glycol · starch · titanium dioxide · zinc stearate
**	**Bayer PM Extra Strength Aspirin with Sleep Aid** Bayer Consumer	caplet	diphenhydramine HCl, 25mg	aspirin, 500mg · colloidal silicon dioxide · dibasic calcium phosphate · dibutyl sebacate · ethylcellulose · FD&C blue#1 lake · FD&C blue#2 lake · hydroxypropyl methylcellulose · oleic acid · propylene glycol · starch · titanium dioxide · zinc stearate
	Compoz Medtech	gelcap · tablet	diphenhydramine HCl, 50mg	
GL	**Doan's P.M. Extra Strength** Novartis Consumer	caplet	diphenhydramine HCl, 25mg	magnesium salicylate tetrahydrate, 580mg · carnauba wax · colloidal silicon dioxide · croscarmellose sodium · microcrystalline cellulose · magnesium stearate · Opadry blue · stearic acid · talc
	Dormarex Republic Drug	capsule	diphenhydramine HCl, 50mg	
	Dormarex 2 Republic Drug	caplet	diphenhydramine HCl, 50mg	
AF GL PU SO	**Dormin** Randob Labs	capsule	diphenhydramine HCl, 25mg	lactose · magnesium stearate · polyethylene glycol · silicon dioxide · talc
** AF	**Excedrin PM** Bristol-Myers Products	geltab	diphenhydramine citrate, 38mg	acetaminophen, 500mg · benzoic acid · corn starch · D&C red#33 lake · D&C yellow#10 · D&C yellow#10 lake · disodium edetate · FD&C blue#1 · FD&C blue#1 lake · gelatin · glycerin · hydroxypropyl methylcellulose · magnesium stearate · methylparaben · mineral oil · polysorbate 20 · povidone · pregelatinized starch · propylene glycol · propylparaben · simethicone emulsion · sorbitan monolaurate · stearic acid · titanium acid
AF GL SO	**Excedrin PM** Bristol-Myers Products	caplet · tablet	diphenhydramine citrate, 38mg	acetaminophen, 500mg · benzoic acid · carnauba wax · corn starch · D&C yellow#10 · D&C yellow#10 aluminum lake · FD&C blue#1 · FD&C blue#1 aluminum lake · hydroxypropyl methylcellulose · magnesium stearate · methylparaben · pregelatinized starch · propylparaben · simethicone emulsion · stearic acid · titanium dioxide · may also contain mineral oil · polysorbate 20 · povidone · sodium citrate · sorbitan monolaurate

See Chapter 10, "Sleep Aid and Stimulant Products," for more information about these products.

SLEEP AID PRODUCTS - continued

	Product Manufacturer/Supplier	Dosage Form	Antihistamine	Other Ingredients
**	**Goody's PM** Goody's Ph'cals	powder	diphenhydramine citrate, 38mg	acetaminophen, 500mg · citric acid · docusate sodium · fumaric acid · glycine · lactose · magnesium stearate · potassium chloride · silica gel · sodium citrate dihydrate
	Legatrin PM Columbia Labs	caplet	diphenhydramine HCl, 50mg	acetaminophen, 500mg · dicalcium phosphate · croscarmellose sodium · stearic acid · microcrystalline cellulose · magnesium stearate · FD&C blue#2 aluminum lake · FD&C red#40 aluminum lake · hydroxypropyl methylcellulose · polyethylene glycol · talc · titanium dioxide
GL SO	**Melatonex** Sunsource	timed-release tablet		pyridoxine HCl, 10mg · melatonin, 3mg · dicalcium phosphate · microcrystalline cellulose · glyceryl monstearate · magnesium stearate
**	**Melatonin** Natrol	softgel		melatonin, 3mg
**	**Melatonin** Natrol	tablet · timed-release tablet		pyridoxine HCl, 10mg (tablet) · melatonin, 3mg
**	**Melatonin** Hudson	timed-release tablet		melatonin, 2mg
**	**Melatonin** Natrol	lozenge		melatonin, 3mg · xylitol · lemon flavoring
** AF	**Melatonin PM Dual Release** Celestial Seasonings	tablet		calcium, 10mg · vitamin B6, 10mg · magnesium, 5mg · niacin, 5mg · melatonin, 3mg · dibasic calcium phosphate · microcrystalline cellulose · maltodextrin · lactose · hydroxypropyl methylcellulose · stearic acid · croscarmellose sodium · magnesium stearate · silica · FD&C blue#1
** AF	**Melatonin PM Fast Acting** Celestial Seasonings	chewable tablet		calcium, 10mg · vitamin B6, 10mg · magnesium, 5mg · niacin, 5mg · melatonin, 3mg · xylitol · sorbitol · mannitol · dextrose · sucrose · magnesium stearate · starch · one or more of: citric acid, malic acid, adipic acid · monoglyceride · diglyceride · silicon dioxide · natural flavors
AF GL SO	**Midol PM Night Time Formula** Bayer Consumer	caplet	diphenhydramine HCl, 25mg	acetaminophen, 500mg
AF	**Nervine Nighttime Sleep-Aid** Bayer Consumer	caplet	diphenhydramine HCl, 25mg	calcium phosphate dibasic · calcium sulfate · carboxymethylcellulose sodium · corn starch · magnesium stearate · microcrystalline cellulose
	NiteGel Republic Drug	liquid-cap	doxylamine succinate, 6.25mg	acetaminophen, 250mg · pseudoephedrine HCl, 30mg · dextromethorphan hydrobromide, 10mg
AF DY	**Nytol** Block Drug	caplet	diphenhydramine HCl, 25mg	cellulose · corn starch · lactose · silica · stearic acid
AF	**Nytol Maximum Strength** Block Drug	softgel	diphenhydramine HCl, 50mg	polyethylene glycol · gelatin · glycerin · sorbitol · water · edible ink
AF GL PU	**Sleep Rite** Hudson	tablet	diphenhydramine HCl, 25mg	

See Chapter 10, "Sleep Aid and Stimulant Products," for more information about these products.

SLEEP AID PRODUCTS - continued

	Product Manufacturer/Supplier	Dosage Form	Antihistamine	Other Ingredients
**	**Sleep-Ettes D** Reese Chemical	caplet	diphenhydramine HCl, 50mg	D&C yellow#10 · di-pac compressed sugar · microcrystalline cellulose · sodium starch glycolate · stearic acid · pregelatinized starch
AF GL SO	**Sleep-eze 3** Medtech	tablet	diphenhydramine HCl, 25mg	croscarmellose sodium · dicalcium phosphate · D&C yellow#10 · FD&C yellow#6 · magnesium stearate · microcrystalline cellulose · stearic acid
AF GL PU SO	**Sleepinal** Thompson Medical	softgel	diphenhydramine HCl, 50mg	D&C yellow#10 · FD&C blue#1 · gelatin · glycerin · polyethylene glycol 400 · povidone 30 · propylene glycol · sorbitol · water · may also contain FD&C green#3
AF GL PU SO	**Sleepinal** Thompson Medical	capsule	diphenhydramine HCl, 50mg	lactose · magnesium stearate · talc
	Snooze Fast BDI Ph'cals	tablet	diphenhydramine HCl, 50mg	FD&C blue#1 aluminum lake
AF	**Sominex Maximum Strength** SmithKline Beecham	caplet	diphenhydramine HCl, 50mg	carnauba wax · crospovidone · dibasic calcium phosphate · FD&C blue#1 aluminum lake · hydroxypropyl methylcellulose · magnesium stearate · microcrystalline cellulose · polyethylene glycol · polysorbate 80 · silicon dioxide · starch · titanium dioxide
AF	**Sominex Original** SmithKline Beecham	tablet	diphenhydramine HCl, 25mg	dibasic calcium phosphate · FD&C blue#1 aluminum lake · magnesium stearate · microcrystalline cellulose · silicon dioxide · starch
AF	**Sominex Pain Relief Formula** SmithKline Beecham	tablet	diphenhydramine HCl, 25mg	acetaminophen, 500mg · colloidal silicon dioxide · corn starch · crospovidone · FD&C blue#1 aluminum lake · stearic acid · pregelatinized starch · povidone
AF DY GL SO	**Tranquil** Alva-Amco Pharmacal	tablet	diphenhydramine HCl, 25mg	lactose microcrystalline cellulose · stearic acid · magnesium stearate
AF DY GL LA SO	**Tranquil Plus** Alva-Amco Pharmacal	caplet	diphenhydramine HCl, 25mg	acetaminophen, 250mg · magnesium salicylate, 250mg · magnesium carbonate · magnesium oxide · calcium carbonate
AF	**Tylenol PM Extra Strength** McNeil Consumer	gelcap · geltab	diphenhydramine HCl, 25mg	acetaminophen, 500mg · benzyl alcohol · butylparaben · castor oil · cellulose · corn starch · edetate calcium disodium · gelatin · hydroxypropyl methylcellulose · magnesium stearate · propylparaben · sodium lauryl sulfate · sodium citrate · sodium propionate · sodium starch glycolate · titanium dioxide · blue#1 · red#28
AF	**Tylenol PM Extra Strength** McNeil Consumer	caplet	diphenhydramine HCl, 25mg	acetaminophen, 500mg · cellulose · corn starch · hydroxypropyl methylcellulose · magnesium stearate or stearic acid · colloidal silicon dioxide · polyethylene glycol · polysorbate 80 · sodium citrate · sodium starch glycolate · titanium dioxide · blue#1 · blue#2
AF GL PU	**Unisom Nighttime Sleep Aid** Pfizer Consumer	tablet	doxylamine succinate, 25mg	microcrystalline cellulose · dibasic calcium phosphate dihydrate · sodium starch glycolate · magnesium stearate · FD&C blue#1 aluminum lake

See Chapter 10, "Sleep Aid and Stimulant Products," for more information about these products.

SLEEP AID PRODUCTS - continued

	Product Manufacturer/Supplier	Dosage Form	Antihistamine	Other Ingredients
AF GL PU SO	**Unisom Pain Relief** Pfizer Consumer	tablet	diphenhydramine HCl, 50mg	acetaminophen, 650mg · corn starch · polyvinylpyrolidone · stearic acid · Opadry blue · Opadry clear · magnesium stearate
	Unisom Sleepgels Pfizer Consumer	softgel	diphenhydramine HCl, 50mg	polyethylene glycol 400 · water · gelatin · sorbitol special glycerin blend 50/50 · glycerin · FD&C blue#1 · pharmaceutical glaze · propylene glycol · titanium dioxide

** New listing

STIMULANT PRODUCTS

Product Manufacturer/Supplier	Dosage Form	Caffeine	Other Ingredients
20/20 Tablets BDI Ph'cals	tablet	200mg	FD&C yellow#6 alum. lake · FD&C red#10 alum. lake · FD&C blue#1 alum. lake · FD&C blue#2 alum. lake
357 Magnum II BDI Ph'cals	tablet	200mg	FD&C red#40 alum. lake · FD&C yellow#6 alum. lake · FD&C blue#1 alum. lake · FD&C blue#2 alum. lake
GL PU SO **Caffedrine** Thompson Medical	caplet	200mg	calcium sulfate · lactose · ethylcellulose · povidone · isopropyl alcohol · stearic acid · magnesium stearate · methyl alcohol · hydroxypropyl methylcellulose · triacetin · FD&C yellow#6 alum. lake · D&C yellow#10 alum. lake · titanium dioxide · propylene glycol
GL PU SO **Enerjets** Chilton Labs	lozenge	75mg	sugar · flavoring
** **High Gear** GumTech	gum	25mg	sorbitol · gum base · sugar · maltitol syrup · cocoa powder · mannitol · glycerin · flavorings · guarana · kola nut · siberian ginseng · aspartame · titanium dioxide · acesulfame potassium
King of Hearts BDI Ph'cals	tablet	200mg	FD&C red#40 aluminum lake · FD&C red#6 aluminum lake
GL SO **No Doz** Bristol-Myers Products	chewable tablet	100mg	aspartame · crospovidone · dicalcium phosphate · ethylcellulose · flavor · magnesium stearate · mannitol · microcrystalline cellulose
GL SO **No Doz Maximum Strength** Bristol-Myers Products	caplet	200mg	benzoic acid · corn starch · FD&C blue#1 · flavor · hydroxypropyl methylcellulose · microcrystalline cellulose · propylene glycol · simethicone emulsion · stearic acid · sucrose · titanium dioxide · water · may also contain: carnauba wax · mineral oil · polysorbate 20 · povidone · sorbitan monolaurate
Overtime BDI Ph'cals	tablet	200mg	
GL SO **Pep-Back** Alva-Amco Pharmacal	tablet	100mg	calcium carbonate
GL SO **Pep-Back Ultra** Alva-Amco Pharmacal	caplet	200mg	calcium carbonate
GL PU SO **Quick-Pep** Thompson Medical	tablet	150mg	dextrose · microcrystalline cellulose · sodium starch glycolate · colloidal silicon dioxide · FD&C yellow#6 alum. lake · D&C yellow#10 alum. lake · stearic acid · magnesium stearate · FD&C red#3 · starch · sucrose · talc
Vivarin SmithKline Beecham	caplet	200mg	carnauba wax · colloidal silicon dioxide · D&C yellow#10 aluminum lake · FD&C yellow#6 aluminum lake · dextrose · hydroxypropyl methylcellulose · magnesium stearate · microcrystalline cellulose · polyethylene glycol · polysorbate 80 · starch · titanium dioxide
Vivarin SmithKline Beecham	tablet	200mg	dextrose · D&C yellow#10 aluminum lake · FD&C yellow#6 aluminum lake · magnesium stearate · microcrystalline cellulose · colloidal silicon dioxide · starch

See Chapter 10, "Sleep Aid and Stimulant Products," for more information about these products.

Acid-Peptic Product Tables

HISTAMINE II RECEPTOR ANTAGONISTS

	Product Manufacturer/Supplier	Dosage Form	Histamine II Receptor Antagonist	Other Ingredients
GL SU	**Axid AR** Whitehall-Robins Healthcare	tablet	nizatidine, 75mg	colloidal silicon dioxide · hydroxypropyl methylcellulose · synthetic iron oxides · magnesium stearate · microcrystalline cellulose · polyethylene glycol · pregelatinized starch · propylene glycol · corn starch · titanium dioxide
**	**Mylanta·AR** Johnson & Johnson·Merck	tablet	famotidine, 10mg	hydroxypropyl cellulose · hydroxypropyl methylcellulose · magnesium stearate · microcrystalline cellulose · starch · talc · titanium dioxide
	Pepcid AC Johnson & Johnson·Merck	tablet	famotidine, 10mg	hydroxypropyl cellulose · hydroxypropyl methylcellulose · red iron oxide · magnesium stearate · microcrystalline cellulose · starch · talc · titanium dioxide
** DY GL PU SO SU	**Tagamet HB 200** SmithKline Beecham	tablet	cimetidine, 200mg	cellulose · corn starch · hydroxypropyl methylcellulose · magnesium stearate · polyethylene glycol · polysorbate 80 · povidone · sodium lauryl sulfate · sodium starch glycolate · titanium dioxide
SO SU	**Zantac 75** Warner-Lambert Consumer	tablet	ranitidine HCl, 84mg (equivalent to ranitidine, 75mg)	hydroxypropyl methylcellulose · magnesium stearate · microcrystalline cellulose · synthetic red iron oxide · titanium dioxide · triacetin

** New listing

ANTIFLATULENT PRODUCTS

Product [a] Manufacturer/Supplier	Dosage Form	Simethicone	Other Ingredients
Alka-Seltzer Anti-Gas Bayer Consumer	gelcap	125mg	D&C red#33 · FD&C blue#1 · FD&C red#40 · gelatin · glycerin · peppermint oil · purified water · sorbitol · titanium dioxide
** DY SU PE **Baby Gasz** Lee Consumer	drops	40mg/0.6ml	purified water · silica · hydrogenated tallow glycerides · polyethylene glycol stearate · potassium sorbate
Beano AkPharma	drops		water · sorbitol · alpha galactosidase enzyme (from aspergillus niger) · salt · disodium citrate · potassium sorbate
Beano AkPharma	tablet		alpha galactosidase enzyme (from aspergillus niger) · corn starch · mannitol · sorbitol · hydrogenated cottonseed oil · invertase · gelatin · magnesium silicate · magnesium stearate
DY GL **Charcoal** Requa	tablet		activated charcoal, 250mg · sugar, 250mg
Charcoal Plus DS Kramer Labs	tablet		activated charcoal, 250mg · eugragit L 30 D · HPMC · PEG-400 · talc · titanium dioxide · red#40 · sorbitol · acacia gum · avicel · silica · magnesium stearate
DY GL SU **CharcoCaps** Requa	capsule		activated charcoal, 260mg
SO **Di-Gel** Schering-Plough Healthcare	liquid	20mg/5ml	aluminum hydroxide, 200mg/5ml · magnesium hydroxide, 200mg/5ml
SO **Di-Gel** Schering-Plough Healthcare	chewable tablet	20mg	calcium carbonate, 280mg · magnesium hydroxide, 128mg · mint or lemon/orange flavor
GL PU SO **Gas-X** Novartis Consumer	chewable tablet	80mg	calcium carbonate · dextrose · maltodextrin · cherry or peppermint creme flavor · red#30
GL PU SO **Gas-X Extra Strength** Novartis Consumer	chewable tablet	125mg	tribasic calcium phosphate · colloidal silicon dioxide · cherry or peppermint creme flavor · dextrose · maltodextrin · silicon dioxide · red#30 · yellow#10
SU **Gas-X Extra Strength** Novartis Consumer	softgel	125mg	blue#1 · gelatin · glycerin · peppermint oil · red#40 · sorbitol · titanium dioxide · water · yellow#10
PU SO **Gelusil** Warner-Lambert Consumer	chewable tablet	25mg	aluminum hydroxide (dried gel), 200mg · magnesium hydroxide, 200mg · flavors · magnesium stearate · mannitol · sorbitol · sugar
SO **Kudrox** Schwarz Pharma	suspension	40mg/5ml	aluminum hydroxide, 500mg/5ml · magnesium hydroxide, 450mg/5ml
DY SO SU PE **Little Tummys Infant Gas Relief** Vetco	drops	20mg/0.3ml	citric acid · purified water · sodium benzoate · microcrystalline cellulose · xanthan gum · natural flavor · acesulfame K
PU **Maalox Antacid Plus Anti-Gas** Novartis Consumer	tablet	25mg	magnesium hydroxide, 200mg · aluminum hydroxide gel, 200mg · D&C red#30 · D&C yellow#10 or D&C red#30 · dextrose · flavors · magnesium stearate · mannitol · saccharin sodium · sorbitol · starch · sugar · talc

See Chapter 11, "Acid-Peptic Products," for more information about these products.

ANTIFLATULENT PRODUCTS - continued

	Product [a] Manufacturer/Supplier	Dosage Form	Simethicone	Other Ingredients
PU	**Maalox Antacid Plus Anti-Gas Extra Strength** Novartis Consumer	tablet	30mg	magnesium hydroxide, 350mg · aluminum hydroxide, 350mg · FD&C blue#1 · D&C yellow#10 · may contain D&C red#30 · dextrose · flavors · glycerin · magnesium stearate · mannitol · saccharin sodium · sorbitol · starch · sugar
GL SO SU SL	**Maalox Antacid/Anti-Gas Extra Strength** Novartis Consumer	suspension	40mg/5ml	aluminum hydroxide, 500mg/5ml (equivalent to dried gel) · magnesium hydroxide, 450mg/5ml · calcium saccharin · flavors · methylparaben · propylparaben · purified water · sorbitol
PU	**Maalox Anti-Gas** Novartis Consumer	tablet	80mg	corn starch · D&C red#30 · D&C yellow#10 or D&C red#27 aluminun lake · flavor · gelatin · mannitol · sucrose · tribasic calcium · phosphate
PU	**Maalox Anti-Gas Extra Strength** Novartis Consumer	tablet	150mg	corn starch · D&C red#30 aluminum lake · D&C yellow#10 or D&C red#27 aluminum lake · flavor · gelatin · mannitol · sucrose · tribasic calcium phosphate
SO	**Mylanta** Johnson & Johnson·Merck	suspension	20mg/5ml	aluminum hydroxide, 200mg/5ml · magnesium hydroxide, 200mg/5ml
	Mylanta Gas Relief Johnson & Johnson·Merck	chewable tablet	80mg	
	Mylanta Gas Relief Maximum Strength Johnson & Johnson·Merck	gelcap	62.5mg	
	Mylanta Gas Relief Maximum Strength Johnson & Johnson·Merck	chewable tablet	125mg	
SO	**Mylanta Maximum Strength** Johnson & Johnson·Merck	suspension	40mg/5ml	aluminum hydroxide, 400mg/5ml · magnesium hydroxide, 400mg/5ml
PE	**Mylicon, Infant's** Johnson & Johnson·Merck	drops	40mg/0.6ml	
	Phazyme Gas Relief Block Drug	tablet	95mg	acacia · carnauba wax · compressible sugar · croscarmellose sodium · FD&C red#40 lake · FD&C yellow#6 lake · hydroxypropyl methylcellulose · microcrystalline cellulose · polyoxyl 40 stearate · povidone · sodium benzoate · sucrose · talc · titanium dioxide · white wax
DY PE	**Phazyme Gas Relief** Block Drug	drops	40mg/0.6ml	carbomer 974P · citric acid · flavor · hydroxypropyl methylcellulose · PEG-8 stearate · sodium benzoate · sodium citrate · water
	Phazyme Gas Relief Maximum Strength Block Drug	chewable tablet	125mg	citric acid · D&C yellow#10 · dextrates · FD&C blue#1 · peppermint flavor · sorbitol · starch · sucrose · talc · tribasic calcium phosphate
	Phazyme Gas Relief Maximum Strength Block Drug	softgel	125mg	FD&C red#40 · gelatin · glycerin · hydrogenated soybean oil · lecithin · methylparaben · polysorbate 80 · propylparaben · soybean oil · titanium dioxide · vegetable shortening · yellow wax

See Chapter 11, "Acid-Peptic Products," for more information about these products.

ANTIFLATULENT PRODUCTS - continued

	Product [a] Manufacturer/Supplier	Dosage Form	Simethicone	Other Ingredients
**	**Phazyme Gas Relief Maximum Strength** Block Drug	liquid	125mg	bentonite · flavor · glycerin · hydrochloric acid · hydroxyethyl cellulose · PEG-40 stearate · sodium benzoate · saccharin sodium · titanium dioxide · water
**	**Phazyme Gas Relief, Cherry or Mint** Block Drug	liquid	62.5mg/5ml	bentonite · flavor · glycerin · hydrochloric acid · hydroxyethyl cellulose · PEG-40 stearate · sodium benzoate · saccharin sodium · titanium dioxide · water
SO SL	**Riopan Plus** Whitehall-Robins Healthcare	suspension	40mg/5ml	magaldrate, 540mg/5ml · mint flavor · glycerin · PEG-8 stearate · potassium citrate · saccharin · sorbitan monostearate · sorbitol · xanthan gum · water · aluminum hydroxide gel · calcium hypochlorite · strong ammonia solution
GL PU SO	**Riopan Plus** Whitehall-Robins Healthcare	chewable tablet	20mg	magaldrate, 480mg · mint flavor · magnesium stearate · polyethylene glycol · silicon dioxide · sorbitol · starch · sucrose · titanium dioxide
GL PU SO	**Riopan Plus Double Strength** Whitehall-Robins Healthcare	chewable tablet	20mg	magaldrate, 1080mg · mint flavor · magnesium stearate · methylcellulose · polyethylene glycol · saccharin · silicon dioxide · sorbitol · starch · titanium dioxide · silica gel · saccharin
SO SL	**Riopan Plus Double Strength, Cherry or Mint** Whitehall-Robins Healthcare	suspension	40mg/5ml	magaldrate, 1080mg/5ml · flavors · glycerin · PEG-8 stearate · potassium citrate · saccharin · sorbitan monostearate · sorbitol · xanthan gum · water · aluminum hydroxide gel · calcium hypochlorite · strong ammonia solution
	Titralac Plus 3M Health Care	chewable tablet	21mg	calcium carbonate, 420mg · glycine · magnesium stearate · saccharin · spearmint oil · starch · may contain croscarmellose sodium
	Titralac Plus 3M Health Care	liquid	20mg/5ml	calcium carbonate, 500mg/5ml · benzyl alcohol · glyceryl laurate · methylparaben · potassium benzoate · propylparaben · saccharin · sorbitol · spearmint flavor · water · xanthan gum
GL PU	**Tums Anti-Gas/Antacid** SmithKline Beecham	chewable tablet	20mg	calcium carbonate, 500mg · adipic acid · corn syrup · D&C red#27 · D&C red#30 · D&C yellow#10 · FD&C blue#1 · FD&C yellow#6 · flavors · glycerin · microcrystalline cellulose · mineral oil · sodium polyphosphate · starch · sucrose · talc · triglycerol monooleate

** New listing

[a] Combination simethicone-antacid products listed in this table are limited to those that contain at least 40mg of simethicone per dose, which is the lowest recommended adult dose (taken 4 times daily) for relief of flatulence. The Antacid and Antireflux Products table lists combination antacid-simethicone products that contain less than 40mg of simethicone per dose.

See Chapter 11, "Acid-Peptic Products," for more information about these products.

ANTACID AND ANTIREFLUX PRODUCTS

Product [a] Manufacturer/Supplier	Dosage Form	Calcium Carbonate	Aluminum Hydroxide	Magnesium Salts	Other Antacids	Other Ingredients
Acid-X BDI Ph'cals	tablet	250mg				acetaminophen, 500mg
Alka-Mints Bayer Consumer	chewable tablet	850mg				dioctyl sodium sulfosuccinate · flavor · hydrolyzed cereal solids · magnesium stearate · polyethylene glycol · sorbitol · sugar (compressible)
Alka-Seltzer Bayer Consumer	gelcap	500mg				FD&C blue#1 · FD&C green#3 · FD&C red#40 · gelatin · glycerin · maltitol · peppermint oil · polyethylene glycol · purified water · titanium dioxide
Alka-Seltzer Bayer Consumer	caplet	380mg				acetaminophen, 500mg · crospovidone · docusate sodium · hydroxypropyl methylcellulose · lecithin · magnesium stearate · polyvinylpyrrolidone · sodium benzoate · sodium hexametaphosphate · sodium starch glycolate · starch · stearic acid
Alka-Seltzer Extra Strength Bayer Consumer	effervescent tablet				sodium bicarbonate, 1985mg (sodium, 588mg)	citric acid, 1000mg · aspirin, 500mg
Alka-Seltzer Gold Bayer Consumer	effervescent tablet				sodium bicarbonate, 958mg (sodium, 311mg) · potassium bicarbonate, 312mg	citric acid, 832mg · tableting aid
Alka-Seltzer Original Bayer Consumer	effervescent tablet				sodium bicarbonate, 1916mg (sodium, 567mg)	citric acid, 1000mg · aspirin, 325mg
Alka-Seltzer, Cherry Bayer Consumer	effervescent tablet				sodium bicarbonate, 1700 mg (sodium, 506mg)	citric acid, 1000mg · aspirin, 325mg · aspartame · flavor · tableting aid

See Chapter 11, "Acid-Peptic Products," for more information about these products.

ANTACID AND ANTIREFLUX PRODUCTS - continued

Product [a] Manufacturer/Supplier	Dosage Form	Calcium Carbonate	Aluminum Hydroxide	Magnesium Salts	Other Antacids	Other Ingredients
PU SU	**Alka-Seltzer, Lemon-Lime** Bayer Consumer	efferverscent tablet				sodium bicarbonate, 1700mg (sodium, 506mg)	citric acid, 1000mg · aspirin, 325mg · aspartame · flavor · tableting aid
	Alkets Lee Consumer	chewable tablet	500mg				dextrose · flavors · magnesium stearate · maltodexrin
	Alkets Extra Strength Lee Consumer	chewable tablet	750mg				dextrose · flavors · magnesium stearate · maltodexrin
GL LA PU SU	**Almora** Forest Ph'cals	chewable tablet			500mg (as gluconate dihydrate) · 2.8mg (as stearate)		starch 1500, 79.22mg · stearic acid hystrene 5016, 1.4mg
SO SU	**ALternaGEL** Johnson & Johnson·Merck	liquid		600mg/5ml			butylparaben · carboxymethyl cellulose sodium · flavors · hydroxypropyl methylcellulose · microcrystalline cellulose · potassium citrate · propylparaben · purified water · simethicone
	Alu-Cap 3M Ph'cals	capsule		400mg			
	Alu-Tab 3M Ph'cals	tablet		500mg			
SO	**Amitone** Menley & James Labs	chewable tablet	350mg				magnesium stearate · mineral oil · powdered peppermint · sodium hexametaphosphate · starch · stearic acid · sucrose · talc
	Amphojel Wyeth-Ayerst Labs	suspension		320mg/5ml			calcium benzoate · glycerin · hydroxypropyl methylcellulose · menthol · peppermint oil · potassium butylparaben · potassium propylparaben · saccharin · simethicone · sorbitol solution · water
	Amphojel Wyeth-Ayerst Labs	tablet		300mg; 600mg			flavors · cellulose · hydrogenated vegetable oil · magnesium stearate · polacrilin potassium · saccharin starch · talc

See Chapter 11, "Acid-Peptic Products," for more information about these products.

ANTACID AND ANTIREFLUX PRODUCTS - continued

	Product [a] Manufacturer/Supplier	Dosage Form	Calcium Carbonate	Aluminum Hydroxide	Magnesium Salts	Other Antacids	Other Ingredients
	Amphojel, Peppermint Wyeth-Ayerst Labs	suspension		320mg/5ml			butylparaben · calcium benzoate · glycerin · hydroxypropyl methylcellulose · methylparaben · propylparaben · saccharin · simethicone · sorbitol solution · water
DY GL LA PU SU	**Arm & Hammer Pure Baking Soda §** Church & Dwight	powder				sodium bicarbonate, 100%	
	Basaljel Wyeth-Ayerst Labs	capsule		500mg			D&C yellow#10 · FD&C blue#1 · FD&C red#40 · FD&C yellow #6 · gelatin · polacrillin potassium · polyethylene glycol · talc · titanium dioxide
	Basaljel Wyeth-Ayerst Labs	tablet		500mg			cellulose · hydrogenated vegetable oil · magnesium stearate · polacrillin potassium · starch · talc
	Basaljel Wyeth-Ayerst Labs	suspension		400mg			flavors · butylparaben · calcium benzoate · glycerin · hydroxypropyl methylcellulose · methylparaben · mineral oil · propylparaben · saccharin · simethicone · sorbitol solution · water
	Bell/ans C. S. Dent	chewable tablet				sodium bicarbonate, 520mg (sodium, 144mg)	wintergreen, ginger flavor · acacia · charcoal · corn starch · gelatin · potato starch · propylene glycol · sucrose · cream mint flavor
	Bromo-Seltzer Warner-Lambert Consumer	granular effervescent				sodium bicarbonate, 2.78mg	acetaminophen, 325mg · citric acid, 2224mg
SO	**Chooz** Schering-Plough Healthcare	gum	500mg				
	Citrocarbonate Roberts Ph'cal	granular effervescent				sodium bicarbonate, 2.34g	sodium citrate · citric acid anhydrous · calcium lactate pentahydrate · sodium chloride · monobasic sodium phosphate anhydrous · dried magnesium sulfate

See Chapter 11, "Acid-Peptic Products," for more information about these products.

ANTACID AND ANTIREFLUX PRODUCTS - continued

	Product [a] Manufacturer/Supplier	Dosage Form	Calcium Carbonate	Aluminum Hydroxide	Magnesium Salts	Other Antacids	Other Ingredients
**	**Creamalin** Lee Consumer	tablet		248mg	75mg (as hydroxide)		corn starch · flavor · magnesium stearate · mannitol · saccharin sodium
DY GL PU SO	**Dicarbosil** BIRA	chewable tablet	500mg				peppermint oil
DY LA PU	**Gaviscon** SmithKline Beecham	chewable tablet		80mg	20mg (as trisilicate)	sodium bicarbonate, 70mg (sodium, 19mg)	alginic acid · calcium stearate · flavor · starch (may contain corn starch) · sucrose
DY LA PU	**Gaviscon Extra Strength** SmithKline Beecham	chewable tablet		160mg	105mg (as carbonate)	sodium bicarbonate	alginic acid · calcium stearate · flavor · sucrose · may contain: stearic acid · sorbitol · mannitol · starch
DY GL LA SU SL	**Gaviscon Extra Strength Liquid** SmithKline Beecham	suspension		762mg/15ml	712.5mg/15ml (as carbonate)		benzyl alcohol · disodium edetate · flavor · glycerin · saccharin sodium · simethicone emulsion · sodium alginate · sorbitol solution · water · xanthan gum
GL LA SU SL	**Gaviscon Liquid** SmithKline Beecham	suspension		95mg/15ml	358mg/15ml (as carbonate)		benzyl alcohol · D&C yellow#10 · disodium edetate · FD&C blue#1 · flavor · glycerin · saccharin sodium · sodium alginate · sorbitol solution · water · xanthan gum
DY LA PU	**Gaviscon-2** SmithKline Beecham	chewable tablet		160mg	40mg (as trisilicate)	sodium bicarbonate, 140mg (sodium, 36.8mg)	alginic acid, 400mg, calcium stearate · flavor · starch (may contain corn starch) · sucrose
DY GL LA SO SU SL	**Maalox** Novartis Consumer	suspension		225mg/5ml	200mg/5ml (as hydroxide)		calcium saccharin · methylparaben · natural flavor · propylparaben · sorbitol · purified water · other ingredients
GL LA SU SL	**Maalox Heartburn Relief** Novartis Consumer	suspension		140mg/5ml	175mg/5ml (as carbonate)	potassium bicarbonate	calcium carbonate · calcium saccharin · FD&C blue#1 · FD&C yellow#5 (tartrazine) · mint flavor · magnesium alginate · methylparaben · propylparaben · sorbitol · purified water

See Chapter 11, "Acid-Peptic Products," for more information about these products.

ANTACID AND ANTIREFLUX PRODUCTS - continued

	Product [a] Manufacturer/Supplier	Dosage Form	Calcium Carbonate	Aluminum Hydroxide	Magnesium Salts	Other Antacids	Other Ingredients
DY GL LA SU SL	**Maalox Therapeutic Concentrate** Novartis Consumer	suspension		600mg/5ml	300mg/5ml (as hydroxide)		flavor · guar gum · methylparaben · propylparaben · sorbitol · purified water
DY GL LA PU SO SU	**Mag-Ox 400** Blaine Ph'cals	tablet			400mg (as oxide)		
	Marblen Fleming	suspension	520mg/5ml		400mg/5ml (as carbonate)		peach/apricot flavor
	Marblen Fleming	tablet	520mg		400mg (as carbonate)		peach/apricot flavor
PR	**Mylanta** Johnson & Johnson·Merck	gelcap	311mg		232mg (as carbonate)		
** PE	**Mylanta Children's Upset Stomach Relief** Johnson & Johnson·Merck	liquid	400mg				
** PE	**Mylanta Children's Upset Stomach Relief, Bubble Gum or Fruit** Johnson & Johnson·Merck	chewable tablet	400mg				citric acid · confectioner's sugar · D&C red#27 · D&C yellow#10 (Fruit Punch) · flavors · magnesium stearate · sorbitol · starch
	Mylanta Double Strength Johnson & Johnson·Merck	chewable tablet	700mg		300mg (as hydroxide)		
SO	**Mylanta Regular Strength** Johnson & Johnson·Merck	chewable tablet	350mg		150mg (as hydroxide)		
	Nephrox Fleming	suspension		320mg/5ml			mineral oil, 10% · watermelon flavor
GL	**Phillips' Milk of Magnesia** Bayer Consumer	chewable tablet			311mg (as hydroxide)		mint flavor · starch · sucrose
AL LA	**Phillips' Milk of Magnesia Concentrate, Strawberry** Bayer Consumer	suspension			800mg/5ml (as hydroxide)		carboxymethlcellulose sodium · citric acid · D&C red#25 · flavor · glycerin · microcrystalline cellulose · propylene glycol · purified water · sorbitol · sugar · xanthan gum
LA	**Phillips' Milk of Magnesia, Cherry or Original Mint** Bayer Consumer	suspension			400mg/5ml (as hydroxide)		flavor · mineral oil · purified water · saccharin sodium

See Chapter 11, "Acid-Peptic Products," for more information about these products.

ANTACID AND ANTIREFLUX PRODUCTS - continued

Product [a] Manufacturer/Supplier	Dosage Form	Calcium Carbonate	Aluminum Hydroxide	Magnesium Salts	Other Antacids	Other Ingredients
LA SO SL **Riopan** Whitehall-Robins Healthcare	suspension				magaldrate, 108mg/ml	potassium citrate · sorbitol · aluminum hydroxide gel · glycerin · xanthan gum · saccharin · flavors · water · calcium · hypochlorite · strong ammonia solution
SO **Rolaids, Asst. Fruit Flavors or Cherry** Warner-Lambert Consumer	chewable tablet	550mg		110mg (as stearate)		flavoring · light mineral oil · magnesium stearate · pregelatinized starch · silicon dioxide · sucrose · blue#1 lake · red#27 lake · red#40 · yellow#5 lake (tartrazine) · yellow#6 lake · microcyrstalline cellulose · polyethylene glycol
Rolaids, Peppermint or Spearmint Warner-Lambert Consumer	chewable tablet	550mg		110mg		pregelatinized starch · flavors · light mineral oil · magnesium stearate · microcrystalline cellulose · polyethylene glycol · silicon dioxide · sucrose
Sodium Bicarbonate Multisource	chewable tablet				sodium bicarbonate, 325mg; 650mg	
SO **Tempo Drops** Thompson Medical	chewable tablet	414mg	133mg	81mg (as hydroxide)		simethicone, 20mg · corn syrup · water · FD&C blue#1 · flavor · sorbitol · soy protein · starch · titanium dioxide
Titralac 3M Health Care	chewable tablet	420mg				glycine · magnesium stearate · saccharin · spearmint flavor · starch
Titralac Extra Strength 3M Health Care	chewable tablet	750mg				glycine · magnesium stearate · saccharin · spearmint flavor · starch
GL LA PU **Tums E-X Extra Strength, Wintergreen or Asst. Fruit Flavors** SmithKline Beecham	chewable tablet	750mg				sucrose · starch · talc · mineral oil · natural and/or artificial flavors · sodium polyphosphate · may also contain: adipic acid · blue#1 lake · yellow#6 lake · yellow#10 lake · red#27 lake · red#30 lake

See Chapter 11, "Acid-Peptic Products," for more information about these products.

ANTACID AND ANTIREFLUX PRODUCTS - continued

	Product [a] Manufacturer/Supplier	Dosage Form	Calcium Carbonate	Aluminum Hydroxide	Magnesium Salts	Other Antacids	Other Ingredients
** SU	**Tums E-X Sugar Free** SmithKline Beecham	chewable tablet	750mg				sorbitol · acacia · natural & artificial flavors · calcium stearate · adipic acid · yellow#6 lake · aspartame
GL LA PU	**Tums Ultra, Fruit or Mint Flavors** SmithKline Beecham	chewable tablet	1000mg				sucrose · starch · talc · mineral oil · natural and/or artificial flavors · sodium polyphosphate · may also contain: adipic acid · blue#1 lake · yellow#6 lake · yellow#10 lake · red#27 lake · red#30 lake
GL LA PU SO	**Tums, Peppermint or Asst. Fruit Flavors** SmithKline Beecham	chewable tablet	500mg				sucrose · starch · talc · mineral oil · natural and/or artificial flavor(s) · sodium polyphosphate · may also contain: adipic acid · blue#1 lake · yellow#6 lake · yellow#10 lake · red#27 lake · red#30 lake
DY GL LA PU SO SU	**Uro-Mag** Blaine Ph'cals	capsule			140mg (as oxide)		
** AF SO	**XS Hangover Relief** Lee Consumer	liquid	350mg/15ml		750mg/15ml (as trisilicate)		calcium citrate, 1250mg/15ml · acetaminophen, 1000mg/15ml · caffeine, 125mg/15ml · glucose · purified water · methylparaben · xanthan gum · glycerin · propylparaben · peppermint oil · FD&C yellow#5 · FD&C blue#1

** New listing

§ Manufacturer/supplier did not confirm information for this edition. Product listing is reprinted from the '96-97 edition.

[a] The Antiflatulent Products table contains combination antacid-simethicone products that contain more than 40mg of simethicone per dose.

See Chapter 11, "Acid-Peptic Products," for more information about these products.

Laxative Product Table

LAXATIVE PRODUCTS

	Product Manufacturer/Supplier	Dosage Form	Stimulant [a]	Bulk	Emollient/ Lubricant	Other Laxatives	Other Ingredients
SL	**Agoral, Marshmallow or Raspberry** Warner-Lambert Consumer	emulsion	phenolphthalein, 0.2g/15ml		mineral oil	glycerin	agar · tragacanth · acacia · benzoic acid · egg albumin · flavors · water · citric acid or sodium hydroxide · D&C red#30 aluminum lake (raspberry) · saccharin sodium · sodium benzoate
GL PU SO	**Alophen** Warner-Lambert Consumer	tablet	phenolphthalein, 60mg				acacia · calcium carbonate · candellila wax · corn starch · compressible sugar · FD&C blue#2 aluminum lake · FD&C red#40 aluminum lake · FD&C yellow#6 aluminum lake · gelatin · kaolin ·microcrystalline cellulose · pregelatinized starch · polyvinylpyrrolidone · sucrose · titanium dioxide · magnesium stearate · sodium benzoate · talc
	Bisacodyl, Enteric Coated Paddock Labs	tablet	bisacodyl, 10mg				
	Caroid Mentholatum	tablet	cascara sagrada extract, 50mg · phenolphthalein, 32.4mg				acacia · beeswax · calcium carbonate · carnauba wax · dicalcium phosphate dihydrate · gelatin · iron oxide · lactose · microcrystalline cellulose · silica · sucrose · magnesium stearate · sodium lauryl sulfate · stearic acid
	Cascara Sagrada Multisource	various	cascara sagrada, 325mg; 450mg				
	Cascara Sagrada Aromatic Fluidextract Multisource	liquid	cascara sagrada				
DY GL LA PU SU	**Ceo-Two** Beutlich, L.P. Ph'cals	suppository				sodium bicarbonate	potassium bitartrate · polyethylene glycol
	Citrucel SmithKline Beecham	powder		methylcellulose, 2g/tbsp			citric acid · FD&C yellow#6 · orange flavor · potassium citrate · riboflavin · sucrose

See Chapter 12, "Laxative Products," for more information about these products.

LAXATIVE PRODUCTS - continued

	Product Manufacturer/Supplier	Dosage Form	Stimulant [a]	Bulk	Emollient/ Lubricant	Other Laxatives	Other Ingredients
SU	**Citrucel Sugar Free** SmithKline Beecham	powder		methylcellulose, 2g/tbsp			aspartame · dibasic calcium phosphate · FD&C yellow#6 · malic acid · maltodextrin · natural & artificial orange flavor · potassium citrate · riboflavin
LA SL	**Colace** Roberts Ph'cal	liquid			docusate sodium, 50mg/5ml		
LA SL	**Colace** Roberts Ph'cal	syrup			docusate sodium, 20mg/5ml		
GL	**Colace** Roberts Ph'cal	capsule			docusate sodium, 50mg; 100mg		
**	**Colace Microenema** Roberts Ph'cal	enema			docusate sodium, 200mg		
	Correctol Schering-Plough Healthcare	caplet · tablet	bisacodyl, 5mg				
	Correctol Herbal Tea, Honey Lemon or Cinnamon Spice Schering-Plough Healthcare	liquid	senna (total sennosides), 30mg/teabag				natural flavors
	Correctol Stool Softener Schering-Plough Healthcare	softgel			docusate sodium, 100mg		
	Dialose Johnson & Johnson·Merck	tablet			docusate sodium, 100mg		
	Dialose Plus Johnson & Johnson·Merck	tablet	yellow phenolphthalein, 65mg		docusate sodium, 100mg		
	Docusate Potassium with Casanthranol Multisource	capsule	casanthranol, 30mg		docusate potassium, 100mg		
** LA SO	**Doxidan** Pharmacia & Upjohn	softgel	casanthranol, 30mg		docusate sodium, 100mg	glycerin	FD&C blue#1 · FD&C red#40 · gelatin · polyethylene glycol · sorbitol · titanium dioxide
LA SO SL	**Dr. Caldwell Senna** Denison Ph'cals	liquid	senna, 166.5mg/5ml				alcohol, 4.9%

See Chapter 12, "Laxative Products," for more information about these products.

LAXATIVE PRODUCTS - continued

	Product Manufacturer/Supplier	Dosage Form	Stimulant [a]	Bulk	Emollient/ Lubricant	Other Laxatives	Other Ingredients
SO	**Dulcolax** Novartis Consumer	tablet	bisacodyl, 5mg				acacia · acetylated monoglyceride · carnauba wax · cellulose acetate phthalate · corn starch · D&C red#30 aluminum lake · D&C yellow#10 aluminum lake · dibutyl phthalate · docusate sodium · gelatin · glycerin · iron oxides · kaolin · lactose · methylparaben · pharmaceutical glaze · povidone · propylparaben · sorbitan monooleate · sucrose · titanium dioxide · white wax · magnesium stearate · polyethylene glycol · sodium benzoate · talc
	Emulsoil Paddock Labs	liquid	castor oil, 95%				flavor · emulsifier
	Epsom Salt Multisource	granule				magnesium sulfate, 40mEq/5mg	
SU	**Evac-Q-Kwik** Savage Labs	liquid				magnesium citrate, 25mEq/30ml	citric acid · potassium citrate · lemon-flavored carbonated base
	Evac-Q-Kwik Savage Labs	suppository	bisacodyl, 10mg				
GL PU GE	**Evac-U-Gen** Walker, Corp. and Co.	chewable tablet	yellow phenolphthalein, 97.2mg				saccharin sodium (sodium, 0.004mEq) · anise oil · corn syrup solids · D&C red#7 · FD&C blue#1 · lactose · confectioner's sugar · magnesium stearate
GL PU	**Ex-Lax Extra Gentle** Novartis Consumer	tablet	yellow phenolphthalein, 65mg		docusate sodium, 75mg		acacia · croscarmellose sodium · dibasic calcium phosphate · colloidal silicon dioxide · microcrystalline cellulose · red#7 · sucrose · titanium dioxide · magnesium stearate · stearic acid · talc

See Chapter 12, "Laxative Products," for more information about these products.

LAXATIVE PRODUCTS - continued

	Product Manufacturer/Supplier	Dosage Form	Stimulant [a]	Bulk	Emollient/ Lubricant	Other Laxatives	Other Ingredients
GL PU	**Ex-Lax Gentle Nature Natural** Novartis Consumer	tablet	sennosides A and B, 20mg				alginic acid · calcium phosphate dibasic · magnesium stearate · microcrystalline cellulose · silicon dioxide · starch · sodium lauryl sulfate · stearic acid
GL PU	**Ex-Lax Maximum Relief Formula** Novartis Consumer	tablet	yellow phenolphthalein, 135mg				acacia · alginic acid · blue#1 · carnauba wax · colloidal silicon dioxide · dibasic calcium phosphate · microcrystalline cellulose · povidone · starch · sucrose · titanium dioxide · magnesium stearate · sodium benzoate · sodium lauryl sulfate · stearic acid · talc
GL PU SO	**Ex-Lax Original Regular Strength Chocolated** Novartis Consumer	tablet	yellow phenolphthalein, 90mg				cocoa · confectioner's sugar · hydrogenated palm kernel oil · nonfat dry milk · vanillin · lecithin
GL PU	**Ex-Lax Regular Strength** Novartis Consumer	tablet	yellow phenolphthalein, 90mg				acacia · alginic acid · carnauba wax · colloidal silicon dioxide · dibasic calcium phosphate · iron oxides · microcrystalline cellulose · starch · sucrose · titanium dioxide · magnesium stearate · sodium benzoate · sodium lauryl sulfate · stearic acid · talc

See Chapter 12, "Laxative Products," for more information about these products.

LAXATIVE PRODUCTS - continued

	Product Manufacturer/Supplier	Dosage Form	Stimulant [a]	Bulk	Emollient/ Lubricant	Other Laxatives	Other Ingredients
** LA PU SU	**Ex-Lax Stool Softener** Novartis Consumer	caplet			docusate sodium, 100mg		alginic acid · blue #1 · microcrystalline cellulose · colloidal silicon dioxide · croscarmellose sodium · dibasic calcium phosphate · hydroxypropyl methylcellulose · magnesium stearate · methylparaben · polydextrose · polyethylene glycol · silicon dioxide · sodium benzoate · stearic acid · talc · titanium dioxide · triacetin · yellow #10
	Feen-A-Mint Schering-Plough Healthcare	tablet	bisacodyl, 5mg				
** DY GL LA SO	**Fiber Naturale** Alva-Amco Pharmacal	caplet		methylcellulose, 300mg · psyllium			oat fiber · apple fiber
GL LA PU SO SU	**FiberCon** Lederle Consumer	tablet		calcium polycarbophil, 625mg			calcium carbonate · caramel · crospovidone · hydroxypropyl methylcellulose · microcrystalline cellulose · povidone · silica gel · magnesium stearate
AL LA PR SO SL PE	**Fleet Babylax** C. B. Fleet	liquid				glycerin	
SO	**Fleet Bisacodyl Enema** C. B. Fleet	enema	bisacodyl, 10mg				
GL PU SO	**Fleet Glycerin Adult Size** C. B. Fleet	suppository				glycerin	
GL PU SO PE	**Fleet Glycerin Child Size** C. B. Fleet	suppository				glycerin	
AL LA PR SO	**Fleet Glycerin Rectal Applicators** C. B. Fleet	liquid				glycerin, 7.5ml	
GL PU	**Fleet Laxative** C. B. Fleet	suppository	bisacodyl, 10mg				
PU	**Fleet Laxative** C. B. Fleet	tablet	bisacodyl, 5mg				

See Chapter 12, "Laxative Products," for more information about these products.

LAXATIVE PRODUCTS - continued

	Product Manufacturer/Supplier	Dosage Form	Stimulant [a]	Bulk	Emollient/ Lubricant	Other Laxatives	Other Ingredients
PR	**Fleet Mineral Oil Enema** C. B. Fleet	enema			mineral oil, 100%		
AL LA PR SO SL	**Fleet Mineral Oil Oral Lubricant** C. B. Fleet	liquid			mineral oil, 100%		
	Fleet Prep Kit 1 C. B. Fleet	liquid; suppository; tablet	bisacodyl, 20mg/4 tablets · bisacodyl, 10mg (suppository)			liquid: sodium phosphate oral solution, 45ml (total sodium, 4950mg/45ml) · glycerin	liquid: flavor · saccharin
SL	**Fleet Prep Kit 2** C. B. Fleet	enema; liquid; tablet	bisacodyl, 20mg/4 tablets			liquid: sodium phosphate oral solution, 45ml (total sodium, 4950mg/45ml) · glycerin	enema: tap water liquid: flavor · saccharin
	Fleet Prep Kit 3 C. B. Fleet	enema; liquid; tablet	bisacodyl, 20mg/4 tablets · bisacodyl, 10mg (enema)			liquid: sodium phosphate oral solution, 45ml (total sodium, 4950mg/45ml) · glycerin	liquid: flavor · saccharin
	Fleet Ready-to-Use Enema C. B. Fleet	enema				monobasic sodium phosphate, 19g/118ml · dibasic sodium phosphate, 7g/118ml (total sodium, 4.4g/118ml)	
PE	**Fleet Ready-to-Use Enema for Children** C. B. Fleet	enema				monobasic sodium phosphate, 9.5g/59ml · dibasic sodium phosphate, 3.5g/59ml (total sodium, 2.2g/59ml)	
AL LA SL PE	**Fletcher's Castoria** Mentholatum	liquid	senna concentrate, 166.5mg/5ml			glycerin	flavor · sucrose · water · sodium benzoate · citric acid · methylparaben · propylbaraben

See Chapter 12, "Laxative Products," for more information about these products.

LAXATIVE PRODUCTS - continued

	Product Manufacturer/Supplier	Dosage Form	Stimulant [a]	Bulk	Emollient/ Lubricant	Other Laxatives	Other Ingredients
LA SL PE	**Fletcher's, Children's Cherry** Mentholatum	suspension	yellow phenolphthalein, 0.3%			glycerin	citric acid · FD&C red#40 · flavor · magnesium aluminum silicate · methylparaben · sucrose · water · xanthan gum · sodium benzoate
SO	**Garfields Tea** Alvin Last	cut plant	senna, 610mg/1/2tsp	psyllium seed husks · buckthorn bark			anise seed · fennel seed
	Gentlax S Blair Labs	tablet	senna concentrate, 8.8mg sennosides		docusate sodium, 50mg		
GL PU SO	**Gentle Laxative** Hudson	tablet	bisacodyl, 5mg				
	Glycerin Multisource	suppository				glycerin	sodium stearate
AL LA	**Haleys M-O, Flavored or Regular** Bayer Consumer	emulsion			mineral oil, 25%	magnesium hydroxide, 6%	D&C red#28 · flavor · purified water · saccharin sodium
** DY LA PU SU	**Herb-Lax** Shaklee	tablet	senna leaf powder, 175mg				alfalfa powder · anise seed powder · blue malva flower powder · buckthorn bark powder · corn syrup solids · culver's root powder · fennel seed powder - karaya gum · licorice root powder · malt extract · barley extract · microcrystalline cellulose · rhubarb root powder
	Hydrocil Instant Solvay Ph'cals	powder		psyllium, 95%			povidone · polyethylene glycol
SO	**Innerclean Herbal** Alvin Last	cut plant · tablet	senna leaves	psyllium seed husks · buckthorn bark			anise seed · fennel seed
AL DY GL LA PR SO SU SL	**Kellogg's Tasteless Castor Oil** BIRA	liquid	castor oil, 100%				
SO	**Kondremul** Novartis Consumer	emulsion			mineral oil, 55%		acacia · benzoic acid · carrageenan · ethyl vanillin · mapleine triple oil · purified water · vanillin · glycerin
SU	**Konsyl** Konsyl Ph'cals	powder		psyllium mucilloid, 100%			sodium, <4mg

See Chapter 12, "Laxative Products," for more information about these products.

LAXATIVE PRODUCTS - continued

	Product Manufacturer/Supplier	Dosage Form	Stimulant [a]	Bulk	Emollient/ Lubricant	Other Laxatives	Other Ingredients
	Konsyl Fiber Konsyl Ph'cals	tablet		calcium polycarbophil, 625mg (polycarbophil, 500mg)			
	Konsyl-D Konsyl Ph'cals	powder		psyllium hydrophilic mucilloid, 50%			dextrose, 50% · sodium, <4mg
	Konsyl-Orange Konsyl Ph'cals	powder		psyllium hydrophilic mucilloid, 28%			sucrose, 67% · sodium, 2.4mg
GL PU SO	**Laxative & Stool Softner** Hudson	softgel	casanthranol, 30mg		docusate sodium, 100mg		
AL LA PR SL	**Liqui-Doss** Ferndale Labs	emulsion			mineral oil		
DY GL LA PU SO SU	**Mag-Ox 400** Blaine Ph'cals	tablet				magnesium oxide, 400mg (elemental magnesium, 241.3mg or 19.86mEq)	
	Magnesium Citrate Multisource	solution				magnesium citrate, 1.74g/oz	
DY LA PU	**Metamucil Fiber Wafer, Apple Crisp or Cinnamon Spice** Procter & Gamble	wafer		psyllium hydrophilic mucilloid, 3.4g/2 wafers			ascorbic acid · brown sugar (Apple Crisp) · cinnamon · corn oil · flavors · fructose · lecithin · modified food starch · molasses · oat hull fiber · sodium bicarbonate · sucrose · nutmeg · oats (Cinnamon Spice) · water · wheat flour
GL LA PU SO	**Metamucil Original Texture, Orange** Procter & Gamble	powder		psyllium hydrophilic mucilloid, 3.4g/tbsp			citric acid · FD&C yellow#6 · flavoring · sucrose
CO DY GL LA PU SU	**Metamucil Original Texture, Regular Flavor** Procter & Gamble	powder		psyllium hydrophilic mucilloid, 3.4g/tsp			dextrose · sodium, 3mg/tsp
GL LA PU SO	**Metamucil Smooth Texture, Orange** Procter & Gamble	powder		psyllium hydrophilic mucilloid, 3.4g/tbsp			citric acid · D&C yellow#10 · FD&C yellow#6 · flavoring · sucrose

See Chapter 12, "Laxative Products," for more information about these products.

LAXATIVE PRODUCTS - continued

	Product Manufacturer/Supplier	Dosage Form	Stimulant [a]	Bulk	Emollient/ Lubricant	Other Laxatives	Other Ingredients
GL LA PU SO SU	**Metamucil Smooth Texture, Sugar Free Orange** Procter & Gamble	powder		psyllium hydrophilic mucilloid, 3.4g/tsp			aspartame · citric acid · D&C yellow#10 · FD&C yellow#6 · flavoring · maltodextrin
GL LA PU SO SU	**Metamucil Smooth Texture, Sugar Free Orange** Procter & Gamble	individual packet		psyllium hydrophilic mucilloid, 3.4g/packet			aspartame · citric acid · D&C yellow#10 · FD&C yellow#6 · flavoring · maltodextrin
DY GL LA PU SO	**Metamucil Smooth Texture, Sugar Free Regular Flavor** Procter & Gamble	powder		psyllium hydrophilic mucilloid, 3.4g/tsp		magnesium sulfate	citric acid, 1% · maltodextrin
LA SO	**Milkinol** Schwarz Pharma	emulsion			mineral oil		butylated hydroxyanisole · emulsifier · color · flavor
	Mineral Oil Multisource	liquid			mineral oil		
** SO	**Mitrolan** Whitehall-Robins Healthcare	chewable tablet		calcium polycarbophil, 500mg			sucrose · citrus and vanilla flavor
	Modane Savage Labs	tablet	phenolphthalein, 130mg				acacia · calcium carbonate · calcium sulfate · corn starch · dibasic calcium phosphate · FD&C red#40 · lactose · magnesium stearate · polyvinyl pyrolidone · shellac · sodium benzoate · titanium dioxide · water · white wax
	Modane Bulk Savage Labs	powder		psyllium hydrophilic mucilloid, 50%			dextrose, 50% · sodium, 2mg/tsp · potassium, 37mg/tsp

See Chapter 12, "Laxative Products," for more information about these products.

LAXATIVE PRODUCTS - continued

	Product Manufacturer/Supplier	Dosage Form	Stimulant [a]	Bulk	Emollient/ Lubricant	Other Laxatives	Other Ingredients
	Modane Plus Savage Labs	tablet	yellow phenolphthalein, 65mg		docusate sodium, 100mg		acacia · calcium carbonate · carnauba wax · cellulose gum · D&C red#7 · dicalcium phosphate · gelatin · iron oxide · magnesium stearate · methylparaben · polyethlene glycol · povidone · propylparaben · silicon dioxide · sodium benzoate · starch · sucrose · talc · titanium dioxide · white wax · may also contain: butylparaben · calcium gluconate · calcium sulfate · wheat flour
	Modane Soft Savage Labs	capsule			docusate sodium, 100mg	glycerin	gelatin · methylparaben · propylene glycol · propylparaben · sorbitol · water · polyethylene glycol 400
	Nature's Remedy Block Drug	tablet	cascara sagrada, 150mg · aloe, 100mg				calcium stearate · FD&C blue#2 · FD&C yellow#6 · hydroxypropyl cellulose · lactose · hydroxypropyl methylcellulose · microcrystalline cellulose · titanium dioxide · polyethylene glycol
	Neoloid Kenwood Labs	oil	castor oil, 36.4%				sodium benzoate, 0.2% · potassium sorbate · mint flavoring
	Perdiem Novartis Consumer	granule	senna (cassia pod concentrate), 0.74g/tsp	psyllium, 3.25g/tsp			sodium, 1.8mg/tsp · potassium, 35.5mg/tsp · acacia · iron oxides · natural flavors · paraffin · sucrose · talc
	Perdiem Fiber Novartis Consumer	granule		psyllium, 4g/tsp			sodium, 1.8mg/tsp · potassium, 36.1mg/tsp · acacia · iron oxides · natural flavors · paraffin · sucrose · titanium dioxide · talc
GL	**Peri-Colace** Roberts Ph'cal	capsule	casanthranol, 30mg		docusate sodium, 100mg		
	Peri-Colace Roberts Ph'cal	syrup	casanthranol, 10mg/5ml		docusate sodium, 20mg/5ml		
GL	**Phillips' Milk of Magnesia** Bayer Consumer	chewable tablet				magnesium hydroxide, 311mg	mint flavor · starch · sucrose

See Chapter 12, "Laxative Products," for more information about these products.

LAXATIVE PRODUCTS - continued

	Product Manufacturer/Supplier	Dosage Form	Stimulant [a]	Bulk	Emollient/ Lubricant	Other Laxatives	Other Ingredients
AL LA	**Phillips' Milk of Magnesia Concentrate, Strawberry** Bayer Consumer	suspension				magnesium hydroxide, 800mg/5ml	flavor
AL LA	**Phillips' Milk of Magnesia; Cherry, Mint, or Original** Bayer Consumer	suspension				magnesium hydroxide, 400mg/5ml	flavor
	Phospho-soda Buffered Saline, Ginger-Lemon or Unflavored C. B. Fleet	liquid				monobasic sodium phosphate, 2.4g/5ml (sodium, 550mg/5ml) · dibasic sodium phosphate, 0.9g/5ml	flavor
LA PR SU SL	**Purge** Fleming	liquid	castor oil, 95%				lemon-flavored base
	Regulace Republic Drug	gelcap	casanthranol, 30mg		docusate sodium, 100mg		
	Regulax SS Republic Drug	gelcap			docusate sodium, 100mg; 250mg		
	Senokot Purdue Frederick	syrup	senna concentrate, 8.8mg/5ml sennosides				alcohol, 7%
	Senokot Purdue Frederick	tablet	senna concentrate, 8.6mg sennosides				sodium, 0.007mEq/dose
	Senokot Purdue Frederick	granule	senna concentrate, 15mg sennosides/tsp				sodium, 0.06mEq/dose
AL PE	**Senokot Children's** Purdue Frederick	syrup	senna concentrate, 8.8mg/5ml sennosides				methylparaben · potassium sorbate · propylparaben · sucrose · water · chocolate flavor
	Senokot-S Purdue Frederick	tablet	senna concentrate, 8.6mg sennosides		docusate sodium, 50mg		sodium, 0.15mEq
	SenokotXTRA Purdue Frederick	tablet	senna concentrate, 17mg sennosides				sodium, 0.014mEq/dose
	Serutan Menley & James Labs	granule		psyllium hydrophilic mucilloid, 2.5mg/tsp			saccharin sodium · sucrose · caramel color · corn starch · invert sugar · oat flour · wheat germ · acacia · carboxymethylcellulose · magnesium stearate

See Chapter 12, "Laxative Products," for more information about these products.

LAXATIVE PRODUCTS - continued

	Product Manufacturer/Supplier	Dosage Form	Stimulant [a]	Bulk	Emollient/ Lubricant	Other Laxatives	Other Ingredients
	Sof·lax C. B. Fleet	gelcap			docusate sodium, 100mg		
	Sof·lax Overnight C. B. Fleet	gelcap	casanthranol, 30mg		docusate sodium, 100mg		
GL PU SO	**Stool Softner** Hudson	softgel			docusate sodium, 100mg		
SO	**Surfak** Pharmacia & Upjohn	softgel			docusate calcium, 240mg	glycerin	alcohol, up to 3% · corn oil · FD&C blue#1 · FD&C red#40 · gelatin · methylparaben · propylparaben · sorbitol
AL LA PR SO SL	**Therevac Plus** Jones Medical	enema			docusate sodium, 283mg	glycerin	benzocaine, 20mg · PEG-400
AL LA PR SL	**Therevac-SB** Jones Medical	enema			docusate sodium, 283mg	glycerin	PEG-400
GL LA SU	**Unilax** B. F. Ascher	capsule	yellow phenolphthalein, 130mg		docusate sodium, 230mg		
DY GL LA PU SO SU	**Uro-Mag** Blaine Ph'cals	capsule				magnesium oxide, 140mg (elemental magnesium, 84.5mg or 6.93mEq)	
	X-Prep Purdue Frederick	liquid	senna concentrate, 3.7g/75ml standardized extract of senna fruit				alcohol, 7%

** New listing

[a] At the time this edition went to press, FDA was still evaluating the safety of stimulant laxative ingredients. In May 1996, the agency announced its intent to reclassify these ingredients from Category I (safe and effective) to Category III (more data needed).

See Chapter 12, "Laxative Products," for more information about these products.

Antidiarrheal Product Tables

ORAL REHYDRATION SOLUTIONS

	Product Manufacturer/Supplier	Osmolarity (mOsm/L)	Carbohydrates (g/L)	Electrolytes (mEq/L)	Other Ingredients
DY GL LA PU	**Infalyte** Mead Johnson Nutritionals	200	rice syrup solids, 30	sodium, 50 · chloride, 45 · citrate, 34 · potassium, 25	
** PE	**Kao Lectrolyte Individual Packets, Flavored or Unflavored** Pharmacia & Upjohn	[a]	dextrose, 5/packet	sodium, 50 · citrate, 30 · potassium, 20 · chloride, 10/packet	aspartame
PE	**Naturalyte, Bubblegum or Unflavored** Unico	270	dextrose, 25	sodium, 45 · chloride, 35 · citrate, 30 · potassium, 20	
PE	**Naturalyte, Fruit Flavored or Grape** Unico	270	dextrose, 20 · fructose, 5	sodium, 45 · chloride, 35 · citrate, 30 · potassium, 20	
PE	**Pedialyte** Ross Products/Abbott Labs	249	dextrose, 25	sodium, 45 · chloride, 35 · citrate, 30 · potassium, 20	water
** PE	**Pedialyte Freezer Pops** Ross Products/Abbott Labs	[a]	dextrose, 25	sodium, 45 · chloride, 35 · citrate, 30 · potassium, 20	water · citric acid · carboxymethylcellulose sodium · asparatame · natural and artificial flavors · artificial coloring
	Rehydralyte Ross Products/Abbott Labs	304	dextrose, 25	sodium, 75 · chloride, 65 · citrate, 30 · potassium, 20	water
PE	**Revital Ice Freezer Pops** PTS Labs	[a]	crystalline fructose, 3	sodium, 45 · chloride, 35 · citrate, 30 · potassium, 20	water · citric acid · carboxymethylcellulose sodium · natural flavors · artificial coloring

** New listing

[a] Osmolarity not determined by manufacturer/supplier.

See Chapter 13, "Antidiarrheal Products," for more information about these products.

ANTIDIARRHEAL PRODUCTS

	Product Manufacturer/Supplier	Dosage Form	Adsorbent	Other Active Ingredients	Other Ingredients
	Dairy Ease [a] Blistex	drops		lactase enzyme	water · glycerol
	Dairy Ease [a] Blistex	caplet		lactase, 3000 FCC untis	colloidal silicon dioxide · dibasic calcium phosphate · magnesium stearate · microcrystalline cellulose · pregelatinized starch
	Dairy Ease [a] Blistex	chewable tablet		lactase, 3000 FCC units	dibasic calcium phosphate · mannitol · colloidal silicon dioxide · magnesium stearate
GL PU SO	**Diar Aid** Thompson Medical	caplet		loperamide HCl, 2mg	corn starch · lactose · magnesium stearate · microcrystalline cellulose
**	**Diarrid** Stellar Health Products	caplet		loperamide HCl, 2mg	dibasic calcium phosphate · magnesium stearate · microcrystalline cellulose · colloidal silicon dioxide · D&C yellow#10
GL PU	**Diasorb** Columbia Labs	tablet	attapulgite, 750mg (activated nonfibrous)		
LA SL	**Diasorb** Columbia Labs	liquid	attapulgite, 750mg/5ml (activated nonfibrous)		
	Donnagel Wyeth-Ayerst Labs	suspension	attapulgite, 600mg/5ml		alcohol, 1.4% · benzyl alcohol · citric acid · FD&C blue#1 · flavors · magnesium aluminum silicate · methylparaben · phosphoric acid · propylene glycol · propylparaben · saccharin sodium · sorbitol · titanium dioxide · water · xanthan gum · carboxymethylcellulose sodium
	Donnagel Wyeth-Ayerst Labs	chewable tablet	attapulgite, 600mg		D&C yellow#10 aluminum lake · FD&C blue#1 aluminum lake · flavors · magnesium stearate · mannitol · saccharin sodium · sorbitol · water
	Equalactin Numark Labs	chewable tablet	polycarbophil, 500mg		citric acid · flavor · magnesium stearate · microcrystalline cellulose · dextrose · crospovidone
	Imodium A-D McNeil Consumer	caplet		loperamide HCl, 2mg	dibasic calcium phosphate · magnesium stearate · microcrystalline cellulose · colloidal silicon dioxide · FD&C blue#1 · D&C yellow#10
	Imodium A-D McNeil Consumer	liquid		loperamide HCl, 1mg/5ml	alcohol, 0.5% · citric acid · flavors · glycerin · purified water · benzoic acid · propylene glycol · sodium benzoate · sorbitol · sucrose
**	**Kao-Paverin** Reese Chemical	liquid	pectin, 65mg/15ml	kaolin, 3g/15ml · bismuth subsalicylate 250mg/15ml	
LA SL	**Kaopectate** Pharmacia & Upjohn	liquid	attapulgite, 750mg/15ml		flavors · glucono-delta-lactone · magnesium aluminum silicate · methylparaben · sorbic acid · sucrose · titanium dioxide · xanthan gum · purified water
GL PU SO	**Kaopectate** Pharmacia & Upjohn	caplet	attapulgite, 750mg		croscarmellose sodium · hydroxypropyl cellulose · hydroxypropyl methylcellulose · methylparaben · pectin · propylene glycol · propylparaben · sucrose · titanium dioxide · zinc stearate · may also contain talc

See Chapter 13, "Antidiarrheal Products," for more information about these products.

ANTIDIARRHEAL PRODUCTS - continued

	Product Manufacturer/Supplier	Dosage Form	Adsorbent	Other Active Ingredients	Other Ingredients
LA SL PE	**Kaopectate, Children's** Pharmacia & Upjohn	liquid	attapulgite, 375mg/7.5ml		FD&C red#40 · flavors · glucono-delta-lactone · magnesium aluminum silicate · methylparaben · sorbic acid · sucrose · titanium dioxide · xanthan gum · purified water
SO SU	**Lactaid [a]** McNeil Consumer	drops		lactase enzyme	glycerin · water
	Lactaid [a] McNeil Consumer	caplet		lactase, 3000 FCC units	mannitol · cellulose · magnesium stearate · dextrose · sodium citrate
	Lactaid Extra Strength [a] McNeil Consumer	caplet		lactase, 4500 FCC units	mannitol · cellulose · magnesium stearate · dextrose · sodium citrate
**	**Lactaid Ultra [a]** McNeil Consumer	caplet		lactase, 9000 FCC units	cellulose · dextrose · sodium citrate · magnesium stearate · colloidal silicon dioxide
	Lactrase [a] Schwarz Pharma	capsule		lactase, 250mg	maltodextrin · magnesium stearate · gelatin · titanium dioxide · yellow iron oxide · red iron oxide
	Parepectolin Rhône-Poulenc Rorer Ph'cals	suspension	attapulgite, 600mg/15ml		flavors · glucono-delta-lactone · magnesium aluminum silicate · methylparaben · sorbic acid · sucrose · titanium dioxide · xanthan gum · purified water
GL PU	**Pepto-Bismol** Procter & Gamble	chewable tablet		bismuth subsalicylate, 262.5mg	calcium carbonate · flavor · magnesium stearate · mannitol · povidone · D&C red#27 aluminum lake · saccharin sodium · talc
	Pepto-Bismol Procter & Gamble	caplet		bismuth subsalicylate, 262mg	calcium carbonate · microcrystalline cellulose · mannitol · sodium starch glycolate · povidone · magnesium stearate · D&C red#27 aluminum lake · silicon dioxide · polysorbate 80
LA SU SL	**Pepto-Bismol Maximum Strength** Procter & Gamble	liquid		bismuth subsalicylate, 1050mg/30ml	benzoic acid · flavor · magnesium aluminum silicate · methylcellulose · D&C red#22 · D&C red#28 · saccharin sodium · salicylic acid · sodium salicylate · sorbic acid · water
LA SU SL	**Pepto-Bismol Original Strength** Procter & Gamble	liquid		bismuth subsalicylate, 525mg/30ml	benzoic acid · flavor · magnesium aluminum silicate · methylcellulose · D&C red#22 · D&C red#28 · saccharin sodium · salicylic acid · sodium salicylate · sorbic acid · water
GL PU	**Pepto-Bismol, Cherry** Procter & Gamble	chewable tablet		bismuth subsalicylate, 262.39mg	adipic acid · calcium carbonate · flavors · magnesium stearate · mannitol · povidone · D&C red#27 aluminum lake · FD&C red#40 aluminum lake · saccharin sodium · talc
DY LA SO SL	**Percy Medicine** Merrick Medicine	liquid		bismuth subnitrate, 959mg/10ml · calcium hydroxide, 21.9mg/10ml · potassium carbonate, 5.6mg/10ml	distilled water · ethyl alcohol, 5% · glycerin · gum arabic · rhubarb fluid extract · sugar · flavors · natural color

See Chapter 13, "Antidiarrheal Products," for more information about these products.

ANTIDIARRHEAL PRODUCTS - continued

	Product Manufacturer/Supplier	Dosage Form	Adsorbent	Other Active Ingredients	Other Ingredients
PU	**Rheaban** Pfizer Consumer	caplet	activated attapulgite, 750mg		carnauba wax · croscarmellose sodium · D&C yellow#10 aluminum lake · D&C blue#1 aluminum lake · hydroxypropyl cellulose · hydroxypropyl methylcellulose · methylparaben · pectin · pharmaceutical glaze · propylene glycol · propylparaben · sucrose · titanium dioxide · zinc stearate · talc
**	**SureLac** Caraco Ph'cal Labs	chewable tablet		lactase, 3000 FCC units	sorbitol · dibasic calcium phosphate · magnesium stearate · colloidal silicon dioxide

** New listing
[a] This preparation can be added to milk products and/or taken with milk to prevent osmotic diarrhea.

See Chapter 13, "Antidiarrheal Products," for more information about these products.

Hemorrhoidal Product Table

HEMORRHOIDAL PRODUCTS

Product Manufacturer/Supplier	Dosage Form	Anesthetic	Vasocon-strictor [a]	Astringent	Protectant	Other Ingredients
Americaine Hemorrhoidal Novartis Consumer	ointment	benzocaine, 20%				benzethonium chloride, 0.1% · polyethylene glycol 300 · polyethylene glycol 3350
Anusol Warner-Lambert Consumer	suppository	benzyl alcohol			topical starch, 51%	partially hydrogenated soy bean oil · sorbitan tristearate · tocopheryl · acetate
Anusol Warner-Lambert Consumer	ointment	pramoxine HCl, 1%		zinc oxide, 12.5%	mineral oil · cocoa butter · kaolin · peruvian balsam	benzyl benzoate · dibasic calcium phosphate · glyceryl monooleate · glyceryl monostearate · polyethylene wax
Balneol Solvay Ph'cals	lotion				mineral oil · lanolin oil	propylene glycol · glyceryl stearate/PEG-100 stearate · PEG-40 stearate · laureth-4, PEG-4 dilaurate · sodium acetate · carbomer 934 · triethanolamine · methylparaben · dioctyl sodium sulfosuccinate · fragrance · acetic acid
Calmol 4 Mentholatum	suppository			zinc oxide, 10%	cocoa butter, 80%	glyceryl stearate · methylparaben · propylparaben · bismuth subgallate
Fleet Medicated Wipes C. B. Fleet	pad			witch hazel, 50%	glycerin, 10%	methylparaben · benzalkonium chloride
Fleet Pain-Relief C. B. Fleet	pad	pramoxine HCl, 1%			glycerin, 12%	
Hemorid for Women Pfizer Consumer	ointment	pramoxine HCl, 1%	phenylephrine HCl, 0.25%		petrolatum, 82.15% · mineral oil, 12.5%	aloe · white wax
Hemorid for Women Pfizer Consumer	cream	pramoxine HCl, 1%	phenylephrine HCl, 0.25%		petrolatum, 30% · mineral oil, 20%	water · stearyl alcohol · cetyl alcohol · methylparaben · propylparaben · polysorbate 80 · aloe vera gel
Hemorid for Women Pfizer Consumer	suppository		phenylephrine HCl, 0.25%	zinc oxide, 231mg	hard fat, 88.25%	aloe
Hydrosal Hemorrhoidal Hydrosal	ointment	benzyl alcohol, 1.4%	ephedrine sulfate, 0.2%	zinc oxide, 5%	lanolin, 14.25% · petrolatum, 22.5% · mineral oil, 14.25%	aloe · water · sorbitan sesquioleate · D&C red#33 · ceresin wax

See Chapter 14, "Hemorrhoidal Products," for more information about these products.

HEMORRHOIDAL PRODUCTS - continued

Product Manufacturer/Supplier	Dosage Form	Anesthetic	Vasocon-strictor [a]	Astringent	Protectant	Other Ingredients
Lanacane Creme Combe	cream	benzocaine, 6%		zinc oxide	glycerin	benzethonium chloride, 0.1% · aloe · chlorothymol · dioctyl sodium sulfosuccinate · ethoxydiglycol · fragrance · glyceryl stearate SE · isopropyl alcohol · methylparaben · propylparaben · sodium borate · stearic acid · sulfated castor oil · triethanolamine - water · zinc oxide · pyrithione zinc
** **Lanacane Maximum Strength** Combe	cream	benzocaine, 20%			dimethicone · mineral oil	benzethonium chloride, 0.2% · acetylated lanolin alcohol · aloe · cetyl acetate · cetyl alcohol · fragrance · glycerin · glyceryl stearate · isopropyl myristate · methylparaben · PEG-100 stearate · propylparaben · sorbitan stearate · stearamidopropyl PG-dimonium chloride phosphate · water · pyrithione zinc
Medicone Merz Consumer	ointment	benzocaine, 20%			light mineral oil · white petrolatum	
Medicone Merz Consumer	suppository		phenylephrine HCl, 0.25%		hard fat, 88.7%	corn starch · methylparaben · propylparaben
Nupercainal Novartis Consumer	suppository			zinc oxide, 0.25g	cocoa butter, 2.1g	acetone sodium bisulfite · bismuth subgallate
Nupercainal Novartis Consumer	ointment	dibucaine, 1%			lanolin · white petrolatum · light mineral oil	acetone · sodium bisulfite · purified water
Pazo Bristol-Myers Products	suppository		ephedrine sulfate, 3.86mg	zinc oxide, 96.5mg	hydrogenated vegetable oil	
Pazo Bristol-Myers Products	ointment	camphor, 2%	ephedrine sulfate, 0.2%	zinc oxide, 5%	lanolin · petrolatum	
** **Peterson's Ointment** Lee Consumer	ointment	phenol · camphor		zinc oxide · tannic acid		
Preparation H Whitehall-Robins Healthcare	suppository		phenylephrine HCl, 0.25%		cocoa butter, 79% · shark liver oil, 3%	methylparaben · propylparaben · corn starch

See Chapter 14, "Hemorrhoidal Products," for more information about these products.

HEMORRHOIDAL PRODUCTS - continued

Product Manufacturer/Supplier	Dosage Form	Anesthetic	Vasocon-strictor [a]	Astringent	Protectant	Other Ingredients
Preparation H Whitehall-Robins Healthcare	ointment		phenylephrine HCl, 0.25%		petrolatum, 71.9% · mineral oil, 14% · shark liver oil, 3% · lanolin · glycerin	benzoic acid · methylparaben · propylparaben · red thyme oil · water · Tenox GT-2 · Tenox 4B · FALBA
Preparation H Whitehall-Robins Healthcare	cream		phenylephrine HCl, 0.250%		petrolatum, 18% · glycerin, 12% · shark liver oil, 3% · lanolin	BHA · carboxymethyl cellulose · cetyl alcohol · citric acid · disodium edetate · methylparaben · propylparaben · sodium benzoate · sodium lauryl sulfate · stearyl alcohol · water · tegacid · Arlacel 186 · Tenox GT-2 · Tenox 2 · medical antifoam emulsion · Rhodigel
Procto Foam Non-Steroid Schwarz Pharma	foam	pramoxine HCl, 1%				butane · cetyl alcohol · glyceryl monostearate · methylparaben · PEG-100 stearate · polyoxyethylene 23 lauryl ether · polyoxyl 40 stearate · propane · propylene glycol · propylparaben · purified water · trolamine
** **Rectacaine** Reese Chemical	ointment				petrolatum 71.9% · mineral oil 14% · shark liver oil 3% · glycerin	beeswax · benzoic acid · BHA · corn oil · lanolin alcohol · methylparaben · paraffin · propylparaben · thyme oil · tocopherol · water
** **Rectacaine** Reese Chemical	suppository		phenylephrine HCl, 0.25%		hard fat 88.7%	corn starch · methylparaben · propylparaben
Tronolane Ross Products/Abbott Labs	cream	pramoxine HCl, 1%		zinc oxide	glycerin	beeswax · cetyl alcohol · cetyl esters wax · methylparaben · propylparaben · sodium lauryl sulfate
Tronolane Ross Products/Abbott Labs	suppository			zinc oxide, 5%	hard fat, 95%	
Tronothane Hydrochloride Abbott Labs	cream	pramoxine HCl, 1%			glycerin	cetyl alcohol · cetyl esters wax · sodium lauryl sulfate · methylparaben · propylparaben
Tucks Warner-Lambert Consumer	pad			witch hazel, 50%	glycerin	alcohol · propylene glycol · sodium citrate · diazolidinyl urea · citric acid · methylparaben · propylparaben · water

See Chapter 14, "Hemorrhoidal Products," for more information about these products.

HEMORRHOIDAL PRODUCTS - continued

Product Manufacturer/Supplier	Dosage Form	Anesthetic	Vasocon- strictor [a]	Astringent	Protectant	Other Ingredients
Tucks Clear Warner-Lambert Consumer	gel	benzyl alcohol		witch hazel, 50%	glycerin, 10%	carbomer 974P · disodium edetate · propylene glycol · sodium hydroxide · water
Vaseline Pure Petroleum Jelly Chesebrough-Pond's	ointment				white petrolatum, 100%	
** **Witch Hazel Hemorrhoidal Pads** T. N. Dickinson	pad			distilled witch hazel, 50%	glycerin	purified water · benzethonium chloride · methylparaben · aloe vera gel
Wyanoids Relief Factor Wyeth-Ayerst Labs	suppository				cocoa butter, 79% · shark liver oil, 3% · glycerin	ascorbyl palmitate · benzoic acid · BHA · corn oil · disodium edetate · methylparaben · PEG-12 dilaurate · propylparaben · tocopherol · water · white wax

** New listing

[a] Patients who are taking monoamine oxidase inhibitors or who have diabetes, hyperthyroidism, hypertension, cardiovascular disease, or difficulty in urination due to prostate enlargement should not use products containing a vasoconstrictor without first consulting a physician.

See Chapter 14, "Hemorrhoidal Products," for more information about these products.

Anthelmintic Product Table

ANTHELMINTIC PRODUCTS

Product Manufacturer/Supplier	Dosage Form	Active Ingredients	Other Ingredients
LA SL	**Antiminth** Pfizer Consumer	suspension	pyrantel pamoate, 250mg/5ml	caramel-currant flavor · citric acid · glycerin · lecithin · magnesium aluminum silicate · polysorbate · povidone · simethicone emulsion · sodium benzoate · sorbitol solution
LA SU PE	**Pin-X** Effcon	liquid	pyrantel pamoate, 50mg/1ml	citric acid · lecithin · methylparaben · povidone · propylparaben · saccharin sodium · sodium benzoate · glycerin · magnesium aluminum silicate · polysorbate 80 · propylene glycol · purified water · simethicone emulsion · sorbitol solution · flavor · color
	Reese's Pinworm Reese Chemical	liquid	pyrantel pamoate, 144mg/ml	
	Reese's Pinworm Reese Chemical	caplet	pyrantel pamoate, 180mg	

See Chapter 15, "Anthelmintic Products," for more information about these products.

Emetic and Antiemetic
Product Tables

EMETIC PRODUCTS

Product Manufacturer/Supplier	Dosage Form	Active Ingredients	Other Ingredients
Ipecac Multisource	syrup	powdered ipecac	alcohol, 1.5-1.75% · glycerin · purified water

See Chapter 16, "Emetic and Antiemetic Products," for more information about these products.

GASTRIC DECONTAMINANT PRODUCTS

Product Manufacturer/Supplier	Dosage Form	Activated Charcoal	Other Ingredients
Actidose with Sorbitol Paddock Labs	liquid	25g/120ml; 50g/240ml	sorbitol
Actidose-Aqua Paddock Labs	liquid	15g/72ml; 25g/120ml; 50g/240ml	
** DY GL SU **CharcoAid G** Requa	granule	15g/120ml	
** **Insta-Char With Cherry Flavor** Frank W. Kerr	suspension	25g/120ml; 50g/240ml	cherry flavor (to be added)
** **Insta-Char With Sorbitol and Cherry Flavor** Frank W. Kerr	suspension	25g/120ml; 50g/240ml	sorbitol, 25g/120ml; 50g/240ml · cherry flavor (to be added)
** **Insta-Char, Unflavored** Frank W. Kerr	suspension	25g/120ml; 50g/240ml	
Liqui Char Jones Medical	liquid	25g/120ml	water
Liqui Char Jones Medical	liquid	25g/120ml	sorbitol, 27g/120ml

** New listing

See Chapter 16, "Emetic and Antiemetic Products," for more information about these products.

ANTIEMETIC PRODUCTS

	Product Manufacturer/Supplier	Dosage Form	Active Ingredients	Other Ingredients
PU	**Bonine** Pfizer Consumer	chewable tablet	meclizine HCl, 25mg	raspberry flavor · corn starch · FD&C red#40 · lactose · magnesium stearate · purified siliceous earth · saccharin · talc
	Calm-X Republic Drug	tablet	dimenhydrinate, 50mg	
	Cola Unico	syrup	phosphoric acid · high fructose corn syrup and/or sucrose	water · caramel color · natural flavors · caffeine
GL PU SO	**Dramamine** Pharmacia & Upjohn	chewable tablet	dimenhydrinate, 50mg	aspartame · citric acid · FD&C yellow#5 · flavor · magnesium stearate · methacrylic acid copolymer · sorbitol · FD&C yellow#6
PU SO	**Dramamine II Less Drowsy Formula** Pharmacia & Upjohn	tablet	meclizine HCl, 25mg	colloidal silicon dioxide · corn starch · lactose · D&C yellow#10 aluminum lake · microcrystalline cellulose · magnesium stearate
GL PU SO	**Dramamine Original** Pharmacia & Upjohn	tablet	dimenhydrinate, 50mg	colloidal silicon dioxide · croscarmellose sodium · lactose · magnesium stearate · microcrystalline cellulose
AL LA SL PE	**Dramamine, Children's** Pharmacia & Upjohn	liquid	dimenhydrinate, 12.5mg/5ml	FD&C red#40 · flavor · glycerin · methylparaben · sucrose · water
**	**Emecheck** Savage Labs	liquid	phosphoric acid, 21.5mg/5ml · dextrose (glucose) 1.87g/5ml · levulose (fructose) 1.87g/5ml	FD&C red#40 · flavors · glycerin · methylparaben · purified water
	Emetrol, Cherry or Lemon Mint Pharmacia & Upjohn	liquid	phosphoric acid, 21.5g/5ml · dextrose, 1.87g/5ml · fructose, 1.87g/5ml	FD&C red#40 (Cherry) · D&C yellow#10 (Lemon Mint)flavors · glycerin · methylparaben · purified water
	Marezine § Martin Himmel	tablet	cyclizine HCl, 50mg	cellulose · lactose · starch · hydrogenated vegetable oil · magnesium stearate · silicon dioxide
DY GL SO SU	**Nauzene** Alva-Amco Pharmacal	tablet	diphenhydramine HCl, 25mg	lactose microcrystalline cellulose · stearic acid · magnesium stearate
** AL	**Rekematol Anti-Nausea** Reese Chemical	liquid	phosphoric acid, 21.5mg/5ml · dextrose, 1.87g/5ml · levulose, 1.87g/5ml	
AL	**Triptone** Del Ph'cals	tablet	dimenhydrinate, 50mg	

** New listing

§ Manufacturer/supplier did not confirm information for this edition. Product listing is reprinted from the '96-97 edition.

See Chapter 16, "Emetic and Antiemetic Products," for more information about these products.

Ostomy Care Product Tables

OSTOMY APPLIANCES

Product Manufacturer/Supplier	Product Form	Size (in)	Quantity	Comments
Active Life Drainable Pouches w/ Stomahesive Skin Barrier § ConvaTec	pouch	10 · 12	10/bx	one piece · stoma opening sizes: 0.75"-2.5"
Adhesive Drainable Pouches Hollister	pouch	12 · 16	50/bx	standard adhesive · transparent odor-barrier film · stoma opening sizes: 1"-3"
Closed-End Adhesive Colostomy Pouches Bard Medical	pouch	5 x 8 · 5.5 x 8 · 6.5 x 10	10/pk	odorproof · rustle free · extra gauge · one piece · rounded corners
Cool Comfort Nu-Support Belts Nu-Hope Labs	belt	width: 3, 4, 6, 9 · circumference: petite/youth 16-27, adult 28-52	1/bx	lightweight, ventilated elastic · hinged horizontally for contoured fit · standard pouch opening: 2 3/8"
Drainable Adhesive Ileostomy Pouches Bard Medical	pouch	mini, 5 x 9 1/4 · regular, 6 x 11 3/16 · wide opening, 6 x 11 13/16	10/pk	odorproof · rustle free · extra gauge · one piece · regular size available in plain or wide opening
Karaya Seal Drainable Pouches Hollister	pouch	9 · 12 · 16	30/bx	Karaya five-seal ring and microporous adhesive · stoma opening sizes: 1"-2" and 1"-3"
PE **Little Ones Active Life Drainable Pouches §** ConvaTec	pouch	6	15/bx	transparent · one piece · stoma opening sizes: 5/16"-2"
PE **Little Ones Sur-Fit Drainable Pouches §** ConvaTec	pouch	6	10/bx	transparent · flange sizes: 1.25" and 1.75"
Nu-Flex Adult Oval or Round Drainable Pouches Nu-Hope Labs	pouch	11	10/bx	transparent · stoma opening sizes: 0.5"-2" (Round) and 0.75" x 1.5"-2.25" x 3.75" trim to fit (Oval)
Nu-Flex Adult Oval or Round Urinary Pouches Nu-Hope Labs	pouch	11	10/bx	one piece · transparent · 3.5" adhesive foam pad (Round) · stoma opening sizes: 0.5"-2" (Round) and 0.75" x 1.5"-2.25" x 3.75" trim to fit (Oval)
Nu-Flex Brief or Mini Urinary Pouches Nu-Hope Labs	pouch	7 (Mini) · 8 (Brief)	10/bx	one piece · transparent · 3" adhesive foam pad · stoma opening sizes: 0.5"-2"
Nu-Self Adult or Brief Drainable Pouches Nu-Hope Labs	pouch	7.5 (Brief) · 11 (Adult)	1/pk	opaque · stoma opening sizes: 0.5"-2" and 3.5" · adhesive foam pad (Adult)
** **Regular One-Piece Colostomy Pouches** Bard Medical	pouch	5.5 x 8 · 6.5 x 10 · 4.5 x 12	10/pk	odor resistant
Sheer Plus Drainable Pouches Smith & Nephew	pouch	11 · 12.25 · 12.5	10/pk	clear or opaque · one piece · 4" x 4" adhesive face plate on free-floating collar with barrier · odor proof · Pre-Fit or Trim 'n' Fit openings
** **Small Drainable One-Piece Pouches** Coloplast	pouch	10	10/bx	odorproof film and simple integral closure · stoma opening sizes: 0.75"-1.625"

See Chapter 17, "Ostomy Care Products," for more information about these products.

OSTOMY APPLIANCES - continued

	Product Manufacturer/Supplier	Product Form	Size (in)	Quantity	Comments
**	**Small Drainable Two-Piece Pouches** Coloplast	pouch	10	10/bx	opaque
**	**Small Urostomy Two-Piece Pouches** Coloplast	pouch	7	10/bx	anti-reflux valve · transparent · stoma opening sizes: up to 1.75"
**	**Standard Drainable One-Piece Pouches** Coloplast	pouch	11	10/bx	odorproof film and simple integral closure · stoma opening sizes: 0.75"-2.375"
**	**Standard Drainable Two-Piece Pouches** Coloplast	pouch	11	10/bx	opaque or transparent
**	**Standard Urostomy Two-Piece Pouches** Coloplast	pouch	10	10/bx	anti-reflux valve · opaque or transparent · stoma opening sizes: up to 2"
	Stoma Urine Bags Bard Medical	bag	adult, 6 x 13.25 · medium, 6.5 x 10.25 · pediatric, 5.5 x 8.5	5/pk	adhesive · one piece
	Sur-Fit Drainable Pouches § ConvaTec	pouch	10 · 12	10/bx	flange sizes: 1.25"-2.75"
	Torbot Belts Torbot	belt	Elastic Web (width from 1 1/8"-45") · Reliabelt (5" width): small, medium, large · Rubber: adjustable, for wet environment · Versatile (2" or 3" width)	1/pk	four types for various sizes and uses
	Torbot Foam Pads Torbot	pad	diameter: 2 11/16 - 4 7/8 · thickness: 1/16 and 1/8	1/pk	use with cement between faceplate and skin for greater comfort · does not allow leakage · available in black or white foam
**	**Torbot PeeWees Pediatric Urine Collection** Torbot	bag	3 x 8	10/pk	non-sterile or sterile
	Torbot Plastic Pouches, Opaque White Torbot	pouch	10 · 12	1/pk	lined · heavy duty · odorproof · reusable; average life of two weeks
	Torbot Plastic Pouches, Transparent Torbot	pouch	9 · 10 · 11	1/pk	lightweight, clear vinyl · reusable; average life of one week
	Torbot Plastic Urinary Pouches, Opaque White Torbot	pouch	10 · 12	1/pk	lined · heavy duty · odorproof · reusable; average life of two weeks · small, narrower spout for special urinal outlet
	Torbot Plastic Urinary Pouches, Transparent Torbot	pouch	pediatric, 6.5 · 9 · 10 · 11	1/pk	lightweight, clear vinyl · includes small spout fitted for urinal valve and stem · reusable; average life of one week
	Torbot Rubber Pouches Torbot	pouch	9 · 10 · 11 · 12	1/pk	recommended for use by ostomates with loose drainage · high quality butyl rubber · for longer term usage · available in black or white, folded or welded seam, and lightweight or medium weight

See Chapter 17, "Ostomy Care Products," for more information about these products.

OSTOMY APPLIANCES - continued

Product Manufacturer/Supplier	Product Form	Size (in)	Quantity	Comments
Torbot Rubber Urinary Pouches Torbot	pouch	pediatric, 5.5 · 9 · 10 · 11 · 12	1/pk	high quality butyl rubber · for longer term usage · small, narrower spout for special urinal outlet · available in black or flesh pink, with metal or plastic valve and stem
Urostomy Pouches Hollister	pouch	12 · 16	20/bx	Karaya five-seal ring · standard adhesive · transparent odor-barrier film · stoma opening sizes: 1"-2"
VPI Non-Adhesive Colostomy Systems VPI	pouch	closed-end: 6 · open-end: 8	2/pk · 10/pk	reusable system · for single patient use only · closed-end set includes pouches, o-ring seal, and belt · open-end set includes pouches, o-ring seal, belt, and drain tail closure · flange sizes: 1 7/8," 2 3/8," 2 7/8"
VPI Non-Adhesive Ileostomy Systems VPI	pouch	300cc · 500cc	1-4/pk	reusable system · for single patient use only · set includes pouch, o-ring seal, belt, and drain tail closure
VPI Non-Adhesive Urostomy Systems VPI	pouch	300cc · 500cc · 800cc · 1100cc	1/pk	reusable system · for single patient use only · set includes pouch, o-ring seal, and belt

** New listing

§   Manufacturer/supplier did not confirm information for this edition. Product listing is reprinted from the '96-97 edition.

See Chapter 17, "Ostomy Care Products," for more information about these products.

OSTOMY ACCESSORIES

Product Manufacturer/Supplier	Ingredients
ADHESIVE DISK PRODUCTS	
A-Ds Transdermal Patch Torbot	medical grade adhesive
Blanchard Karaya Wafers Blanchard	karaya gum powder, 70% · glycerin, 30%
Lan-Tex Torbot	hydrophilic polymer combined with synthetic rubber polymer
** **Nu-Hope Adhesive** Nu-Hope Labs	natural rubber · hexane
Universal Adhesive Gaskets Smith & Nephew	rubber-based adhesive
CEMENT PRODUCTS	
Liquid Cement Perry Products	rubber base · ethyl ether, 24% · alcohol, 5% · nitromersol, 0.005%
Mastisol Ferndale Labs	gum mastic
Skin-Bond Cement Smith & Nephew	natural rubber · hexane · fillers
SOLVENT PRODUCTS	
Detachol Ferndale Labs	paraffin hydrocarbons
Remove Adhesive Remover Smith & Nephew	C10-11 isoparaffin · dipropylene glycol methyl ether · aloe extract · benzyl alcohol · fragrance
Torbot Adhesive Remover Torbot	naphtha petroleum
Uni-Solve Adhesive Remover Smith & Nephew	isopropyl alcohol · C10-11 isoparaffin · dipropylene glycol methyl ether · aloe extract · fragrance
APPLIANCE DEODORIZER PRODUCTS	
Banish II Liquid Deodorant Smith & Nephew	dipropylene glycol · zinc ricinoleate · water · FD&C blue#1
** **Devko Tablets** Parthenon	bismuth subgallate, 200mg · activated charcoal
Liquid Deodorant Perry Products	water · alcohol · fragrance
Odo-Way Appliance Deodorant Tablets Smith & Nephew	dicalcium phosphate · starch · sodium dichloro-s-triazinetrione · magnesium stearate · stearic acid
Super Banish Appliance Deodorant Smith & Nephew	triethylene glycol · water · ethylene thiourea · silver nitrate · FD&C yellow#5 · FD&C blue#1 · sodium chloride · sodium sulfate

See Chapter 17, "Ostomy Care Products," for more information about these products.

OSTOMY ACCESSORIES - continued

Product Manufacturer/Supplier	Ingredients
INTERNAL DEODORIZER PRODUCTS	
Charcoal Tablets Requa	activated charcoal, 250mg
CharcoCaps Caplets or Capsules Requa	activated charcoal, 260mg · sugar, 300mg
** **Derifil Tablets** Menley & James Labs	chlorophyllin copper complex · sodium · dextrose · hydrogenated vegetable oil · hydroxypropyl methylcellulose · microcrystalline cellulose · peppermint powder · polyethylene glycol · sodium chloride
Devrom Chewable Tablets Parthenon	bismuth subgallate, 200mg
SKIN PROTECTIVE PRODUCTS	
Barri-Care Topical Antimicrobial Ointment Care-Tech Labs	chloroxylenol, 0.8% · vitamins A, D3, and E · mineral oil · petrolatum · milk protein · propylparaben · paraffin · methylparaben · propylene glycol · potassium hydroxide
** **Carbo Zinc Powder** Nu-Hope Labs	karaya powder · zinc oxide · corn starch · petrolatum
Care-Creme Antimicrobial Cream Care-Tech Labs	chloroxylenol, 0.8% · cetyl alcohol · cod liver oil · lanolin oil · lanolin alcohol · propylene glycol · vitamins A, D3, and E
Formula A Stretchable Karaya Washers & Sheets Smith & Nephew	karaya gum powder · propylene glycol
** **Orchid Fresh II Liquid** Care-Tech Labs	benzethonium chloride, 0.1% · water · amphoteric 2 · DMDM hydantoin · fragrance · citric acid
Pro Cute Ferndale Labs	stearic acid · cetyl alcohol · forlan-LM · ceraphyl 230 · glycerin · triethanolamine · deltyl prime · PVP · sorbic acid · silicone · perfume · menthol · dowicil 200
** **Protective Barrier Film Wipes** Bard Medical	isopropanol · butyl methacrylate · dimethyl phthalate
Skin-Prep Protective Dressing Smith & Nephew	isopropyl alcohol · butyl ester of PVM/MA copolymer · acetyl tributyl citrate
Tincture of Benzoin Multisource	tincture of benzoin
** **Torbot Healskin Powder** Torbot	karaya powder
Triple Care Cream Smith & Nephew	water · petrolatum · zinc oxide · cetearyl alcohol · PEG-40 castor oil · polysorbate 20 · octyl palmitate · sodium cetearyl sulfate · octyl stearate · dioctyl adipate · vitamin E acetate · methylparaben · allantoin · clove oil · o-phenylphenol · aloe
Triple Care Extra Protective Cream Smith & Nephew	petrolatum · zinc oxide · karaya · water · carboxymethylcellulose sodium · methyl glucose dioleate · mineral oil · glycerin · triethanolamine · chloroxylenol · tocopheryl acetate · butylparaben
Uni-Salve Ointment Smith & Nephew	petrolatum · benzethonium chloride · chloroxylenol · propylparaben · butylated hydroxyanisole · fragrance · vitamin A palmitate · vegetable oil · vitamin D3 · D&C green#6
Velvet Fresh Powder Care-Tech Labs	corn starch · tricalcium phosphate · fragrance

See Chapter 17, "Ostomy Care Products," for more information about these products.

Diabetes Care Products and Monitoring Devices Tables

INSULIN PREPARATIONS

Product Manufacturer/Supplier	Species Source [a]	Onset (h)	Peak (h)	Dura- tion (h)	Preser- vative	Purity (ppm of proin- sulin)	Stability at Room Temp. (mo)	Zinc (mg/ 100 U)	Protein (mg/ 100 U)
RAPID ACTING									
Humulin R (Regular Human Insulin) Eli Lilly	h	0.5-1	1-3	5-7	metacresol	<1	1	0.01-0.04	
Novolin R (Regular Human Insulin) Novo Nordisk Ph'cals	h	0.5	2.5-5	8	metacresol	<1	1, in use	trace	
Novolin R PenFill (Regular Human Insulin, 1.5ml cartridge) Novo Nordisk Ph'cals	h	0.5	2.5-5	8	metacresol	<1	1, in use	trace	
Novolin R Prefilled (Reg. Human Insulin, 1.5ml syringe) Novo Nordisk Ph'cals	h	0.5	2.5-5	8	metacresol	<1	1, in use	trace	
Regular (Purified Pork) Novo Nordisk Ph'cals	p	0.5	2.5-5	8	phenol	<1	1, in use	trace	
Regular Iletin I Eli Lilly	b · p	0.5-1	1-3	5-7	metacresol	<10	1	0.01-0.04	
Regular Iletin II (Purified Pork) Eli Lilly	p	0.5-1	1-3	5-7	metacresol	<1	1	0.01-0.04	
Velosulin BR (Buffered Reg. Human Insulin, semi-synthetic) Novo Nordisk Ph'cals	h	0.5	1-3	8	metacresol	<1	1, in use	trace	
INTERMEDIATE ACTING									
Humulin L (Lente Human Insulin Zinc Suspension) Eli Lilly	h	2-4	8-10	18-24	methylparaben	<1	1	0.12-0.25	
Humulin N (NPH Human Insulin Isophane Suspension) Eli Lilly	h	1-3	8-10	18-24	phenol · metacresol	<1	1	0.01-0.04	protamine, 0.32-0.44
Iletin I Lente (Zinc Suspension) Eli Lilly	b · p	2-4	8-10	18-24	methylparaben	<10	1	0.12-0.25	
Iletin I NPH (Isophane Suspension) Eli Lilly	b · p	1-3	8-10	18-24	phenol · metacresol	<10	1	0.01-0.04	protamine, 0.32-0.44
Iletin II Lente (Zinc Suspension, Purified Pork) Eli Lilly	p	2-4	8-10	18-24	methylparaben	<1	1	0.12-0.25	

See Chapter 18, "Diabetes Care Products and Monitoring Devices," for more information about these products.

INSULIN PREPARATIONS - continued

Product Manufacturer/Supplier	Species Source [a]	Onset (h)	Peak (h)	Dura-tion (h)	Preser-vative	Purity (ppm of proin-sulin)	Stability at Room Temp. (mo)	Zinc (mg/ 100 U)	Protein (mg/ 100 U)
Iletin II NPH (Isophane Suspension, Purified Pork) Eli Lilly	p	1-3	8-10	18-24	phenol · metacresol	<1	1	0.01-0.04	protamine, 0.32-0.44
Lente (Zinc Suspension, Purified Pork) Novo Nordisk Ph'cals	p	2.5	7-15	22	methylparaben	<1	1, in use	0.15 (approx.)	
Novolin L (Lente Human Insulin Zinc Suspension) Novo Nordisk Ph'cals	h	2.5	7-15	22	methylparaben	<1	1, in use	0.15 (approx.)	
Novolin N (NPH Human Insulin Isophane Suspension) Novo Nordisk Ph'cals	h	1.5	4-12	24	phenol · metacresol	<1	1, in use	trace	protamine, 0.35 (approx.)
Novolin N PenFill (NPH Human Insulin Isophane Susp., 1.5ml) Novo Nordisk Ph'cals	h	1.5	4-12	24	phenol · metacresol	<1	0.25 (7 days), in use	trace	protamine, 0.35 (approx.)
Novolin N Prefilled (NPH Human Insulin Iso. Susp., 1.5ml) Novo Nordisk Ph'cals	h	1.5	4-12	24	phenol · metacresol	<1	0.25 (7 days), in use	trace	protamine, 0.35 (approx.)
NPH (Isophane, Purified Pork) Novo Nordisk Ph'cals	p	1.5	4-12	24	phenol · metacresol	<1	1, in use	trace	protamine, 0.35 (approx.)
MIXED (INTERMEDIATE/RAPID ACTING)									
Humulin 50/50 (50% NPH Isophane Suspension, 50% Regular) Eli Lilly	h	0.5-1	2-12	up to 24	phenol · metacresol	<1	1	0.01-0.04	protamine, 0.16-0.18
Humulin 70/30 (70% NPH Isophane Suspension, 30% Regular) Eli Lilly	h	0.5-1	2-12	up to 24	phenol · metacresol	<1	1	0.01-0.04	protamine, 0.22-0.26
Novolin 70/30 (70% NPH Human Iso. Susp., 30% Regular Human) Novo Nordisk Ph'cals	h	0.5	2-12	24	phenol · metacresol	<1	1, in use	trace	protamine, 0.25 (approx.)
Novolin 70/30 PenFill (70% NPH Human, 30% Reg. Human; 1.5ml) Novo Nordisk Ph'cals	h	0.5	2-12	24	phenol · metacresol	<1	0.25 (7 days), in use	trace	protamine, 0.25 (approx.)

See Chapter 18, "Diabetes Care Products and Monitoring Devices," for more information about these products.

INSULIN PREPARATIONS - continued

Product Manufacturer/Supplier	Species Source [a]	Onset (h)	Peak (h)	Dura-tion (h)	Preser-vative	Purity (ppm of proin-sulin)	Stability at Room Temp. (mo)	Zinc (mg/ 100 U)	Protein (mg/ 100 U)
Novolin 70/30 Prefilled (70% NPH Human, 30% Reg Hum.; 1.5ml) Novo Nordisk Ph'cals	h	0.5	2-12	24	phenol · metacresol	<1	0.25 (7 days), in use	trace	protamine, 0.25 (approx.)
LONG ACTING									
Humulin U (Ultralente Human Insulin Extended Zinc Susp.) Eli Lilly	h	4-6	8-14	24-28	methylparaben	<1	1	0.12-0.25	

[a] b=beef, p=pork, h=human insulin derived through recombinant DNA biotechnology. Insulins with a combination of beef and pork contain 70% beef and 30% pork.

See Chapter 18, "Diabetes Care Products and Monitoring Devices," for more information about these products.

INSULIN SYRINGES AND RELATED PRODUCTS

Product Manufacturer/Supplier	Comments
SYRINGES	
Autopen Owen Mumford	pen-like injection device · 6" long, 7 oz. in weight · uses a prefilled, replaceable, 1.5ml cartridge of insulin · two models: delivers 2 to 32 units in 2-unit increments, or delivers 1 to 16 units in 1-unit increments · dial-a-dose selector offers both visual and audio indication of setting · one-handed insulin delivery button
B-D Micro-Fine IV Syringe § Becton Dickinson Consumer	28 gauge, disposable · 3/10, 1/2, or 1cc · for U-100 insulin · packages of 10 in boxes of 100 · capped at both needle and plunger ends for sterility and protection · single scale, single unit markings for precise dosage measurement · large bold numbers · lubricated needle · zero dead space · flat plunger tip
**	**B-D Pen §** Becton Dickinson Consumer	pen-shaped insulin delivery device · uses 1.5ml cartridges of insulin · uses B-D Ultra Fine 29-gauge pen needles, available in Original (1/2") and Short (5/16") lengths
**	**B-D Ultra-Fine II Short Needle Syringe §** Becton Dickinson Consumer	30 gauge, disposable · 3/10 or 1/2cc · needle is 37% shorter than standard length · for U-100 insulin · packages of 10 in boxes of 100 · capped at both needle and plunger ends for sterility and protection · single scale, single unit markings for precise dosage measurement · large bold numbers · lubricated needle · zero dead space · flat plunger tip
B-D Ultra-Fine Syringe § Becton Dickinson Consumer	29 gauge, disposable · 3/10, 1/2, or 1cc · for U-100 insulin · packages of 10 in boxes of 100 · capped at both needle and plunger ends for sterility and protection · single scale, single unit markings for precise dosage measurement · large bold numbers · lubricated needle · zero dead space · flat plunger tip
Monoject Ultra Comfort 29 Syringe Can-Am Care	29 gauge, disposable · 3/10, 1/2, or 1cc · for U-100 insulin · individually packaged in tamper-evident, sterile peel packs of five; 30 or 100 count boxes · bold numbers · zero dead space · flat plunger tip · permanently attached, advanced laser-welded needle · improved lubricant
Monoject Ultra Comfort Syringe Can-Am Care	28 gauge, disposable · 1/2 or 1cc · for U-100 insulin · individually packaged in tamper-evident, sterile peel packs of five; 30 or 100 count boxes · bold numbers · zero dead space · flat plunger tip · permanently attached, advanced laser-welded needle · improved lubricant
NovoFine 30 Needle Novo Nordisk Ph'cals	30 gauge, disposable · beveled needle tip · siliconized throughout the length · ensures minimal friction with skin · 1/3 inch (8mm) long · for single use only, 100/box · disposable needles specifically designed for use with NovoNordisk insulin delivery systems · protective outer cap, smooth plastic needle cap, and a protective tab · should not be used if protective tab is missing or damaged
NovoPen 1.5 Novo Nordisk Ph'cals	lightweight, durable dial-a-dose insulin delivery device · made from stainless steel and high-impact plastic · 6" long, 1.4 oz. in weight · uses 1.5ml cartridges of Novolin human insulin · delivers 1 to 40 units in 1-unit increments · uses the NovoFine 30 disposable needle
**	**Sure-Dose Plus Syringe** Terumo Medical	29 gauge, disposable · 1/2 or 1cc · for U-100 insulin · individually wrapped for sterility in boxes of 100 · 1/2cc has single unit scale markings · 1cc has scale markings every two units · large, bold numbers · lubricated needle · zero dead space · tapered hub/flush fit plunger tip · latex free
**	**Sure-Dose Syringe** Terumo Medical	28 gauge, disposable · 1/2 or 1cc · for U-100 insulin · individually wrapped for sterility in boxes of 100 · 1/2cc has single unit scale markings · 1cc has scale markings every two units · large, bold numbers · lubricated needle · zero dead space · tapered hub/flush fit plunger tip · latex free
Terumo Insulin Syringe Terumo Medical	29 gauge, disposable · 1/4cc · for U-100 insulin · individually wrapped for sterility in boxes of 100 · the only insulin syringe available with 1/2 unit scale markings · large, bold scale markings · lubricated needle · zero dead space · tapered hub/flush fit plunger tip · latex free
RELATED PRODUCTS	
Autoject Owen Mumford	plastic spring-loaded syringe injector to be positioned over skin · press device against injection site, then push button to simultaneously insert needle and inject insulin · fits most brands and sizes of disposable fixed-needle syringes
Autoject 2 Owen Mumford	plastic spring-loaded syringe injector to be positioned over skin · press device against injection site then push button to simultaneously insert needle and inject insulin · fits B-D 1/2, 1, and 2cc disposable syringes, plus Terumo 1/4, 1/2, and 1cc disposable syringes · two models: for use with fixed-needle and nonfixed-needle syringes · can be adjusted for depth of needle penetration · internal syringe cocking device · observation window shows when injection is complete · safety lock prevents accidental discharge

See Chapter 18, "Diabetes Care Products and Monitoring Devices," for more information about these products.

INSULIN SYRINGES AND RELATED PRODUCTS - continued

Product Manufacturer/Supplier	Comments
B-D Home Sharps Container § Becton Dickinson Consumer	container for safe disposal of syringes, needles, and lancets · leak-proof, puncture-resistant plastic with snap-on lid · red-colored with biohazard symbol · small opening for depositing of syringes and lancets helps prevent children from reaching inside · compact size for easy storage
B-D Magni-Guide § Becton Dickinson Consumer	magnifies entire syringe scale calibrations 2 times to make them easier to read · helps guide syringe needle into insulin vial · syringe is slipped into curved channel of Magni-Guide · insulin vial is snapped into collar at opposite end
B-D Safe-Clip § Becton Dickinson Consumer	clips and stores more than one year's supply of used syringe needles for safe and easy disposal
** **Blue Needle Box Sharps Disposal System** Bio-Oxidation	a service providing a mail-back sharps container to be purchased, filled, and returned for safe disposal of used syringes, needles, and lancets · when returned, the container of medical waste is processed via electric bi-oxidation to leave behind only sterile inorganic residue · a confirmation letter is mailed to patients assuring them of complete waste disposal
Count-a-Dose Jordan Medical	syringe filling device · empty B-D Lo-Dose 1/2cc syringe is secured in easy-to-locate platform · click wheel activates slide to ensure accurate dosage in 1-unit increments · slide moves syringe plunger to control insulin intake · "click" heard and felt as each insulin unit is filled · holds 1 insulin vial, or 2 vials for mixing insulins
Inject-Ease Palco Labs	plastic spring-loaded syringe injector to be positioned over skin · press device against site, push button to simultaneously insert needle and inject insulin · fits most brands and sizes of disposable syringes · can be adjusted for depth of needle penetration
Instaject Jordan Medical	combination insulin injector and blood lancet device · button-activated · self-contained as injector · fits most brands and sizes of disposable insulin syringes · can be adjusted for depth of needle penetration
Insuflon Chronimed	small, flexible teflon catheter to be inserted subcutaneously · allows the patient to inject insulin for several days without repeated skin punctures
Insul-eze Palco Labs	syringe loading device with magnifier · assists patients with impaired vision or decreased hand coordination · magnifies syringe calibration · sits on any flat surface, horizontally or vertically · holds all types of insulin bottles
** **Insul-Guide** Stat Medical	syringe loading device · assists patients with impaired vision or decreased hand coordination · funnel-shaped design guides syringe into insulin bottle · internal collar allows more insulin to be extracted from the bottle
Load-Matic Palco Labs	syringe loading device · allows visually-impaired patients to measure dosage by touch alone · using B-D 1cc syringe, dosage may be set in single-unit or ten-unit increments; dosage may then be used repeatedly without further adjustment
Monoject Injectomatic Can-Am Care	metal spring-loaded syringe injector · press device against selected injection site to insert needle, then press syringe plunger to inject insulin · increases injection-site alternatives · 1/2cc size for 1/2cc and 3/10cc syringes, 1cc size for 1cc syringes · used only with Monoject disposable syringes and a 90-degree injection angle
TruHand Whittier Medical	syringe/vial holder with magnifier · easy-to-use device · click sound is heard when insulin vial is locked in place · user fills the syringe while reading enlarged scale markings · insulin vials may be interchanged to allow for mixed dosages
Wright Prefilled Syringe Case LLW Enterprises	impact-resistant polypropylene case for carrying one prefilled insulin syringe · resembles a fountain pen with clip · holds most types of disposable syringes · case interior holds syringe's plunger in personalized preset position · 90-day product replacement warranty

** New listing

§ Manufacturer/supplier did not confirm information for this edition. Product listing is reprinted from the '96-97 edition.

See Chapter 18, "Diabetes Care Products and Monitoring Devices," for more information about these products.

GLUCOSE AND KETONE TEST PRODUCTS

Product Manufacturer/Supplier	Product Form	Biological Fluid Tested	Active Ingredients
Acetest Bayer Diagnostics	tablet	urine · blood	nitroprusside-glycine · buffer
Albustix Bayer Diagnostics	strip	urine	tetrabromphenol blue · buffer
Bili-Labstix Bayer Diagnostics	stick	urine	see Multistix 10 SG
Chemstrip 2GP Boehringer Mannheim	strip	urine	glucose: tetramethylbenzidine · glucose oxidase · peroxidase · protein: tetrachlorophenol · tetrabromosulfophthalein
Chemstrip 2LN Boehringer Mannheim	strip	urine	see Chemstrip 10 with SG
Chemstrip 4 the OB Boehringer Mannheim	strip	urine	see Chemstrip 10 with SG
Chemstrip 6 Boehringer Mannheim	strip	urine	see Chemstrip 10 with SG
Chemstrip 7 Boehringer Mannheim	strip	urine	see Chemstrip 10 with SG
Chemstrip 8 Boehringer Mannheim	strip	urine	see Chemstrip 10 with SG
Chemstrip 9 Boehringer Mannheim	strip	urine	see Chemstrip 10 with SG
Chemstrip 10 with SG Boehringer Mannheim	strip	urine	specific gravity: EGTA · ethyleneglycol-bis (aminoethylether) tetraacetic acid · bromthymol blue · pH: bromthymol blue · methyl red · phenolphthalein · leukocytes: indoxylcarbonic acid ester · diazonium salt · nitrite: 3-hydroxy-1,2,3,4-tetrahydro-7,8-benzoquinoline · sulfanilamide · protein: tetrachlorophenol-tetrabromosulfophthalein · glucose: tetramethylbenzidine · glucose oxidase · peroxidase · ketones: sodium nitroferricyanide · glycine · urobilinogen: 4-methoxybenzene-diazonium-tetrafluoroborate · bilirubin: 2,6-dichlorobenzene-diazonium-tetrafluoroborate · blood: tetramethylbenzidine · 2,5-dimethyl-2,5-dihydroperoxthexane
Chemstrip bG Boehringer Mannheim	strip	blood	glucose oxidase · peroxidase · o-tolidine · tetramethylbenzidine
Chemstrip K Boehringer Mannheim	strip	urine	sodium nitroferricyanide · glycine
Chemstrip uG Boehringer Mannheim	strip	urine	glucose oxidase (aspergillus niger) · peroxidase (horseradish) · tetramethylbenzidine
Chemstrip uGK Boehringer Mannheim	strip	urine	glucose oxidase (aspergillus niger) · peroxidase (horseradish) · tetramethylbenzidine · sodium nitroferricyanide · glycine
Clinistix Bayer Diagnostics	strip	urine	glucose oxidase · peroxide o-tolidine
Clinitest Bayer Diagnostics	tablet	urine	copper reduction

See Chapter 18, "Diabetes Care Products and Monitoring Devices," for more information about these products.

Indication of Product Deterioration	Test Time (sec)	Drug Interference	Comments [a]
tan-to-brown discoloration or darkening	30	some false (+)	tests for ketones · requires dropper and clean, white paper
discoloration or darkening of reagent area	60	some false (+) · some masking of color development	
discoloration or darkening of test area	see Multistix 10 SG	see Multistix 10 SG	tests for glucose, protein, pH, blood, ketones, and bilirubin
discoloration of test area	60 (dip & read)	phenazopyridine	tests for glucose and protein
discoloration of test area	60 (dip & read)	see Chemstrip 10 with SG	tests for leukocytes and nitrite
discoloration of test area	60 (dip & read)	see Chemstrip 10 with SG	tests for leukocytes, protein, glucose, and blood
discoloration of test area	60 (dip & read)	see Chemstrip 10 with SG	tests for leukocytes, pH, protein, glucose, ketones, and blood
discoloration of test area	60 (dip & read)	see Chemstrip 10 with SG	tests for leukocytes, pH, protein, glucose, ketones, bilirubin, and blood
discoloration of test area	1-60 (dip & read)	see Chemstrip 10 with SG	tests for leukocytes, pH, protein, glucose, ketones, urobilinogen, bilirubin, and blood
discoloration of test area	see Chemstrip 10 with SG	see Chemstrip 10 with SG	tests for leukocytes, nitrite, pH, protein, glucose, ketones, urobilinogen, bilirubin, and blood
discoloration of test area	60 (dip & read)	see package insert for details	tests for specific gravity, pH, leukocytes, nitrite, protein, glucose, ketones, urobilinogen, bilirubin, and blood
darkening of test area when compared to "unused" color block on side of vial	120	false (-) from dopamine or methyldopa in concentration of 10mg/dL · see package insert for details	tests for glucose in capillary blood · requires drop of blood on both zones of the test strip · requires cotton ball to wipe off blood after 60 seconds · can be read visually after 60 additional seconds or used with an Accu-Chek II, IIm, or III meter
discoloration of test area	60 (dip & read)	mesna · see package insert for details	tests for ketones
discoloration of test area	60 (dip & read)		tests for glucose
discoloration of test area	60 (dip & read)	mesna	tests for glucose and ketones
tan or dark test area	10	no false (+) · some false (-) (levodopa, ascorbic acid, aspirin)	tests for glucose · convenient for type II diabetics · not quantitative
deep blue tablet	15	false (+) in presence of reducing agents · no false (-)	tests for glucose · use either 2-drop or 5-drop method · for use by type I diabetics · most reliable at high glucose levels · use for "sliding scale" · packaged with water dropper and test tube

GLUCOSE AND KETONE TEST PRODUCTS - continued

Product Manufacturer/Supplier	Product Form	Biological Fluid Tested	Active Ingredients
Combistix Bayer Diagnostics	strip	urine	see Hema-Combistix
Dextrostix Bayer Diagnostics	strip	blood	see Clinistix
Diastix Bayer Diagnostics	strip	urine	glucose oxidase · peroxidase · potassium iodide · chromogen
** **GLUCOchek Visual Blood Glucose Test** Clinical Diagnostics	strip	blood	glucose oxidase · peroxidase · tetramethylbenzidine
Glucofilm § Bayer Diagnostics	strip	blood	glucose oxidase · peroxidase · tetramethylbenzidine
Glucostix Bayer Diagnostics	strip	blood	glucose oxidase · peroxidase · ortho-tolidine dihydrochloride
Hema-Combistix Bayer Diagnostics	strip	urine	pH: methyl red · bromthymol blue · protein: tetrabromphenol blue · buffer · glucose: glucose oxidase · peroxidase · potassium iodide · buffer · blood: disopropylbenzene dihydroperoxide · 3,3′ 5,5′-tetramethylbenzidine · buffer
Keto-Diastix Bayer Diagnostics	strip	urine	glucose oxidase · nitroprusside
Ketostix Bayer Diagnostics	strip	urine	nitroprusside
Labstix Bayer Diagnostics	strip	urine	glucose: glucose oxidase · peroxidase · potassium iodide · buffer · ketone: sodium nitroprusside · buffer · blood: disopropylbenzene dihydroperoxide · 3.3′, 5.5′-tetramethylbenzidine · buffer · pH: methyl red · bromthymol blue · protein: tetrabromphenol blue · buffer
Micral Boehringer Mannheim	strip	urine	anti-human albumin IgG (mouse) · labeled with colloidal gold · fixed albumin
Multistix Bayer Diagnostics	strip	urine	see Multistix 10 SG
Multistix 2 Bayer Diagnostics	stick	urine	see Multistix 10 SG
Multistix 7 Bayer Diagnostics	stick	urine	see Multistix 10 SG
Multistix 8 SG Bayer Diagnostics	stick	urine	see Multistix 10 SG
Multistix 9 SG Bayer Diagnostics	stick	urine	see Multistix 10 SG

See Chapter 18, "Diabetes Care Products and Monitoring Devices," for more information about these products.

Indication of Product Deterioration	Test Time (sec)	Drug Interference	Comments [a]
discoloration or darkening of test area	see Hema-Combistix	see Hema-Combistix	tests for glucose, protein, and pH
test area does not resemble "O" on color chart	60	no false (+) · some false (-)	tests for glucose · useful in screening · accurate if read by Dextrometer · can use to correlate blood and urine levels
variation from light blue or "neg" on color chart	30	no false (+) · some complete false (-) (levodopa, ascorbic acid, aspirin)	tests for glucose · under-reading possible at high glucose levels · for use by both type I and type II diabetics
discoloration of test area	90		tests for glucose
discoloration or darkening of reagent areas	60	some slightly lower results	tests for glucose
discoloration or darkening of reagent area	120	some slightly lower results	tests for glucose · blot after 30 seconds, read after 90 additional seconds
discoloration or darkening of test area	proper read time is critical for optimal results · glucose: 30 · blood: 60 · protein and pH: up to 120	no false (+) for glucose · some false (+) · some false (-) · color may be masked · false (-) for blood may be caused by Capoten	tests for glucose, pH, protein, and blood
green glucose area; darkened ketone area	15-30	no false (+) for glucose · some false (-)	tests for glucose and ketones
tan or brown	15	false (+) possible but rare (levodopa)	tests for acetoacetic acid · useful in determining whether or not a diabetic is developing ketoacidosis
discoloration of test area	proper read time is critical for optimal results · glucose: 30 · ketone: 40 · blood: 60 · protein and pH: up to 120	no false (+) for glucose · some false (+) · some false (-) · color may be masked · false (+) for ketone with levodopa and mesna (free sulfhydryl groups) · false (-) for blood may be caused by Capoten	tests for blood, pH, glucose, ketones, and protein
` variation from white to red	5 (dip) · 60 (read)	oxytetracycline	tests for human albumin
discoloration or darkening of test area	see Multistix 10 SG	see Multistix 10 SG	tests for glucose, protein, pH, bilirubin, and urobilinogen
discoloration or darkening of test area	see Multistix 10 SG	see Multistix 10 SG	tests for nitrite and leukocytes
discoloration or darkening of test area	see Multistix 10 SG	see Multistix 10 SG	tests for glucose, protein, pH, blood, ketones, nitrite, and leukocytes
discoloration or darkening of test area	see Multistix 10 SG	see Multistix 10 SG	tests for glucose, protein, pH, blood, ketones, nitrite, leukocytes, and specific gravity
discoloration or darkening of test area	see Multistix 10 SG	see Multistix 10 SG	tests for glucose, protein, pH, blood, ketones, bilirubin, nitrite, and specific gravity

GLUCOSE AND KETONE TEST PRODUCTS - continued

Product Manufacturer/Supplier	Product Form	Biological Fluid Tested	Active Ingredients
Multistix 10 SG Bayer Diagnostics	strip	urine	glucose: glucose oxidase · peroxidase · potassium iodide · buffer · bilirubin: 2,4-dichloroaniline diazonium salt · buffer · ketone: sodium nitroprusside · buffer · specific gravity: bromthymol blue · poly (methyl vinyl ether/maleic anhydride) · sodium hydroxide · blood: disopropylbenzene dihydroperoxide · 3,3', 5,5'-tetramethylbenzidine · buffer · pH: methyl red · bromthymol blue · protein: tetrabromphenol blue · buffer · urobilinogen: p-diethylaminobenzaldehyde · nitrite: p-arsanilic acid · 1,2,3,4-tetrahydrobenzo(h)-quinolin-3-ol · buffer · leukocytes: derivatized pyrrole amino acid ester · diazonium salt · buffer
Multistix SG Bayer Diagnostics	stick	urine	see Multistix 10 SG
N-Multistix Bayer Diagnostics	strip	urine	see Multistix 10 SG
N-Multistix SG Bayer Diagnostics	stick	urine	see Multistix 10 SG
Uristix Bayer Diagnostics	strip	urine	see Multistix 10 SG
Uristix 4 § Bayer Diagnostics	strip	urine	see Multistix 10 SG

** New listing
[a] Protect all products from light, heat, and moisture.

See Chapter 18, "Diabetes Care Products and Monitoring Devices," for more information about these products.

Indication of Product Deterioration	Test Time (sec)	Drug Interference	Comments [a]
discoloration or darkening of test area	proper read time is critical for optimal results · glucose and bilirubin: 30 · ketone: 40 · specific gravity: 45 · urobilinogen, blood, and nitrite: 60 · leukocytes: 120 · protein and pH: up to 120	no false (+) for glucose · some false (+) · some false (-) · color may be masked · false (+) for bilirubin with Lodine · false (+) for ketone with levodopa and mesna (free sulfhydryl groups) · false (-) for blood may be caused by Capoten · false (+) for urobilinogen with sulfonamides and p-aminosalicylic acid · false (-) for leukocytes with Keflex, Keflin, and tetracycline	test for glucose, bilirubin, ketones, specific gravity, blood, pH, protein, urobilinogen, nitrite, and leukocytes
discoloration or darkening of test area	see Multistix 10 SG	see Multistix 10 SG	tests for glucose, protein, pH, blood, ketones, bilirubin, urobilinogen, leukocytes, and specific gravity
discoloration or darkening of test area	see Multistix 10 SG	see Multistix 10 SG	tests for glucose, protein, pH, blood, ketones, bilirubin, and nitrite
discoloration or darkening of test area	see Multistix 10 SG	see Multistix 10 SG	tests for glucose, protein, pH, blood, ketones, bilirubin, urobilinogen, nitrite, and specific gravity
discoloration of test area	30-60 (dip & read)	no false (+) for glucose · some false (-)	tests for glucose and protein; useful to determine if protein is in urine (diabetic nephropathy)
discoloration of test area	30-60 (dip & read)	no false (+) for glucose · some false (-)	tests for glucose, protein, nitrite, and leukocytes

BLOOD GLUCOSE METERS

Product Manufacturer/Supplier	Test Strip	Method	Test Time (sec)	Range (mg/dL)
Accu-Chek Advantage Boehringer Mannheim	Accu-Chek Advantage	no timing, no wiping, no cleaning	40	20-600
Accu-Chek Easy Boehringer Mannheim	Accu-Chek Easy	no timing, no wiping, visual confirmation	15-60	20-500
Accu-Chek III Boehringer Mannheim	Chemstrip bG	wiping required, visual confirmation	120	20-500
Accu-Chek Instant Boehringer Mannheim	Accu-Chek Instant Glucose Test Strips	no timing, no wiping, visual confirmation	12	20-500
Accu-Chek Instant DM Boehringer Mannheim	Accu-Chek Instant Glucose	no timing, no wiping, visual confirmation	12	20-600
** **Accu-Chek InstantPlus** Boehringer Mannheim	Accu-Chek Instant Glucose; Accu-Chek Instant Plus Cholesterol	no timing, no wiping, visual confirmation	12 (glucose); 180 (cholesterol)	20-600 (glucose); 150-300 (cholesterol)
CheckMate Plus Cascade Medical	CheckMate Plus	no timing, no wiping	30-70	25-500
Diascan Partner Home Diagnostics	Diascan	wipe	90	10-600
Diascan-S Home Diagnostics	Diascan	wipe, visual confirmation	90	10-600
ExacTech Card Model MediSense	ExacTech	no timing, no wiping, no cleaning, 3-step process	30	40-450
** **ExacTech R·S·G** MediSense	ExacTech R·S·G	no calibration, no timing, no wiping, 3-step process	30	40-450
** **GLUCOchek PocketLab** Clinical Diagnostics	GLUCOchek PocketLab	wipe	90	40-450
Glucometer Elite Bayer Diagnostics	Glucometer Elite	no timing, no wiping	30	40-500
MediSense 2 Card Model MediSense	MediSense 2	no timing, no wiping, no cleaning	20	20-600
MediSense 2 Pen Model MediSense	MediSense 2	no timing, no wiping	20	20-600
One Touch Basic LifeScan	Genuine One Touch	no timing, no wiping, 3-step process	45	0-600

See Chapter 18, "Diabetes Care Products and Monitoring Devices," for more information about these products.

Memory Capacity	Calibration	Warranty	Battery	Dimensions (in) (L x W x H)	Weight (oz)	Comments
100 tests; with time and date	lot-specific code chip	3 years	(2) 3-volt lithium	3.6 x 2.4 x 0.6	3	shows time and date
350 tests; with time and date, ave./min./max. event markers	lot-specific code chip	3 years	6-volt alkaline	4.5 x 2.5 x 0.75	3.4	shows time and date · 7-day test average · event markers · 7-day max./min. value · control marker
20 tests; with time and date	lot-specific code strip	2 years	6-volt alkaline	5.5 x 2.7 x 0.8	5.4	shows time and date · test strips may also be read visually
9 tests	push-button	3 years	(4) 1.5-volt alkaline	4 x 2.2 x 0.6	1.76	
500 tests	lot-specific strip	3 years	9-volt	6.2 x 3.2 x 1	8.4	shows time, date, and up to 4 of 29 event markers · insulin dosage is entered on numeric keypad · graphic display of 48-hour trend graph, 7-day trend graph, and insulin graph
50 tests (glucose); 15 tests (cholesterol)	calibration strip	3 years	(3) 1.5-volt AAA	4.6 x 2.5 x .7	3.75	
255 tests; with time and date	automatic	lifetime	(2) 3-volt lithium	6.3 x 1.1 x 0.7	1.8	built-in lancing device · activity markers code test results · word prompts in 6 languages · data port for CheckLink software · low-cost test strips
10 tests				3.1 x 8.4 x 0.61	7.8	voice instructions guide user through test procedure · error codes announced · minimal cleaning required
10 tests	single button	2 years	J-type 6-volt alkaline (1,500 tests)	3.1 x 5.2 x 0.6	4.8	extreme temperature warnings
1 test	2 steps with calibrator bar	4 years	non-replaceable (4,000 tests)	2.15 x 3.65 x 0.375	1.5	credit card size
1 test	none required	4 years	non-replaceable (4000 tests)	3.5 x 2.1 x 0.5	1.4	credit card size · extra large display · low-cost test strips
15 tests	9 codes	2 years	(3) 1.3-volt lithium	5 x 2 x 0.7	3.3	low-cost test strips
20 tests	code strip	5 years	(2) 3-volt lithium (DL or CR 2032)	3.38 x 2.5 x 0.5	1.75	after blood touches the test strip, the blood is drawn into a chamber within the strip for automatic sampling
125 downloadable tests, 10 recallable tests	1 step with calibrator bar	4 years	non-replaceable (4,000 tests)	2.15 x 3.65 x 0.375	1.5	credit card size
125 downloadable tests, 10 recallable tests	1 step with calibrator bar	4 years	non-replaceable (4,000 tests)	5.4 x 0.1	1.1	pen shape/size
1 test	built-in single button	3 years	J-type 6-volt alkaline	4.75 x 2.63 x 1.06	4.8	prompts in English or Spanish · alerts user when the meter requires cleaning

BLOOD GLUCOSE METERS - continued

Product Manufacturer/Supplier	Test Strip	Method	Test Time (sec)	Range (mg/dL)
One Touch Profile LifeScan	Genuine One Touch	no timing, no wiping, 3-step process	45	0-600
Precision Q·I·D MediSense	Precision Q·I·D	no timing (automatic start), no wiping, 2-step process	20	20-600
** **Prestige** Home Diagnostics	Prestige	no timing, no wiping	20	25-600
Supreme Chronimed	Supreme	no timing, no wiping	55	40-400
** **Supreme II** Chronimed	Supreme	no timing, no wiping	50	30-600
** **SureStep** LifeScan	SureStep touchable strip with confirmation dot	no timing, no wiping, 3-step process	15-30	0-500
Ultra+ Home Diagnostics	Ultra+	no timing, no wiping, visual confirmation	45	0-600

** New listing

See Chapter 18, "Diabetes Care Products and Monitoring Devices," for more information about these products.

Memory Capacity	Calibration	Warranty	Battery	Dimensions (in) (L x W x H)	Weight (oz)	Comments
250 tests; with time and date, 14- and 30-day averages by time of day or activity	built-in single button	5 years	(2) AAA alkaline	4.3 x 2.6 x 1.2	4.5	shows time and date · 15 event labels · screen prompts, in any one of 19 languages, alert user in response to test results · alerts user when the meter requires cleaning · records insulin type/dosage and carbohydrates · In Touch diabetes management software available, IBM Windows format
125 downloadable tests, 10 recallable tests	1 step with calibrator bar	4 years	non-replaceable (4,000 tests)	3.82 x 1.89 x 0.57	1.4	extra large display · test strip ensures correct blood sampling · Precision Link diabetes management software available, Windows format
40 tests	single button	2 years	J-type 6-volt alkaline	4.5 x 3.1 x 1.3	4.4	offers a choice of blood application methods: apply blood to strip either before or after strip is inserted in meter
	single button	3 years	J-type 6-volt alkaline	5 x 2.25 x 0.75	4.5	color chart may serve as a visual-read backup
100 tests	self-calibrated	3 years	J-type · 6-volt	4.75 x 2.5 x 1.25	4.7	color chart may serve as a visual read backup
10 tests	single button	3 years	(2) AA alkaline	3.5 x 2.4 x 8	3.8	test strip displays blue dot to confirm that enough blood has been applied · simple application of blood sample aids patients who have shaky hands, vision impairment, or who are inexperienced testers · extra large display
2 tests	single button	2 years	J-type 6-volt alkaline	2.8 x 3.9 x 1.2	4.7	

BLOOD SUGAR ELEVATING PRODUCTS

Product Manufacturer/Supplier	Dosage Form	Comments
B-D Glucose § Becton Dickinson Consumer	chewable tablet	glucose, 5g; 19cal · orange flavor
DEX4 Glucose Can-Am Care	chewable tablet	dextrose, 4g; 15cal · grape, lemon, orange, or raspberry flavor · vitamin C · convenient plastic tube of 10 tablets or bottle of 50 tablets
DextroEnergy Glucose Aero Assemblies	chewable tablet	dextrose, 3g; 12.5cal · vitamin C · black currant, lemon, orange, original, or raspberry flavor · 14 tablets/pack
DY **Glutose** Paddock Labs	gel	glucose, 15g (dextrose solution, 40%); 60cal · lemon flavor · tube of 15g (single dose) or 45g (3 doses)
DY **Glutose** Paddock Labs	chewable tablet	glucose, 5g; 20cal · lemon flavor
GL **Insta-Glucose** ICN Ph'cals	gel	carbohydrate, 24g; 96cal · cherry flavor · convenient plastic tube of one unit dose
Monojel Glucose Can-Am Care	gel	glucose, 10g (dextrose, 40%); 46cal · orange flavor · individual foil packet

§ Manufacturer/supplier did not confirm information for this edition. Product listing is reprinted from the '96-97 edition.

See Chapter 18, "Diabetes Care Products and Monitoring Devices," for more information about these products.

MISCELLANEOUS DIABETES PRODUCTS

Product Manufacturer/Supplier	**Comments**
CARRYING CASES	
Control Injection Monitor Kit **IMK-1A** Mustang	carrying case holds a one-week supply of syringes and swabs, plus two insulin vials and a needle break-off disk · is also a syringe storage box for patient to verify if shots have been taken · dimensions: 12" x 8" x 1.75"
Control Injection Monitor Kit **IMK-1B** Mustang	carrying case designed for use by physically/visually impaired patients · holds a one-week supply of prefilled syringes, plus swabs and a needle break-off disk · is also a syringe storage box for patient to verify if shots have been taken · dimensions: 12" x 8" x 1.75"
Daily Organizer Medport	compact version of Travel Organizer · organizes a three-day supply · includes one refreezable ice pack · can be attached to a belt or carried by the strap · dimensions: 6.75" x 5.5" x 2.5"
Dia-Pak Jr. § Atwater Carey	compact version of Dia-Pak Original · optional adjustable waist belt · dimensions: 6" x 5" x 1.5"
Dia-Pak Mini § Atwater Carey	smallest version of Dia-Pak Original · semi-rigid case protects two pre-drawn insulin syringes, a small glucose meter, and a few additional supplies; compatible with all insulin pen systems · optional refreezable cold gel packs · clips to belt · dimensions: 2" x 6" x 1"
Dia-Pak Original § Atwater Carey	water-resistant, nylon carrying case for daily supplies · organizes a two-week supply · optional refreezable cold gel packs with insulating insert · optional adjustable waist belt or adjustable shoulder strap · dimensions: 6" x 8" x 2.5"
Diabetic's Traveler, Traveler II, **or Traveler III** • Entry 21	insulated, water-resistant, nylon-vinyl carrying case for daily supplies · keeps insulin cold for up to 10 hours · includes refreezable ice pack · Traveler (with adjustable shoulder strap) dimensions: 12" x 10" x 2 1/4" · Traveler II dimensions: 10 7/8" x 10" x 2" · Traveler III dimensions: 3 3/4" x 9 7/8" x 1 7/16"
Insul-Tote Palco Labs	foam-insulated nylon carrying case for daily supplies · includes refreezable gel pack to keep insulin cool · available in four models: back-opening and top-opening (with shoulder strap) dimensions: 7" x 7" x 3," Junior (with adjustable hip strap) dimensions: 6" x 4.5" x 3," and Pen-tote (zippered) dimensions: 4" x 7"
Insulin Protector Medicool	insulated nylon carrying case for daily supplies · keeps insulin cool for up to 16 hours · cooler component may be prerefrigerated to keep insulin cool, or unrefrigerated to prevent insulin from freezing in extremely cold conditions · comes with two refreezable cooler packs · dimensions: 7.75" x 4" x 2.5"
ProtectAll Medicool	insulated nylon carrying case for daily supplies · removable cooler compartment accommodates two insulin vials or a pen system and two pen vials, keeping them cool for up to 12 hours · additional storage compartments and pockets · may be carried either around waist or over shoulder with strap that adjusts up to 52 inches
Thermakit Jordan Medical	thermal styrofoam case for insulin · holds two insulin vials and two insulin syringes · dimensions: 2" x 6" x 2"
Travel Organizer Medport	insulated, water-resistant carrying case for daily supplies · available in nylon or simulated leather · organizes a two-week supply · includes two refreezable ice packs · one side of case keeps insulin cool, the other side keeps meter and supplies at room temperature · includes removable pouch used for safe storage of medical waste until disposal · carried by handle · dimensions: 9" x 6" x 2.5"
Wallet Organizer Medport	smallest version of Travel Organizer · rigid case protects four pre-drawn insulin syringes, a small glucose meter, and a few additional supplies · includes one refreezable ice pack · dimensions: 9" x 3" x 0.75"
COMPUTER SOFTWARE	
** **Balance PC** MediLife	requires IBM-compatible PC with Windows and eight megabytes of memory · allows users, working with their healthcare professionals, to personalize their treatment plan · features include Interview for planning, Calendar for event tracking plus glucose meter data transfer, Managers for reporting and analysis, Library for extensive medication and nutrition reference, and Personal Medical Record for reporting health history and status to health care providers · allows users direct access to MediLife Diabetes Center on the Internet
Diabetes Works ITA Software	requires IBM-compatible PC with Windows · five computer programs packaged together: Insulin Therapy Analysis v2.1 pharmacologically predicts user's glucose results, Diabetes Easy Internet Access v1.0 uses Internet service providers, Glucose Plotter v1.4 manages data from daily blood glucose testing, Diabetes Diet Analyzer v1.1 examines nine meals/snacks per day, and Dear Diary v2.5 accepts personal journaling of graphs/tables and events/comments

See Chapter 18, "Diabetes Care Products and Monitoring Devices," for more information about these products.

MISCELLANEOUS DIABETES PRODUCTS - continued

Product

Manufacturer/Supplier | **Comments**

	Product / Manufacturer/Supplier	Comments
**	**Healthmate** MedData Interactive	requires Apple Newton hand-held computer · this software/hardware combination provides a portable means of tracking and managing data · memory stores more than a year of treatment records · includes an expandable nutrient database, automated insulin dosage and timing computations, graphical data analysis functions · reports can be produced via most Apple and PC printers
**	**In Touch** LifeScan	requires IBM-compatible 486 (or higher) PC with Windows and eight megabytes of memory · also requires 640 x 480 resolution VGA monitor · uploads data from LifeScan meters · creates graphs and tables · includes on-line diabetes education and monitoring information
	Level HealthWare	Windows-based software · uploads data from One Touch II and One Touch Profile meters · provides detailed graphing of numerous trends all on a single page (shows many interrelationships) · provides total health profile including exercise history, caloric intake, mental stress level, illness, etc. · three data fields are left available for tracking data of personal choice
	Mellitus Manager MetaMedix	requires IBM-compatible 386 (or higher) PC with Windows and at least four megabytes of memory · uploads data from Accu-Chek, MediSense, and One Touch meters; it can also be customized to either Disetronic or Mini-Med insulin pumps · creates graphs and tables

LANCETS AND LANCING DEVICES

	Product / Manufacturer/Supplier	Comments
	Auto-Lancet Palco Labs	lancing device with adjustable tip · adjustable tip matches different skin types: soft skin 1-2, average skin 2-3, and tougher skin 4-5
	Autolet Lite Owen Mumford	lancing device · cocks lancet automatically when the hinge top is closed · mechanized lancet ejection eliminates risk of accidental injury · uses shallow, regular, and deep penetration platforms
	Autolet Lite Clinisafe Owen Mumford	professional lancing device for clinically safer blood sampling · ejection of both Unilet lancet and platform after each use at the push of a button · shallow, regular, and deep penetration platforms
**	**Autolet Mini** Owen Mumford	compact lancing device · fits in palm for discreet blood sampling · compatible with most lancets
	B-D Lancet Device § Becton Dickinson Consumer	lancing device · pen shape · uses B-D Ultra-Fine lancets and others
	B-D Ultra Fine Lancet § Becton Dickinson Consumer	lancet · 28-gauge needle · fits most lancing devices · boxes of 100 and 200
	Carelet Safety § Gainor Medical	lancet · needle automatically retracts after use/exposure · single use only
	Cleanlet § Gainor Medical	lancet · 25-gauge needle · snap-on protective cap virtually eliminates accidental needle sticks · needle tip snaps securely into protective cap for safe disposal after a single use
**	**Cleanlet §** Gainor Medical	lancet · 28-gauge needle
PE	**Cleanlet Kids §** Gainor Medical	lancet · 25-gauge (0.5mm) needle · snap-on protective cap virtually eliminates accidental needle sticks · needle tip snaps securely into protective cap for safe disposal after a single use · comes in six bright colors per box
	Dialet Home Diagnostics	lancing device · pen shape · comes with one regular, one deep puncture endcap · for safety, blue dot appears when device is armed
	E-Z Ject Can-Am Care	lancet · needle has a comfortable "junior" lite angle · fits most lancing devices · boxes of 100 and 200 · ivory-colored or assorted colors
	EZ-Let Palco Labs	lancet · 21-gauge, tri-beveled needle point · fits most lancing devices · boxes of 100 and 200
**	**EZ-Let II** Palco Labs	lancing device · gentle puncture model for regular blood flow, deep puncture model for large blood flow
**	**EZ-Let Thin** Palco Labs	lancet · 25-gauge, tri-beveled needle point · fits most lancing devices · boxes of 100 and 200

See Chapter 18, "Diabetes Care Products and Monitoring Devices," for more information about these products.

MISCELLANEOUS DIABETES PRODUCTS - continued

Product Manufacturer/Supplier	Comments
Gentle-let 1 Lukens Medical	lancing device · needle retracts automatically for disposal after single use · normal or extra spring pressure
Gentle-let, GP style Lukens Medical	lancet · fits most lancing devices
Gentle-let-PC Lukens Medical	lancing device · pen shape
Glucolet Bayer Diagnostics	lancing device with clip · pen shape · regular and deep penetration endcaps
Haemolance Chronimed	lancing device · 21-gauge needle · built-in needle protection · needle retracts automatically for disposal after single use
Lady Lite Medicore	lancet · delicate, fine needle tip, designed for the feminine fingertip · cap is rose-shaped · fits most lancing devices · boxes of 200
Medi-Lance II Medicore	lancet · fits most lancing devices · boxes of 200
Medi-Let Medicore	lancing device · patented lancet ejector arm · uses platforms with two penetration depths
MediSense Lancing Device MediSense	lancing device · pen shape · uses Ultra TLC lancets · provides controlled depth of penetration
Monoject Monojector Can-Am Care	lancing device with clip · pen shape
Monolet Can-Am Care	lancet · the original "universal fit" design · tri-beveled needle point · boxes of 100 and 200
Penlet II LifeScan	lancing device · pen shape · "hands-off" lancet removal system to minimize possibility of accidental lancet needle sticks · comes with LifeScan lancets and two different endcaps to control the depth of penetration
** **Qwik-Let** Stat Medical	lancing device · pen shape, yet ergonomical instead of cylindrical · internal mechanism automatically cocks device while lancet is being loaded · compatible with most lancets
** **Soft Touch Lancet** Boehringer Mannheim	lancet · 28-gauge needle point
Soft Touch Lancet Device Boehringer Mannheim	lancing device · pen shape · adjustable penetration depth with five depth settings
Softclix Boehringer Mannheim	lancing device · pen shape · adjustable dial allows for six lancet penetration depths · device's design reduces the lancet's lateral motion when entering the skin · uses Softclix 21-gauge lancets
** **tenderfoot** Biocare	lancing device for heel incision · safety clip prevents premature blade release · blade retracts automatically into its case, preventing accidental injury · three models available: tenderfoot for full-term to six-month-old babies (1mm penetration depth), preemie for babies weighing less than 3.25 lbs. (0.85mm depth), and toddler for older infants and toddlers (3mm depth)
** **Tenderlett** Biocare	lancing device · contoured shape matches finger shape, minimizing skin indentation · blade retracts automatically into its case, preventing accidental injury · three models available: Adult for older children and adults (1.75mm penetration depth), Jr. for children (1.25mm depth), and Toddler for older infants and toddlers (0.85mm depth)
Unilet and Unilet G.P. Owen Mumford	lancet · 21-gauge, 0.81mm diameter needle · Unilet G.P. (short body length) fits more lancing devices than Unilet (long body length) · Unilet in 200-count boxes · Unilet G.P. in boxes of 100 and 200
Unilet Superlite and Unilet G.P. Superlite Owen Mumford	lancet · 23-gauge, 0.66mm diameter needle · Unilet G.P. Superlite (short body length) fits more lancing devices than Unilet Superlite (long body length) · boxes of 100 and 200
Unilet Universal ComforTouch Owen Mumford	lancet · 26-gauge, 0.45mm diameter needle · fits all major lancing devices except Softclix and Soft Touch · cap fits back over needle tip for safe disposal after a single use · boxes of 100 and 200

See Chapter 18, "Diabetes Care Products and Monitoring Devices," for more information about these products.

MISCELLANEOUS DIABETES PRODUCTS - continued

Product Manufacturer/Supplier	Comments
Unistik 2 Owen Mumford	lancing device · lancet is concealed before and after use · self-contained lancet needle automatically retracts for disposal after single use · provides controlled depth of lancet penetration (regular or deep) · boxes of 50 and 100

MEDICAL IDENTIFICATION

Goldware Jewelry Goldware	bracelets, pendants, and watch charm with medical insignia on the front · 14K gold or sterling silver · custom engraved on the back with emergency medical information
Identi-Find Iron-on Labels Identi-Find	permanent · pre-printed with custom emergency medical information
** **Identi-Find Medic-ID Card** Identi-Find	accommodates a large amount of personal identification information · two-sided, unfolds to five sections · includes vinyl case
Medic Alert Emblem and Emergency Information Service Medic Alert	bracelets, neck chains/tags with medical insignia on the front · stainless steel, sterling silver, gold-filled, or 14K gold · custom engraved on the back with patient's emergency medical information and company's 24-hour hotline telephone number · around-the-world service available · membership fee starts at $35
MediCheck Identification MediCheck	stainless steel bracelets and neck tags, plus aluminum wallet cards · custom engraved with emergency medical information · $15 donation requested
** **Protect Your Life Card** Apothecary Products	wallet card with medical emblem on front and space for writing personal medical information on back
** **Protect Your Life Keychain** Apothecary Products	two styles: key ring with leather holder for stainless steel medical emblem, metal key ring labeled with medical emblem

METER ACCESSORIES

Digi-Voice Deluxe and Mini-DV Science Products	voice module which talks user through glucose meter self-test procedure · plugs into the datajack of the One Touch Profile meter · repeat feature · comes with earphones and audio cassette tape instructions · the Mini-DV is a smaller version
Smart Dot Pharmacy Counter	aid for patients who are visually impaired and/or who have hand tremors · blood collector-dropper places a droplet from the finger onto the target area of the glucose meter's test strip · attaches to the One Touch Basic, One Touch II, and One Touch Profile meters
Transfer-Ease Transfer-Ease	pipette transfers blood sample from the finger to the target area of the glucose meter's test strip · unbreakable, disposable · packaged with easy-to-follow directions

** New listing
§ Manufacturer/supplier did not confirm information for this edition. Product listing is reprinted from the '96-97 edition.

See Chapter 18, "Diabetes Care Products and Monitoring Devices," for more information about these products.

Nutritional Product Tables

VITAMIN PRODUCTS

	Product Manufacturer/Supplier	Vitamin A (IU)	Vitamin D (IU)	Vitamin E (IU)	Ascorbic Acid (C) (mg)	Thiamine (B1) (mg)	Riboflavin (B2) (mg)	Niacin (mg)
** PE	**A Kid's Companion Wafers** Natrol	1250 (as beta carotene and palmitate)	200	15	30	1.25	1.25	niacinamide, 10
DY GL LA PU SO SU	**A-D-E with Selenium Tablets** Freeda Vitamins	10000	400	100				
GL PU	**ABC Plus Tablets** Hudson	5000 (as acetate and beta carotene)	400	30	60	1.5	1.7	niacinamide, 20
GL PU	**Adavite-M Tablets** Hudson	5000 (as acetate and beta carotene)	400	30	90	3	3.4	20
** DY GL LA PU SO SU	**Adeks Chewable Tablets** Scandipharm	4000 (as beta carotene)	400	150	60	1.2	1.3	10
** AL DY GL LA SL PE	**Adeks Drops** Scandipharm	500/ml (as beta carotene)	400/ml	40/ml	45/ml	0.5/ml	0.6/ml	6/ml
GL PU SU	**Akorn Antioxidants Caplets** Akorn	5000		200	400			
	Allbee C-800 + Iron Tablets Selfcare			45	800	15	17	100

See Chapter 19, "Nutritional Products," for more information about these products.

Pyridox-ine HCl	Cyanoco-balamin	Folic Acid	Panto-thenic	Elemental Iron (mg)	Elemental Calcium (mg)	Phos-phorus (mg)	Magne-sium (mg)	Other Ingredients
1.25	5	200	6.25	2.5 (as gluconate)	100 (as carbonate)		25 (as oxide)	zinc, 1.25mg · manganese, 0.5mg · potassium, 0.5mg · copper, 100mcg · biotin, 75mcg · iodine, 75mcg · vitamin K, 12.5mcg · chromium, 5mcg · selenium, 2.5mcg
								selenium, 50mcg
2	6	400	10 (as d-calcium pantothenate)	18 (as fumarate)	162 (as dicalcium phosphate)	109	100 (as oxide)	boron, 150mg · potassium, 40mg · chloride, 36.3mg · zinc, 15mg · manganese, 2.5mg · copper, 2mg · silicon, 2mg · iodine, 150mcg · biotin, 30mcg · chromium, 25mcg · molybdenum, 25mcg · vitamin K, 25mcg · selenium, 20mcg · tin, 10mcg · vanadium, 10mcg · nickel, 5mcg
3	9	400	10 (as d-calcium pantothenate)	27 (as fumarate)	40 (as calcium phosphate)	31	100 (as oxide)	zinc, 15mg · chloride, 7.5mg · potassium, 7.5mg · manganese, 5mg · copper, 2mg · iodine, 150mcg · biotin, 30mcg · molybdenum, 15mcg · chromium, 15mcg · selenium, 10mcg
1.5	12	200	10					zinc oxide, 7.5mg · vitamin K, 150mcg · biotin, 50mcg
0.6/ml	4/ml		3/ml					zinc, 5mg/ml · vitamin K, 100mcg/ml · biotin, 1.5mcg/ml
								zinc, 40mg · l-glutathione, 5mg · sodium pyruvate, 3mg · copper, 2mg · selenium, 40mcg · cellulose · stearic acid · magnesium stearate · silicon dioxide
25	12	400	25	27				modified starch · hydrolyzed protein · hydroxypropyl methylcellulose · stearic acid · povidone · silicon dioxide · artificial color · lactose · magnesium stearate · polyethylene glycol 400 or 4000 · vanillin · gelatin · polysorbate 20 or 80 · sorbic acid · sodium benzoate · may also contain: hydroxypropyl cellulose · propylene glycol

VITAMIN PRODUCTS - continued

	Product Manufacturer/Supplier	Vitamin A (IU)	Vitamin D (IU)	Vitamin E (IU)	Ascorbic Acid (C) (mg)	Thiamine (B1) (mg)	Riboflavin (B2) (mg)	Niacin (mg)
	Allbee C-800 Tablets Selfcare			45	800	15	17	100
	Allbee with C Caplets Selfcare				300	15	10.2	50
**	**Anti-Oxidant Take One Capsules or Tablets** Natrol	12500 (as beta carotene)		200	200			
GL PU SO SU	**Antioxidant Formula Softgels** Hudson	25000 (as beta carotene)		400	500			
GL PU SO SU	**Antioxidant Vitamin & Mineral Formula Softgels** Hudson	20000 (as beta carotene)		250	400			
	Apatate Liquid (with Flouride) Kenwood Labs					15		
	Apatate Liquid or Tablets Kenwood Labs					15		
	Avail Tablets Menley & James Labs	5000	400	30	90	2.25	2.55	niacinamide, 20
SU	**B 50 Complex Capsules or Tablets** Sundown					50	50	50
SU	**B Complex Maxi Tablets** Sundown					15	17	200
** GL LA SO SU GE	**B-C-Bid Caplets** Lee Consumer				300	15	10.2	50

See Chapter 19, "Nutritional Products," for more information about these products.

Pyridox-ine HCl	Cyanoco-balamin	Folic Acid	Panto-thenic	Elemental Iron (mg)	Elemental Calcium (mg)	Phos-phorus (mg)	Magne-sium (mg)	Other Ingredients
25	12		25					modified starch · hydrolyzed protein · hydroxypropyl methylcellulose · stearic acid · artificial color · silicon dioxide · lactose · magnesium stearate · povidone · polyethylene glycol 400 or 4000 · vanillin · gelatin · polysorbate 20 or 80 · sorbic acid · sodium benzoate · may also contain: hydroxypropyl cellulose · propylene glycol
5			10					microcrystalline cellulose · corn starch · hydroxypropyl methylcellulose · magnesium stearate · silicon dioxide · propylene glycol · lactose · methacrylic acid · triethyl citrate · titanium dioxide · polysorbate 20 · artificial flavor · saccharin sodium · sodium sorbate
								flavonoid complex, 150mg · green tea extract, 30mg · zinc, 10mg · selenium, 50mcg
								selenium, 50mcg
								carrot powder, 1mg · broccoli powder, 1mg · spinach powder, 1mg · selenium, 50mcg
0.5	25							sodium fluoride, 0.5mg
0.5	25							
3	9	400		18	400		100	zinc, 22.5mg · iodine, 150mcg · chromium, 15mcg · selenium, 15mcg
50	50	400	500					biotin, 50mcg · PABA · inositol · choline · rice bran · watercress · parsley · lecithin (capsules) · alfalfa (tablets)
20	60	400	10					choline · inositol complex · PABA
5			10					

VITAMIN PRODUCTS - continued

	Product Manufacturer/Supplier	Vitamin A (IU)	Vitamin D (IU)	Vitamin E (IU)	Ascorbic Acid (C) (mg)	Thiamine (B1) (mg)	Riboflavin (B2) (mg)	Niacin (mg)
	Beminal-500 Tablets Selfcare				500	25	12.5	niacinamide, 100
GL PU SO SU	**Brewers Yeast Tablets** Hudson					0.06	0.02	0.2
SU	**Buffered C Tablets** Sundown				500			
PU SO PE	**Bugs Bunny Complete Vitamins Plus Minerals Chewable Tablets** Bayer Consumer	5000 (as acetate and beta carotene)	400	30	60	1.5	1.7	20
PU SO PE	**Bugs Bunny Plus Iron Chewable Tablets** Bayer Consumer	2500 (as acetate and beta carotene)	400	15	60	1.05	1.2	13.5
PU SO PE	**Bugs Bunny with Extra C Children's Chewable Tablets** Bayer Consumer	2500 (as acetate and beta carotene)	400	15	250	1.05	1.2	13.5
GL PU SO SU	**C & E Softgels** Hudson			400	500			
DY GL LA PU SO SU	**C Vitamin Tablets** Freeda Vitamins				100; 250; 500; 1000			
DY GL LA PU SO SU	**C Vitamin Timed-Release Tablets** Freeda Vitamins				500; 1000			
GL PU	**Calcet Plus Tablets** Mission Pharmacal	5000 (as acetate)	400	30	500 (as calcium ascorbate and ascorbic acid)	2.25	2.55	niacinamide, 30
	Cecon Solution Abbott Labs				100/ml			
GL PU	**Ceebevim Caplets** Hudson				300	15	10.2	niacinamide, 50

See Chapter 19, "Nutritional Products," for more information about these products.

Pyridox-ine HCl	Cyanoco-balamin	Folic Acid	Panto-thenic	Elemental Iron (mg)	Elemental Calcium (mg)	Phos-phorus (mg)	Magne-sium (mg)	Other Ingredients
10	5		20 (as calcium pantothenate)					calcium carboxymethyl cellulose · ethylcellulose · FD&C blue#2 lake · FD&C red#40 lake · FD&C yellow#6 · flavor · iron oxide · lactose · magnesium stearate · mannitol · microcrystalline cellulose · pharmaceutical glaze · polyethylene glycol · starch · talc · titanium dioxide
					25			rose hips
2	6	400	10	18	100	100	20	zinc, 15mg · copper, 2mg · biotin, 40mcg · iodine, 150mcg
1.05	4.5	300		15				sorbitol · flavor
1.05	4.5	300						sorbitol · aspartame · xylitol · flavor
								rose hips powder, 20mg
3	9	800	15 (as d-calcium pantothenate)	18 (as fumarate)	152.8 (as ascorbate and carbonate)			zinc, 15mg (zinc sulfate, dried) · sugar · povidone · color · magnesium stearate · croscarmellose · food glaze · carnauba wax · beeswax · sodium benzoate
								propylene glycol
5			10 (as d-calcium pantothenate)					

VITAMIN PRODUCTS - continued

	Product Manufacturer/Supplier	Vitamin A (IU)	Vitamin D (IU)	Vitamin E (IU)	Ascorbic Acid (C) (mg)	Thiamine (B1) (mg)	Riboflavin (B2) (mg)	Niacin (mg)
DY GL LA SL	**Centrum High Potency Liquid** Lederle Consumer	2500/15ml	400/15ml	30/15ml	60/15ml	1.5/15ml	1.7/15ml	20/15ml
GL PU SO SU	**Centrum High Potency Tablets** Lederle Consumer	5000	400	30	60	1.5	1.7	20
GL PU SO PE	**Centrum Jr. Shamu and His Crew + Extra C Chew. Tablets** Lederle Consumer	5000	400	30	300	1.5	1.7	20
GL PU SO PE	**Centrum Jr. Shamu and His Crew + Extra Calcium Chew. Tablets** Lederle Consumer	5000	400	30	60	1.5	1.7	20

See Chapter 19, "Nutritional Products," for more information about these products.

Pyridox-ine HCl	Cyanoco-balamin	Folic Acid	Panto-thenic	Elemental Iron (mg)	Elemental Calcium (mg)	Phos-phorus (mg)	Magne-sium (mg)	Other Ingredients
2/15ml	6/15ml		10/15ml	9/15ml				zinc, 3mg/15ml · manganese, 2.5mg/15ml · biotin, 300mcg/15ml · iodine, 150mcg/15ml · chromium, 25mcg/15ml · molybdenum, 25mcg/15ml · alcohol, 6.7% · flavors · BHA · citric acid · edetic acid · glycerin · polysorbate 80 · sodium benzoate · sucrose
2	6	400	10	18	162	109	100	potassium 80mg · chloride, 72mg · zinc, 15mg · manganese, 3.5mg · copper, 2mg · silicon, 2mg · molybdenum, 160mcg · iodine, 150mcg · boron, 150mcg · chromium, 65mcg · biotin, 30mcg · vitamin K, 25mcg · selenium, 20mcg · tin, 10mcg · vanadium, 10mcg · nickel, 5mcg · microcrystalline cellulose · gelatin · crospovidone · hydroxypropyl methylcellulose · titanium dioxide · magnesium stearate · stearic acid · silicon dioxide · triethyl citrate · polysorbate 80 · FD&C yellow#6 · lactose
2	6	400	10	18	108	50	40	zinc, 15mg · copper, 2mg · manganese, 1mg · iodine, 150mcg · biotin, 45mcg · molybdenum, 20mcg · chromium, 20mcg · vitamin K, 10mcg · sugar · sorbitol · microcrystalline cellulose · citric acid · food starch · monoglyceride · diglyceride · gelatin · modified food starch · stearic acid · artificial flavors · FD&C red#40 · FD&C yellow#6 · FD&C blue#2 · aspartame · silicon dioxide · magnesium stearate · partially hydrogenated coconut oil · dextrose · lactose · acacia
2	6	400	10	18	160	50	40	zinc, 15mg · copper, 2mg · manganese, 1mg · iodine, 150mcg · biotin, 45mcg · molybdenum, 20mcg · chromium, 20mcg · vitamin K, 10mcg · sugar · sorbitol · food starch · microcrystalline cellulose · citric acid · monoglyceride · diglyceride · gelatin · modified food starch · stearic acid · artificial flavors · FD&C red#40 · FD&C yellow#6 · FD&C blue#2 · silicon dioxide · aspartame · magnesium stearate · partially hydrogenated coconut oil · dextrose · lactose · acacia

VITAMIN PRODUCTS - continued

	Product Manufacturer/Supplier	Vitamin A (IU)	Vitamin D (IU)	Vitamin E (IU)	Ascorbic Acid (C) (mg)	Thiamine (B1) (mg)	Riboflavin (B2) (mg)	Niacin (mg)
GL PU SO PE	**Centrum Jr. Shamu and His Crew + Iron Chew. Tablets** Lederle Consumer	5000	400	30	60	1.5	1.7	20
GL LA PU SO GE	**Centrum Silver for Adults 50+** Lederle Consumer	5000	400	45	60	1.5	1.7	20
** GL SO SU GE	**Cevi-Bid Tablets** Lee Consumer				500			
GL PU SU	**Chelated Calcium Magnesium Tablets** Hudson							
GL PU SU	**Chelated Calcium Magnesium Zinc Tablets** Hudson							
** GL LA SO PE	**Chewy Bears Citrus Free Vitamin C Chewable Wafers** American Health				60			

Pyridox-ine HCl	Cyanoco-balamin	Folic Acid	Panto-thenic	Elemental Iron (mg)	Elemental Calcium (mg)	Phos-phorus (mg)	Magne-sium (mg)	Other Ingredients
2	6	400	10	18	108	50	40	zinc, 15mg · copper, 2mg · manganese, 1mg · iodine, 150mcg · biotin, 45mcg · vitamin K, 10mcg · molybdenum, 20mcg · chromium, 20mcg · sugar · sorbitol · citric acid · food starch · microcrystalline cellulose · monoglyceride · diglyceride · gelatin · stearic acid · artificial flavors · modified food starch · FD&C red#40 · FD&C yellow#6 · FD&C blue#2 · aspartame · silicon dioxide · magnesium stearate · partially hydrogenated coconut oil · dextrose · lactose · acacia
3	25	400	10	4	200	48	100	potassium, 80 mg · chloride, 72mg · zinc, 15mg · manganese, 3.5mg · copper, 2mg · silicon, 2mg · molybdenum, 160mcg · iodine, 150mcg · boron, 150mcg · chromium, 130mcg · biotin, 30mcg · selenium, 20mcg · vanadium, 10mcg · vitamin K, 10mcg · nickel, 5mcg · microcrystalline cellulose · gelatin · modified food starch · maltodextrin · crospovidone · hydroxypropyl methylcellulose · titanium dioxide · magnesium stearate · stearic acid · silicon dioxide · dextrose · triethyl citrate · polysorbate 80 · FD&C blue#2 · FD&C yellow#6 · FD&C red#40
								dicalcium phosphate · methylcellulose · stearic acid · talc · magnesium stearate · silicon dioxide · polyethylene glycol · carnauba wax
					500 (as carbonate and oyster shell)		250 (as oxide and gluconate)	
					333.3		133.3	zinc, 8.3mg
								black currant juice · apricots · peaches · rose hips · acerola · fructose

VITAMIN PRODUCTS - continued

	Product Manufacturer/Supplier	Vitamin A (IU)	Vitamin D (IU)	Vitamin E (IU)	Ascorbic Acid (C) (mg)	Thiamine (B1) (mg)	Riboflavin (B2) (mg)	Niacin (mg)
** PE	**Chewy Bears Complete Chewable Tablets** American Health	2500 (beta carotene, 1250; palmitate, 1250)	200	15	60	0.75	0.85	niacinamide, 10
**	**Chewy Bears Multi-Vitamins with Calcium Chewable Wafers** American Health	2500 (as beta carotene and palmitate)	200	151	60	0.75	0.85	niacinamide, 10
GL PU SO PE	**Children's Chewable Vitamins with Extra C Tablets** Hudson	2500 (as acetate and beta carotene)	400	15	250 (as ascorbic acid and sodium ascorbate)	1.05	1.2	niacinamide, 13.5
** PE	**Children's Multi-Vitamin Liquid** Natrol	1250/5ml (as beta carotene)	200/5ml	15/5ml	50/5ml	0.5/5ml	0.5/5ml	niacinamide, 10/5ml
PE	**Circus Chews Complete Chewable Tablets** Sundown	5000 (beta carotene, 2500)	400	30	60	1.5	1.7	20
PE	**Circus Chews with Beta Carotene Chewable Tablets** Sundown	2500 (beta carotene, 1250)	400	15	60	1.05	1.2	13.5
PE	**Circus Chews with Calcium Chewable Tablets** Sundown	2500 (beta carotene, 1250)	400	15	60	1.05	1.2	13.5
PE	**Circus Chews with Extra Vitamin C Tablets** Sundown	2500 (beta carotene, 1250)	400	15	250	1.05	1.2	13.5
CA PE	**Circus Chews with Iron** Sundown	2500 (beta carotene, 1250)	400	15	60	1.05	1.2	13.5
** DY GL LA SO SU	**Clinical Nutrients for Men Tablets** PhytoPharmica	5833	34	67	100	20	20	niacinamide, 30

See Chapter 19, "Nutritional Products," for more information about these products.

Pyridox- ine HCl	Cyanoco- balamin	Folic Acid	Panto- thenic	Elemental Iron (mg)	Elemental Calcium (mg)	Phos- phorus (mg)	Magne- sium (mg)	Other Ingredients
1	3	200	5	2 (as fumarate)	100 (as ascorbate, carbonate, citrate)		50 (as oxide)	zinc, 3.8mg · copper, 0.5mg · biotin, 150mcg · iodine, 37.5mcg · chromium, 7.5mcg · selenium, 7.5mcg · boron, 5mcg · molybdenum, 5mcg · vanadium, 2.5mcg · nickle, 1mcg · tin, 1mcg · vitamin K1, 1mcg
1	3	200	5		125 (as ascorbate, carbonate, and citrate)			biotin, 50mcg · rose hips · acerola · black currant and raspberry juice concentrates · dried apricots · dried peaches · dried dates · fructose
1.05	4.5	300						
0.7/5ml	1.25/5ml	50/5ml	3/5ml (as d-calcium pantothenate)					hesperidin, 5mg · biotin, 10mcg
2	6	0.4	10	18	100	100	20	zinc, 15mg · copper, 2mg · iodine, 150mcg · biotin, 40mcg · flavor · sucrose · dextrose · aspartame
1.05	4.5	0.3						dextrose
1.05	4.5	0.3			200			flavor · sucrose · dextrose · aspartame
1.05	4.5	0.3						flavor · sucrose · dextrose
1.05	4.5	0.3		15				flavor · dextrose · sucrose
20	267	267	20	9	67		133	potassium, 33mg · alfalfa juice, 17mg · flavonoids, 17mg · choline bitartrate, 10mg · ginger root extract, 10mg · green tea extract, 10mg · inositol, 10mg · korean ginseng, 5mg · muira puama extract, 10mg · PABA, 10mg · saw palmetto berry, 10mg · zinc, 10mg · carotenes, 1.5mg · manganese, 1.5mg · boron, 667mcg · copper, 334mcg · biotin, 200mcg · iodine, 100mcg · chromium, 67mcg · selenium, 67mcg · vitamin K, 20mcg · vanadium, 17mcg · molybdenum, 8mcg

VITAMIN PRODUCTS - continued

	Product Manufacturer/Supplier	Vitamin A (IU)	Vitamin D (IU)	Vitamin E (IU)	Ascorbic Acid (C) (mg)	Thiamine (B1) (mg)	Riboflavin (B2) (mg)	Niacin (mg)
** DY GL LA SO SU	**Clinical Nutrients for Women Tablets** PhytoPharmica	5833	34	67	100	20	20	niacinamide, 30
** DY GL LA SU	**Coldvac Lozenges** Alva-Amco Pharmacal				60			
** GL PU	**Compete Tablets** Mission Pharmacal	5000 (as acetate)	400	43	90	2	2.6	niacinamide, 30
GL PU SO SU	**Daily Plus Iron & Calcium Tablets** Hudson	5000 (as acetate and beta carotene)	400	30	60	1.5	1.7	niacinamide, 20
GL PU SO SU	**Daily Vitamins Plus Minerals Tablets** Hudson	5000 (as acetate and beta carotene)	400	30	60	1.5	1.7	20
	Dayalets Filmtabs Tablets Abbott Labs	5000	400	30	60	1.5	1.7	20
	Dayalets Plus Iron Filmtabs Tablets Abbott Labs	5000	400	30	60	1.5	1.7	20
	Dexatrim Caffeine Free Plus Vitamins Thompson Medical	caplet: 5000 (as acetate and beta carotene)	caplet: 400	caplet: 30	caplet: 60 timed-release caplet: 180	caplet: 1.5	caplet: 1.7	caplet: niacinamide, 20

See Chapter 19, "Nutritional Products," for more information about these products.

Pyridox-ine HCl	Cyanoco-balamin	Folic Acid	Panto-thenic	Elemental Iron (mg)	Elemental Calcium (mg)	Phos-phorus (mg)	Magne-sium (mg)	Other Ingredients
30	267	267	10	9	134		100	potassium, 33mg · zinc, 7mg · alfalfa juice · flavonoids, 17mg · choline bitartrate, 10mg · dong quai, 10mg · inositol, 10mg · licorice root extract, 10mg · PABA, 10mg · chaste tree berry extract, 5mg · fennel seed extract, 5mg · carotenes, 1.5mg · manganese, 1.5mg · boron, 1mg · copper, 334mcg · silica, 300mcg · biotin, 200mcg · iodine, 100mcg · chromium, 67mcg · selenium · vitamin K, 20mcg · vanadium, 17mcg · molybdenum, 8mcg
								zinc, 13.3mg (as citrate) · glycine · sorbitol
20	9	400		27 (as gluconate)				zinc sulfate, 25mg · microcrystalline cellulose · sugar · calcium carbonate · magnesium stearate · color · croscarmellose sodium · povidone · yellow#6 lake · food glaze · carnauba wax · white beeswax · sodium benzoate
2	6	400	10 (as d-calcium pantothenate)	27 (as fumarate)	450 (as carbonate)			zinc, 15mg · zinc oxide
2	6	400	10 (as d-calcium pantothenate)	18 (as fumarate)	130 (as dicalcium phosphate)	100	100 (as oxide)	potassium, 37.5mg · chloride, 34mg · zinc, 15mg · manganese, 2.5mg · copper, 2mg · iodine, 150mcg · biotin, 30mcg · chromium, 10mcg · molybdenum, 10mcg · selenium, 10mcg
2	6	400						cellulose · hydroxypropyl methylcellulose · povidone · hydroxypropyl cellulose · magnesium stearate · FD&C red#40 · silicon dioxide · FD&C yellow#6 · vanillin
2	6	400		18				cellulose · hydroxypropyl methylcellulose · povidone · hydroxypropyl cellulose · FD&C yellow#6 · magnesium stearate · silicon dioxide · FD&C blue#2 · vanillin · titanium dioxide
caplet: 2	caplet: 6	caplet: 400	caplet: 10 (as calcium pantothenate)	caplet: 18 (as fumarate)	caplet: 162 (as dicalcium phosphate)		caplet: 100 (as oxide)	caplet: zinc, 15mg · copper, 2mg · potassium iodide, 150mcg timed-release caplet: phenylpropanolamine HCl, 75mg

VITAMIN PRODUCTS - continued

	Product Manufacturer/Supplier	Vitamin A (IU)	Vitamin D (IU)	Vitamin E (IU)	Ascorbic Acid (C) (mg)	Thiamine (B1) (mg)	Riboflavin (B2) (mg)	Niacin (mg)
DY GL PU SU	**DiabeVite Tablets** R & D Labs	625 (as beta carotene)	100	100	250	1.5	1.7	20
	DiaVite Plus Caplets Jordan Medical	2000 (beta carotene, 10000)	600	800	500	1.5	1.7	niacinamide, 20
** GL SO SU	**Diostate D Tablets** Lee Consumer		133					
GL PU SO	**Dolomite Tablets** Hudson							
**	**Ester-C Capsules** Natrol				500 (from calcium ascorbate)			
**	**Ester-C Liquid** Natrol				125/5ml (from calcium ascorbate)			
**	**Ester-C Softgels** Natrol				200 (from calcium ascorbate)			
GL PU SO SU	**Eye-Vites Tablets** Hudson	5000 (as beta carotene)		30	60			
	Femiron Multivitamins and Iron Tablets Menley & James Labs	5000	400	15	60	1.5	1.7	20
PU SO PE	**Flintstones Children's Chewable Tablets** Bayer Consumer	2500 (as acetate and beta carotene)	400	15	60	1.05	1.2	13.5
PU SO PE	**Flintstones Complete Chewable Tablets** Bayer Consumer	5000 (as acetate and beta carotene)	400	30	60	1.5	1.7	20
PE	**Flintstones Plus Extra C Children's Chewable Tablets** Bayer Consumer	2500 (as acetate and beta carotene)	400	15	250	1.05	1.2	13.5
PU SO PE	**Flintstones Plus Iron Chewable Tablets** Bayer Consumer	2500 (as acetate and beta carotene)	400	15	60	1.05	1.2	13.5

See Chapter 19, "Nutritional Products," for more information about these products.

Pyridox-ine HCl	Cyanoco-balamin	Folic Acid	Panto-thenic	Elemental Iron (mg)	Elemental Calcium (mg)	Phos-phorus (mg)	Magne-sium (mg)	Other Ingredients
2	6	800	10				100	zinc, 15mg · manganese, 2.5mg · copper, 2mg · biotin, 300mcg · chromium, 200mcg · selenium, 25mcg
2	6	400	10	15	80	20	400	citrus bioflavonoids, 50mg · inositol, 50mg · zinc, 15mg · vanadyl sulfate, 6.5mg · manganese, 2.5mg · copper, 2mg · iodine, 150mcg · chromium, 50mcg · biotin, 30mcg · vitamin K, 25mcg · molybdenum, 25mcg · selenium, 25mcg
					33	230		microcrystalline cellulose · stearic acid · magnesium stearate
					130	78		
					50 (from calcium ascorbate)			
					12.5/5ml (from calcium ascorbate)			pure bioflavonoids, 5mg/5ml · purified water · brown rice syrup · honey · vanilla bean extract · citric acid · sodium benzoate
					25 (from calcium ascorbate)			citrus bioflavonoid complex, 100mg · gelatin · glycerin · water · soybean oil
								zinc, 40mg · copper, 2mg · selenium, 40mcg
2	6	400	10	20				FD&C red#40 · FD&C blue#2 · calcium carbonate · microcrystalline cellulose · starch · alginic acid
1.05	4.5	300						sucrose
2	6	400	10	18	100	100	20	zinc, 15mg · copper, 2mg · iodine, 150mcg · biotin, 40mcg · sorbitol
1.05	4.5	300						sucrose · fructose
1.05	4.5	300		15				sucrose

VITAMIN PRODUCTS - continued

	Product Manufacturer/Supplier	Vitamin A (IU)	Vitamin D (IU)	Vitamin E (IU)	Ascorbic Acid (C) (mg)	Thiamine (B1) (mg)	Riboflavin (B2) (mg)	Niacin (mg)
GL PU	**Fosfree Tablets** Mission Pharmacal	1500 (as acetate)	150		50	4.5	2	niacinamide, 10.5
DY GL LA PU SO SU	**Freedavite Tablets** Freeda Vitamins	5000 (with beta carotene)	400	3	60	5	3	niacinamide, 25
DY GL LA PU SO SU	**Fruit C Chewable Tablets** Freeda Vitamins				100; 200; 500			
PE	**Garfield Complete Vitamins with Minerals Chewable Tablets** Menley & James Labs	5000	400	30	60	1.5	1.7	20
PE	**Garfield Regular Vitamins Chewable Tablets** Menley & James Labs	2500	400	15	60	1.05	1.2	13.5
PE	**Garfield Vitamins Plus Extra C Chewable Tablets** Menley & James Labs	2500	400	15	250	1.05	1.2	13.5
PE	**Garfield Vitamins Plus Iron Chewable Tablets** Menley & James Labs	2500	400	15	60	1.05	1.2	13.5
DY GL LA PU SO SU GE	**Geri-Freeda Tablets** Freeda Vitamins	10000 (with beta carotene)	400	15	150	15	15	niacinamide, 50
SO SU GE	**Gerimed Tablets** Fielding	5000	400	30	120	3	3	25

See Chapter 19, "Nutritional Products," for more information about these products.

Pyridox-ine HCl	Cyanoco-balamin	Folic Acid	Panto-thenic	Elemental Iron (mg)	Elemental Calcium (mg)	Phos-phorus (mg)	Magne-sium (mg)	Other Ingredients
2.5	2		1 (as d-calcium pantothenate)	14.5 (as gluconate)	175.5 (as lactate, gluconate, and carbonate)			sugar · polyethylene glycol · color · croscarmellose sodium · povidone · food glaze · magnesium stearate · yellow#5 lake · carnauba wax · white beeswax · sodium benzoate
2	2		5 (as calcium pantothenate)	9.9	50 (as dicalcium phosphate)	50		choline, 10mg · inositol, 10mg · potassium gluconate, 5mg · manganese gluconate, 2mg · magnesium gluconate, 2mg · copper gluconate, 0.2mg · zinc gluconate, 0.2mg · potassium iodide, 0.1mg · selenium, 35mcg
2	6	400	10	18	100	100	20	zinc, 15mg · copper, 2mg · iodine, 150mcg · biotin, 40mcg · FD&C red#40 · FD&C blue#2 · FD&C yellow#6 · calcium phosphate · sorbitol · aspartame · flavors · gelatin · talc
1.05	4.5	300						FD&C red#40 · FD&C yellow#6 · FD&C blue#2 · FD&C blue#1 · sucrose · talc · flavors · gelatin · lactose · starch
1.05	4.5	300						FD&C red#40 · FD&C yellow#6 · FD&C blue#2 · FD&C blue#1 · sucrose · talc · flavors · gelatin · lactose · starch
1.05	4.5	300		15				FD&C red#40 · FD&C yellow#6 · FD&C blue#2 · FD&C blue#1 · sucrose · talc · flavors · gelatin · lactose
15	15	100	15 (as calcium pantothenate)	15 (as fumarate)	100 (as tricalcium phosphate)		10 (as gluconate)	choline, 50 mg · inositol, 50mg · PABA, 30mg · potassium gluconate, 30mg · l-lysine, 25mg · hesperidin complex, 10mg · betaine, 10mg · copper gluconate, 10mg · zinc gluconate, 10mg · iodine, 0.15mg · selenium, 35mcg
2	6				200	600		zinc, 15mg

VITAMIN PRODUCTS - continued

	Product Manufacturer/Supplier	Vitamin A (IU)	Vitamin D (IU)	Vitamin E (IU)	Ascorbic Acid (C) (mg)	Thiamine (B1) (mg)	Riboflavin (B2) (mg)	Niacin (mg)
	Geritol Complete Tablets SmithKline Beecham	6000	400	30	60	1.5	1.7	20
	Geritol Extend Caplets SmithKline Beecham	3333	200	15	60	1.2	1.4	15
	Geritol Liquid SmithKline Beecham					2.5/15ml	2.5/15ml	50/15ml
DY GL LA SO SL GE	**Gevrabon Liquid** Selfcare					5/ml	2.5/ml	50/ml
GL PU SO	**Gevral T Tablets** Selfcare	5000	400	45	90	2.25	2.6	30
	Glutofac Caplets Kenwood Labs	5000	400	75	300	15	10	50
	Halls Vitamin C Lozenges Warner-Lambert Consumer				60			
	Hepacolin Capsules Kenwood Labs						2.5	niacinamide, 10

See Chapter 19, "Nutritional Products," for more information about these products.

Pyridox-ine HCl	Cyanoco-balamin	Folic Acid	Panto-thenic	Elemental Iron (mg)	Elemental Calcium (mg)	Phos-phorus (mg)	Magne-sium (mg)	Other Ingredients
2	6	400	10	18	162	125	100	potassium, 40mg · chloride, 35mg · zinc, 15mg · manganese, 2.5mg · copper, 2mg · iodine, 150mcg · silicon, 80mcg · biotin, 45mcg · vitamin K, 25mcg · chromium, 15mcg · molybdenum, 15mcg · selenium, 15mcg · tin, 10mcg · vanadium, 10mcg · nickel, 5mcg · microcrystalline cellulose · gelatin · hydrolyzed protein · stearic acid · crospovidone · hydroxypropyl methylcellulose · stearic acid glyceride · palmitic acid glyceride · polyethylene glycol · FD&C blue#2 · FD&C red#40 · FD&C yellow#6
2	2	200		10	130	100	35	zinc, 15mg · iodine, 150mcg · vitamin K, 80mcg · selenium, 70mcg · microcrystalline cellulose · stearic acid · croscarmellose sodium · silicon dioxide
0.5/15ml			2/15ml	18mg/15ml				methionine, 25mg/15ml · choline bitartrate, 50mg/15ml · invert sugar · purified water · alcohol, 12% · caramel color · citric acid · benzoic acid · natural flavors · artificial flavors · sodium hydroxide
1/ml	1/ml		10/ml	15/ml			2/ml	choline, 100mg · manganese, 2mg · zinc, 2mg · iodine, 100mcg · alcohol · citric acid · glycerin · sherry wine · sucrose
3	9	400		27	162	125	100	zinc, 22.5mg · copper, 1.5mg · iodine, 225mcg · BHA · BHT · blue#2 · gelatin · hydrolyzed protein · hydroxypropyl methylcellulose · lactose · magnesium stearate · methylparaben · microcrystalline cellulose · modified food starch · monoglyceride · diglyceride · polacrilin · polysorbate 60 · potassium sorbate · propylparaben · PVPP · red#40 · silica gel · sodium benzoate · sodium lauryl sulfate · sorbic acid · stearic acid · sucrose · titanium dioxide
50	12	400	20		50	40	100	zinc, 5mg · copper, 1mg · chromium, 200mcg · selenium, 25mcg
								sugar · citric acid · sodium ascorbate · natural flavoring · red#40 · glucose syrup · yellow#5 · yellow#6
2			1.5					choline bitartrate, 240mg · di-methionine, 110mg · inositol, 83mg · desiccated liver, 56mg · liver concentrate, 30mg · cobalamin concentrate, 1.5mcg

VITAMIN PRODUCTS - continued

	Product Manufacturer/Supplier	Vitamin A (IU)	Vitamin D (IU)	Vitamin E (IU)	Ascorbic Acid (C) (mg)	Thiamine (B1) (mg)	Riboflavin (B2) (mg)	Niacin (mg)
GL LA SO SU	**Herpetrol Tablets** Alva-Amco Pharmacal	313		3.75	15		4	
GL PU SO	**Hexavitamin Tablets** Upsher-Smith Labs	5000	400		75	2	3	20
	I.L.X. B12 Caplets Kenwood Labs				120	2	2	niacinamide, 20
	I.L.X. B12 Elixir Kenwood Labs					5	2	
SU	**I.L.X. B12 Sugar Free Elixir** Kenwood Labs					5	2	
	I.L.X. Elixir Kenwood Labs					5	2	
	Iberet Filmtab Tablets Abbott Labs				150	6	6	niacinamide, 30
	Iberet Liquid Abbott Labs				112.5/15ml	4.5/15ml	4.5/15ml	niacinamide, 22.5/15ml
	Iberet-500 Filmtab Tablets Abbott Labs				500	6	6	niacinamide, 30
	Iberet-500 Liquid Abbott Labs				375/15ml	4.5/15ml	4.5/15ml	niacinamide, 22.5/15ml
	ICAPS Plus Tablets CIBA Vision/Novartis	600 (as beta carotene)		60	200			
	ICAPS Timed-Release Tablets CIBA Vision/Novartis	7000 (as beta carotene)		100	200		20	
GL PU	**Iromin-G Tablets** Mission Pharmacal	4000 (as acetate)	400		100	4.8	2	niacinamide, 10

See Chapter 19, "Nutritional Products," for more information about these products.

Pyridox-ine HCl	Cyanoco-balamin	Folic Acid	Panto-thenic	Elemental Iron (mg)	Elemental Calcium (mg)	Phos-phorus (mg)	Magne-sium (mg)	Other Ingredients
					19 (as sulfate)			lysine HCl, 315mg · zinc, 2mg (as oxide)
	12			37.5 (micronized)				desiccated liver, 130mg
	10			102				liver fraction, 98mg · nicotinamide, 10mg
	10			102				liver fraction, 98mg · nicotinamide, 10mg
				70				liver concentrate, 98mg · nicotinamide, 10mg
5	25		10 (as calcium pantothenate)	105 (as sulfate)				castor oil · cellulosic polymers · corn starch · FD&C red#40 · FD&C yellow#6 · magnesium stearate · methyl acrylate-methyl methacrylate copolymers · polyethylene glycol · povidone · stearic acid · talc · titanium dioxide · vanillin
3.75/15ml	18.75/15ml			78.75/15ml (as sulfate)				dexpanthenol, 7.5mg/15ml · sorbitol · methylparaben · propylparaben · alcohol, 1% · natural and artificial flavor · water
5	25		10 (as calcium pantothenate)					castor oil · cellulose polymers · corn starch · FD&C red#40 · FD&C yellow#6 · magnesium stearate · methyl acrylate-methyl methacrylate copolymers · polyethylene glycol · propylene glycol · povidone · stearic acid · talc · titanium dioxide · vanillin
3.75/15ml	18.75/15ml			78.75/15ml (as sulfate)				dexpanthenol, 7.5mg/15ml · sorbitol · methylparaben · propylparaben · artificial flavor · glycerin · propylene glycol · sodium bicarbonate · sucrose · water
								zinc acetate, 40mg · copper, 2mg
								zinc, 40mg · copper, 2mg
20	2	800	1 (as d-calcium pantothenate)	30 (as gluconate)	57 (as gluconate, lactate, and carbonate)			sugar · microcrystalline cellulose · color · croscarmellose sodium · magnesium stearate · povidone · red#40 lake · food glaze · carnauba wax · sodium benzoate · white beeswax · yellow#6 lake

VITAMIN PRODUCTS - continued

	Product Manufacturer/Supplier	Vitamin A (IU)	Vitamin D (IU)	Vitamin E (IU)	Ascorbic Acid (C) (mg)	Thiamine (B1) (mg)	Riboflavin (B2) (mg)	Niacin (mg)
DY GL LA PU SO SU PE	**Jets Chewable Tablets** Freeda Vitamins				25	10		
AL SU	**Kenwood Therapeutic Liquid** Kenwood Labs	10000	400	4.5	150	6	3	niacinamide, 6
AL DY GL LA SO SU SL PE	**Kovitonic Liquid** Freeda Vitamins					5/15ml		
DY GL LA PU SO SU	**KPN (Key Prenatal) Tablets** Freeda Vitamins	2667 (with beta carotene)	133.3	10	33.3	2	2	niacinamide, 10
	Liqui-Lea Liquid Shaklee	5000/5ml	400/5ml	15/5ml		2.1/5ml	1.8/5ml	20/5ml
AL DY GL LA SO SU SL PE	**LKV (Liquid Kiddie** **Vitamins) Drops** Freeda Vitamins	2500/0.6ml	400/0.6ml	5/0.6ml	50/0.6ml	1/0.6ml	1/0.6ml	niacinamide, 10/0.6ml
**	**Magna II Timed-Release** **Tablets** American Health	10000 (beta carotene, 5000; fish oil, 5000)	1000	150	250	100	100	niacinamide, 100
**	**Magna One Timed-Release** **Tablets** American Health	5000 (as beta carotene and fish liver oil)	400	100	40	50	50	niacinamide, 50

See Chapter 19, "Nutritional Products," for more information about these products.

Pyridox-ine HCl	Cyanoco-balamin	Folic Acid	Panto-thenic	Elemental Iron (mg)	Elemental Calcium (mg)	Phos-phorus (mg)	Magne-sium (mg)	Other Ingredients
5	25							l-lysine, 300mg · sorbitol base
1			6 (as calcium pantothenate)		38	29	6	potassium, 5mg · manganese, 1mg
10/15ml	30/15ml	100/15ml		350/15ml (as pyrophosphate) equivalent to 42				l-lysine, 10mg · sorbitol solution
0.83	2	266.6	3.3 (as calcium pantothenate)	9.6 (as fumarate)	333.3		33.3 (as oxide)	hesperidin-citrus bioflavonoids, 21.7mg · zinc (from gluconate), 6.6mg · potassium gluconate, 2mg · copper gluconate, 0.03mg · manganese gluconate, 0.033mg · iodine, 0.01mg
2/5ml	9/5ml		5/ml	18/5ml				biotin, 300mcg/5ml
1/0.6ml	4/0.6ml							panthenol, 3mg/0.6ml · biotin, 75mcg/0.6ml
100	100	400	100	18 (as fumarate)	50 (as carbonate)		25 (as oxide)	choline, 100mg · inositol, 100mg · PABA, 100mg · lemon bioflavonoid comples, 50mg · rutin, 50mg · betaine hydrochloride, 30mg · hesperidin complex, 10mg · zinc, 15mg · potassium, 10mg · manganese, 6mg · copper, 0.5mg · iodine, 150mcg · biotin, 100mcg · chromium, 50mcg · selenium, 2mcg
50	200		50 (as calcium panthothenate)	18 (as fumarate)	150 (as carboante)		100 (as oxide)	choline, 50mg · betaine HCl, 30mg · PABA, 25mg · rutin, 25mg · hesperidin, 10mg · inositol, 10mg · lemon bioflavonoid complex, 10mg · potassium, 10mg · zinc, 10mg · manganese, 5mg · copper, 2mg · iodine, 225mcg · biotin, 50 mcg · chromium, 25mcg · selenium, 25mcg

VITAMIN PRODUCTS - continued

	Product Manufacturer/Supplier	Vitamin A (IU)	Vitamin D (IU)	Vitamin E (IU)	Ascorbic Acid (C) (mg)	Thiamine (B1) (mg)	Riboflavin (B2) (mg)	Niacin (mg)
SU GE	**Mature Complete Tablets** Sundown	6000 (as beta carotene)	400	30	60	1.5	1.7	20
	Megaplex Tablets Legere Ph'cals	833	66	33	100	16	16	16
GL PU	**Mission Prenatal F.A. Tablets** Mission Pharmacal	4000 (as acetate)	400		100	5	2	niacinamide, 10
GL PU	**Mission Prenatal H.P. Tablets** Mission Pharmacal	4000 (as acetate)	400		100	4	2	niacinamide, 10
GL PU	**Mission Prenatal Tablets** Mission Pharmacal	4000 (as acetate)	400		100	5	2	niacinamide, 10
DY GL LA PU SO SU	**Monocaps Tablets** Freeda Vitamins	10000 (with beta carotene)	400	15	125	15	15	niacinamide, 41
** GL LA SU	**More Than a Multiple Tablets** American Health	3333.3 (as beta carotene)	133.3	66.7	166.7	12.5	12.5	niacinamide, 12.5
GL PU SU	**Multi-Mineral Tablets** Hudson							
**	**Multi-Vitamin Liquid** Natrol	5000/5ml	200/5ml	50/5ml	100/5ml	3.75/5ml	4.25/5ml	niacinamide, 10/5ml
	Multimin Tablets Republic Drug	5000	400	30	60	1.5	17	20

See Chapter 19, "Nutritional Products," for more information about these products.

Pyridox-ine HCl	Cyanoco-balamin	Folic Acid	Panto-thenic	Elemental Iron (mg)	Elemental Calcium (mg)	Phos-phorus (mg)	Magne-sium (mg)	Other Ingredients
2	6	400	10	18	162	125	100	potassium, 37.5mg · chloride, 34mg · zinc, 15mg · manganese, 2.5mg · copper, 2mg · iodine, 150mcg · silicon, 80mcg · biotin, 45mcg · vitamin K, 25mcg · chromium, 15mcg · molybdenum, 15mcg · selenium, 15mcg · tin, 10mcg · vanadium, 10mcg · nickel, 15mcg
16	83		16	2.5	66	16	33	choline, 116mg · potassium, 16.5mg · biotin, 16mg ·
10	2	800	1 (as d-calcium pantothenate)	30 (as gluconate)	50 (as gluconate, lactate, and carbonate)			zinc sulfate, 15mg · sugar · microcrystalline cellulose · color · magnesium stearate · croscarmellose · food glaze · povidone · carnauba wax · sodium benzoate · beeswax
20	2	800	1 (as d-calcium pantothenate)	30 (as gluconate)	50 (as gluconate, lactate, and carbonate)			sugar · microcrystalline cellulose · color · magnesium stearate · croscarmellose sodium · food glaze · povidone · yellow#5 lake · blue#1 lake · carnauba wax · sodium benzoate ·white beeswax · yellow#6 lake
3	2	400	1 (as d-calcium pantothenate)	30 (as gluconate)	50 (as gluconate, lactate, and carbonate)			microcrystalline cellulose · sugar · color · povidone · croscarmellose · magnesium stearate · food glaze · carnauba wax · beeswax · sodium benzoate
15	15	100	15 (as calcium pantothenate)	14	40 (as carbonate)		100 (as oxide)	magnesium oxide, 100mg · l-lysine, 15mg · zinc gluconate, 12mg · manganese gluconate, 10mg · PABA, 10mg · l-linoleic acid, 10mg · potassium gluconate, 10mg · copper gluconate, 1mg · iodine, 0.15mg · selenium, 35mcg · biotin, 15mcg
12.5	12.5	66.7	12.5	5	166.7		83.3	bioflavonoids, 50mg · potassium, 16.5mg · PABA, 12.5mg · hesperidin, 8.3 · rutin, 8.3mg · zinc, 5mg · manganese, 1.67mg · iodine, 25mcg · chromium, 16.7mcg · selenium, 16.7mcg · biotin, 12.5mcg · boron, 0.3mcg · copper, 0.3mcg · lipotropic factors · enzyme factors · amino acids · food factors
				3 (as gluconate)	166.7	75.7	66.7 (as oxide)	potassium, 12.5mg · manganese, 8.3mg · zinc, 2.5mg · copper, 0.33mg · iodine, 25mcg
8.5/5ml	25/5ml		200/5ml (as d-calcium pantothenate)					flavonoids complex, 25mg/5ml · inositol, 12.5mg/5ml
2	6	400	10	18	162	125	100	potassium, 40mg · biotin, 30mcg · minerals

VITAMIN PRODUCTS - continued

	Product Manufacturer/Supplier	Vitamin A (IU)	Vitamin D (IU)	Vitamin E (IU)	Ascorbic Acid (C) (mg)	Thiamine (B1) (mg)	Riboflavin (B2) (mg)	Niacin (mg)
**	**My Favorite Multiple Take One Tablets** Natrol	1000	400	100	100	15	17	20
**	**My-B-Tabs Tablets** Legere Ph'cals							
GL SO	**Myadec High-Potency Multivitamin/Multimineral Tablets** Warner-Lambert Consumer	5000	400	30mg	60	1.7	2	20
DY GL LA PU SU	**Natalins Tablets** Mead Johnson Nutritionals	4000 (preformed vitamin A, 2667; beta carotene, 1333)	400	15	70	1.5	1.6	17
DY GL PU	**Nephro-Vite Tablets** R & D Labs				60	1.5	1.7	20
SU	**Nestabs Tablets** Fielding	5000	400	30	120	3	3	20
** GL LA SU	**Nutri-Mega Softgels** American Health	5000 (beta carotene, 1000; fish liver oil, 4000)	200	150	150	25	25	niacinamide, 25
	Ocuvite Extra Tablets Storz Ophthalmics	6000 (as beta carotene)		50	200		3	niacinamide, 40

See Chapter 19, "Nutritional Products," for more information about these products.

Pyridox-ine HCl	Cyanoco-balamin	Folic Acid	Panto-thenic	Elemental Iron (mg)	Elemental Calcium (mg)	Phos-phorus (mg)	Magne-sium (mg)	Other Ingredients
17	50	400	50	18	25		10	flavonoid complex, 100mg · ultragreen, 100mg · choline, 50mg · lecithin, 50mg · inositol, 25mg · PABA, 25mg · zinc, 15mg · silica, 10mg · manganese, 5mg · potassium, 5mg · boron, 3mg · copper, 2mg · biotin, 300mcg · iodine, 150mcg
	50	10						adenosine monophosphate, 50mg
3	6	400	10	18	162	125	100	zinc, 15mg · biotin, 30mcg · vitamin K, 25mcg · chromium · copper · iodine · potassium · manganese · molybdenum · selenium · chloride · nickel · tin · silicon · vanadium · boron
2.6	2.5	500		30	200		100	acacia · zinc, 15mg · copper, 1.5mg · povidone · microcrystalline cellulose · polacrilin potassium · hydroxypropyl methylcellulose · polyethylene glycol · magnesium stearate · hydroxypropyl cellulose · silicon dioxide
12.2	6	800	10 (as calcium pantothenate)		10		<0.30	d-biotin · lactose · cellulose · silicon dioxide · stearic acid
3	8	800		36	80			zinc, 15mg · iodine, 150mcg
25	25	200	25	9 (as fumarate)	100 (as bone meal and eggshell)	25 (as bone meal)	25 (as oxide)	lecithin, 40mg · choline, 25mg · PABA, 25mg · bioflavonoids, 15mg · manganese, 15mg · potassium, 15mg · zinc, 7.5mg · rutin, 5mg · royal jelly, 2.5mcg · copper, 1mg · DNA, 1mg · RNA, 1mg · boron, 0.5mg · iodine, 75mcg · Co-Q-10, 50mcg · biotin, 25mcg · inositol, 25mg · chromium, 12.5mcg · selenium, 12.5mcg · octacosanol, 5mcg
								zinc, 40mg · copper, 2mg · manganese, 5mg · selenium, 40mcg · l-glutathione, 5mg · dibasic calcium phosphate · FD&C yellow#6 · hydroxypropyl methylcellulose · magnesium stearate · microcrystalline cellulose · mineral oil · polysorbate 80 · polyvinylpyrrolidone · silica gel · sodium lauryl sulfate · stearic acid · titanium dioxide · triethyl citrate

VITAMIN PRODUCTS - continued

	Product Manufacturer/Supplier	Vitamin A (IU)	Vitamin D (IU)	Vitamin E (IU)	Ascorbic Acid (C) (mg)	Thiamine (B1) (mg)	Riboflavin (B2) (mg)	Niacin (mg)
	Ocuvite Tablets Storz Ophthalmics	5000 (as beta carotene)		30	60			
** GL LA PU	**Oncovite Tablets** Mission Pharmacal	1000 (as acetate and beta carotene)	400	200	500	0.37	0.5	niacinamide, 5
	One Daily Plus Iron Tablets Multisource	5000	400	30	60	1.5	1.7	20
	One-A-Day 50 Plus Tablets Bayer Consumer	600 (as acetate and beta carotene)	400	60	120	4.5	3.4	20
	One-A-Day Antioxidant Plus Softgels Bayer Consumer	5000 (as beta carotene)		200	250			
PU SO	**One-A-Day Essential Tablets** Bayer Consumer	5000 (as acetate and beta carotene)	400	30	60	1.5	1.7	20
	One-A-Day Extras Antioxidant Softgels Bayer Consumer	5000 (as beta carotene)		200	250			
PU SO	**One-A-Day Maximum Formula Tablets** Bayer Consumer	5000 (as acetate and beta carotene)	400	30	60	1.5	1.7	20
	One-A-Day Men's Tablets Bayer Consumer	5000 (as acetate and beta carotene)	400	45	200	2.25	2.55	20
	One-A-Day Women's Tablets Bayer Consumer	5000 (as acetate and beta carotene)	400	30	60	1.5	1.7	20

See Chapter 19, "Nutritional Products," for more information about these products.

Pyridox-ine HCl	Cyanoco-balamin	Folic Acid	Panto-thenic	Elemental Iron (mg)	Elemental Calcium (mg)	Phos-phorus (mg)	Magne-sium (mg)	Other Ingredients
								zinc, 40mg · copper, 2mg · selenium, 40mcg · dibasic calcium phosphate · FD&C yellow#6 · hydroxypropyl methylcellulose · magnesium stearate · microcrystalline cellulose · polysorbate 80 · polyvinyl-pyrrolidone · silica gel · sodium lauryl sulfate · stearic acid · titanium dioxide · triethyl citrate
25	1.5	400	2.5					zinc oxide (zinc, 7.5mg) · calcium carbonate · sugar · croscarmellose sodium · color · magnesium stearate · povidone · ethylcellulose · food glaze · carnauba wax · white beeswax
2	6	400	10	18				
6	25	400	20		220		100	vitamin B6 · biotin · vitamin K · iodine · copper · zinc · chromium · selenium · molybdenum · manganese · potassium · chloride · FD&C yellow#6
								zinc, 7.5mg · manganese, 1.5mg · copper, 1mg · selenium, 15mcg · gelatin · glycerin · soybean oil · lecithin · vegetable oil (partially hydrogenated cottonseed and soybean oils) · yellow beeswax · titanium dioxide · FD&C yellow#5 tartrazine
2	6	400	10					
								zinc · copper · selenium · manganese
2	6	400	10	18	130	100	100	zinc, 15mg · biotin, 30mcg · chloride · chromium · copper · iodine · potassium · manganese · molybdenum · selenium
3	9	400	10					calcium carbonate · gelatin · starch · cellulose · calcium silicate · hydroxypropyl methylcellulose · magnesium stearate · FD&C yellow#6 · lecithin · sodium hexametaphosphate
2	6	400	10	27	450			acacia · gelatin · microcrystalline cellulose · hydroxypropyl methylcellulose · zinc, 15mg · modified cellulose gum · magnesium stearate · FD&C yellow#5 · FD&C yellow#6 · hydroxypropyl cellulose · starch · lecithin · sodium hexametaphosphate

VITAMIN PRODUCTS - continued

	Product Manufacturer/Supplier	Vitamin A (IU)	Vitamin D (IU)	Vitamin E (IU)	Ascorbic Acid (C) (mg)	Thiamine (B1) (mg)	Riboflavin (B2) (mg)	Niacin (mg)
	Optilets-500 Filmtab Tablets Abbott Labs	5000	400	30	500	15	10	niacinamide, 100
	Optilets-M-500 Filmtab Tablets Abbott Labs	5000	400	30	500	15	10	niacinamide, 100
GL LA PU SO SU	**Os-Cal Fortified Tablets** SmithKline Beecham		125	0.8	50	1.7 (as mononitrate)	1.7	15
DY GL LA PU SO SU	**Oxi-Freeda Tablets** Freeda Vitamins	5000 (as beta carotene)		150	100	20	20	niacinamide, 40
	Palmitate-A 5,000 Tablets Akorn	5000						
	Palmitate-A Tablets Akorn	15000						
DY GL LA PU SO SU	**Parvlex Tablets** Freeda Vitamins				50	20	20	niacinamide, 20
GL LA PU SO SU	**Peridin-C Tablets** Beutlich, L.P. Ph'cals				200			
GL LA PU PE	**Poly-Vi-Sol Chewable Vitamins** Mead Johnson Nutritionals	2500	400	15	60	1.05	1.2	13.5
AL GL LA SO SU SL PE	**Poly-Vi-Sol Vitamin Drops** Mead Johnson Nutritionals	1500/ml	400/ml	5/ml	35/ml	0.5/ml	0.6/ml	8/ml

See Chapter 19, "Nutritional Products," for more information about these products.

Pyridox-ine HCl	Cyanoco-balamin	Folic Acid	Panto-thenic	Elemental Iron (mg)	Elemental Calcium (mg)	Phos-phorus (mg)	Magne-sium (mg)	Other Ingredients
5	12		20 (as calcium pantothenate)					cellulosic polymers · corn starch · D&C yellow#10 · FD&C yellow#6 · iron oxide · polyethylene glycol · povidone · stearic acid · talc · titanium dioxide · vanillin
5	12		20 (as calcium pantothenate)	20			80	zinc, 1.5mg · copper, 2mg · iodine, 0.15mg · manganese, 1mg · polyethylene glycol · propylene glycol · povidone · cellulosic · polymers · colloidal silicon dioxide · corn starch · D&C red#7 · FD&C blue#1 · titanium dioxide · iron oxide · magnesium stearate · microcrystalline cellulose · sorbic acid
2				5 (as fumarate)	250 (as oyster shell powder)		3 (as oxide)	zinc, 0.5 (as sulfate) · manganese, 0.5 (as sulfate) · corn syrup solids · hydroxypropyl methylcellulose · calcium stearate · corn starch · mineral oil · titanium dioxide · polysorbate 80 · methylparaben · yellow#10 lake · blue#1 lake · propylparaben · carnauba wax · edetate disodium
20	10		20 (as calcium pantothenate)					l-cysteine, 75mg · glutathione, 40mg · zinc, 15mg · oceanic selenium, 50mcg
								cellulose · stearic acid · magnesium stearate · silicon dioxide
								cellulose · stearic acid · magnesium stearate · silicon dioxide
10	50	400	1 (as calcium pantothenate)	29 (as fumarate)				copper, 1.5mg · manganese gluconate, 1mg
								hesperidin complex, 150mg · hesperidin methyl chalcone, 50mg
1.05	4.5	300						dextrates · sugar · magnesium stearate · silicon dioxide · artificial flavor · artificial color · salt
0.4/ml	2/ml							glycerin · water · polysorbate 80 · ferrous sulfate · artificial flavor · color

VITAMIN PRODUCTS - continued

	Product Manufacturer/Supplier	Vitamin A (IU)	Vitamin D (IU)	Vitamin E (IU)	Ascorbic Acid (C) (mg)	Thiamine (B1) (mg)	Riboflavin (B2) (mg)	Niacin (mg)
GL LA PU PE	**Poly-Vi-Sol with Iron Chewable Vitamins & Minerals Tablets** Mead Johnson Nutritionals	2500	400	15	60	1.05	1.2	13.5
AL GL LA SO SU SL PE	**Poly-Vi-Sol with Iron Vitamin Drops** Mead Johnson Nutritionals	1500/ml	400/ml	5/ml	35/ml	0.5/ml	0.6/ml	8/ml
DY GL SO	**Pro-Pep Chewable Tablets** Alva-Amco Pharmacal	375	30	2.16	5	0.17	0.12	1.375
GL PU SO	**Progen Caplets** Legere Ph'cals	12500		15	500			
GL LA PU SO SU	**Protegra Antioxidant Softgels** Selfcare	5000 (as beta carotene)		200	250			
DY GL LA PU SO SU	**Quintabs-M Tablets** Freeda Vitamins	10000 (with beta carotene)	400	50	300	30	30	niacinamide, 150
GL	**Rejuvex for the Mature Woman Caplets** Sunsource			30		2	2	10
**	**Releaf Menopause Formula Tablets** Lake Consumer	5000	400	30	200	30	4	30
**	**Releaf Stress Formula Tablets** Lake Consumer			30	500	10	10	100

See Chapter 19, "Nutritional Products," for more information about these products.

Pyridox-ine HCl	Cyanoco-balamin	Folic Acid	Panto-thenic	Elemental Iron (mg)	Elemental Calcium (mg)	Phos-phorus (mg)	Magne-sium (mg)	Other Ingredients
1.05	4.5	300		12				zinc, 8mg · copper, 0.8mg · dextrates · sugar · magnesium stearate · stearic acid · silicon dioxide · artificial flavor · color · salt
0.4/ml				10/ml				glycerin · water · artificial flavor · color · polysorbate 80
0.17	0.5	30	0.78	1.2				chromium, 7.5mcg (as picolinate) · zinc, 1mg · copper, 0.14mg · biotin, 23mcg · iodine, 9mcg · dextrose · maltodextrin · sorbitol
5							20	garlic, 75mg · zinc, 50mg · selenium, 50mcg
								zinc, 7.5mg · manganese, 1.5mg · copper, 1mg · selenium, 15mcg · gelatin · cottonseed oil · glycerin · sorbitol · calcium phosphate · lecithin · beeswax · soybean oil · FD&C red#40 · titanium dioxide · FD&C blue#1 ·
30	30	400	30 (as calcium pantothenate)	15 (as fumarate)			18	PABA, 30mg · potassium gluconate, 30mg · zinc gluconate, 30mg · manganese gluconate, 15mg · copper gluconate, 2mg · potassium iodide, 0.15mg · selenium, 35mcg
10			10 (as d-calcium pantothenate)				500 (as oxide)	dong quai, 200mg · boron, 3mg · manganese, 2mg · selenium, 25mcg · raw glandular powders from bovine source · microcrystalline cellulose · croscarmellose sodium · colloidal silica · stearic acid · magnesium stearate
20	10	400	10	20	100	100	100	potassium, 15mg · zinc, 15mg · manganese, 5mg · copper, 2mg · iodine, 150mcg · biotin, 30mcg · chromium, 15mcg · molybenum, 15mcg · selenium, 10mcg
5	12	400	20					zinc, 23.9mg · copper, 3mg · biotin, 45mcg · dicalcium phosphate · cellulose · stearic acid · magnesium stearate · silicon dioxide · pharmaceutical glaze · talc

VITAMIN PRODUCTS - continued

	Product Manufacturer/Supplier	Vitamin A (IU)	Vitamin D (IU)	Vitamin E (IU)	Ascorbic Acid (C) (mg)	Thiamine (B1) (mg)	Riboflavin (B2) (mg)	Niacin (mg)
	Secran B Vitamin Supplement Liquid Scherer Labs					5ml		5ml
PE	**Sesame Street Complete Vitamins & Minerals Chewable Tablets** McNeil Consumer	2750 (as acetate and beta carotene, 495)	200	10	40	0.75	0.85	niacinamide, 10
PE	**Sesame Street Vitamins Plus Extra C Chewable Tablets** McNeil Consumer	2750 (as acetate and beta carotene, 500)	200	10	80	0.75	0.85	niacinamide, 10
PE	**Sesame Street Vitamins Plus Iron Chewable Tablets** McNeil Consumer	2750 (as acetate and beta carotene, 500)	200	10	40	0.75	0.85	niacinamide, 10
	Sigtab-M Tablets Lee Consumer	6000	400	45		5	5	niacinamide, 25
	Sigtabs Tablets Lee Consumer	5000 (as acetate)	400	15		10.3	10	100
	Stress Formula Plus Iron Tablets Multisource			30	500	10	10	100
	Stress Formula Tablets Multisource			30	500	15	10	niacinamide, 100
	Stress Formula with Zinc Tablets Multisource			30	500	15	10	niacinamide, 100
	Stress-600 Tablets Upsher-Smith Labs			30	600	15	15	100

See Chapter 19, "Nutritional Products," for more information about these products.

Pyridox-ine HCl	Cyanoco-balamin	Folic Acid	Panto-thenic	Elemental Iron (mg)	Elemental Calcium (mg)	Phos-phorus (mg)	Magne-sium (mg)	Other Ingredients
	5ml							alcohol, 15% · sodium citrate · sugar · glycerin · sherry wine concentrate · FD&C red#40 · citric acid
0.7	3	200	5 (as d-calcium pentothenate)	10 (as fumarate)	80 (as dicalcium phosphate)		20	iodine, 75mcg · biotin, 15mcg · zinc, 8mg · copper, 1mg · sucrose · natural flavors · talc · stearic acid glyceride · palmitic acid glyceride · starch · silicon dioxide · gelatin · natural coloring · lactose · potassium iodide · d-biotin
0.7	3	200	5 (as d-calcium pantothenate)					sucrose · talc · natural flavors · stearic acid glyceride · palmitic acid glyceride · gelatin · silicon dioxide · starch · magnesium stearate · natural coloring · dicalcium phosphate · lactose
0.7	3	200	5 (as d-calcium pantothenate)	10 (as fumarate)				sucrose · talc · natural flavors · stearic acid glyceride · palmitic acid glyceride · gelatin · silicon dioxide · magnesium stearate · starch · natural coloring · dicalcium phosphate · lactose
3	18	400	0.015	18	200	150	100	potassium chloride, 40mg · chloride, 36.3mg · zinc, 15mg · manganese sulfate, 5mg · copper, 2mg · boron, 150mcg · iodine, 150mcg · biotin, 45mcg · vitamin K1, 25mcg · chromium, 25mcg · molybdenum, 25mcg · selenium, 25mcg · vanadium, 19mcg · tin, 10mcg · nickel, 5mcg · silicon, 2mcg · microcrystalline cellulose · stearic acid · croscarmellose sodium · magnesium stearate · hydroxypropyl methylcellulose · propylene glycol
6	18	400	20 (as calcium pantothenate)					sucrose · calcium sulfate · gelatin · povidone · lacca · magnesium stearate · silica · sodium benzoate · polyethylene glycol · carnauba wax · sesame seed oil · titanium dioxide
5	12	400	20	27				biotin, 45mcg
5	12	400	20					biotin, 45mcg
5	12	400	20					zinc, 23.9mg · copper, 3mg · biotin, 45mcg
5	12	400	20					biotin, 45mcg

VITAMIN PRODUCTS - continued

Product Manufacturer/Supplier	Vitamin A (IU)	Vitamin D (IU)	Vitamin E (IU)	Ascorbic Acid (C) (mg)	Thiamine (B1) (mg)	Riboflavin (B2) (mg)	Niacin (mg)
GL PU SO **Stress-600 with Zinc Tablets** Upsher-Smith Labs			30	600	20	10	100
GL LA PU SO SU **Stresstabs High Potency Stress Formula + Iron Tablets** Selfcare			30	500	10	10	100
GL LA PU SO SU **Stresstabs High Potency Stress Formula Plus Zinc Tablets** Selfcare			30	500	10	10	100
GL LA PU SO SU **Stresstabs High Potency Stress Formula Tablets** Selfcare			30	500	10	10	100
Stuart Prenatal Tablets Wyeth-Ayerst Labs	4000 (as acetate and beta carotene)	400	11	100	1.5	1.7	18
GL PU SO PE **Sunkist Multivitamins Complete Tablets** Novartis Consumer	5000	400	30	60	1.5	1.7	20
GL PU SO PE **Sunkist Multivitamins Plus Extra C Tablets** Novartis Consumer	2500 (as beta carotene)	400	15	250	1.1	1.2	14

See Chapter 19, "Nutritional Products," for more information about these products.

Pyridox-ine HCl	Cyanoco-balamin	Folic Acid	Panto-thenic	Elemental Iron (mg)	Elemental Calcium (mg)	Phos-phorus (mg)	Magne-sium (mg)	Other Ingredients
5	12	400	25					zinc, 23.9mg · copper, 3mg · biotin, 45mcg
5	12	400	20	18				biotin, 45mcg · microcrystalline cellulose · calcium carbonate · modified food starch · stearic acid · magnesium stearate · silicon dioxide · mineral oil · FD&C yellow#6 · FD&C red#40
5	12	400	20					zinc, 23.9mg · copper, 3mg · biotin, 45mcg · microcrystalline cellulose · calcium carbonate · modified food starch · mineral oil · silicon dioxide · stearic acid · magnesium stearate · FD&C yellow#6
5	12	400	20					biotin, 45mcg · microcrystalline cellulose · calcium carbonate · modified food starch · mineral oil · magnesium stearate · silicon dioxide · FD&C yellow#6 · stearic acid
2.6	4	800		60	200			zinc, 25mg · croscarmellose sodium · hydroxypropyl methylcellulose · microcrystalline cellulose · pregelatinized starch · red iron oxide · titanium dioxide
2	6	400	10	18	100	78	20	iodine, 150mcg · biotin, 40mcg · vitamin K1, 10mcg · zinc, 10mg · manganese, 1mg · copper, 2mg · sorbitol · dicalcium phosphate · monoglyceride · diglyceride · natural flavors · stearic acid · carrageenan · starch · hydrolyzed protein · citric acid · yellow#6 · gelatin · sucrose · magnesium stearate · red#40 · yellow#5 · aspartame · silica · calcium silicate · cellulose · hydrogenated vegetable oils · beta carotene
1	5	300						vitamin K1, 5mcg · sorbitol · flavors · monoglyceride · diglyceride · starch · stearic acid · hydrolyzed protein · aspartame · hydrogenated vegetable oils · yellow#6 · silica · red#40 · cellulose · yellow#5 · gelatin · magnesium stearate · calcium silicate · sucrose · ascorbyl palmitate

VITAMIN PRODUCTS - continued

	Product Manufacturer/Supplier	Vitamin A (IU)	Vitamin D (IU)	Vitamin E (IU)	Ascorbic Acid (C) (mg)	Thiamine (B1) (mg)	Riboflavin (B2) (mg)	Niacin (mg)
GL PU SO PE	**Sunkist Multivitamins Plus Iron Tablets** Novartis Consumer	2500	400	15	60	1.1	1.2	niacinamide, 13.5
GL PU SO PE	**Sunkist Multivitamins Regular Tablets** Novartis Consumer	2500	400	15	60	1.1	1.2	niacinamide, 13.5
	Sunkist Vitamin C Chewable Tablets Novartis Consumer				60; 250; 500			
DY GL LA PU SO SU	**Super A&D Tablets** Freeda Vitamins	25000	1000					
DY GL LA PU SO SU	**Super Dec B-100 Coated Tablets** Freeda Vitamins					100	100	niacinamide, 100
SU	**Super Multiple 42 with Beta Carotene Softgels** Sundown	5000 (with beta carotene)	200	15	250	7.5	8.5	50
DY GL LA PU SO SU	**Super Quints-50 Tablets** Freeda Vitamins					50	50	niacinamide, 50

See Chapter 19, "Nutritional Products," for more information about these products.

Pyridox-ine HCl	Cyanoco-balamin	Folic Acid	Panto-thenic	Elemental Iron (mg)	Elemental Calcium (mg)	Phos-phorus (mg)	Magne-sium (mg)	Other Ingredients
1	5	300		15				vitamin K1, 5mcg · sorbitol · natural flavors · monoglyceride · diglyceride · starch · stearic acid · carrageenan · hydrolyzed protein · aspartame · magnesium stearate · hydrolyzed vegetable oils · red#40 · silica · yellow#5 · yellow#6 · cellulose · gelatin · beta carotene
1	5	300						vitamin K1, 5mcg · sorbitol · natural flavors · monoglyceride · diglyceride · starch · stearic acid · hydrolyzed protein · carrageenan · hydrogenated vegetable oils · magnesium stearate · citric acid · aspartame · silica · yellow#6 · red#40 · cellulose · yellow#5 · gelatin · beta carotene
								fructose (250mg · 500mg) · sorbitol · sucrose · natural flavors · citrus bioflavonoids · hydrogenated vegetable oil (250mg) · dextrin · magnesium stearate · modified food starch · silica hydrogel · lactose
100	100	400	100 (as calcium pantothenate)					PABA, 100mg · inositol, 100mg · d-biotin, 100mcg
10	30	200	12.5	5.4	8	4.5		potassium, 75mg · choline bitartrate, 50mg · desiccated liver, 25mg · citrus bioflavonoids, 12.5mg · PABA, 12.5mg · zinc, 7.5mg · amino acids, 5mg · hesperidin, 5mg · manganese, 2mg · acerola, 1mg · copper, 0.4mg · inositol, 150mcg · iodine, 75mcg · biotin, 25mcg · selenium, 12.5mcg · papaya · fish liver oil · rose hips · magnesium gluconate · lecithin · yeast
50	50	400	50 (as calcium pantothenate)					inositol, 50mg · PABA, 30mg · d-biotin, 50mcg · l-lysine · glycine · l-glutamine · l-glutamic acid

VITAMIN PRODUCTS - continued

	Product Manufacturer/Supplier	Vitamin A (IU)	Vitamin D (IU)	Vitamin E (IU)	Ascorbic Acid (C) (mg)	Thiamine (B1) (mg)	Riboflavin (B2) (mg)	Niacin (mg)
	Surbex Filmtab Tablets Abbott Labs					6	6	niacinamide, 30
	Surbex With C Filmtab Tablets Abbott Labs				250	6	6	niacinamide, 30
	Surbex-750 with Iron Filmtab Tablets Abbott Labs			30	750	15	15	niacinamide, 100
	Surbex-750 with Zinc Abbott Labs			30	750	15	15	100
	Surbex-T Filmtab Tablets Abbott Labs				500	15	10	niacinamide, 100
GL LA PU SU	**Theragran High Potency Multivitamin Caplets** Mead Johnson Nutritionals	5000 (as acetate and beta carotene)	400	30mg	90	3	3.4	20
AL DY GL LA SL	**Theragran High Potency Multivitamin Liquid** Mead Johnson Nutritionals	5000/5ml	400/5ml		200/5ml	10/5ml	10/5ml	100/5ml
GL LA PU SU	**Theragran Stress Formula High Potency Multivitamin Caplets** Mead Johnson Nutritionals			30	600	15	15	100

See Chapter 19, "Nutritional Products," for more information about these products.

Pyridox-ine HCl	Cyanoco-balamin	Folic Acid	Panto-thenic	Elemental Iron (mg)	Elemental Calcium (mg)	Phos-phorus (mg)	Magne-sium (mg)	Other Ingredients
2.5	5		10 (as calcium pantothenate)					cellulosic polymers · corn starch · D&C yellow#10 · dibasic calcium phosphate · FD&C yellow#6 · magnesium stearate · polyethylene glycol · povidone · propylene glycol · stearic acid · titanium dioxide · vanillin
2.5	5		10 (as calcium pantothenate)					cellulosic polymers · corn starch · D&C yellow#10 · FD&C yellow#6 · lactose · magnesium stearate · polyethylene glycol · microcrystalline cellulose · povidone · propylene glycol · titanium dioxide · vanillin
25	12	400	20 (as calcium pantothenate)	27 (as sulfate)				cellulosic polymers · colloidal silicon dioxide · FD&C red#3 · corn starch · iron oxide · magnesium stearate · microcrystalline cellulose · polyethylene glycol · povidone · vanillin
20	12	400	20					zinc, 22.5mg · cellulose · povidone · talc · magnesium stearate · titanium dioxide · polyethylene glycol · colloidal silicon dioxide · vanillin · iron oxide
5	10		20 (as calcium pantothenate)					cellulosic polymers · corn starch · D&C yellow#10 · FD&C yellow#6 · magnesium stearate · microcrystalline cellulose · polyethylene glycol · povidone · stearic acid · titanium dioxide · vanillin
3	9	400	10					biotin, 30mcg · lactose · microcrystalline cellulose · hydroxypropyl methylcellulose · povidone · silicon dioxide · magnesium stearate · polyethylene glycol · triacetin · stearic acid · titanium dioxide · annatto · red#40 lake · blue#2 lake · yellow#6 lake
4.1/5ml	5/5ml		21.4/5ml					sucrose · water · glycerin · propylene glycol · polysorbate 80 · carboxymethyl cellulose sodium · flavors · sodium benzoate · methylparaben · ferric ammonium citrate
25	12	400	20	27				biotin, 45mcg · lactose · crospovidone · povidone · hydroxypropyl methylcellulose · magnesium stearate · silicon dioxide · stearic acid · polyethylene glycol · triacetin · titanium dioxide · red#40 lake · blue#2 lake · yellow#6 lake ·

VITAMIN PRODUCTS - continued

	Product Manufacturer/Supplier	Vitamin A (IU)	Vitamin D (IU)	Vitamin E (IU)	Ascorbic Acid (C) (mg)	Thiamine (B1) (mg)	Riboflavin (B2) (mg)	Niacin (mg)
GL LA PU SU	**Theragran-M High Potency Vitamins with Minerals Caplets** Mead Johnson Nutritionals	5000	400	30	90	3	3.4	20
GL PU SO	**Therapeutic B Complex with Vitamin C Capsules** Upsher-Smith Labs				300	15	10.2	50
GL PU SO	**Therapeutic Multiple with Minerals Tablets** Upsher-Smith Labs	5500	400	30	120	3	3.4	30
GL PU SO	**Therapeutic Multivitamin Tablets** Upsher-Smith Labs	5500	400	30	120	3	3.4	30
**	**Thex Forte Caplets** Lee Consumer				500	25	15	niacinamide, 100
** SU	**Total Antioxidant Softgels** Celestial Seasonings			30	60			
AL GL LA SU SL PE	**Tri-Vi-Sol Vitamins A,D+C Drops** Mead Johnson Nutritionals	1500/ml	400/ml		35/ml			
AL GL LA SU SL PE	**Tri-Vi-Sol With Iron Vitamin A,D+C Drops** Mead Johnson Nutritionals	1500/ml	400/ml		35/ml			

See Chapter 19, "Nutritional Products," for more information about these products.

Pyridox-ine HCl	Cyanoco-balamin	Folic Acid	Panto-thenic	Elemental Iron (mg)	Elemental Calcium (mg)	Phos-phorus (mg)	Magne-sium (mg)	Other Ingredients
3	9	400	10	18	40	31	100	zinc, 15mg · chloride, 7.5mg · potassium, 7.5mg · manganese, 3.5mg · copper, 2mg · silicon, 2mg · boron, 150mcg · iodine, 150mcg · molybdenum, 32mcg · biotin, 30mcg · vitamin K, 28mcg · chromium, 26mcg · selenium, 21mcg · tin, 10mcg · vanadium, 10mcg · nickel, 5mcg · lactose · crospovidone · hydroxypropyl methylcellulose · povidone · magnesium stearate · stearic acid · polyethylene glycol · triacetin · red#40 lake · titanium dioxide · blue#2 lake · silica gel · microcrystalline cellulose
5			10					
3	9	400	10	27	40		100	zinc, 15mg · potassium, 7.5mg · chloride, 7.5mg · manganese, 5mg · copper, 2mg · iodine, 150mcg · biotin, 15mcg · chromium, 15mcg · molybdenum, 15mcg · selenium, 10mcg
3	9	400	10					biotin, 15mcg
5			10					
								tumeric extract, 30mg · alpha lipoic acid, 20mg · green tea extract, 30mg · grape seed extract, 10mg · rosemary extract, 15mg · coenzyme Q10, 10mg · selenium, 25mg
								glycerin · water · polysorbate 80 · artificial flavor · color
			•					
				10/ml				glycerin · water · propylene · glycol · polysorbate 80 · artificial flavor · color

VITAMIN PRODUCTS - continued

	Product Manufacturer/Supplier	Vitamin A (IU)	Vitamin D (IU)	Vitamin E (IU)	Ascorbic Acid (C) (mg)	Thiamine (B1) (mg)	Riboflavin (B2) (mg)	Niacin (mg)
DY GL LA PU SO SU	**Ultra-Freeda Tablets** Freeda Vitamins	3333.3 (as palmitate and beta carotene, 833.3)	133.3	66.7	333.3	16.7	16.7	8.3 · niacinamide, 25
	Unicap Tablets Pharmacia & Upjohn	5000	400	15	60	1.5	1.7	20
PE	**Unicap Jr. Chewable Tablets** Pharmacia & Upjohn	5000	400	15	60	1.5	1.7	20
	Unicap M Tablets Pharmacia & Upjohn	5000	400	30	60	1.5	1.7	20
	Unicap Plus Iron Tablets Pharmacia & Upjohn	5000	400	30	60	1.5	1.7	20
GE	**Unicap Senior Tablets** Pharmacia & Upjohn	5000	200	15	60	1.2	1.4	16
	Unicap Softgels Pharmacia & Upjohn	5000	400	30	60	1.5	1.7	20
	Unicap T Tablets Pharmacia & Upjohn	5000	400	30	500	10	10	100
DY GL LA PU SO SU	**Unilife-A Gelcaps** Chronimed	15000 (as palmitate)						
GL PU	**Variplex-C Tablets** Hudson				500	15	10	niacinamide, 100
LA PE	**Vi-Daylin ADC Vitamins Drops** Ross Products/Abbott Labs	1500/ml	400/ml		35/ml			
LA PE	**Vi-Daylin ADC Vitamins Plus Iron Drops** Ross Products/Abbott Labs	1500/ml	400/ml		35/ml			
GL PE	**Vi-Daylin Multi-Vitamin Chewable Tablets** Ross Products/Abbott Labs	2500	400	15	60	1.05	1.2	13.5
LA PE	**Vi-Daylin Multi-Vitamin Drops** Ross Products/Abbott Labs	1500/ml	400/ml	5/ml	35/ml	0.5/ml	0.6/ml	8/ml

See Chapter 19, "Nutritional Products," for more information about these products.

Pyridox-ine HCl	Cyanoco-balamin	Folic Acid	Panto-thenic	Elemental Iron (mg)	Elemental Calcium (mg)	Phos-phorus (mg)	Magne-sium (mg)	Other Ingredients
16.7	33.3	266.7	33.3	5	66.7		33.3	bioflavonoids complex, 33.3mg · choline citrate, 33.3mg · i-inosital, 33.3mg · PABA, 16.7mg · potassium, 11mg · zinc, 7.5mg · manganese, 3.3mg · biotin, 100mcg · chromium, 66.7mcg · iodine, 44.3mcg · selenium, 33.3mcg · molybdenum, 4.2mcg
2	6	400						
2	6	400						sucrose · mannitol · flavor
2	6	400	10	18	60	45		zinc, 15mg · potassium, 5mg · copper, 2mg · manganese, 1mg · iodine, 150mcg · tartrazine
2	6	400	10	22.5	100			
2.2	3	400	10	10	100	77	30	zinc, 15mg · potassium, 5mg · copper, 2mg · manganese, 1mg · iodine, 150mcg
2	6	400						
6	18	400	25	18				zinc, 15mg · potassium, 5mg · copper, 2mg · manganese, 1mg · iodine, 150mcg · selenium, 10mcg
5	10		20					
								flavor · propylene glycol · polysorbate 80 · glycerin · water · methylparaben · propylparaben · caramel color
				10/ml				flavor · glycerin · water · polysorbate 80 · benzoic acid · methylparaben · caramel color
1.05	4.5	300						sucrose · flavor · dextrins · colors
0.4/ml	1.5/ml							alcohol, < 0.5% · flavor · glycerin · water · benzoic acid · methylparaben · disodium edetate · ferric ammonium citrate

VITAMIN PRODUCTS - continued

	Product Manufacturer/Supplier	Vitamin A (IU)	Vitamin D (IU)	Vitamin E (IU)	Ascorbic Acid (C) (mg)	Thiamine (B1) (mg)	Riboflavin (B2) (mg)	Niacin (mg)
LA	**Vi-Daylin Multi-Vitamin Liquid** Ross Products/Abbott Labs	2500/5ml	400/5ml	15/ml	60/5ml	1.05/5ml	1.2/5ml	13.5/5ml
GL PE	**Vi-Daylin Multi-Vitamin Plus Iron Chewable Tablets** Ross Products/Abbott Labs	2500	400	15	60	1.05	1.2	13.5
LA PE	**Vi-Daylin Multi-Vitamin Plus Iron Drops** Ross Products/Abbott Labs	1500/ml	400/ml	5/ml	35/ml	0.5/ml	0.6/ml	8/ml
LA	**Vi-Daylin Multi-Vitamin Plus Iron Liquid** Ross Products/Abbott Labs	2500/5ml	400/5ml	15/5ml	60/5ml	1.05/5ml	1.2/5ml	13.5/5ml
GL	**Vi-Zac Capsules** UCB Pharma	5000		50	500			
	Vicon C Capsules UCB Pharma				300	20	10	100
GL	**Vicon Plus Capsules** UCB Pharma	4000		50	150	10	5	25
GL PU	**Vioday Tablets** Hudson	5000 (as acetate and beta carotene)	400	30	60	1.5	1.7	niacinamide, 20
**	**Vita ACES+ Gum** GumTech	1250 (as beta carotene)		15	30			
PE	**Vita-Lea for Children Tablets** Shaklee	2500 (as palmitate)	400	30	60	1.5	1.7	20
PE	**Vita-Lea for Infants & Toddlers Powder** Shaklee	1250/5ml	100/5ml	5/5ml	20/5ml	0.35/5ml	0.4/5ml	4.5/5ml

See Chapter 19, "Nutritional Products," for more information about these products.

Pyridox-ine HCl	Cyanoco-balamin	Folic Acid	Panto-thenic	Elemental Iron (mg)	Elemental Calcium (mg)	Phos-phorus (mg)	Magne-sium (mg)	Other Ingredients
1.05/5ml	4.5/5ml							alcohol, < 0.5% · glucose · sucrose · flavor · color · benzoic acid · methylparaben · cysteine HCl
1.05	4.5	300		12				sucrose · flavor · dextrins · mannitol · FD&C yellow#6
0.4/ml				10/ml				alcohol, < 0.5% · flavor · glycerin · water · color · benzoic acid · methylparaben
1.05/5ml	4.5/5ml			10/5ml				alcohol, < 0.5% · flavor · glucose · sucrose · propylparaben · benzoic acid · methylparaben · cysteine HCl
								zinc, 18mg
5			20				7	zinc, 18mg
2			10				7	zinc, 18mg · manganese, 1.8mg
2	6	400	10 (as d-calcium pantothenate)					
								grape extract, 5mg · selenium, 9mcg · sorbitol · gum base · maltitol syrup · glycerin · natural flavors · mannitol · lecithin · citric acid · acesulfame potassium · FD&C red#10
2	6	400	10	10	200 (as dicalcium phosphate)	160	80 (as oxide)	zinc, 10mg · manganese, 1.5mg · copper, 1mg · biotin, 300mcg · iodine, 90mcg · chromium, 50mcg · molybdenum, 50mcg · selenium, 20mcg · vitamin K, 10mcg · sorbitol · fructose · natural flavors · vegetable juice extracts · citric acid · inositol · choline bitartrate · mixed tocopherols · rice bran powder · rose hips powder · alfalfa powder · acerola extract · grapefruit bioflavonoid · hesperidin complex · lemon bioflavonoid · orange bioflavonoid · sea kelp powder
0.35/5ml	1.5/5ml	100/5ml	2.5/5ml	5/5ml	80/5ml		20/5ml	zinc, 4mg · copper, 500mcg · manganese, 500mcg · biotin, 75mcg · iodine, 35mcg · molybdenum, 12.5mcg · chromium, 10mcg · selenium, 10mcg · vitamin K, 5mcg · dextrose · trace mineral rice protein hydrolysate · inositol · choline bitartrate · acerola extract · mixed tocopherols

VITAMIN PRODUCTS - continued

Product Manufacturer/Supplier	Vitamin A (IU)	Vitamin D (IU)	Vitamin E (IU)	Ascorbic Acid (C) (mg)	Thiamine (B1) (mg)	Riboflavin (B2) (mg)	Niacin (mg)
Vita-Lea, with or without Iron, Tablets Shaklee	5000 (as palmitate)	400	60	120	1.5	1.7	20
DY GL LA PU SO SU PE · **Vitalets Chewable Tablets, Flavored or Unflavored** Freeda Vitamins	5000 (with beta carotene)	400	5	60	2.5	0.9	niacinamide, 20
AL DY GL LA SO SU SL · **Vitalize Liquid** Scot-Tussin Pharmacal					10/5ml		
Z-Bec Tablets Whitehall-Robins Healthcare			45	600	15	10.2	100
Zymacap Capsules Lee Consumer	5000 (as palmitate)	400	15	90	2.25	2.6	niacinamide, 30

** New listing

See Chapter 19, "Nutritional Products," for more information about these products.

Pyridox-ine HCl	Cyanoco-balamin	Folic Acid	Panto-thenic	Elemental Iron (mg)	Elemental Calcium (mg)	Phos-phorus (mg)	Magne-sium (mg)	Other Ingredients
2	6	400	10	18 (as fumarate) or 0	450 (as dicalcium phosphate)	350	200 (as oxide)	zinc, 15mg · manganese, 3.5mg · copper, 2mg · boron, 1mg · biotin, 300mcg · molybdenum, 160mcg · iodine, 150mcg · chromium, 130mcg · vitamin K, 80mcg · selenium, 70mcg · nickel, 15mcg · tin, 10mcg · vanadium, 2mcg
2	5		3 (as calcium pantothenate)	10 (as fumarate)	61.5			zinc, 5mg · manganese gluconate, 1mg · biotin, 25mcg
5/5ml	25/5ml			100/5ml (as pyrophosphate) equivalent to 22mg				l-lysine monohydrochloride, 100mg/5ml · methylparaben · propylparaben · cherry-strawberry flavor · potassium benzoate · glycerin
10	6		25					zinc (elemental), 22.5mg · microcrystalline cellulose · hydroxypropyl methylcellulose · stearic acid · propylene glycol · titanium dioxide · FD&C blue#1 · aluminium lake · methylparaben · propylparaben · xanthan gum · sodium citrate · potassium sorbate · silicon dioxide · polysorbate 20 · magnesium stearate · polyvinyl pyrrolidone · vanillin
3	9	400	15					soybean oil · gelatin · glycerin · lecithin · corn oil · titanium dioxide · ethyl vanillin

CALCIUM PRODUCTS

	Product Manufacturer/Supplier	Dosage Form	Elemental Calcium	Vitamin D	Other Ingredients
GL PU SO	**Calcet** Mission Pharmacal	tablet	150mg (as gluconate, lactate, and carbonate)	100 IU	sugar · polyethylene glycol · croscarmellose sodium · color · povidone · magnesium stearate · yellow#5 lake · carnauba wax · white beeswax · sodium benzoate
DY GL PU	**Calci-Caps** Nion Labs	tablet	125mg (as gluconate and dicalcium phosphate)	66.7 IU	lactose · starch · cellulose · magnesium silicate · hydrogenated vegetable oil · croscarmellose sodium · calcium carbonate sugar · titanium dioxide · wax · food shellac
DY GL LA PU SU	**Calci-Caps Super** Nion Labs	tablet	400mg (as oyster shell, bone meal, gluconate, and dicalcium phosphate)	400 IU	croscarmellose sodium · hydrogenated vegetable oil · stearic acid · titanium dioxide · magnesium silicate · wax · hydroxypropyl methylcellulose
GL PU SO	**Calci-Caps with Iron** Nion Labs	tablet	125mg (as gluconate and dicalcium phosphate)	66.7 IU	ferrous gluconate, 7.4mg · starch · cellulose · magnesium silicate · calcium carbonate sugar · titanium dioxide · FD&C blue#1 · FD&C yellow#5 (tartrazine) · wax
GL PU SO	**Calci-Chew; Cherry, Lemon, or Orange** R & D Labs	chewable tablet	500mg (as carbonate)		sugar · citric acid · stearic acid · silica · magnesium stearate · flavoring
DY GL LA PU SO SU	**Calci-Mix** R & D Labs	capsule	500mg (as carbonate)		
**	**Calcium and Magnesium with Zinc** American Health	tablet	333.3mg (as carbonate and gluconate)		magnesium, 133.3mg (as oxide and gluconate) · zinc, 8.3mg (as gluconate and citrate)
	Calcium Carbonate 600 Republic Drug	tablet	1200mg (as carbonate)		
DY GL LA PU SU	**Calcium Complex** Shaklee	tablet	400mg		magnesium, 13.3mg · zinc, 0.5mg · manganese, 0.5mg · copper, 0.07mg · ground limestone · modified cellulose gum · carbohydrate gum
DY GL PR PU	**Calcium Complex** Shaklee	chewable tablet	333.3mg		magnesium, 13.3mg · zinc, 0.5mg · manganese, 0.5mg · copper, 0.07mg · corn syrup solids · non-fat dry milk · acacia gum · flavors
DY LA PU SU	**Calcium Magnesium** Shaklee	tablet	162.5mg	50 IU	phosphorus, 125mg · magnesium, 100mg · modified cellulose gum · dried yeast · ground limestone · modified food starch
** LA SU	**Calcium with Vitamins A&D** American Health	wafer	500mg (as carbonate)	200 IU	vitamin A, 200 IU · sorbitol · mannitol · cellulose · acacia · vegetable sterates · natural lemon and mint flavors · silica
GL LA PU SO SU	**Caltrate 600 High Potency** Lederle Consumer	tablet	600mg (as carbonate)		maltodextrin · cellulose · mineral oil · hydroxypropyl methylcellulose · titanium dioxide · sodium lauryl sulfate · gelatin · crospovidone · stearic acid · magnesium stearate

See Chapter 19, "Nutritional Products," for more information about these products.

CALCIUM PRODUCTS - continued

	Product Manufacturer/Supplier	Dosage Form	Elemental Calcium	Vitamin D	Other Ingredients
GL LA PU SO SU	**Caltrate 600 High Potency+ D** Lederle Consumer	tablet	600mg (as carbonate)	200 IU	maltodextrin · cellulose · mineral oil · hydroxypropyl methylcellulose · titanium dioxide · sodium lauryl sulfate · FD&C yellow#6 · gelatin · crospovidone · stearic acid · magnesium stearate
GL LA PU SO SU	**Caltrate Plus** Lederle Consumer	tablet	600mg	200 IU	magnesium, 40mg · zinc, 7.5mg · manganese, 1.8mg · copper, 1mg · boron, 250mcg · maltodextrin · cellulose · mineral oil · hydroxypropyl methylcellulose · titanium dioxide · sodium lauryl sulfate · FD&C red#40 · FD&C yellow#6 · FD&C blue#1 · gelatin · crospovidone · stearic acid · magnesium stearate
	Caltrate Plus Nutrient Enriched, Asst. Fruit Flavors Lederle Consumer	chewable tablet	600mg	200 IU	magnesium, 40mg · zinc, 7.5mg · manganese, 1.8mg · copper, 1mg · boron, 250mcg · dextrose · mineral oil · magnesium stearate · maltodextrin · adipic acid · modified food starch · cellulose · artificial flavors · sucrose · FD&C red#40 · FD&C yellow#6 · FD&C blue#2 · gelatin · crospovidone · stearic acid
GL LA PU SO	**Caltrate Plus Nutrient Enriched, Spearmint** Lederle Consumer	chewable tablet	500 mg	200 IU	magnesium, 40mg · zinc, 7.5mg · manganese, 1.8mg · copper, 1mg · boron, 250mcg · dextrose · mineral oil · magnesium stearate · maltodextrin · cellulose · modified food starch · FD&C yellow#5 · sucrose · FD&C blue#1 · natural spearmint flavor · gelatin · crospovidone · stearic acid
** PE	**Chewy Bears Chewable Calcium** American Health	wafer	250mg (as carbonate and citrate)		lactose, 300 FCC units · malted goat milk · fructose · fruit juice solids · dried honey · vegetable gums · pectin
DY GL LA PU SO SU	**Citracal** Mission Pharmacal	tablet	200mg (as citrate)		polyethylene glycol · croscarmellose sodium · HPMC · magnesium stearate · color · talc
DY GL LA PU SO SU	**Citracal + D** Mission Pharmacal	caplet	315mg (as citrate)	200 IU	polyethylene glycol · croscarmellose sodium · HPMC · magnesium stearate · color · talc
DY GL LA PU SU	**Citracal Liquitab** Mission Pharmacal	effervescent tablet	500mg (as citrate)		citric acid · adipic acid · saccharin sodium · orange flavor · cellulose gum · aspartame
GL PU SO	**Citron** Legere Ph'cals	caplet	1000mg (as citrate carbonate)		boron, 3mg (as chelate aspartate)

See Chapter 19, "Nutritional Products," for more information about these products.

CALCIUM PRODUCTS - continued

	Product Manufacturer/Supplier	Dosage Form	Elemental Calcium	Vitamin D	Other Ingredients
	Dical-D Abbott Labs	tablet	117mg	133 IU	phosphorus, 90mg · microcrystalline cellulose · sodium starch glycolate · corn starch · hydrogenated vegetable oil wax · magnesium stearate · talc
DY GL LA PU SO SU	**Fem Cal** Freeda Vitamins	tablet	250mg	100 IU	magnesium, 100mg · silicon, 2.5mg · manganese, 5mg · boron, 0.5mg
	Florical Mericon	tablet	145.6mg (as carbonate, 364mg)		fluoride, 3.75mg (as sodium fluoride, 8.3mg)
GL PU SU	**Florical** Mericon	capsule	145.6mg (as carbonate and oyster shell, 364mg)		fluoride, 3.75mg (as sodium fluoride, 8.3mg)
DY GL LA PU SO SU	**Mag/Cal Mega** Freeda Vitamins	tablet	133.3mg		magnesium, 266.6mg
SU	**Monocal** Mericon	tablet	250mg (as carbonate, 625mg)		fluoride, 3mg (as sodium mono-fluorophosphate, 22.75mg)
	Neo-Calglucon Novartis Consumer	syrup	115mg/5ml (as gluconate)		sucrose · saccharin · citric acid · benzoic acid · sorbitol · flavors
DY GL PU SU	**Nephro-Calci** R & D Labs	tablet	600mg (as carbonate)		magnesium stearate · cellulose, <0.2mg
	One-A-Day Calcium Plus Bayer Consumer	chewable tablet	500mg	100 IU	magnesium, 50mg · sorbitol · maltodextrin · xylitol · starch · stearic acid · aspartame · flavors · polyethylene glycol · gelatin · polydextrose · poloxamer 407 · docusate sodium · vitamin D3
GL LA PU SO SU	**Os-Cal 250 + D** SmithKline Beecham	tablet	250mg (as oyster shell)	125 IU	oyster shell powder · talc · corn syrup solids · hydroxypropyl methylcellulose · corn starch · polysorbate 80 · titanium dioxide · polyethylene glycol · propylparaben · methylparaben · simethicone · yellow#10 lake · blue#1 lake · carnauba wax · edetate sodium
GL LA PU SO	**Os-Cal 500** SmithKline Beecham	tablet	500mg (as oyster shell)		oyster shell powder · talc · corn syrup solids · hydroxypropyl methylcellulose · corn starch · polysorbate 80 · titanium dioxide · polyethylene glycol · propylparaben · methylparaben · polydextrose · triacetin · yellow#10 lake · blue#1 lake · carnauba wax
AF DY GL LA PU SU	**Os-Cal 500** SmithKline Beecham	chewable tablet	500mg (as carbonate)		dextrose monohydrate · maltodextrin · microcrystalline cellulose · magnesium stearate · artificial flavors · sodium chloride

See Chapter 19, "Nutritional Products," for more information about these products.

CALCIUM PRODUCTS - continued

	Product Manufacturer/Supplier	Dosage Form	Elemental Calcium	Vitamin D	Other Ingredients
GL LA PU SO	**Os-Cal 500 + D** SmithKline Beecham	tablet	500mg	125 IU	oyster shell powder · talc · corn syrup solids · hydroxypropyl methylcellulose · corn starch · polysorbate 80 · titanium dioxide · polyethylene glycol · propylparaben · methylparaben · polydextrose · triacetin · yellow#10 lake · blue#1 lake · carnauba wax
GL PU SO SU	**Oyster Calcium** Hudson	tablet	375mg (as carbonate and oyster shell)	200 IU	vitamin A, 800 IU (as acetate)
GL PU SO SU	**Oyster Calcium 500 + D** Hudson	tablet	500mg (as oyster shell)	125 IU	
GL PU SU	**Oystercal 500** Hudson	tablet	500mg (as oyster shell)		
GL PU SO SU	**Oystercal-D 250** Hudson	tablet	250mg (as oyster shell powder)	125 IU	
DY GL LA PU SO SU	**Parvacal 500** Freeda Vitamins	tablet	500mg	200 IU	
GL	**Posture** Selfcare	tablet	600mg (as tribasic phosphate)		croscarmellose sodium · ethylcellulose · magnesium stearate · microcrystalline cellulose · polyethylene glycol · sodium lauryl sulfate
GL	**Posture-D** Selfcare	tablet	600mg (as tribasic phosphate)	125 IU	croscarmellose sodium · ethylcellulose · magnesium stearate · microcrystalline cellulose · polyethylene glycol · povidone · sodium lauryl sulfate
**	**Releaf Osteoporosis Formula** Lake Consumer	tablet	100mg	0.83mcg	magnesium, 50mg · zinc, 1.67mg
DY GL LA PU SO SU	**Super Cal/Mag** Freeda Vitamins	tablet	333.3mg		magnesium, 166.6mg
GL LA PU SO	**Tums 500; Asst. Fruit or Peppermint** SmithKline Beecham	chewable tablet	500mg (as carbonate)		sucrose · corn starch · talc · mineral oil · natural & artificial flavors · sodium polyphosphate · adipic acid (Fruit) · yellow#6 lake (Fruit) · yellow#10 lake (Fruit) · blue#1 lake (Fruit) · red#27 lake · red#30 lake
DY GL LA PU	**Vita-Cal** Shaklee	chewable tablet	250mg	66.7 IU	phosphorus, 166.7mg · thiamine, 1mg · riboflavin, 1mg · ground limestone · fructose · mannitol · sorbitol · primary grown yeast · spearmint oil · peppermint oil

See Chapter 19, "Nutritional Products," for more information about these products.

IRON PRODUCTS

	Product Manufacturer/Supplier	Dosage Form	Elemental Iron	Vitamins & Nutrients	Other Ingredients
	Fe-50 Extended Release Northampton Medical	caplet	50mg		corn starch · glyceryl monostearate · polyethylene glycol · titanium dioxide
	Femiron Daily Iron Supplement Menley & James Labs	tablet	20mg (as fumarate)		alginic acid · calcium phosphate · FD&C red#40 · starch · magnesium stearate · stearic acid · silicon dioxide · polyethylene glycol · white wax · carnauba wax
	Feosol SmithKline Beecham	elixir	44mg/5ml (as sulfate)		alcohol, 5% · purified water · sucrose · glucose · citric acid · saccharin sodium · FD&C yellow#6 · flavors
**	**Feosol** SmithKline Beecham	caplet	50mg		lactose · sorbitol · hydroxypropyl methylcellulose · polydextrose · crospovidone · polyethylene glycol · magnesium stearate · stearic acid · triacetin · titanium dioxide · maltodextrin · FD&C blue#2 · FD&C red#40 · FD&C yellow#6
	Feosol SmithKline Beecham	tablet	65mg (as sulfate)		calcium sulfate · starch · glucose · hydroxypropyl methylcellulose · talc · stearic acid · polyethylene glycol · sodium lauryl sulfate · mineral oil · titanium dioxide · D&C yellow#10 · FD&C blue#2
AL DY GL LA SL	**Feostat** Forest Ph'cals	suspension	33mg/5ml (as fumarate)		sucrose, 1917.5mg/5ml · sorbitol solution · methylparaben · veegum · flavor
AL DY GL LA SL	**Feostat** Forest Ph'cals	drops	15mg/0.6ml (as fumarate)		sucrose · sorbitol · methylparaben · veegum · isoascorbic acid · flavor
GL LA PU SU	**Feostat** Forest Ph'cals	chewable tablet	33mg (as fumarate)		magnesium stearate · stearic acid hystrene · saccharin sodium · flavor
DY GL LA SL PE	**Fer-In-Sol** Mead Johnson Nutritionals	syrup	18mg/5ml (as sulfate)		alcohol, 5% · sugar · water · sorbitol · citric acid · salt · artificial flavor · sodium bisulfite
DY GL LA SL PE	**Fer-In-Sol** Mead Johnson Nutritionals	drops	15mg/0.6ml (as sulfate)		alcohol, 0.2% · sugar · sorbitol · water · citric acid · sodium bisulfite · natural flavors
GL PU SO	**Feratab** Upsher-Smith Labs	tablet	60mg; 300mg (as sulfate)		
GL SO	**Fergon** Bayer Consumer	tablet	36mg (as gluconate)		
	Fero-Grad-500 Filmtabs Abbott Labs	tablet	105mg (as sulfate)	sodium ascorbate, 500mg	cellulosic polymers · D&C red#7 · castor oil · magnesium stearate · methyl acrylate-methyl methacrylate copolymers · polyethylene glycol · povidone · pregelatinized starch (contains corn starch) · propylene glycol · talc · titanium dioxide · vanillin

See Chapter 19, "Nutritional Products," for more information about these products.

IRON PRODUCTS - continued

	Product Manufacturer/Supplier	Dosage Form	Elemental Iron	Vitamins & Nutrients	Other Ingredients
	Fero-Gradumet Filmtabs Abbott Labs	tablet	105mg (as sulfate)		castor oil · cellulosic polymers · FD&C red#40 · FD&C yellow#6 · magnesium stearate · methyl acrylate-methyl methacrylate copolymers · polyethylene glycol · povidone · propylene glycol · titanium dioxide · vanillin
GL PU SU	**Ferro-Sequels** Selfcare	timed-release tablet	50mg (as fumarate)		lactose · microcrystalline cellulose · hydroxypropyl methylcellulose · docusate sodium · magnesium stearate · sodium benzoate · silicon dioxide · mineral oil · titanium dioxide · yellow#10 · blue#1 · sodium lauryl sulfate
	Ferrous Fumarate Multisource	tablet	106mg (as fumarate)		
GL PU SO	**Ferrous Gluconate** Upsher-Smith Labs	tablet	34mg; 300mg (as gluconate)		
	Ferrous Gluconate Multisource	capsule	38mg (as gluconate)		
	Ferrous Sulfate Multisource	capsule	30mg (as sulfate)		
GL PU	**Hytinic** Hyrex Ph'cals	capsule	150mg (as polysaccharide-iron complex)		sodium, 0.2mEq
	I.L.X. B12 Elixir Kenwood Labs	liquid	102mg	nicotinamide, 10mg · B1, 5mg · B2, 2mg · B12, 10mcg	liver fraction, 98mg
	I.L.X. B12 Elixir (Sugar Free) Kenwood Labs	liquid	102mg	nicotinamide, 10mg · B1, 5mg · B2, 2mg · B12, 10mcg	liver fraction, 98mg
	I.L.X. Elixir Kenwood Labs	liquid	70mg	nicotinamide, 10mg · B1, 5mg · B2, 2mg	liver concentrate, 98mg
	Ircon Kenwood Labs	tablet	200mg (as fumarate)		
SL	**Ircon FA** Kenwood Labs	tablet	250mg (as fumarate)	folic acid, 800mcg	
DY GL LA PU SU	**Iron Plus Vitamin C** Shaklee	tablet	18mg	calcium, 136mg · phosphorus, 97mg · ascorbic acid, 60mg	maltodextrin · modified cellulose gum · beet powder · acacia gum · spinach powder · barley flour · locust bean gum · agar-agar
SU	**Irospan** Fielding	tablet	65mg	ascorbic acid, 150mg	
	Irospan Fielding	capsule	65mg	ascorbic acid, 150mg	
GL PU SO	**Nephro-Fer** R & D Labs	tablet	115mg (as fumarate)		whey · stearic acid · hydrogenated vegetable oil · cellulose · silicon dioxide
DY LA SU	**Niferex** Schwarz Pharma	elixir	20mg/ml (as polysaccharide-iron complex)		alcohol, 10%

See Chapter 19, "Nutritional Products," for more information about these products.

IRON PRODUCTS - continued

	Product Manufacturer/Supplier	Dosage Form	Elemental Iron	Vitamins & Nutrients	Other
	Niferex Schwarz Pharma	tablet	50mg (as polysaccharide-iron complex)		
LA	**Niferex with Vitamin C** Schwarz Pharma	tablet	50mg (as polysaccharide-iron complex)	sodium ascorbate, 168.75mg · ascorbic acid, 100mg	
LA	**Niferex-150** Schwarz Pharma	capsule	150mg (as polysaccharide-iron complex)		
GL PU SO	**Slow Fe** Novartis Consumer	tablet	50mg (as sulfate)		cetostearyl alcohol · hydroxypropyl methylcellulose · lactose · magnesium stearate · polysorbate 80 · talc · titanium dioxide · yellow iron oxide · blue#2
	Slow Fe + Folic Acid Novartis Consumer	tablet	50mg (as sulfate)	folic acid, 400mcg	cetostearyl alcohol · hydroxypropyl methylcellulose · lactose · magnesium stearate · polysorbate 80 · talc · titanium dioxide · yellow iron oxide
GL	**Vitron-C** Novartis Consumer	tablet	66mg (as fumarate)	ascorbic acid, 125mg	colloidal silicon dioxide · flavor · glycine · hydroxypropyl methylcellulose · iron oxides · magnesium stearate · microcrystalline cellulose · polyethylene glycol · polysorbate 80 · povidone · saccharin sodium · talc · titanium dioxide

** New listing

See Chapter 19, "Nutritional Products," for more information about these products.

MISCELLANEOUS MINERAL PRODUCTS

	Product Manufacturer/Supplier	Dosage Form	Elemental Mineral(s)	Other Ingredients
**	**Chroma Trim** GumTech	gum	calcium, 50mg · chromium, 60mcg (as nicotinate) · selenium, 9mcg	vitamin D, 50 IU · vitamin E, 4 IU · creatine, 62.5mg · blue-green algae, 10mg · siberian ginseng, 7.5mg · vitamin B12, 5mcg · sorbitol · gum base · maltitol syrup · glycerin · natural flavors · lecithin · acesulfame potassium · carmine
**	**Chromemate** Natrol	capsule	chromium, 200mcg (as polynicotinate)	l-arginine, 50mg · l-lysine, 50mg · vitamin B6, 3mg
	Chromium Picolinate Sundown	tablet	chromium, 200mcg (as picolinate, 1.6mg)	
**	**Chromium Picolinate** Natrol	capsule	chromium, 200mcg (as picolinate)	
** GL LA SO SU	**Chromium Picolinate** American Health	tablet	chromium, 200mcg (as picolinate)	dicalcium phosphate · silica · vegetable magnesium stearate · vegetable stearic acid
DY GL LA PU SO SU	**Chromium, Organic** Freeda Vitamins	tablet	chromium, 200mcg; 400mcg	
** GL LA	**Dr. Powers Colloidal Mineral Source** American Health	liquid	magnesium, 100mg · calcium, 25mg · potassium, 10mg · zinc, 10mg · manganese, 5mg · selenium, 50mcg · chromium, 50mcg	cyanocobalamin, 1100mcg · silica, 1000mcg · biotin, 200mcg
DY GL LA PU SO SU	**Manganese Chelate** Sundown	tablet	manganese, 50mg (as gluconate)	
DY GL LA PU SO SU	**Maxi-Minerals** Freeda Vitamins	tablet	calcium, 300mg (as carbonate) · magnesium, 175mg (as oxide) · zinc, 50mg (as gluconate) · manganese, 20mg (as gluconate) · iron, 19.6mg (as fumarate) · potassium, 10mg (as gluconate) · copper, 8mg (as gluconate) · iodine, 0.1mg · selenium, 10mcg	
**	**Mineral Complex** Natrol	tablet	calcium, 166.7%mg · magnesium, 66.7%mg · potassium, 33mg · zinc, 10mg · manganese, 3.3mg · copper, 0.7mg · boron, 66.7mcg · chromium, 66.7mcg · selenium, 66.7mcg · iodine, 50mcg · molybdenum, 16.7mcg · vanadium, 16.7mcg	fruitbase, 200mcg
	Orazinc 110 Mericon	tablet	zinc, 25mg (as sulfate)	
	Orazinc 220 Mericon	capsule	zinc, 50mg (as sulfate)	

See Chapter 19, "Nutritional Products," for more information about these products.

MISCELLANEOUS MINERAL PRODUCTS - continued

	Product Manufacturer/Supplier	Dosage Form	Elemental Mineral(s)	Other Ingredients
	Permathene Maximum Strength Chromium Picolinate § CCA Industries	softgel	chromium, 200mcg (as picolinate) · zinc oxide	phenylpropanolamine HCl, 75mg · beeswax · gelatin · glycerin · lecithin · soybean oil · vegetable oil · water
DY GL LA PU SO SU	**Selenium, Oceanic** Freeda Vitamins	tablet	selenium, 50mcg; 100mcg; 200mcg	
** DY GL SU	**Verazinc** Forest Ph'cals	capsule	zinc, 50mg (as sulfate monohydrate, 139mg)	lactose · starch · magnesium stearate
**	**Zinc** Natrol	tablet	zinc, 30mg	fruitbase, 60mg
DY GL LA PU SO SU	**Zinc** Freeda Vitamins	tablet	zinc, 8.5mg; 30mg (as gluconate)	
	Zinc 15 Mericon	tablet	zinc, 15mg (as sulfate)	

** New listing

§ Manufacturer/supplier did not confirm information for this edition. Product listing is reprinted from the '96-97 edition.

See Chapter 19, "Nutritional Products," for more information about these products.

ENTERAL FOOD SUPPLEMENT PRODUCTS

	Product Manufacturer/Supplier	Dosage Form	Calories (per mL)	Protein [a] (g)	Carbohy- drate [a] (g)	Fat [a] (g)	Vitamins & Minerals	Comments
GL LA	**Advera** Ross Products/Abbott Labs	liquid	1.28	14.2/8fl oz	51.1/8fl oz	5.4/8fl oz	taurine, 0.05g/8fl oz · l- carnitine, 0.03g/8fl oz	for dietary management of patients with HIV infection or AIDS
	Alitra Q Ross Products/Abbott Labs	individual packet	1	15.8/packet	49.5/packet	4.65/packet	various [b,c,d] · glutamine · arginine · carnitine · taurine	elemental nutrition with glutamine · 300 calories/packet · 5 servings = 100% vitamin USRDA
	Amin-Aid Instant Drink R & D Labs	individual packet	665kcal/packet	6.6/packet (as amino acids)	124.3/packet	15.7/packet		low protein formula for patients with acute or chronic renal failure
GL LA	**Boost** Mead Johnson Nutritionals	liquid	1.01	43	174	17.5	various [b,c]	volume to meet 100% USRDA is 1180ml · should be used by persons with galactosemia
LA	**Broth Plus** Novartis Nutrition	powder	0.68	39.5	125	2.3		prepare with water
	Carnation Instant Breakfast Carnation Nutritional	liquid	0.73	12.5/10fl oz	36/10fl oz	3.25/10fl oz	various [b,c,d]	
	Carnation Instant Breakfast Carnation Nutritional	individual packet	1.2	12.5	39	12	various [b,c,d]	prepare with whole milk
	Carnation Instant Breakfast Carnation Nutritional	individual packet	0.92	12.5	39	1.3	various [b,c,d]	prepare with skim milk
DY GL LA PU SU	**Casec** Mead Johnson Nutritionals	powder	380/100g	90/100g		2/100g		calcium caseinate · soy lecithin
DY GL LA	**Choice dm** Mead Johnson Nutritionals	liquid	1.06	45	106	51	various [b,c,d]	vanilla flavor · volume to meet 100% USRDA is 1000ml
CO GL LA	**Citrotein** Novartis Nutrition	powder	0.66	41	122	1.6	various [b,c,d]	orange and punch flavors
LA	**Compleat Modified Formula** Novartis Nutrition	liquid	1.07	43	140	37	various [b,c,d]	contains fiber · contains blenderized traditional foods: beef, vegetables, fruits

See Chapter 19, "Nutritional Products," for more information about these products.

ENTERAL FOOD SUPPLEMENT PRODUCTS - continued

	Product Manufacturer/Supplier	Dosage Form	Calories (per mL)	Protein [a] (g)	Carbohy- drate [a] (g)	Fat [a] (g)	Vitamins & Minerals	Comments
** GL LA PE	**Compleat Pediatric** Novartis Nutrition	liquid	1	38	126	39	various [b,c,d]	blenderized formula from traditional foods · fiber, 4.2g
	Compleat Regular Formula Novartis Nutrition	liquid	1.07	43	130	43	various [b,c,d]	milk base · contains fiber · contains blenderized traditional foods: beef, vegetables, fruits
** CO GL LA	**Comply** Mead Johnson Nutritionals	liquid	1.5	60	180	61	various [b,c]	volume to meet 100% USRDA is 830ml
CA DY GL LA SU	**Criticare HN** Mead Johnson Nutritionals	liquid	1.06	38	220	5.3	various [b,c]	volume to meet 100% USRDA is 1890ml
CO DY GL LA SU	**Deliver 2.0** Mead Johnson Nutritionals	liquid	2	75	200	101	various [b,c]	volume to meet 100% USRDA is 1000ml
LA SU	**DiabetiSource** Novartis Nutrition	liquid	1	50	90	49	various [b,c,d]	fructose sweetened · includes traditional food ingredients · fiber content: fruits and vegetables
	Egg Nog Novartis Nutrition	powder	1.2	62.3	154	37.5	various [b]	prepare with whole milk
GL LA	**Ensure** Ross Products/Abbott Labs	liquid	1.06	9/8fl oz	40/8fl oz	6/8fl oz	various [b,c,d]	4 cans = 100% USRDA
GL LA	**Ensure** Ross Products/Abbott Labs	pudding	250	6.8/5oz	34.0/5oz	9.7/5oz	various [b,c,d]	
GL LA	**Ensure** Ross Products/Abbott Labs	powder	1.06	8.8/8fl oz	34.3/8fl oz	8.8/8fl oz	various [b,c,d]	
GL LA	**Ensure High Protein** Ross Products/Abbott Labs	liquid	0.95	12/8fl oz	30.8fl oz	6/8fl oz	various [b,c,d]	
GL LA	**Ensure Light** Ross Products/Abbott Labs	liquid	0.84	10/8fl oz	33/8fl oz	3/8fl oz	various [b,c,d]	chocolate, strawberry, and vanilla flavors
GL LA	**Ensure Plus** Ross Products/Abbott Labs	liquid	1.5	13/8fl oz	47.3/8fl oz	12.6/8fl oz	various [b,c,d]	high calorie

See Chapter 19, "Nutritional Products," for more information about these products.

ENTERAL FOOD SUPPLEMENT PRODUCTS - continued

	Product Manufacturer/Supplier	Dosage Form	Calories (per mL)	Protein [a] (g)	Carbohy- drate [a] (g)	Fat [a] (g)	Vitamins & Minerals	Comments
GL LA	**Ensure Plus HN** Ross Products/Abbott Labs	liquid	1.5	14.8/8fl oz	47.3/8fl oz	11.8/8fl oz	various [b,c,d] · l-carnitine, 0.038g/8fl oz · taurine, 0.038g/8fl oz	high nitrogen · high calorie
GL LA	**Ensure with Fiber** Ross Products/Abbott Labs	liquid	1.06	8.8/8fl oz	43.8/8fl oz	6.1/8fl oz	various [b,c,d]	dietary fiber, 3.6oz/8fl oz
LA	**Fibersource** Novartis Nutrition	liquid	1.2	43	170	41	various [b,c,d]	contains fiber
LA	**Fibersource HN** Novartis Nutrition	liquid	1.2	53	160	41	various [b,c,d]	contains fiber
GL LA	**Forta Drink** Ross Products/Abbott Labs	powder	77/0.8oz mix	5/0.8oz mix	13/0.8oz mix	<1/0.8oz mix	various [b,c,d]	suitable for clear liquid diets
	Forta Shake Ross Products/Abbott Labs	powder	140/1.4oz mix	9/1.4oz mix	24/1.4oz mix	<1/1.4oz mix	various [b,c,d]	milk base
LA	**Gelatin Plus** Novartis Nutrition	powder	1.3	101.7	220	3.32		prepare with water
GL LA	**Glucerna** Ross Products/Abbott Labs	liquid	1	9.9/8fl oz	22.8/8fl oz	12.9/8fl oz	various [b,c,d] · l-carnitine · taurine · m-inositol	for patients with abnormal glucose tolerance · dietary fiber, 3.4g/8fl oz
	Health Shake (Frozen) Novartis Nutrition	liquid	1.58	51	271	34	various [b,c]	
	Health Shake, Aspartame Sweetened (Frozen) Novartis Nutrition	liquid	1.6	67.8	226	51	various [b,c]	soluble dietary fiber, 3g/6fl oz serving; 2g/4fl oz serving
GL LA SU	**Impact** Novartis Nutrition	liquid	1	56	130	28	various [b,c,d]	contains arginine, dietary nucleotides, and fish oil
GL LA SU	**Impact 1.5** Novartis Nutrition	liquid	1.5	80	140	69	various [b,c,d]	calorically dense · contains arginine, dietary nucleotides, and fish oil
GL LA SU	**Impact with Fiber** Novartis Nutrition	liquid	1	56	140	28	various [b,c,d]	contains RNA, arginine, and fish oil · fiber content: soy fiber and partially hydrolyzed guar gum

See Chapter 19, "Nutritional Products," for more information about these products.

ENTERAL FOOD SUPPLEMENT PRODUCTS - continued

	Product Manufacturer/Supplier	Dosage Form	Calories (per mL)	Protein [a] (g)	Carbohy-drate [a] (g)	Fat [a] (g)	Vitamins & Minerals	Comments
	Instant Breakfast Novartis Nutrition	liquid	1.06	51	140	34	various [b]	
	Instant Breakfast Novartis Nutrition	powder	1.2	63.5	156.8	38	various [b]	prepare with whole milk
CO DY GL LA SU	**Isocal** Mead Johnson Nutritionals	liquid	1.06	34	135	44	various [b,c]	volume to meet 100% USRDA is 1890ml
CO DY GL LA SU	**Isocal HN** Mead Johnson Nutritionals	liquid	1.06	44	124	45	various [b,c]	volume to meet 100% USRDA is 1180ml
LA	**IsoSource** Novartis Nutrition	liquid	1.2	43	170	41	various [b,c,d]	
GL LA	**IsoSource 1.5 Cal** Novartis Nutrition	liquid	1.5	68	170	65	various [b,c,d]	fiber content: soy fiber and partially hydrolyzed guar gum
LA	**IsoSource HN** Novartis Nutrition	liquid	1.2	53	160	41	various [b,c,d]	
GL LA SU	**IsoSource VHN** Novartis Nutrition	liquid	1	62	130	29	various [b,c,d]	fiber content: soy fiber and partially hydrolyzed guar gum
GL LA	**Isotein HN** Novartis Nutrition	powder	1.19	68	160	34	various [b,c,d]	
GL LA	**Jevity** Ross Products/Abbott Labs	liquid	1.06	10.5/8fl oz	36.4/8fl oz	8.2/8fl oz	various [b,c,d] · l-carnitine, 0.027g/8fl oz · taurine, 0.027g/8fl oz	high nitrogen · dietary fiber, 3.4g/8fl oz
CO DY GL LA	**Lipisorb** Mead Johnson Nutritionals	liquid	1.35	57	161	57	various [b,c]	volume to meet 100% USRDA is 1180ml
DY GL LA PU	**Lipisorb** Mead Johnson Nutritionals	powder	4.7/g	16.5/100g	54/100g	23/100g	various [b]	volume to meet 100% USRDA is 2000ml at 30cal/30ml or 1480ml at 40cal/30ml
**	**Lipomul** Lee Consumer	liquid	270/45ml			30/45ml		

See Chapter 19, "Nutritional Products," for more information about these products.

ENTERAL FOOD SUPPLEMENT PRODUCTS - continued

	Product Manufacturer/Supplier	Dosage Form	Calories (per mL)	Protein [a] (g)	Carbohy- drate [a] (g)	Fat [a] (g)	Vitamins & Minerals	Comments
** CO DY GL LA	**Magnacal Renal** Mead Johnson Nutritionals	liquid	2	75	200	101	various [b,c]	volume to meet 100% USRDA (except Vitamin D, phosphorus, and magnesium) is 1000ml
CO DY GL LA SO SU	**MCT Oil** Mead Johnson Nutritionals	oil	8.3/g			1/g		
GL	**Meritene** Novartis Nutrition	powder	1.06	69	120	34	various [b,c,d]	milk base · chocolate, milk chocolate, strawberry, and vanilla flavors; also plain-unflavored
** CO DY GL LA SO SU	**Microlipid** Mead Johnson Nutritionals	oil	4.5			510		
	Milk Shake Novartis Nutrition	powder	1.2	38	174	38	various [b]	prepare with whole milk
	Milk Shake Plus Novartis Nutrition	powder	1.2	63.5	157	38	various [b]	prepare with whole milk
CO DY GL LA PU SU	**Moducal** Mead Johnson Nutritionals	powder	3.8/g		0.95/g			maltodextrin
GL LA	**Nepro** Ross Products/Abbott Labs	liquid	2	16.6/8fl oz	51.1/8fl oz	22.7/8fl oz	various [b,c,d] · l-carnitine, 0.062g/8fl oz · taurine, 0.038g/8fl oz	for dialyzed patients with renal failure
** CO GL LA	**NuBasics** Nestlé Clinical Nutrition	liquid	1	8.75/250ml	33.1/250ml	9.2/250ml	various [b,c,d]	chocolate, strawberry, and vanilla flavors
** CO GL LA	**NuBasics Plus** Nestlé Clinical Nutrition	liquid	1.5	13.1/250ml	44.1/250ml	16.2/250ml	various [b,c,d]	high calorie · chocolate, strawberry, and vanilla flavors
** CO GL LA	**NuBasics VHP** Nestlé Clinical Nutrition	liquid	1	15.6/250ml	28.2/250ml	8.3/250ml	various [b,c,d]	high protein · vanilla flavor

See Chapter 19, "Nutritional Products," for more information about these products.

ENTERAL FOOD SUPPLEMENT PRODUCTS - continued

	Product Manufacturer/Supplier	Dosage Form	Calories (per mL)	Protein [a] (g)	Carbohy- drate [a] (g)	Fat [a] (g)	Vitamins & Minerals	Comments
** CO GL LA	**NuBasics with Fiber** Nestlé Clinical Nutrition	liquid	1	8.75/250ml	33.1/250ml	9.2/250ml	various [b,c,d]	dietary fiber, 3.5g/250ml · vanilla flavor
	Nutra Start Slim Fast Foods	liquid	0.89	10/8fl oz	40/8fl oz	2.5/8fl oz	various [b,c,d]	chocolate and vanilla flavors
** GL LA	**Nutren 1.0 Complete** Nestlé Clinical Nutrition	liquid	1	40	127	38	various [b,c,d] · carnitine · taurine	volume to meet 100% USRDA is 1500ml
** GL LA	**Nutren 1.0 with Fiber Complete** Nestlé Clinical Nutrition	liquid	1	40	127	38	various [b,c,d] · carnitine · taurine	dietary fiber, 14g/L · volume to meet 100% USRDA is 1500ml
** GL LA	**Nutren 1.5 Complete** Nestlé Clinical Nutrition	liquid	1.5	60	169.2	67.6	various [b,c,d] · carnitine · taurine	high calorie · volume to meet 100% USRDA is 1000ml
** GL LA	**Nutren 2.0 Complete** Nestlé Clinical Nutrition	liquid	2	80	196	106	various [b,c,d] · carnitine · taurine	calorically dense · volume to meet 100% USRDA is 750ml
	Nutritious Pudding Novartis Nutrition	powder	1.7	61	236.5	54	various [b]	prepare with whole milk
	Nutritious Pudding (Frozen) Novartis Nutrition	pudding	1.7	61	236	54	various [b]	
GL LA	**Osmolite** Ross Products/Abbott Labs	liquid	1.06	8.8/8fl oz	35.6/8fl oz	8.2/8fl oz	various [b,c,d] · l-carnitine, 0.019g/8fl oz · taurine, 0.019g/8fl oz	isotonic
GL LA	**Osmolite HN** Ross Products/Abbott Labs	liquid	1.06	10.5/8fl oz	33.9/8fl oz	8.2/8fl oz	various [b,c,d] · l-carnitine, 0.027g/8fl oz · taurine, 0.027g/8fl oz	high nitrogen · isotonic
** GL LA	**Peptamen Complete** Nestlé Clinical Nutrition	liquid	1	40	127	39	various [b,c,d] · carnitine · taurine	isotonic elemental peptide-based diet · volume to meet 100% USRDA is 1500ml

See Chapter 19, "Nutritional Products," for more information about these products.

ENTERAL FOOD SUPPLEMENT PRODUCTS - continued

	Product Manufacturer/Supplier	Dosage Form	Calories (per mL)	Protein [a] (g)	Carbohy-drate [a] (g)	Fat [a] (g)	Vitamins & Minerals	Comments
** GL LA PE	**Peptamen Junior Complete** Nestlé Clinical Nutrition	liquid	1	30	137.5	38.5	various [b,c,d] · carnitine · taurine	for children 1-10 years of age · elemental peptide-based diet · volume to meet 100% NAS-NRC RDA is 1000ml
** GL LA	**Peptamen VHP Complete** Nestlé Clinical Nutrition	liquid	1	62.5	104.5	39	various [b,c,d]	very high protein · elemental peptide-based diet · volume to meet 100% USRDA is 1500ml
GL LA	**Perative** Ross Products/Abbott Labs	liquid	1.3	15.8/8fl oz	42.0/8fl oz	8.8/8fl oz	various [b,c,d] · l-carnitine, 0.031g/8fl oz · taurine, 0.031g/8fl oz	for management of metabolically stressed patients · 1500 calories = 100% USRDA
GL LA	**Polycose** Ross Products/Abbott Labs	liquid	2		500			glucose polymers to supply carbohydrate calories
GL LA	**Polycose** Ross Products/Abbott Labs	powder	380/100g		940			glucose polymers to supply carbohydrate calories
	Pro Mod Ross Products/Abbott Labs	powder	28/6.6g (scoop)	5/6.6g (scoop)	0.67/6.6g (scoop)	0.6/6.6g (scoop)		protein supplement
** GL LA GE	**ProBalance Complete** Nestlé Clinical Nutrition	liquid	1.2	54	156	40.6	various [b,c,d] · carnitine · taurine	geriatric care · dietary fiber, 10g/L · volume to meet 100% USRDA is 1000ml
GL LA	**Promote** Ross Products/Abbott Labs	liquid	1	14.8/8fl oz	30.8/8fl oz	6.2/8fl oz	various [b,c,d] · l-carnitine, 0.036g/8fl oz · taurine, 0.036g/8fl oz	high protein
** CO DY GL LA	**Protain XL** Mead Johnson Nutritionals	liquid	1	57	129	30	various [b,c]	volume to meet 100% USRDA is 1250ml
GL LA	**Pulmocare** Ross Products/Abbott Labs	liquid	1.5	14.8/8fl oz	25/8fl oz	22.1/8fl oz	various [b,c,d] · l-carnitine, 0.036g/8fl oz · taurine, 0.036g/8fl oz	for pulmonary patients

See Chapter 19, "Nutritional Products," for more information about these products.

ENTERAL FOOD SUPPLEMENT PRODUCTS - continued

	Product Manufacturer/Supplier	Dosage Form	Calories (per mL)	Protein [a] (g)	Carbohy- drate [a] (g)	Fat [a] (g)	Vitamins & Minerals	Comments
** GL LA	**Renalcal Diet** Nestlé Clinical Nutrition	liquid	2	34.4	290.4	82.4	various [b,c,d] · carnitine · taurine	for patients with renal failure · includes arginine and histidine · elemental peptide-based diet · volume to meet 100% USRDA is 1000ml
** GL LA	**Replete Complete** Nestlé Clinical Nutrition	liquid	1	62.5	113	34	various [b,c,d]	high protein · volume to meet 100% USRDA is 1000ml
** GL LA	**Replete with Fiber Complete** Nestlé Clinical Nutrition	liquid	1	62.5	113	34	various [b,c,d]	high protein · dietary fiber, 14g/L · volume to meet 100% USRDA is 1000ml
CO LA	**ReSource** Novartis Nutrition	liquid	1.06	37	152	25	various [b,c,d]	chocolate, strawberry, and vanilla flavors
**	**ReSource Bar** Novartis Nutrition	bar	170/1.66oz bar	11.1/1.66oz bar	23/1.66oz bar	5/1.66oz bar	various [b,c,d]	chocolate-coconut and chocolate-peanut flavors
CO GL LA	**ReSource Crystals** Novartis Nutrition	powder	1.06	37	140	37	various [b,c,d]	vanilla flavor
GL LA SU	**ReSource Diabetic** Novartis Nutrition	liquid	1.06	63	99	47	various [b,c,d]	1.0L and 1.5L closed system container for tube feeding
CO LA	**ReSource Fruit Beverage** Novartis Nutrition	liquid	0.76	37	150	0	various [b,c,d]	orange, peach, wild berry, and lemon iced tea flavors
GL LA PE	**ReSource Just for Kids** Novartis Nutrition	liquid	1	30	110	50	various [b,c,d]	renal solute load: 190mOsm/1000ml · chocolate, strawberry, and vanilla flavors
	ReSource Nutritious Juice Drink (Frozen) Novartis Nutrition	liquid	1.07	33.9	231	1	various [b,c]	
CO LA	**ReSource Plus** Novartis Nutrition	liquid	1.5	55	220	46	various [b,c,d]	chocolate, strawberry, and vanilla flavors
	ReSource Shake Novartis Nutrition	liquid	1.5	51	254	33.9	various [b]	<1g of lactose/serving

See Chapter 19, "Nutritional Products," for more information about these products.

ENTERAL FOOD SUPPLEMENT PRODUCTS - continued

	Product Manufacturer/Supplier	Dosage Form	Calories (per mL)	Protein [a] (g)	Carbohy- drate [a] (g)	Fat [a] (g)	Vitamins & Minerals	Comments
	ReSource Shake Plus (Frozen) Novartis Nutrition	liquid	1.7	63.6	246	51	various [b]	
	ReSource Shake Thickened (Frozen) Novartis Nutrition	liquid	1.5	51	254	34	various [b]	
** GL LA	**ReSource Yogurt Flavored Beverage** Novartis Nutrition	liquid	1.06	37	186	18	various [b,c,d]	peach flavor
DY GL LA	**Respalor** Mead Johnson Nutritionals	liquid	1.52	76	148	71	various [b,c]	volume to meet 100% USRDA is 1420ml
GL LA SU	**SandoSource Peptide** Novartis Nutrition	liquid	1	50	160	17	various [b,c,d]	semi-elemental peptide-based diet with supplemental arginine
** CO GL PU	**Scandishake** Scandipharm	individual packet	1.85	8.23/100g	68/100g	25/100g	various [c]	for weight maintenance or weight gain · prepare with whole milk
** CO GL PU	**Scandishake (Sweetened with Aspartame)** Scandipharm	individual packet	1.85	8.23/100g	68/100g	25/100g	various [c]	for weight maintenance or weight gain · prepare with whole milk
CO LA PU	**Scandishake Lactose Free** Scandipharm	individual packet	1.6	8/100g	65/100g	25/100g	calcium	high calorie · for weight maintenance or weight gain · prepare with low lactose milk, or juice, or water
GL LA	**Suplena** Ross Products/Abbott Labs	liquid	2	7.1/8fl oz	60.6/8fl oz	22.7/8fl oz	various [b,c,d] · l-carnitine, 0.038g/8fl oz · taurine, 0.038g/8fl oz	for dietary management of renal patients prone to uremia · 1900 calories = 100% USRDA
DY GL PU	**Sustacal** Mead Johnson Nutritionals	powder	1.09	79	180	2.6	various [b]	mix with skim milk · vanilla flavor · volume to meet 100% USRDA is 840ml
GL PU	**Sustacal** Mead Johnson Nutritionals	pudding	1.67/g	6.8/5oz	32/5oz	9.5/5oz	various [b]	milk base · butterscotch, chocolate, and vanilla flavors

See Chapter 19, "Nutritional Products," for more information about these products.

ENTERAL FOOD SUPPLEMENT PRODUCTS - continued

	Product Manufacturer/Supplier	Dosage Form	Calories (per mL)	Protein [a] (g)	Carbohy- drate [a] (g)	Fat [a] (g)	Vitamins & Minerals	Comments
GL LA	**Sustacal** Mead Johnson Nutritionals	liquid	1.01	61	139	23	various [b]	chocolate, egg nog, strawberry, and vanilla flavors · volume to meet 100% USRDA is 1060ml
CO GL LA	**Sustacal Basic** Mead Johnson Nutritionals	liquid	1.06	38	146	38	various [b,c]	chocolate, strawberry, and vanilla flavors · volume to meet 100% USRDA is 1890ml
CO GL LA PU	**Sustacal Plus** Mead Johnson Nutritionals	liquid	1.52	61	190	57	various [b,c]	chocolate, egg nog, strawberry, and vanilla flavors · volume to meet 100% USRDA is 1180ml
CO GL LA	**Sustacal with Fiber** Mead Johnson Nutritionals	liquid	1.06	46	139	35	various [b]	chocolate, strawberry, and vanilla flavors · volume to meet 100% USRDA is 1420ml
CO GL LA	**Tolerex** Novartis Nutrition	powder	1	21	230	1.5	various [b,c,d]	elemental diet · contains 100% free amino acids
DY GL LA PU	**TraumaCal** Mead Johnson Nutritionals	liquid	1.5	82	142	68	various [b,c]	vanilla flavor · volume to meet 100% USRDA is 2000ml
** GL LA	**Travasorb HN** Nestlé Clinical Nutrition	powder	1	45	175	13.5	various [b,c,d]	high nitrogen · high protein · elemental peptide-based diet · prepare with water · volume to meet 100% USRDA is 2000ml
** GL LA	**Travasorb MCT** Nestlé Clinical Nutrition	powder	1	49.6	122.8	33	various [b,c,d]	high protein · prepare with water · volume to meet 100% USRDA is 2000ml
** GL LA	**Travasorb STD** Nestlé Clinical Nutrition	powder	1	30	190	13.5	various [b,c,d]	elemental peptide-based diet · prepare with water · volume to meet 100% USRDA is 2000ml
GL LA	**Two Cal HN** Ross Products/Abbott Labs	liquid	2	19.8/8fl oz	51.4/8fl oz	21.5/8fl oz	various [b,c,d]	high calorie · high nitrogen

See Chapter 19, "Nutritional Products," for more information about these products.

ENTERAL FOOD SUPPLEMENT PRODUCTS - continued

	Product Manufacturer/Supplier	Dosage Form	Calories (per mL)	Protein [a] (g)	Carbohy- drate [a] (g)	Fat [a] (g)	Vitamins & Minerals	Comments
CO DY LA PU	**Ultracal** Mead Johnson Nutritionals	liquid	1.06	44	123	45	various [b,c]	vanilla flavor · volume to meet 100% USRDA is 1180ml
GL LA	**Vital High Nitrogen** Ross Products/Abbott Labs	individual packet	1	12.5/packet	55.4/packet	3.25/packet	various [b,c,d]	for patients with limited digestion, absorption · 300 calories/packet
CO GL LA SU PE	**Vivonex Pediatric** Novartis Nutrition	powder	0.8	24	130	24	various [b,c,d]	100% elemental diet for children ages 1-10 · contains 100% free amino acids and free glutamine
CO GL SU	**Vivonex Plus** Novartis Nutrition	powder	1	45	190	6.7	various [b,c,d]	100% elemental high nitrogen diet · contains 100% free amino acids and free glutamine
CO GL LA SU	**Vivonex T.E.N.** Novartis Nutrition	powder	1	38	210	2.8	various [b,c,d]	elemental diet · contains 100% free amino acids and free glutamine

** New listing

[a] Unless otherwise specified, content given in grams per liter. Powder products must be added to liquid according to package directions.

[b] Includes vitamins A, D, E, ascorbic acid, thiamine, riboflavin, niacin, pyridoxine HCl, cyanocobalamin, and/or various other substances having vitamin activity

[c] Includes iron, calcium, phosophorus, iodine, magnesium, copper, zinc, potassium, sodium, manganese, chromium, selenium, and/or molybdenum

[d] Includes choline, biotin, inositol, and/or folic acid

See Chapter 19, "Nutritional Products," for more information about these products.

This page intentionally left blank.

Infant Formula Product Table

INFANTS' AND CHILDREN'S FORMULA PRODUCTS

	Product Manufacturer/Supplier	Dosage Form	Kcal (per oz) [b]	Protein Type	Protein (g/L)	Carbo- hydrate Type	Carbo- hydrate (g/L)	Fat Type
	NATURAL MILKS							
	Cow Milk, Whole Cows	liquid	20	casein, 80% · whey, 20%	31	lactose	49	cow milk fat
	Human Breast Milk, Mature Mother	liquid	21	casein, 40% · whey, 60%	9	lactose	68	human milk fat
	MILK-BASED FORMULAS							
PE	**Carnation Follow-Up** Carnation Nutritional	concentrate · powder · ready-to- feed	20	nonfat milk	18	lactose · corn syrup	89.2	palm olein · soy oil · coconut oil · high- oleic safflower oil
DY GL PU SU PE	**Enfamil** Mead Johnson Nutritionals	concentrate · powder · ready-to- feed	20	nonfat milk, whey- predominant	14.5	lactose	73	palm olein · soy oil · coconut oil · high- oleic sunflower oil
GL PU SU PE	**Enfamil Next Step** Mead Johnson Nutritionals	concentrate · powder · ready-to- feed	20	nonfat milk	17.6	corn syrup solids · lactose	75	palm olein · soy oil · coconut oil · high oleic sunflower oil
DY GL PU SU PE	**Enfamil with Iron** Mead Johnson Nutritionals	concentrate · powder · ready-to- feed	20	nonfat milk, whey- predominant	14.5	lactose	73	palm olein · soy oil · coconut oil · high- oleic sunflower oil
DY GL PU SU PE	**Gerber Baby Formula Low Iron** Gerber Products	powder	20	nonfat milk, casein- predominant	14.3	lactose	74	palm olein · soy oil · coconut oil · high- oleic sunflower oil
DY GL PU SU PE	**Gerber Baby Formula with Iron** Gerber Products	concentrate · powder	20	nonfat milk, casein- predominant	14.3	lactose	74	palm olein · soy oil · coconut oil · high- oleic sunflower oil
DY GL LA PU PE	**Kindercal** Mead Johnson Nutritionals	ready-to-feed	31.3	calcium caseinate · sodium caseinate · milk protein concentrate	34	maltodextrin · sucrose	135	canola oil · MCT oil · high oleic sunflower oil
DY GL LA PU SU PE	**Lactofree** Mead Johnson Nutritionals	concentrate · powder · ready-to- feed	20	milk protein isolate, casein- predominant	14.3	corn syrup solids	74	palm olein · soy oil · coconut oil · high- oleic sunflower oil
PE	**Similac** Ross Products/Abbott Labs	concentrate · powder · ready-to- feed	20	nonfat milk, casein- predominant	14.5	lactose	72.3	soy oil · coconut oil

See Chapter 20, "Infant Formula Products," for more information about these products.

Fat (g/L)	Sodium (mEq/L)	Potassium (mEq/L)	Calcium (mg/L)	Phosphorus (mg/L)	Ca:P Ratio	Iron (mg/L)	Osmolality (mOsm/kg)	Renal Solute Load (mOsm/L)	Comments [c]
38	21	39	1200	920	1.3:1	0.5	288	308	
40	7	13	340	150	2.3:1	0.5	300	93	
27.7	11.5	23.4	912.6	609	1.5:1	13	326	122	for babies 4-12 months and older eating cereal and other baby foods
36	8	18.7	530	360	1.47:1	4.7	300	132	
34	12.2	23	810	570	1.43:1	12.2	270	168	alternative to cow milk for toddlers
36	8	18.7	530	360	1.47:1	12.2	300	132	
36	8.7	18.7	530	360	1.47:1	4.7	320	132	
36	8.7	18.7	530	360	1.47:1	12.2	320	132	
44	16.1	34	850	850	1:1	10.6	310	290	volume to meet 100% USRDA for 1-10 yr. olds is 950ml (1.06 kcal/ml)
36	8.7	18.9	550	370	1.49:1	12.2	200	132	
36.5	8	18.1	493	380	1.3:1	1.5	300	96.3	

INFANTS' AND CHILDREN'S FORMULA PRODUCTS - continued

	Product Manufacturer/Supplier	Dosage Form	Kcal (per oz) [b]	Protein Type	Protein (g/L)	Carbo- hydrate Type	Carbo- hydrate (g/L)	Fat Type
PE	**Similac Toddler's Best; Berry, Chocolate, or Vanilla** Ross Products/Abbott Labs	ready-to-feed	20	nonfat milk, casein- predominant	23.3	sucrose · lactose	73.4	high-oleic safflower oil · coconut oil · soy oil
PE	**Similac with Iron** Ross Products/Abbott Labs	concentrate · powder · ready-to- feed	20	nonfat milk, casein- predominant	14.5	lactose	72.3	soy oil · coconut oil
	SOY-BASED THERAPEUTIC FORMULAS							
PE	**Carnation Alsoy** Carnation Nutritional	concentrate · powder · ready-to- feed	20	soy protein isolate	19	corn maltodextrin · sucrose	75	palm olein · soy oil · coconut oil · high oleic safflower oil
PE	**Carnation Follow-Up Soy** Carnation Nutritional	powder	20	soy protein isolate	21	corn maltodextrin · sucrose	81	palm olein · soy oil · coconut oil · high oleic safflower oil
DY GL LA PE	**Enfamil Next Step Soy** Mead Johnson Nutritionals	concentrate	20	soy protein isolate · L- methionine	20	corn syrup · sucrose	68	palm olein · soy oil · coconut oil · high- oleic sunflower oil
GL LA PE	**Enfamil Next Step Soy** Mead Johnson Nutritionals	powder	20	soy protein isolate · L- methionine	22	corn syrup solids · sucrose	80	palm olein · soy oil · coconut oil · high- oleic sunflower oil
DY GL PE	**Gerber Soy Baby Formula** Gerber Products	concentrate · powder	20	soy protein isolate	20	corn syrup · sucrose	68	palm olein · soy oil · coconut oil · high- oleic sunflower oil
LA PE	**Isomil** Ross Products/Abbott Labs	concentrate · powder · ready-to- feed	20	soy protein isolate · L- methionine	18	corn syrup · sucrose	68.3	soy oil · coconut oil
LA PE	**Isomil DF** Ross Products/Abbott Labs	ready-to-feed	20	soy protein isolate · L- methionine	18	corn syrup solids · sucrose · soy fiber	68.3	soy oil · coconut oil
LA PE	**Isomil SF** Ross Products/Abbott Labs	concentrate	20	soy protein isolate · L- methionine	18	glucose polymers	68.3	soy oil · coconut oil
DY GL LA SU PE	**ProSobee** Mead Johnson Nutritionals	concentrate · powder · ready-to- feed	20	soy protein isolate · L- methionine	17.3	corn syrup solids	73	palm olein · soy oil · coconut oil · high- oleic sunflower oil

See Chapter 20, "Infant Formula Products," for more information about these products.

Fat (g/L)	Sodium (mEq/L)	Potassium (mEq/L)	Calcium (mg/L)	Phosphorus (mg/L)	Ca:P Ratio	Iron (mg/L)	Osmolality (mOsm/kg)	Renal Solute Load (mOsm/L)	Comments [c]
31.3	12.6	25.6 (Berry, Vanilla); 38.7 (Chocolate)	1040	747	1.4:1	12	[d]	175	for toddlers over 12 months
36.5	8	18.1	493	380	1.3:1	12	300	96.3	
33.5	9.7	20.1	710	412	1.72:1	12.17	270	118	for milk-free feeding during baby's first year
30	12.3	20.4	912.6	608.4	1.5:1	12.17	270	130	for babies 4-12 months and older eating cereal and other baby foods, and who require milk-free or lactose-free feeding
36	10.4	21	710	560	1.27:1	12.2	230	179	alternative to cow milk for toddlers
30	13	26	780	610	1.28:1	12.2	260	200	alternative to cow milk for toddlers
36	10.4	21	710	560	1.27:1	12.2	230	179	
36.9	13	18.7	710	510	1.4:1	12	280	115.6	
36.9	13	18.7	710	510	1.4:1	12	240	115.3	for dietary management of diarrhea in infants and toddlers · total dietary fiber, 6g/L
36.9	13	18.7	710	510	1.4:1	12	180	115.6	
37	10.4	21	710	560	1.27:1	12.2	200	179	

INFANTS' AND CHILDREN'S FORMULA PRODUCTS - continued

	Product Manufacturer/Supplier	Dosage Form	Kcal (per oz) [b]	Protein Type	Protein (g/L)	Carbo- hydrate Type	Carbo- hydrate (g/L)	Fat Type
LA PE	**RCF (Ross Carbohydrate Free)** Ross Products/Abbott Labs	concentrate	12 (diluted 1:1 with water, no carbohydrates added)	soy protein isolate · L-methionine	20	selected by physician	0.04	soy oil · coconut oil

OTHER THERAPEUTIC FORMULAS

	Product Manufacturer/Supplier	Dosage Form	Kcal (per oz) [b]	Protein Type	Protein (g/L)	Carbo- hydrate Type	Carbo- hydrate (g/L)	Fat Type
PE	**Carnation Good Start** Carnation Nutritional	concentrate · powder · ready-to-feed	20	enzymatically hydrolyzed reduced minerals whey	16	lactose · maltodextrin	74.4	palm olein · soy oil · coconut oil · high-oleic safflower oil
DY GL LA PU SU PE	**Lofenalac** Mead Johnson Nutritionals	powder	20	casein hydrolysate with L-tyrosine, L-tryptophan, L-histidine HCl, L-methionine (see comments)	22	corn syrup solids · modified tapioca starch	88	corn oil
DY GL LA PU SU PE	**Nutramigen** Mead Johnson Nutritionals	concentrate · powder · ready-to-feed	20	casein hydrolysate supplemented with L-cystine, L-tyrosine, and L-tryptophan	19	corn syrup solids · modified corn starch	74	palm olein · soy oil · coconut oil · high oleic sunflower oil
DY GL LA PU PE	**Portagen** Mead Johnson Nutritionals	powder	20	sodium caseinate	24	corn syrup solids · sucrose	78	medium chain triglyceride oil · corn oil
DY GL LA PU SU PE	**Pregestimil** Mead Johnson Nutritionals	nursette bottle · ready-to-feed	24	casein hydrolysate supplemented with L-cystine, L-tyrosine, and L-tryptophan	23	corn syrup solids · modified corn starch	83	medium chain triglycerides · soy oil · high-oleic safflower oil

See Chapter 20, "Infant Formula Products," for more information about these products.

Fat (g/L)	Sodium (mEq/L)	Potassium (mEq/L)	Calcium (mg/L)	Phosphorus (mg/L)	Ca:P Ratio	Iron (mg/L)	Osmolality (mOsm/kg)	Renal Solute Load (mOsm/L)	Comments [c]
36	13	18.7	700	500	1.4:1	1.5	74	123.6	carbohydrate-free base · carbohydrate must be added before feeding
34.5	7	17	433	243	1.8:1	10	265	99.3	hydrolyzed whey formula intended for routine feeding of healthy full-term infants
26	13.9	17.6	640	470	1.34:1	12.7	360	186	protein is incomplete; it contains inadequate levels of phenylalanine needed for normal growth
34	13.9	18.9	640	430	1.49:1	12.2	320	172	for protein sensitivity, food allergies, and severe diarrhea
32	16.1	22	640	470	1.34:1	12.7	230	200	for malabsorption problems and pancreatic insufficiency · higher amounts of vitamins added · infants with cholestatic disease may require supplementation of linoleic acid if Portagen is used as the sole or major food
45	16.5	23	930	610	1.53:1	15.2	320	210	for fat malabsorption, severe diarrhea, GI immaturity, and protein intolerance

INFANTS' AND CHILDREN'S FORMULA PRODUCTS - continued

	Product Manufacturer/Supplier	Dosage Form	Kcal (per oz) [b]	Protein Type	Protein (g/L)	Carbo-hydrate Type	Carbo-hydrate (g/L)	Fat Type
DY GL LA PU SU PE	**Pregestimil** Mead Johnson Nutritionals	nursette bottle · ready-to-feed	20	casein hydrolysate supplemented with L-cystine, L-tyrosine, and L-tryptophan	19	corn syrup solids · modified corn starch	69	medium chain triglycerides · soy oil · high-oleic safflower oil
DY GL LA PU SU PE	**Pregestimil** Mead Johnson Nutritionals	powder	20	casein hydrolysate supplemented with L-cystine, L-tyrosine, and L-tryptophan	19	corn syrup solids · modified corn starch · dextrose	69	medium chain triglycerides · corn oil · soy oil · high-oleic safflower oil
PE	**Similac PM 60/40** Ross Products/Abbott Labs	powder	20	whey protein · sodium caseinate	15.8	lactose	69	soy oil · coconut oil
	FORMULAS FOR PREMATURE INFANTS							
DY GL PU SU PE	**Enfamil Premature Formula** Mead Johnson Nutritionals	nursette bottle · ready-to-feed	20	nonfat milk, whey-predominant	20	corn syrup solids · lactose	75	medium chain triglycerides · soy oil · coconut oil
DY GL PU SU PE	**Enfamil Premature Formula** Mead Johnson Nutritionals	nursette bottle · ready-to-feed	24	nonfat milk, whey-predominant	24	corn syrup solids · lactose	90	medium chain triglycerides · soy oil · coconut oil
DY GL PU SU PE	**Enfamil Premature Formula with Iron** Mead Johnson Nutritionals	nursette bottle · ready-to-feed	20	nonfat milk, whey-predominant	20	corn syrup solids · lactose	75	medium chain triglycerides · soy oil · coconut oil
DY GL PU SU PE	**Enfamil Premature Formula with Iron** Mead Johnson Nutritionals	nursette bottle · ready-to-feed	24	nonfat milk, whey-predominant	24	corn syrup solids · lactose	90	medium chain triglycerides · soy oil · coconut oil
PE	**Similac Special Care 24 with Iron** Ross Products/Abbott Labs	ready-to-feed	24	nonfat milk, whey-predominant	22	lactose · glucose polymer	86.1	medium chain triglycerides · soy oil · coconut oil
	MISCELLANEOUS PRODUCTS							
DY GL PU SU PE	**Enfamil Human Milk Fortifier** Mead Johnson Nutritionals	powder	14	whey protein · sodium caseinate	0.7	corn syrup solids · lactose	2.7	

See Chapter 20, "Infant Formula Products," for more information about these products.

Fat (g/L)	Sodium (mEq/L)	Potassium (mEq/L)	Calcium (mg/L)	Phosphorus (mg/L)	Ca:P Ratio	Iron (mg/L)	Osmolality (mOsm/kg)	Renal Solute Load (mOsm/L)	Comments [c]
38	13.9	18.9	780	510	1.53:1	12.7	280	174	for fat malabsorption, severe diarrhea, GI immaturity, and protein intolerance
38	11.3	18.9	640	430	1.49:1	12.7	320	169	for fat malabsorption, severe diarrhea, GI immaturity, and protein intolerance
37.6	7	14.8	380	190	2:1	1.5	280	96.3	low in sodium, potassium, and minerals
35	11.3	17.9	1120	560	2:1	1.7	260	175	
41	13.9	21	1340	670	2:1	2	310	210	
35	11.3	17.9	1120	560	2:1	12.2	260	175	
41	13.9	21	1340	670	2:1	14.6	310	210	
44.1	15.2	26.9	1460	730	2:1	15	280	148.7	
<0.1	0.3	0.4	90	45	2:1		120		values are listed for 4 packets of fortifier only, before mixing with breast milk · adequate nutrients only when added to breast milk

INFANTS' AND CHILDREN'S FORMULA PRODUCTS - continued

	Product Manufacturer/Supplier	Dosage Form	Kcal (per oz) [b]	Protein Type	Protein (g/L)	Carbo-hydrate Type	Carbo-hydrate (g/L)	Fat Type
DY GL LA PU SU PE	**MSUD Diet** Mead Johnson Nutritionals	powder	20	amino acids (see comments)	11.5	corn syrup solids · modified tapioca starch	91	corn oil
PE	**PediaSure** Ross Products/Abbott Labs	ready-to-feed	30	low lactose whey protein · sodium caseinate	30	hydrolyzed corn starch · sucrose	110	high-oleic safflower and soy oils · medium chain triglycerides
GL PE	**PediaSure with Fiber** Ross Products/Abbott Labs	ready-to-feed	30	low lactose whey protein · sodium caseinate	30	hydrolyzed corn starch · sucrose · soy fiber	114	high-oleic safflower and soy oils · medium chain triglycerides
DY GL LA PU PE	**Phenyl-Free** Mead Johnson Nutritionals	powder	25	amino acids (see comments)	42	sucrose · corn syrup solids · modified tapioca starch	137	corn oil · coconut oil

[a] Refer to the text of Chapter 13, "Antidiarrheal Products," for information about fluid and electrolyte replacement products.
[b] Unless otherwise noted, calorie content and other nutritional information pertain to ready-to-feed formula.
[c] Formulas contain appropriate range of vitamins, minerals, and trace elements unless noted otherwise in "Comments" section.
[d] Osmolality not determined by manufacturer/supplier.

See Chapter 20, "Infant Formula Products," for more information about these products.

Fat (g/L)	Sodium (mEq/L)	Potassium (mEq/L)	Calcium (mg/L)	Phosphorus (mg/L)	Ca:P Ratio	Iron (mg/L)	Osmolality (mOsm/kg)	Renal Solute Load (mOsm/L)	Comments [c]
28	11.3	17.9	700	380	1.84:1	12.7	330	122	protein is incomplete; it contains inadequate levels of leucine, isoleucine, and valine needed for normal growth
50	16.5	33.5	970	800	1.2:1	14	310	198.5	liquid nutrition for children 1-6 years of age · tube or oral feeding
50	16.5	33.5	970	800	1.2:1	14	345	198.5	liquid nutrition for children 1-6 years of age · tube or oral feeding · total dietary fiber, 1.2g/8fl oz
14.2	37	74	1690	1690	1:1	25	790	460	not recommended for use with infants · protein is incomplete; it contains no phenylalanine

Weight Control Product Table

APPETITE SUPPRESSANT PRODUCTS

	Product Manufacturer/Supplier	Dosage Form	Phenylpropa- nolamine HCl	Other Ingredients
GL PU SO	**Acutrim 16 Hour Steady Control** Novartis Consumer	timed-release tablet	75mg	cellulose acetate · hydroxypropyl methylcellulose · stearic acid
GL PU SO	**Acutrim Late Day Strength** Novartis Consumer	timed-release tablet	75mg	cellulose acetate · FD&C yellow#6 · hydroxypropyl methylcellulose · isopropyl alcohol · propylene glycol · riboflavin · stearic acid · titanium dioxide
GL PU SO	**Acutrim Maximum Strength** Novartis Consumer	timed-release tablet	75mg	cellulose acetate · D&C yellow#10 · FD&C blue#1 · FD&C yellow#6 · hydroxypropyl methylcellulose · povidone · propylene glycol · stearic acid · titanium dioxide
GL PU SO	**Amfed T.D.** Legere Ph'cals	capsule	75mg	
GL PU SO	**Dexatrim Caffeine Free Extended Duration** Thompson Medical	timed-release tablet	75mg	calcium sulfate · D&C yellow#10 aluminum lake · ethylcellulose · FD&C yellow#6 aluminum lake · hydroxypropyl methylcellulose · iron oxide · magnesium stearate · propylene glycol · povidone · stearic acid · titanium dioxide · triacetin · carnauba wax
GL PU SO	**Dexatrim Caffeine Free Maximum Strength** Thompson Medical	timed-release caplet	75mg	stearic acid · magnesium stearate · D&C yellow#10 aluminum lake · FD&C yellow#6 aluminum lake · hydroxypropyl methylcellulose · iron oxide · polyethylene glycol · titanium dioxide · carnauba wax · microcrystalline cellulose · polysorbate 80 · povidone · silicon dioxide
	Dexatrim Caffeine Free Plus Vitamins Thompson Medical	caplet · timed-release caplet	timed-release caplet, 75mg	caplet: vitamins A, D, E, C, B6, B2, B1, B12 · dibasic calcium phosphate · magnesium oxide · niacinamide · ferrous fumarate · zinc · calcium pantothenate · copper · folic acid · potassium iodide timed-release caplet: ascorbic acid, 180mg · croscarmellose sodium · ethylcellulose · FD&C red#40 aluminum lake · FD&C yellow#6 aluminum lake · hydroxypropyl methylcellulose · magnesium stearate · polyethylene glycol · polysorbate 80 · stearic acid · titanium dioxide · may also contain: calcium sulfate dihydrate · carnauba wax · FD&C blue#1 aluminum lake · lactose · microcrystalline cellulose · povidone · silicon dioxide
GL PU SO	**Dexatrim Caffeine Free with Vitamin C** Thompson Medical	timed-release caplet	75mg	ascorbic acid, 180mg · FD&C blue#1 aluminum lake · FD&C red#40 aluminum lake · FD&C yellow#6 aluminum lake · hydroxypropyl methylcellulose · magnesium stearate · microcrystalline cellulose · povidone · stearic acid · silicon dioxide · carnauba wax
GL PU SO	**Dieutrim T.D.** Legere Ph'cals	capsule	75mg	benzocaine, 9mg
	Mini Slims BDI Ph'cals	timed-release capsule	75mg	
**	**Mini Thin Diet Aid** BDI Ph'cals	timed-release capsule	75mg	

See Chapter 21, "Weight Control Products," for more information about these products.

APPETITE SUPPRESSANT PRODUCTS - continued

Product Manufacturer/Supplier	Dosage Form	Phenylpropa-nolamine HCl	Other Ingredients
Permathene Maximum Strength Chromium Picolinate § CCA Industries	softgel	75mg	chromium, 200mcg (as picolinate) · beeswax · gelatin · glycerin · lecithin · soybean oil · vegetable oil · water · zinc oxide
Permathene with Calcium § CCA Industries	tablet	25mg	calcium · croscarmellose · lactose ANH · magnesium stearate · microcrystalline cellulose · stearic acid
Permathene-12 § CCA Industries	timed-release caplet	75mg	dicalcium phosphate · FD&C red#40 · FD&C yellow#6 · lactose D/C · magnesium stearate · microcrystalline cellulose · primellose · stearic acid
Permathene-12 Maximum Strength with Vitamin C § CCA Industries	timed-release caplet	75mg	ascorbic acid · dicalcium phosphate · FD&C yellow#10 · lactose D/C · magnesium stearate · microcrystalline cellulose · primellose · stearic acid
Permathene-16 § CCA Industries	timed-release caplet	75mg	D&C yellow#10 · dicalcium phosphate · FD&C blue#1 · lactose D/C · magnesium stearate · microcrystalline cellulose · primellose · stearic acid
Protrim Legere Ph'cals	caplet	37.5mg	benzocaine, 9mg
GL PU SO **Protrim S.R.** Legere Ph'cals	caplet	75mg	
Super Odrinex Fox Pharmacal	tablet	25mg	cellulose · dicalcium phosphate · magnesium stearate · stearic acid · yellow#6
LA SO **Thinz Back-To-Nature** Alva-Amco Pharmacal	timed-release tablet	75mg	dicalcium phosphate · natural oat bran · wheat bran · apple fiber · fillers · coating
GL LA SO **Thinz-Span** Alva-Amco Pharmacal	timed-release capsule	75mg	

** New listing

§ Manufacturer/supplier did not confirm information for this edition. Product listing is reprinted from the '96-97 edition.

See Chapter 21, "Weight Control Products," for more information about these products.

Ophthalmic Product Tables

ARTIFICIAL TEAR PRODUCTS

	Product / Manufacturer/Supplier	Dosage Form	Viscosity Agent	Preservative	pH	Other Ingredients
PU	**Adsorbotear** / Alcon Labs	drops	povidone, 1.67% · hydroxyethyl cellulose, 0.41%	thimerosal, 0.004%	7.1-7.6	
PU	**Akwa Tears** / Akorn	drops	polyvinyl alcohol, 1.4%	benzalkonium chloride, 0.01%	5.21	sodium chloride · dibasic sodium phosphate · monobasic sodium phosphate · purified water · disodium edetate
PR PU	**Akwa Tears** / Akorn	ointment	white petrolatum · mineral oil · lanolin		5.21	
	AquaSite / CIBA Vision/Novartis	drops	Dextran 70, 0.1% · polycarbophil	sorbic acid, 0.2%	6.5-7	PEG-400, 0.2% · purified water · sodium chloride · sodium hydroxide · disodium edetate
PR PU	**Bion Tears** / Alcon Labs	drops	hydroxypropyl methylcellulose, 0.3% · Dextran 70, 0.1%		6-9	sodium chloride · potassium chloride · sodium bicarbonate · magnesium chloride · calcium chloride · zinc chloride
PR	**Celluvisc** / Allergan	drops	carboxymethylcellulose sodium, 1%		6.2-6.8	calcium chloride · potassium chloride · purified water · sodium chloride · sodium lactate
	Comfort Tears / Allergan	liquid	hydroxyethyl cellulose	benzalkonium chloride, 0.005%	6.7-7.2	disodium edetate, 0.02% · sodium chloride
	Dry Eye Therapy / Bausch & Lomb	drops	glycerin, 0.3%			calcium chloride · magnesium chloride · potassium chloride · sodium chloride · sodium citrate · sodium phosphate · zinc chloride
	Duolube / Bausch & Lomb	ointment	white petrolatum, 80% · mineral oil, 20%			
	DuraTears Naturale / Alcon Labs	ointment	petrolatum · mineral oil · lanolin			
	GenTeal Lubricant / CIBA Vision/Novartis	drops	hydroxypropyl methylcellulose	sodium perborate		boric acid · sodium chloride · potassium chloride · phosphoric acid · purified water
	Hypo Tears / CIBA Vision/Novartis	drops	polyvinyl alcohol, 1% · polyethylene glycol 400	benzalkonium chloride, 0.01%	6.6	dextrose · purified water
PR	**Hypo Tears** / CIBA Vision/Novartis	ointment	white petrolatum · light mineral oil			
PR	**Hypo Tears PF** / CIBA Vision/Novartis	drops	polyvinyl alcohol, 1% · polyethylene glycol 400		5-7.5	dextrose · purified water · disodium edetate
PU	**Isopto Alkaline** / Alcon Labs	drops	hydroxypropyl methylcellulose, 1%	benzalkonium chloride, 0.01%	6.0-7.8	
PU	**Isopto Tears** / Alcon Labs	drops	hydroxypropyl methylcellulose, 0.5%	benzalkonium chloride, 0.01%	6.0-7.8	
PR	**Lacri-Lube N.P.** / Allergan	ointment	white petrolatum, 57.3% · mineral oil, 42.5% · lanolin alcohol			
	Lacri-Lube S.O.P. / Allergan	ointment	white petrolatum, 56.8% · mineral oil, 42.5% · lanolin alcohol	chlorobutanol		

See Chapter 22, "Ophthalmic Products," for more information about these products.

ARTIFICIAL TEAR PRODUCTS - continued

	Product Manufacturer/Supplier	Dosage Form	Viscosity Agent	Preservative	pH	Other Ingredients
PU	**Liquifilm Tears** Allergan	drops	polyvinyl alcohol, 1.4%	chlorobutanol, 0.5%	3.3-7	sodium chloride · purified water · may contain hydrochloric acid or sodium hydroxide
	Moisture Drops Bausch & Lomb	drops	hydroxypropyl methylcellulose, 0.5% · glycerin, 0.2% · povidone, 0.1%	benzalkonium chloride, 0.01%		sodium chloride · potassium chloride · sodium borate · boric acid · disodium edetate
PU	**Murine Tears Lubricant** Ross Products/Abbott Labs	drops	povidone, 0.6% · polyvinyl alcohol, 0.5%	benzalkonium chloride	6-7.3	dextrose · potassium chloride · sodium bicarbonate · sodium chloride · sodium citrate · sodium phosphate · purified water · disodium edetate
	Murocel Lubricant Ophthalmic Bausch & Lomb	solution	methylcellulose, 1% · propylene glycol	methylparaben, 0.023% · propylparaben, 0.01%		sodium chloride · boric acid · sodium borate
	Ocucoat Lubricating Storz Ophthalmics	drops	hydroxypropyl methylcellulose, 0.8% · Dextran 70, 0.1%	benzalkonium chloride, 0.01%	5.5-7.8	monobasic sodium phosphate · dibasic sodium phosphate · potassium chloride · dextrose · purified water · may also contain hydrochloric acid and/or sodium hydroxide
PR	**Ocucoat PF Lubricating** Storz Ophthalmics	drops	hydroxypropyl methylcellulose, 0.8% · Dextran 70, 0.1%		5.5-7.8	monobasic sodium phosphate · dibasic sodium phosphate · potassium chloride · dextrose · purified water · may also contain hydrochloric acid and/or sodium hydroxide
**	**Ocurest Tears Formula Lubricant** Ocurest Labs	drops	hydroxypropyl methylcellulose, 0.4%	benzalkonium chloride, 0.01%	6.0-7.8	dibasic sodium phosphate · monobasic sodium phosphate · potassium chloride · sodium chloride · purified water · disodium edetate
	Puralube Tears E. Fougera	drops	polyvinyl alcohol, 1% · polyethylene glycol 400, 1%	benzalkonium chloride		dextrose · purified water · disodium edetate
PR PU	**Refresh** Allergan	drops	polyvinyl alcohol, 1.4% · povidone, 0.6%		5.5-6.5	sodium chloride · purified water · may contain hydrochloric acid and/or sodium hydroxide
PR	**Refresh P.M.** Allergan	ointment	white petrolatum, 56.8% · mineral oil, 41.5% · lanolin alcohols			purified water · sodium chloride
PR PU	**Refresh Plus** Allergan	drops	carboxymethylcellulose sodium, 0.5%		6-7	calcium chloride · magnesium chloride · potassium chloride · purified water · sodium chloride · sodium lactate · may contain hydrochloric acid and/or sodium hydroxide
	Stye Sterile Lubricant Del Ph'cals	ointment	petrolatum, 55% · mineral oil, 32%			
	Tearisol CIBA Vision/Novartis	drops	hydroxypropyl methylcellulose, 0.5%	benzalkonium chloride, 0.01%	7.5	boric acid · potassium chloride · sodium carbonate

See Chapter 22, "Ophthalmic Products," for more information about these products.

ARTIFICIAL TEAR PRODUCTS - continued

	Product Manufacturer/Supplier	Dosage Form	Viscosity Agent	Preservative	pH	Other Ingredients
PU	**Tears Naturale** Alcon Labs	drops	hydroxypropyl methylcellulose, 0.3% · Dextran 70, 0.1%	benzalkonium chloride, 0.01%	6.6-7.8	potassium chloride · sodium chloride · sodium hydroxide · purified water · disodium edetate
PR PU	**Tears Naturale Free** Alcon Labs	drops	hydroxypropyl methylcellulose, 0.3% · Dextran 70, 0.1%		6.0-8.0	sodium chloride · potassium chloride · sodium borate · sodium HCl and/or sodium hydroxide · purified water
PU	**Tears Naturale II** Alcon Labs	drops	hydroxypropyl methylcellulose, 0.3% · Dextran 70, 0.1%	polyquad, 0.001%	6.5-8.0	potassium chloride · sodium chloride · sodium borate · hydrochloric acid and/or sodium hydroxide · purified water
PU	**Tears Plus** Allergan	drops	polyvinyl alcohol, 1.4% · povidone, 0.6%	chlorobutanol, 0.5%	3.5-7	purified water · sodium chloride · may contain hydrochloric acid or sodium hydroxide
PU	**Tears Renewed** Akorn	drops	hydroxypropyl methylcellulose 2906, 0.3% · Dextran 70, 0.1%	benzalkonium chloride, 0.01%	6.7-7.3	sodium chloride · potassium chloride · hydrochloric acid and/or sodium hydroxide · purified water · disodium edetate
PR	**Tears Renewed** Akorn	ointment	white petrolatum · light mineral oil			
PU	**Ultra Tears** Alcon Labs	drops	hydroxypropyl methylcellulose, 1%	benzalkonium chloride, 0.01%	6.0-7.8	
	Visine Lubricating Pfizer Consumer	drops	hydroxypropyl methylcellulose, 0.2% · glycerin, 0.2%	sodium borate · boric acid	6.3-6.5	disodium edetate

** New listing

See Chapter 22, "Ophthalmic Products," for more information about these products.

OPHTHALMIC DECONGESTANT PRODUCTS

	Product Manufacturer/Supplier	Dosage Form	Viscosity Agent	Vasoconstrictor	Preservative	Buffer	pH	Other Ingredients
PU	**AK-Nefrin** Akorn	drops	polyvinyl alcohol, 1.4%	phenylephrine HCl, 0.12%	benzalkonium chloride, 0.005%	monobasic sodium phosphate · dibasic sodium phosphate · hydrochloric acid and/or sodium hydroxide	6.2-6.8	sodium chloride · purified water · disodium edetate
	Allerest Eye Drops Novartis Consumer	drops		naphazoline HCl, 0.012%	benzalkonium chloride	boric acid · sodium borate	5.5-6.3	water · EDTA
PU	**Clear eyes ACR Allergy Cold Relief** Ross Products/Abbott Labs	drops	glycerin, 0.2%	naphazoline HCl, 0.012%	benzalkonium chloride	boric acid · sodium citrate	5.5-6.3	zinc sulfate, 0.25% · sodium chloride · purified water · disodium edetate
PU	**Clear eyes Lubricating Eye Redness Reliever Extra Relief** Ross Products/Abbott Labs	drops	glycerin, 0.2%	naphazoline HCl, 0.012%	benzalkonium chloride	boric acid · sodium borate	5.5-6.3	purified water · disodium edetate
	Collyrium Fresh Wyeth-Ayerst Labs	drops	glycerin, 1%	tetrahydrozoline HCl, 0.05%	benzalkonium chloride, 0.01%	boric acid · sodium borate · hydrochloric acid		disodium edetate, 0.01%
PU	**Estivin II** Alcon Labs	drops	hydroxypropyl methylcellulose, 0.3% · Dextran 70, 0.1%	naphazoline HCl, 0.012%	benzalkonium chloride, 0.01%		5.5-6.5	
	Eye-Sed Scherer Labs	drops		tetrahydrozoline HCl, 0.05%	benzalkonium chloride	sodium borate · boric acid	5.8-7	zinc sulfate, 0.25% · sodium chloride · disodium edetate
	EyeSine Akorn	drops		tetrahydrozoline HCl, 0.05%	benzalkonium chloride, 0.01%	boric acid · sodium borate	5.8-6.5	sodium chloride · purified water · disodium edetate
PU	**Isopto-Frin** Alcon Labs	drops	hydroxypropyl methylcellulose, 0.5%	phenylephrine HCl, 0.12%	benzalkonium chloride, 0.01%	sodium citrate · sodium phosphate · sodium biphosphate	4.0-7.5	
PU	**Murine Tears Plus Lubricant Redness Reliever** Ross Products/Abbott Labs	drops	povidone, 0.6% · polyvinyl alcohol, 0.5%	tetrahydrozoline HCl, 0.05%	benzalkonium chloride	sodium phosphate	6-7.3	dextrose · potassium chloride · purified water · sodium bicarbonate · sodium chloride · disodium edetate
PU	**Naphcon** Alcon Labs	drops		naphazoline HCl, 0.012%	benzalkonium chloride, 0.01%	boric acid	5.5-7.0	sodium chloride · potassium chloride · disodium edetate

See Chapter 22, "Ophthalmic Products," for more information about these products.

OPHTHALMIC DECONGESTANT PRODUCTS - continued

	Product Manufacturer/Supplier	Dosage Form	Viscosity Agent	Vasoconstrictor	Preservative	Buffer	pH	Other Ingredients
PU	**Naphcon A** Alcon Labs	solution		naphazoline HCl, 0.025%	benzalkonium chloride, 0.01%	boric acid · sodium borate · hydrochloric acid and/or sodium hydroxide	5-7	pheniramine maleate, 0.3% · disodium edetate · sodium chloride · purified water
	Ocu Clear Schering-Plough Healthcare	drops		oxymetazoline HCl, 0.025%	benzalkonium chloride, 0.01%	sodium hydroxide	6.4	EDTA
	OcuHist Pfizer Consumer	drops		naphazoline HCl, 0.025%	benzalkonium chloride, 0.01%	boric acid · sodium borate · hydrochloric acid and/or sodium hydroxide	5.5-6.5	pheniramine maleate, 0.3% · disodium edetate, 0.1% · purified water
**	**Ocurest Redness Reliever Lubricant** Ocurest Labs	drops	polyethylene glycol 400, 1%	tetrahydrozoline HCl, 0.05%	benzalkonium chloride, 0.013%	boric acid · sodium borate	5.8-6.5	disodium edetate · sodium chloride · purified water
	Opcon-A Bausch & Lomb	drops	hydroxypropyl methylcellulose, 0.5%	naphazoline HCl, 0.027%	benzalkonium chloride, 0.01%	boric acid · sodium borate	5.5-6.3	pheniramine maleate, 0.315% · disodium edetate, 0.1% · sodium chloride · purified water
PU	**Prefrin Liquifilm** Allergan	drops	polyvinyl alcohol, 1.4%	phenylephrine HCl, 0.12%	benzalkonium chloride, 0.005%	monobasic sodium phosphate · dibasic sodium phosphate · may contain hydrochloric acid or sodium hydroxide	6.3-7.1	disodium edetate · purified water · sodium acetate · sodium thiosulfate
PR PU	**Relief** Allergan	drops	polyvinyl alcohol, 1.4%	phenylephrine HCl, 0.12%		monobasic sodium phosphate · dibasic sodium phosphate · may contain hydrochloric acid and/or sodium chloride	6.3-7.1	disodium edetate · purified water · sodium acetate · sodium thiosulfate
	Sensitive Eyes Redness Reliever Lubricant Bausch & Lomb	drops	polyethylene glycol 300, 0.2%	naphazoline HCl, 0.012%	benzalkonium chloride, 0.01%	boric acid · sodium borate		sodium chloride · disodium edetate
	Sensitive Eyes Redness Reliever Lubricant Maximum Strength Bausch & Lomb	drops	hydroxypropyl methylcellulose, 0.5%	naphazoline HCl, 0.03%	benzalkonium chloride, 0.01%	boric acid · sodium borate		sodium chloride · disodium edetate
PU	**Soothe** Alcon Labs	drops	povidone, 1.67% · polyethylene glycol	tetrahydrozoline HCl, 0.05%	benzalkonium chloride, 0.004%	boric acid · sodium borate · hydrochloric acid and/or sodium hydroxide	5.8-6.5	sodium chloride · disodium edetate

See Chapter 22, "Ophthalmic Products," for more information about these products.

OPHTHALMIC DECONGESTANT PRODUCTS - continued

	Product Manufacturer/Supplier	Dosage Form	Viscosity Agent	Vasoconstrictor	Preservative	Buffer	pH	Other Ingredients
	Vaso Clear CIBA Vision/Novartis	drops	polyvinyl alcohol	naphazoline HCl, 0.02%	benzalkonium chloride, 0.01%		5.5-7	PEG-8000 · EDTA
	Vaso Clear A CIBA Vision/Novartis	drops	polyvinyl alcohol, 0.25%	naphazoline HCl, 0.02%	benzalkonium chloride, 0.005%		5.5-6.6	zinc sulfate, 0.25% · PEG-8000 · EDTA
	Vasocon-A CIBA Vision/Novartis	drops		naphazoline HCl, 0.05%	benzalkonium chloride		5.5-6.3	antazoline phosphate, 0.5%
PU	**Visine Allergy Relief** Pfizer Consumer	drops		tetrahydrozoline HCl, 0.05%	benzalkonium chloride, 0.01%	boric acid · sodium citrate	6.3-6.5	zinc sulfate, 0.25% · EDTA, 0.1% · sodium chloride
PU	**Visine L.R.** Pfizer Consumer	drops		oxymetazoline HCl, 0.025%	benzalkonium chloride, 0.01%	boric acid · sodium borate	6.3-6.5	EDTA, 0.1% · sodium chloride
PU	**Visine Moisturizing** Pfizer Consumer	drops	polyethylene glycol 400, 1%	tetrahydrozoline HCl, 0.05%	benzalkonium chloride, 0.013%	boric acid · sodium borate	6.3-6.5	EDTA, 0.1% · sodium chloride
PU	**Visine Original Formula** Pfizer Consumer	drops		tetrahydrozoline HCl, 0.05%	benzalkonium chloride, 0.01%	boric acid · sodium borate	6.3-6.5	EDTA, 0.1% · sodium chloride
	Zincfrin Alcon Labs	drops		phenylephrine HCl, 0.12%	benzalkonium chloride, 0.01%	citric acid · sodium citrate	7.0-7.8	zinc sulfate, 0.25%

** New listing

See Chapter 22, "Ophthalmic Products," for more information about these products.

MISCELLANEOUS OPHTHALMIC PRODUCTS

Product Manufacturer/Supplier	Dosage Form	Buffer	pH	Preservative	Other Ingredients
IRRIGANTS					
Collyrium for Fresh Eyes Wyeth-Ayerst Labs	solution	boric acid · sodium borate		benzalkonium chloride	water
Dacriose CIBA Vision/Novartis	liquid	sodium phosphate		benzalkonium chloride, 0.01%	disodium edetate, 0.3% · sodium hydroxide, 0.01% · sodium chloride · potassium chloride
Eye Wash Bausch & Lomb	liquid	borate		sorbic acid, 0.1%	EDTA, 0.025% · sodium chloride
PU **Eye-Stream** Alcon Labs	liquid	sodium acetate, 0.39% · sodium citrate, 0.17% · sodium hydroxide and/or hydrochloric acid	6.5-7.5	benzalkonium chloride, 0.013%	potassium chloride, 0.075% · sodium chloride, 0.64% · calcium chloride, 0.048% · magnesium chloride, 0.03%
Lavoptik Eye Wash Lavoptik	liquid	sodium phosphate	7	benzalkonium chloride, 0.005%	sodium chloride, 0.49%
HYPEROSMOTICS					
PU **Adsorbonac** Alcon Labs	solution	sodium phosphate · sodium hydroxide and/or hydrochloric acid		thimerosal, 0.004%	sodium chloride, 2%; 5% · polyethylene glycol · hydroxythethyl cellulose · povidone · disodium edetate
PR **AK-NaCl** Akorn	ointment		6-8		sodium chloride, 5% · lanolin oil · mineral oil · white petrolatum · purified water
AK-NaCl Akorn	solution	boric acid · sodium borate · sodium hydroxide and/or hydrochloric acid	6-8	methylparaben, 0.023% · propylparaben, 0.017%	sodium chloride, 5% · hydroxypropyl methylcellulose 2906 · propylene glycol · purified water
Muro 128 Bausch & Lomb	ointment				sodium chloride, 5%
Muro 128 Bausch & Lomb	solution				sodium chloride, 2%
EYE LID SCRUBS					
Eye-Scrub CIBA Vision/Novartis	liquid			benzyl alcohol	PEG-200 glyceryl monotallowate · disodium laureth sulfosuccinate · cocoamido propyl amine oxide · PEG-78 glyceryl monococoate · EDTA
PR PU **Lid Wipes-SPF** Akorn	pad	sodium phosphate · monobasic sodium hydroxide · phosphoric acid	6-7.6		PEG-200 glyceryl tallowate · PEG-80 glyceryl cocoate · laureth-23 · cocoamido propyl amine oxide · sodium chloride · glycerin · water

PROSTHESIS LUBRICANT/CLEANSER

See Chapter 22, "Ophthalmic Products," for more information about these products.

MISCELLANEOUS OPHTHALMIC PRODUCTS - continued

Product Manufacturer/Supplier	Dosage Form	Buffer	pH	Preservative	Other Ingredients
PU **Enuclene** Alcon Labs	solution		6.1-6.8	benzalkonium chloride, 0.02%	hydroxypropyl methylcellulose, 0.85% · tyloxapol, 0.25%

See Chapter 22, "Ophthalmic Products," for more information about these products.

Contact Lens Product Tables

HARD LENS PRODUCTS

	Product Manufacturer/Supplier	Product Form	Use	Viscosity Agent	Preservative	Other Ingredients
PU	**Adapettes Sensitive Eyes** Alcon Labs	liquid	lubricating · rewetting		sorbic acid, 0.2%	disodium edetate, 0.1% · boric acid · sodium borate · sodium chloride
PU	**Adapt** Alcon Labs	liquid	wetting · rewetting	hydroxyethyl cellulose	thimerosal, 0.004%	poloxamer · povidone · sodium phosphate · sodium chloride · disodium edetate
PU	**Blairex Hard Lens Cleaner** Blairex Labs	liquid	cleaning			miracare 2MCA, 20% · water
	Blairex Sterile Contact Lens Cleaner Blairex Labs	liquid	cleaning		benzalkonium chloride, 0.01%	disodium edetate, 0.1% · cocoamphodiacetate · glycols
	Blairex Sterile Contact Lens Conditioning Blairex Labs	solution	wetting · soaking · disinfecting		benzalkonium chloride, 0.01%	disodium edetate, 0.1%
	Clean-N-Soak Allergan	liquid	cleaning · soaking		phenylmercuric nitrate, 0.004%	cleaning agent
PU	**Clerz 2** Alcon Labs	drops	lubricating · rewetting	hydroxyethyl cellulose	sorbic acid, 0.2%	disodium edetate, 0.1% · sodium chloride · potassium chloride · sodium borate
	LC-65 Daily Contact Lens Cleaner Allergan	liquid	cleaning	cocoamphocarboxygly-cinate		sodium lauryl sulfate · hexylene glycol · sodium chloride · sodium phosphate · EDTA
	Lens Fresh Allergan	drops	rewetting · lubricating	hydroxyethyl cellulose	sorbic acid, 0.1%	EDTA, 0.2% · sodium chloride · boric acid · sodium borate
	Lens Lubricant Bausch & Lomb	liquid	rewetting · lubricating	povidone	thimerosal, 0.004%	EDTA, 0.1% · polyoxyethylene
	Liquifilm Allergan	solution	wetting	hydroxypropyl methylcellulose · polyvinyl alcohol	benzalkonium chloride, 0.004%	sodium chloride · potassium chloride · EDTA
PU	**Opti-Clean Daily Cleaner** Alcon Labs	liquid	cleaning	hydroxyethyl cellulose	thimerosal, 0.004%	disodium edetate, 0.1% · nylon 11 · polysorbate 21 · boric acid · sodium borate · sodium chloride
PU	**Opti-Clean II Daily Cleaner for Sensitive Eyes** Alcon Labs	liquid	cleaning	hydroxyethyl cellulose	polyquaternium-1	nylon 11 · polysorbate 21 · boric acid · sodium borate · sodium chloride · disodium edetate
PU	**Opti-Free Daily Cleaner** Alcon Labs	liquid	cleaning	hydroxyethyl cellulose	polyquaternium-1	disodium EDTA
	Opti-Zyme Enzymatic Cleaner Alcon Labs	tablet	weekly protein cleaning			pancreatin
PU	**Soaclens** Alcon Labs	liquid	soaking · wetting	hydroxyethyl cellulose · polyvinyl alcohol	thimerosal, 0.004%	disodium edetate, 0.1% · sodium chloride · sodium phosphate · polyvinyl alcohol
	Total All-In-One Contact Lens Allergan	solution	wetting · cleaning · soaking	polyvinyl alcohol	benzalkonium chloride	EDTA

See Chapter 23, "Contact Lens Products," for more information about these products.

RIGID GAS-PERMEABLE LENS PRODUCTS

	Product Manufacturer/Supplier	Product Form	Use	Viscosity Agent	Preservative	Other Ingredients
	Blairex Sterile Contact Lens Cleaner Blairex Labs	liquid	cleaning		benzalkonium chloride, 0.01%	disodium edetate, 0.1% · cocoamphodiacetate · glycols
	Blairex Sterile Contact Lens Conditioning Blairex Labs	solution	wetting · soaking · disinfecting		benzalkonium chloride, 0.01%	disodium edetate, 0.1%
PR	**Boston Advance Cleaner** Bausch & Lomb	liquid	cleaning			alkyl ether sulfate · ethoxylated alkyl phenol · triquaternary cocoa-based phospholipid · silica gel
	Boston Advance Comfort Formula Conditioning Solution Bausch & Lomb	solution	wetting · soaking · disinfecting	cellulosic viscosifier	chlorhexidine gluconate, 0.003% · polyaminopropyl biguanide, 0.0005%	disodium edetate, 0.05% · cationic cellulose derivative polymer · derivatized polyethylene glycol · polyvinyl alcohol
PR	**Boston Cleaner** Bausch & Lomb	liquid	cleaning			alkyl ether sulfate · silica gel · titanium dioxide · fragrance
	Boston Conditioning Solution Bausch & Lomb	solution	wetting · soaking · disinfecting	hydroxyethyl cellulose	chlorhexidine gluconate, 0.006%	disodium edetate, 0.05% · polyvinyl alcohol · cationic cellulose derivatives
	Boston Rewetting Drops Bausch & Lomb	drops	lubricating · rewetting	hydroxyethyl cellulose	chlorhexidine gluconate, 0.006%	disodium edetate, 0.05% · polyvinyl alcohol · cationic cellulose derivatives
	Boston Simplicity Bausch & Lomb	solution	cleaning · rinsing · disinfecting · conditioning	cellulosic viscosifier	chlorhexidine gluconate, 0.003% · polyaminopropyl biguanide, 0.0005%	disodium edetate, 0.05% · PEO sorbitan monolaurate · betaine surfactant · silicone glycol copolymer · derivatized polyethylene glycol
**	**ComfortCare GP Comfort Drops** Allergan	drops	lubricating · rewetting	hydroxyethyl cellulose	potassium sorbate, 0.13%	disodium edetate, 0.1% · oxtylphenoxy (oxyethylene) ethanol · sodium chloride
**	**ComfortCare GP Dual Action** Allergan	tablets	daily protein cleaning			subtilisin · poloxamer 338 · potassium carbonate · citric acid · sodium benzoate · povidone
**	**ComfortCare GP Wetting & Soaking** Allergan	solution	wetting · chemical disinfecting · storing	polyvinyl alcohol	chlorhexidine gluconate	octylphenoxy (oxyethylene) ethanol · povidone · disodium edetate
	Concentrated Cleaner Bausch & Lomb	liquid	cleaning			sodium chloride · sulfate surfactant
PU	**Opti-Clean II Daily Cleaner for Sensitive Eyes** Alcon Labs	liquid	cleaning	hydroxyethyl cellulose	thimerosal, 0.004%	EDTA, 0.1% · polysorbate 21 · cleaning agent · boric acid · sodium borate · sodium chloride · sodium hydroxide · purified water

See Chapter 23, "Contact Lens Products," for more information about these products.

RIGID GAS-PERMEABLE LENS PRODUCTS - continued

	Product Manufacturer/Supplier	Product Form	Use	Viscosity Agent	Preservative	Other Ingredients
PU	**Opti-Free Daily Cleaner** Alcon Labs	liquid	cleaning	hydroxyethyl cellulose	polyquaternium-1	nylon 11 · polysorbate 21 · sodium borate · boric acid · hydrochloric acid and/or sodium hydroxide · purified water · disodium EDTA
	Opti-Zyme Enzymatic Cleaner Alcon Labs	tablet	weekly protein cleaning			pancreatin
	Pro Free/GP Weekly Enzymatic Cleaner [a] Allergan	tablet	weekly protein cleaning			sodium chloride · sodium carbonate · sodium borate · papain · disodium edetate
	Resolve/GP Daily Cleaner Allergan	liquid	cleaning	cocoamphocarboxygly-cinate		fatty acid amide · surfactants · sodium lauryl sulfate · hexylene glycol · alkyl ether sulfate
	Wet & Soak Allergan	drops	rewetting · lubricating	hydroxyethyl cellulose	WSCP (poly [oxyethylene (dimethyliminio) ethylene (dimethyliminio) ethylene dichloride]), 0.006%	borate
	Wet-N-Soak Plus Allergan	solution	wetting · soaking	polyvinyl alcohol	benzalkonium chloride, 0.003%	EDTA
	Wetting & Soaking Solution Bausch & Lomb	solution	rinsing · disinfecting · storage	polyvinyl alcohol · hydroxyethyl cellulose	chlorhexidine gluconate, 0.006%	EDTA, 0.05%

** New listing
[a] Tablet must be dissolved in water

See Chapter 23, "Contact Lens Products," for more information about these products.

SOFT LENS PRODUCTS

	Product Manufacturer/Supplier	Product Form	Use	Viscosity Agent	Preservative	Other Ingredients
	MULTIPURPOSE SOLUTIONS					
	Complete Multi-Purpose Allergan	solution	cleaning · rinsing · disinfecting · storing		polyhexamethylene biguanide	sodium chloride · tromethamine · tyloxapol · EDTA
PU	**Opti-Free Express** Alcon Labs	solution	cleaning · rinsing · disinfecting · storing		polyquaternium-1	sodium citrate · sodium chloride · citric acid · disodium edetate
PU	**Opti-One Multi-Purpose** Alcon Labs	solution	rinsing · chemical disinfecting · storing		polyquaternium-1, 0.001%	disodium EDTA, 0.05% · citric acid · sodium citrate · sodium chloride · sodium hydroxide and/or hydrochloric acid · purified water
	ReNu Multi-Purpose Bausch & Lomb	solution	cleaning · rinsing · chemical disinfecting · storing · enzyme diluent		polyaminopropyl biguanide	sodium chloride · sodium borate · boric acid · poloxamine · EDTA
**	**SOLO·care** CIBA Vision/Novartis	solution	cleaning · rinsing · disinfecting · storing		polyhexanide, 0.0001%	disodium edetate dihydrate, 0.025% · sodium chloride · polyoxyethylene polypropylene · block copolymer · dibasic sodium phosphate · monobasic sodium phosphate
	SURFACE ACTIVE CLEANSERS					
	Ciba Vision Cleaner CIBA Vision/Novartis	liquid	cleaning	cocoamphocarboxyglycinate	sorbic acid, 0.1%	EDTA, 0.2% · sodium lauryl sulfate · hexylene glycol
	Daily Cleaner Bausch & Lomb	liquid	cleaning	hydroxyethyl cellulose · polyvinyl alcohol	thimerosal, 0.004%	EDTA, 0.2% · tyloxapol · sodium phosphate · sodium chloride
	DURAcare II Blairex Labs	liquid	cleaning		sorbic acid, 0.1%	disodium edetate, 0.25% · block copolymers of ethylene and propylene oxide · octylphenoxy polyethoxyethanol
	LC-65 Daily Contact Lens Cleaner Allergan	liquid	cleaning	cocoamphocarboxyglycinate		sodium lauryl sulfate · hexylene glycol · sodium chloride · sodium phosphate · EDTA
	Lens Clear Cleaner Allergan	liquid	cleaning	cocoamphocarboxyglycinate	sorbic acid, 0.1%	EDTA, 0.2% · sodium lauryl sulfate · hexylene glycol
	Lens Plus Daily Cleaner Allergan	liquid	cleaning	cocoamphocarboxyglycinate		sodium lauryl sulfate · hexylene glycol · sodium chloride · sodium phosphate
	MiraFlow Extra Strength CIBA Vision/Novartis	liquid	cleaning			isopropyl alcohol, 20% · poloxamer 407 · amphoteric 10
PU	**Opti-Clean Daily Cleaner** Alcon Labs	liquid	cleaning	hydroxyethyl cellulose	thimerosal, 0.004%	disodium edetate, 0.1% · nylon 11 · polysorbate 21 · boric acid · sodium borate · sodium chloride
PU	**Opti-Clean II Daily Cleaner for Sensitive Eyes** Alcon Labs	liquid	cleaning	hydroxyethyl cellulose	polyquaternium-1	nylon 11 · polysorbate 21 · boric acid · sodium borate · sodium chloride · disodium edetate

See Chapter 23, "Contact Lens Products," for more information about these products.

SOFT LENS PRODUCTS - continued

	Product / Manufacturer/Supplier	Product Form	Use	Viscosity Agent	Preservative	Other Ingredients
PU	**Opti-Free Daily Cleaner** Alcon Labs	liquid	cleaning	hydroxyethyl cellulose	polyquaternium-1	nylon 11 · polysorbate 21 · sodium borate · boric acid · hydrochloric acid and/or sodium hydroxide · purified water · disodium EDTA
PU	**Opti-Soak Conditioning** Alcon Labs	solution	cleaning	hydroxyethyl cellulose · polyvinyl alcohol	polyquaternium-1	sodium phosphate · sodium chloride · polysorbate 80 · disodium edetate
PU	**Opti-Soak Daily Cleaner** Alcon Labs	liquid	cleaning	hydroxyethyl cellulose	polyquaternium-1	nylon 11 · polysorbate 21 · sodium borate · boric acid · sodium chloride · disodium edetate
PU	**Pliagel** Alcon Labs	solution	cleaning		sorbic acid, 0.25%	trisodium edetate, 0.5% · poloxamer 407 · potassium chloride · sodium chloride
PU	**Preflex for Sensitive Eyes** Alcon Labs	liquid	cleaning	hydroxyethyl cellulose · polyvinyl alcohol	sorbic acid, 0.2%	EDTA, 0.2% · sodium chloride · sodium phosphate · tyloxapol · sodium chloride
	Pure Eyes 1 Cleaner/Rinse CIBA Vision/Novartis	liquid	cleaning · rinsing			boric acid · sodium borate · sodium perborate · phosphoric acid · pluronic surfactant
	Sensitive Eyes Daily Cleaner Bausch & Lomb	liquid	cleaning	hydroxypropyl methylcellulose	sorbic acid, 0.25%	EDTA, 0.5% · sodium chloride · borate buffer · surfactant

ENZYMATIC CLEANERS

	Product / Manufacturer/Supplier	Product Form	Use	Viscosity Agent	Preservative	Other Ingredients
PU	**Alcon Enzymatic Cleaner** Alcon Labs	tablet	weekly protein cleaning			citric acid · sodium bicarbonate · sucrose
	Complete Weekly Enzymatic Cleaner Allergan	tablet	weekly protein cleaning			subtilisin A
PU	**Opti-Free Enzymatic Cleaner for Sensitive Eyes** Alcon Labs	tablet	weekly protein cleaning	povidone		pancreatin · citric acid · sodium bicarbonate · polyethylene glycol · dehydrated alcohol · compressible sugar
** PR PU	**Opti-Free SupraClens Daily Protein Remover** Alcon Labs	liquid	daily protein cleaning			highly purified porcine pancreatin enzymes · polyethylene glycol · sodium borate
	Opti-Zyme Enzymatic Cleaner Alcon Labs	tablet	weekly protein cleaning			pancreatin
	ReNu 1 Step Enzymatic Cleaner Bausch & Lomb	tablet	weekly protein cleaning			subtilisin · sodium carbonate · sodium chloride · boric acid
	ReNu Effervescent Enzymatic Bausch & Lomb	tablet	weekly protein cleaning			subtilisin PEG · sodium carbonate · sodium chloride · tartaric acid
	ReNu Thermal Enzymatic Bausch & Lomb	tablet	weekly protein cleaning			subtilisin PEG · sodium carbonate · sodium chloride · boric acid

See Chapter 23, "Contact Lens Products," for more information about these products.

SOFT LENS PRODUCTS - continued

	Product Manufacturer/Supplier	Product Form	Use	Viscosity Agent	Preservative	Other Ingredients
	Sensitive Eyes Effervescent Enzymatic Bausch & Lomb	tablet	weekly protein cleaning			subtilisin PEG · sodium carbonate · sodium chloride · tartaric acid
	Ultrazyme Enzymatic Cleaner Allergan	tablet	weekly protein cleaning			subtilisin A · effervescing agents · buffers
	CHEMICAL DISINFECTING PRODUCTS					
	Disinfecting Solution Bausch & Lomb	solution	rinsing · chemical disinfecting · storing		chlorhexidine gluconate, 0.005% · thimerosal, 0.001%	EDTA, 0.1% · sodium chloride · sodium borate · boric acid
PU	**Flex-Care for Sensitive Eyes** Alcon Labs	liquid	rinsing · chemical disinfecting		chlorhexidine gluconate, 0.005%	EDTA, 0.1% · sodium chloride · sodium borate · boric acid
PU	**Opti-Free for Disinfection** Alcon Labs	solution	rinsing · chemical disinfecting · storing		polyquaternium-1, 0.001%	EDTA, 0.05% · citrate buffer · sodium chloride
	HYDROGEN PEROXIDE DISINFECTING PRODUCTS AND RINSING/NEUTRALIZING PRODUCTS					
	AO SEPT CIBA Vision/Novartis	liquid	disinfecting			hydrogen peroxide, 3% · sodium chloride, 0.85% · sodium stannate · phosphate buffers · phosphoric acid
**	**Consept 1** Allergan	liquid	cleaning · disinfecting			hydrogen peroxide, 3% · sodium stannate · sodium nitrate · phosphate buffers · polyoxyl 40 stearate
**	**Consept 2** Allergan	solution	rinsing · neutralizing		chlorhexidine gluconate, 0.001%	sodium chloride, 0.5% · borate buffers · disodium edetate
PU	**Mirasept Step 1** Alcon Labs	solution	disinfecting			hydrogen peroxide · sodium stannate · sodium nitrate
PU	**Mirasept Step 2** Alcon Labs	solution	rinsing · neutralizing		sorbic acid	boric acid · sodium borate · sodium pyruvate · disodium edetate
	Oxysept 1 Disinfecting Allergan	solution	disinfecting			hydrogen peroxide, 3% · sodium stannate · sodium nitrate · phosphate buffers
	Oxysept 2 Neutralizing Allergan	tablet	neutralizing			catalase · buffering agents · tableting agents
	Oxysept 2 Rinse and Neutralizer Allergan	liquid	rinsing · neutralizing			catalase · sodium chloride · monobasic sodium phosphate · dibasic sodium phosphate
	Pure Eyes 2 Disinfectant/Soaking CIBA Vision/Novartis	solution	disinfecting · soaking · neutralizing			hydrogen peroxide, 3% · sodium chloride, 0.85% · sodium stannate · phosphate buffers · phosphoric acid · packaged with a plastic lens case with built-in neutralizer
	Quick CARE System, Finishing CIBA Vision/Novartis	solution	rinsing · soaking · storing			hydrogen peroxide, 0.006% · sodium borate · boric acid · phosphoric acid

See Chapter 23, "Contact Lens Products," for more information about these products.

SOFT LENS PRODUCTS - continued

	Product Manufacturer/Supplier	Product Form	Use	Viscosity Agent	Preservative	Other Ingredients
	Quick CARE System, Starting CIBA Vision/Novartis	solution	cleaning · disinfecting · neutralizing			purified water · polyoxypropylene · polyoxyethylene block copolymer · disodium lauroamphodiacetate · isopropanol · sodium chloride
	Ultracare Disinfecting Solution/Neutralizer [a] Allergan	solution · tablet	disinfecting · neutralizing	tablet: hydroxypropyl methylcellulose		solution: hydrogen peroxide, 3% · sodium stannate · sodium nitrate · phosphates · purified water · tablet: catalase
	REWETTING PRODUCTS					
PU	**Clerz 2** Alcon Labs	drops	lubricating · rewetting	hydroxyethyl cellulose	boric acid, 0.2%	disodium edetate, 0.1% · sodium chloride · potassium chloride · sodium borate
	Lens Drops CIBA Vision/Novartis	drops	lubricating · rewetting		sorbic acid, 0.15%	EDTA, 0.2% · sodium chloride · borate buffer · carbamide · poloxamer 407
	Lens Fresh Allergan	drops	lubricating · rewetting	hydroxyethyl cellulose	sorbic acid, 0.1%	EDTA, 0.2% · sodium chloride · boric acid · sodium borate
	Lens Lubricant Bausch & Lomb	liquid	lubricating · rewetting	povidone	thimerosal, 0.004%	EDTA, 0.1% · polyoxyethylene
	Lens Plus Allergan	drops	rewetting			sodium chloride · boric acid
PU	**Opti-Free** Alcon Labs	drops	rewetting		polyquaternium-1, 0.001%	citric acid · sodium citrate · sodium chloride
PU	**Opti-Soak Soothing** Alcon Labs	drops	rewetting	hydroxypropyl methylcellulose · Dextran	polyquaternium-1	sodium chloride · potassium chloride · disodium edetate
PU	**Opti-Tears Soothing** Alcon Labs	drops	lubricating · rewetting	hydroxypropyl methylcellulose · Dextran 70	polyquaternium-1, 0.001%	EDTA, 0.1% · sodium chloride · potassium chloride · sodium hydroxide and/or HCl · purified water
	ReNu Rewetting Bausch & Lomb	drops	rewetting		sorbic acid, 0.15%	borate buffer · EDTA
	Sensitive Eyes Plus Lubricating Bausch & Lomb	drops	lubricating	hydroxypropyl methylcellulose	sorbic acid	poloxamine · sodium chloride · disodium edetate
	Sensitive Eyes Rewetting Bausch & Lomb	drops	rewetting		sorbic acid, 0.1%	borate buffer · EDTA
	SALINE PRODUCTS					
PR	**Blairex Sterile Saline** Blairex Labs	solution	rinsing · thermal disinfecting · storing			sodium chloride, 0.7% · boric acid · sodium borate
	Ciba Vision Saline CIBA Vision/Novartis	liquid	rinsing · storing			sodium chloride · boric acid
	Lens Plus Sterile Saline Allergan	solution	rinsing · thermal disinfecting · storing			sodium chloride · boric acid
PU	**Opti-Soft** Alcon Labs	solution	rinsing · thermal disinfecting · storing		polyquaternium-1, 0.001%	EDTA, 0.1% · sodium chloride · borate buffer

See Chapter 23, "Contact Lens Products," for more information about these products.

SOFT LENS PRODUCTS - continued

	Product Manufacturer/Supplier	Product Form	Use	Viscosity Agent	Preservative	Other Ingredients
	Preserved Saline Bausch & Lomb	solution	rinsing · thermal disinfecting · storing		thimerosal, 0.001%	boric acid · sodium chloride · EDTA
	ReNu Saline Bausch & Lomb	liquid	rinsing · thermal disinfecting · storing · enzyme diluent		polyaminopropyl biguanide	sodium chloride · boric acid · EDTA
	Sensitive Eyes Plus Saline Bausch & Lomb	solution	rinsing · thermal disinfecting · storing · enzyme diluent		polyaminopropyl biguanide	sodium chloride · potassium chloride
	Sensitive Eyes Saline Bausch & Lomb	solution	rinsing · thermal disinfecting · storing · enzyme diluent		sorbic acid, 0.1%	sodium chloride · borate buffer · EDTA
	Sensitive Eyes Saline Bausch & Lomb	aerosol spray	rinsing · thermal disinfecting · storing · enzyme diluent			sodium chloride · boric acid · sodium borate
	Sensitive Eyes Saline/Cleaning Bausch & Lomb	solution	cleaning · rinsing · thermal disinfecting · storing		sorbic acid	sodium chloride · borate buffer · surfactant · EDTA
	SoftWear Saline CIBA Vision/Novartis	liquid	rinsing · storing			sodium chloride · sodium borate · boric acid · sodium perborate
	Sterile Preserved Saline Blairex Labs	solution	rinsing · chemical disinfecting · storing		sorbic acid, 0.1%	sodium chloride · disodium edetate
	Sterile Saline Bausch & Lomb	liquid	rinsing · thermal disinfecting · storing			sodium chloride · borate buffer · EDTA
PR PU	**Unisol 4 Saline** Alcon Labs	solution	rinsing · thermal disinfecting · storing			sodium chloride · sodium borate · boric acid · purified water

** New listing
[a] Disinfects and neutralizes in one step

See Chapter 23, "Contact Lens Products," for more information about these products.

Otic Product Table

OTIC PRODUCTS

Product Manufacturer/Supplier	Dosage Form	Anti-infective	Other Ingredients
Auro Del Ph'cals	drops	carbamide peroxide, 6.5%	anhydrous glycerin
Auro-Dri Del Ph'cals	drops	isopropyl alcohol, 97.25%	
Aurocaine Republic Drug	drops	carbamide peroxide	chlorobutanol, 0.5% · glycerin · propylene glycol
Aurocaine 2 Republic Drug	drops	boric acid, 2.75% · isopropyl alcohol	
Debrox SmithKline Beecham	drops	carbamide peroxide, 6.5%	citric acid · glycerin · propylene glycol · sodium stannate · water
Dent's Ear Wax Drops C. S. Dent	drops	carbamide peroxide	glycerin
E.R.O. Drops Scherer Labs	drops	carbamide peroxide, 6.5%	anhydrous glycerin
E.R.O. Ear Wax Removal System Scherer Labs	drops	carbamide peroxide, 6.5%	anhydrous glycerin · packaged with syringe
Ear Wax Removal System Bausch & Lomb	drops	carbamide peroxide, 6.5%	anhydrous glycerin base
Ear-Dry Scherer Labs	drops	isopropyl alcohol, 95%	anhydrous glycerin, 5%
Earsol-HC Parnell Ph'cals	drops	alcohol	hydrocortisone, 1% · propylene glycol · benzyl benzoate · water · yerba santa · fragrance
Murine Ear Wax Removal System Ross Products/Abbott Labs	drops	carbamide peroxide, 6.5% · alcohol, 6.3%	glycerin · polysorbate 20
Swim-EAR E. Fougera	drops	isopropyl alcohol, 95%	anhydrous glycerin, 5%

See Chapter 24, "Otic Products," for more information about these products.

Oral Health Product Tables

ORAL DISCOMFORT PRODUCTS

	Product Manufacturer/Supplier	Dosage Form	Anesthetic/ Analgesic	Debriding Agent/ Wound Cleanser	Other Ingredients
AL	**Amosan §** Oral-B Labs	powder		sodium peroxyborate monohydrate	sodium bitartrate · saccharin · peppermint, menthol, and vanilla flavors
	Anbesol Whitehall-Robins Healthcare	liquid	benzocaine, 6.4% · phenol, 0.5%		alcohol, 70% · camphor · glycerin · menthol · potassium iodide · povidone iodine
	Anbesol Whitehall-Robins Healthcare	gel	benzocaine, 6.3% · phenol, 0.5%		alcohol, 70% · camphor · carbomer 934P · D&C red#33 · D&C yellow#10 · FD&C blue#1 · FD&C yellow#6 · flavor · glycerin
AL PE	**Anbesol Baby, Grape** Whitehall-Robins Healthcare	gel	benzocaine, 7.5%		benzoic acid · carbomer 934P · D&C red#33 · disodium edetate · FD&C blue#1 · flavor · glycerin · methylparaben · polyethylene glycol · propylparaben · purified water · saccharin
AL PE	**Anbesol Baby, Original** Whitehall-Robins Healthcare	gel	benzocaine, 7.5%		carbomer 934P · clove oil · D&C red#33 · disodium edetate · glycerin · glycerin · polyethylene glycol · purified water · saccharin
	Anbesol Maximum Strength Whitehall-Robins Healthcare	gel · liquid	benzocaine, 20%		alcohol, 60% · carbomer 934P (gel) · D&C yellow#10 · FD&C blue#1 · FD&C red#40 · flavor · polyethylene glycol · saccharin
** AL SU PE	**Baby Gumz** Lee Consumer	gel	benzocaine, 10%		polyethylene glycol 8 and 32
	Benzodent Denture Analgesic [a] Chattem	ointment	benzocaine, 20%		8-hydroxyquinoline sulfate · petrolatum · carboxymethylcellulose sodium · eugenol · color
	Blistex Lip Medex Blistex	ointment	camphor, 1% · menthol, 1% · phenol, 0.5%		petrolatum · cocoa butter · flavor · lanolin · mixed waxes · oil of cloves
	Blistex Medicated Blistex	ointment	menthol, 0.6% · camphor, 0.5% · phenol, 0.5%		water · mixed waxes · mineral oil · petrolatum · lanolin
AL	**Campho-phenique [b]** Bayer Consumer	gel	camphor, 10.8% · phenol, 4.7%		eucalyptus oil
	Cankaid Merz Consumer	liquid		carbamide peroxide, 10%	citric acid monohydrate · sodium citrate dihydrate · disodium edetate
	Carmex Lip Balm Carma Labs	ointment	menthol · camphor · salicylic acid · phenol		alum · fragrance · petrolatum · lanolin · cocoa butter · wax
	ChapStick Medicated Lip Balm Whitehall-Robins Healthcare	stick	camphor, 1% · menthol, 0.6% · phenol, 0.5%		petrolatum 41% · paraffin wax · mineral oil · cocoa butter · 2-octyl dodecanol · arachidyl propionate · polyphenylmethylsiloxane 556 · white wax · isopropyl lanolate · carnauba wax · isopropyl myristate · lanolin · fragrance · methylparaben · propylparaben · oleyl alcohol · cetyl alcohol
	ChapStick Medicated Lip Balm, Jar or Squeeze Tube Whitehall-Robins Healthcare	ointment	camphor, 1% · menthol, 0.6% · phenol, 0.5%		petrolatum 60% (Jar) · petrolatum, 67% (Squeeze Tube) · microcrystalline wax · mineral oil · cocoa butter · lanolin · paraffin wax (Jar) · fragrance · methylparaben · propylparaben

See Chapter 25, "Oral Health Products," for more information about these products.

ORAL DISCOMFORT PRODUCTS - continued

	Product Manufacturer/Supplier	Dosage Form	Anesthetic/ Analgesic	Debriding Agent/ Wound Cleanser	Other Ingredients
	Dent's 3 In 1 Toothache Relief C. S. Dent	drops · gel · gum	benzocaine, 20% (drops · gum); 5% (gel)		drops: denatured alcohol, 74% · chlorobutanol anhydrous, 0.09% · propylene glycol · FD&C red#40 · eugenol gel: distilled water · methylparaben · propylparaben · propylene glycol · carbopol 934-P · methyl salicylate · FD&C red#40 · 2.2' iminodiethanol gum: petrolatum · cotton and wax base · beeswax · FD&C red#40 aluminum lake · eugenol
	Dent's Double-Action Kit C. S. Dent	drops · tablet	benzocaine, 20% (drops) · acetaminophen, 325mg (tablet)		drops: denatured alcohol, 74% · chlorobutanol anhydrous, 0.09% · propylene glycol · FD&C red#40 · eugenol
	Dent's Extra Strength Toothache Gum C. S. Dent	gum	benzocaine, 20%		petrolatum · cotton and wax base · beeswax · FD&C red#40 aluminum lake · eugenol
	Dent's Maxi-Strength Toothache Treatment C. S. Dent	drops	benzocaine, 20%		denatured alcohol, 74% · chlorobutanol anhydrous, 0.09% · propylene glycol · FD&C red#40 · eugenol
DY	**Dent-Zel-Ite Oral Mucosal Analgesic** Alvin Last	liquid	benzocaine, 5% · camphor		alcohol, 81% · wintergreen · glycerin
	Dent-Zel-Ite Temporary Dental Filling Alvin Last	liquid	camphor		alcohol, 55% · sandarac gum · methyl salicylate
	Dent-Zel-Ite Toothache Relief Alvin Last	drops	eugenol, 85% · camphor		alcohol, 13.5% · wintergreen
** AL	**Dentapaine** Reese Chemical	gel	benzocaine, 20%		glycerin · oil of cloves · saccharin sodium · methylparaben · polyethylene glycol 400 and 4000 · water
** AL DY GL SU SL	**Dentemp Temporary Filling Mix** Majestic Drug	liquid; powder	eugenol		zinc oxide
** PE	**Dr. Hand's Teething** Lee Consumer	gel · lotion	menthol		SD alcohol 38B, 10% (gel) · SD alcohol 38B, 11% (lotion) · sterilized water · carbomer 940 · witch hazel · polysorbate 80 · sodium hydroxide · simethicone · D&C red#33 · FD&C red#3
	Gly-Oxide SmithKline Beecham	liquid		carbamide peroxide, 10%	citric acid · flavor · glycerin · propylene glycol · sodium stannate · water
	Herpecin-L Cold Sore Lip Balm Chattem	stick			allantoin, 0.5% · padimate O, 7% · titanium dioxide
DY GL SL	**Hurricane, Wild Cherry [a]** Beutlich, L.P. Ph'cals	aerosol spray	benzocaine, 20%		polyethylene glycol · saccharin · flavoring · alcohol

See Chapter 25, "Oral Health Products," for more information about these products.

ORAL DISCOMFORT PRODUCTS - continued

	Product / Manufacturer/Supplier	Dosage Form	Anesthetic/ Analgesic	Debriding Agent/ Wound Cleanser	Other Ingredients
AL DY GL SL	**Hurricaine, Wild Cherry or Pina Colada [a]** Beutlich, L.P. Ph'cals	liquid	benzocaine, 20%		polyethylene glycol · saccharin · flavoring
AL DY GL SL	**Hurricaine; Wild Cherry, Pina Colada, or Watermelon [a]** Beutlich, L.P. Ph'cals	gel	benzocaine, 20%		polyethylene glycol · saccharin · flavoring
	Kank-A Professional Strength [a] Blistex	liquid	benzocaine, 20%		benzoin tincture compound · cetylpyridinium chloride · ethylcellulose · SD alcohol, 24% · dimethyl isosorbide · castor oil · flavor · tannic acid · propylene glycol · saccharin · benzyl alcohol
**	**Lip-Ex** Lee Consumer	ointment	phenol · camphor · salicylic acid · menthol		cherry flavor · petrolatum
** DY GL SL	**Lipmagik** Reese Chemical	liquid	benzocaine, 6.3% · phenol, 0.5%		alcohol, 70%
AL DY SO SU PE	**Little Teethers Oral Pain Relief** Vetco	gel	benzocaine, 7.5%		carbomer · glycerin · flavor · potassium sorbate · acesulfame K · PEGs
	Lotion-Jel C. S. Dent	gel	benzocaine, 5%		distilled water · methylparaben · propylparaben · propylene glycol · carbopol 934-P · methyl salicylate · FD&C red#40 · 2.2' iminodiethanol
	Medadyne Vetco	liquid	benzocaine, 10% · benzyl alcohol · menthol · camphor		benzalkonium chloride · tannic acid · flavors · SD alcohol · thymol
	Numzident Adult Strength Block Drug	gel	benzocaine, 10%		PEG-400 · glycerin · PEG-3350 · saccharin sodium · purified water · cherry vanilla flavor
	Numzit Teething Block Drug	gel	benzocaine, 7.5%		PEG-400 · PEG-3350 · saccharin sodium · clove oil · peppermint oil · purified water
CA GL	**Numzit Teething** Block Drug	lotion	benzocaine, 0.2%		alcohol · glycerin · kelgin MV · saccharin sodium · methylparaben · FD&C red#40 · FD&C blue#1
	Orabase Colgate-Palmolive	gel	benzocaine, 15%		ethanol · propylene glycol · hydroxypropyl cellulose · tannic acid · salicylic acid · flavor · saccharin sodium
AL PE	**Orabase Baby [a]** Colgate-Palmolive	gel	benzocaine, 7.5%		glycerin · PEG · carbopol · preservative · sweetener · flavor
AL	**Orabase Lip Cream** Colgate-Palmolive	cream	benzocaine, 5% · menthol, 0.5% · camphor · phenol		allantoin, 1% · carboxymethylcellulose sodium · veegum · Tween 80 · phenonip · PEG · biopure · talc · kaolin · lanolin · petrolatum · oil of clove · hydrated silica

See Chapter 25, "Oral Health Products," for more information about these products.

ORAL DISCOMFORT PRODUCTS - continued

	Product Manufacturer/Supplier	Dosage Form	Anesthetic/ Analgesic	Debriding Agent/ Wound Cleanser	Other Ingredients
AL	**Orabase Plain [a]** Colgate-Palmolive	paste			pectin · gelatin · carboxymethylcellulose sodium · polyethylene · mineral oil · flavors · preservative · guar · tragacanth
AL	**Orabase-B with Benzocaine [a]** Colgate-Palmolive	paste	benzocaine, 20%		plasticized hydrocarbon gel · guar · carboxymethylcellulose · tragacanth · pectin · preservatives · flavors
SL	**Oragesic** Parnell Ph'cals	solution	benzyl alcohol, 2% · menthol		water · sorbitol · sodium chloride · yerba santa · saccharin · flavor
** AL PE	**Orajel Baby** Del Ph'cals	liquid	benzocaine, 7.5%		
AL PE	**Orajel Baby** Del Ph'cals	gel	benzocaine, 7.5%		FD&C red#40 · flavor · glycerin · polyethylene glycols · saccharin sodium · sorbic acid · sorbitol
AL PE	**Orajel Baby Nighttime Formula** Del Ph'cals	gel	benzocaine, 10%		FD&C red#40 · flavor · glycerin · polyethylene glycols · saccharin sodium · sorbic acid · sorbitol
	Orajel CoverMed, Tinted Light or Medium Del Ph'cals	cream	dyclonine HCl, 1.0%		allantoin, 0.5%
	Orajel Denture [a] Del Ph'cals	gel	benzocaine, 10%		chlorothymol · FD&C red#40 · flavor · polyethylene glycols · purified water · saccharin sodium · sorbic acid · eugenol
	Orajel Maximum Strength Del Ph'cals	gel	benzocaine, 20%		clove oil · flavor · polyethylene glycols · saccharin sodium · sorbic acid
	Orajel Mouth-Aid Del Ph'cals	liquid	benzocaine, 20% · phenol, 0.5%		cetylpyridinium chloride, 0.1% · ethylcellulose
	Orajel Mouth-Aid Del Ph'cals	gel	benzocaine, 20%		zinc chloride, 0.1% · benzalkonium chloride, 0.02% · allantoin · carbomer · disodium edetate · peppermint oil · polyethylene glycol · polysorbate 60 · propyl gallate · propylene glycol · purified water · povidone · saccharin sodium · sorbic acid · stearyl alcohol
**	**Orajel P.M.** Del Ph'cals	gel	benzocaine, 20%		
	Orajel Perioseptic Spot Treatment Oral Cleanser Del Ph'cals	liquid		carbamide peroxide, 15%	citric acid · disodium edetate · flavor · methylparaben · propylene glycol · purified water · sodium chloride · saccharin sodium
**	**Orajel Perioseptic Super Cleaning Oral Rinse** Del Ph'cals	solution		hydrogen peroxide, 1.5%	ethyl alcohol, 4%
	Orajel Regular Strength Del Ph'cals	gel	benzocaine, 10%		clove oil · flavor · polyethylene glycols · saccharin sodium · sorbic acid

See Chapter 25, "Oral Health Products," for more information about these products.

ORAL DISCOMFORT PRODUCTS - continued

	Product Manufacturer/Supplier	Dosage Form	Anesthetic/ Analgesic	Debriding Agent/ Wound Cleanser	Other Ingredients
GL SL	**Peroxyl Hygienic Dental Rinse** Colgate-Palmolive	liquid		hydrogen peroxide, 1.5%	alcohol, 5% · pluronic F108 · sorbitol · saccharin sodium · dye · polysorbate 20 · mint flavor
GL SU	**Peroxyl Oral Spot Treatment** Colgate-Palmolive	gel		hydrogen peroxide, 1.5%	ethyl alcohol, 5% · mint flavor · pluronic F108 · polysorbate 20 · sorbitol · saccharin sodium · dye · pluronic F127
AL DY GL SU	**Probax [b]** Fischer Ph'cals	ointment			propolis, 2% · petrolatum · mineral oil
** DY GL SU	**Proxigel [b]** Block Drug	gel	menthol	carbamide peroxide, 10%	glycerin · carbomer · phosphoric acid · triethanolamine
	Red Cross Canker Sore Medication [b] Mentholatum	ointment	benzocaine, 20% · phenol		carbomer 974P · mineral oil · petrolatum · propylparaben
	Red Cross Toothache Medication Mentholatum	drops	eugenol, 85%		sesame oil
**	**Retre-Gel [b]** Triton Consumer	gel	benzocaine, 5% · menthol, 1%		glycerin, 20%
AL	**SensoGARD [b]** Dentco	gel	benzocaine, 20%		methylparaben · polycarbophil · polyethylene glycol 600 · propylparaben · sorbitan monooleate
	Tanac Del Ph'cals	stick	benzocaine, 7.5%		benzalkonium chloride, 0.125%
	Tanac Medicated Del Ph'cals	gel	dyclonine HCl, 1.0%		allantoin, 0.5%
	Tanac No Sting Del Ph'cals	liquid	benzocaine, 10%		benzalkonium chloride, 0.125% · saccharin
	Vaseline Lip Therapy Chesebrough-Pond's	ointment	camphor, 0.8% · menthol, 0.8% · phenol, 0.5%		white petrolatum, 93.8% · borage seed oil · sunflower seed oil · tocopheryl acetate · bisabolol · retinyl palmitate · panthenol · aloe extract · kukui nut oil · lecithin · stearic acid · corn oil · soya sterol · salicylic acid · zinc sulfate · methyl salicylate · flavor
**	**Viractin [b]** Schering-Plough Healthcare	cream · gel	tetracaine HCl, 2%		
GL	**Zilactin** Zila Ph'cals	gel	benzyl alcohol, 10%		
** AL DY GL PE	**Zilactin Baby** Zila Ph'cals	gel	benzocaine, 10%		
GL	**Zilactin-B** Zila Ph'cals	gel	benzocaine, 10%		

See Chapter 25, "Oral Health Products," for more information about these products.

ORAL DISCOMFORT PRODUCTS - continued

	Product Manufacturer/Supplier	Dosage Form	Anesthetic/ Analgesic	Debriding Agent/ Wound Cleanser	Other Ingredients
GL	**Zilactin-L** Zila Ph'cals	liquid	lidocaine, 2.5%		

** New listing

§ Manufacturer/supplier did not confirm information for this edition. Product listing is reprinted from the '96-97 edition.

[a] Carries American Dental Association (ADA) seal indicating safety and efficacy

[b] For cold sore treatment only

See Chapter 25, "Oral Health Products," for more information about these products.

ORAL HYGIENE PRODUCTS

	Product Manufacturer/Supplier	Dosage Form	Antiseptic	Other Ingredients
	Astring-O-Sol Mentholatum	liquid	SD alcohol 38-B, 75.6% · methyl salicylate	water · myrrh extract · zinc chloride · citric acid
	Betadine Mouthwash/Gargle Purdue Frederick	liquid	alcohol, 8.8%	povidone-iodine, 0.5% · glycerin · saccharin sodium · flavors
GL SU	**Cepacol Mouthwash/Gargle** J. B. Williams	liquid	alcohol, 14% · cetylpyridinium chloride, 0.05%	disodium edetate · colors · flavors · glycerin · polysorbate 80 · saccharin · sodium biphosphate · sodium phosphate · water
GL SU	**Cepacol Mouthwash/Gargle, Mint** J. B. Williams	liquid	alcohol, 14.5% · cetylpyridinium chloride, 0.05%	colors · flavors · glucono delta-lactone · glycerin · poloxamer-407 · saccharin sodium · sodium gluconate · water
	DentSure Denture Rinse, Peppermint Pfizer Consumer	liquid	alcohol, 14.4%	water · glycerin · tetrapotassium pyrophosphate · benzoic acid · poloxamer 407 · sodium benzoate · saccharin sodium
DY GL	**Dr. Tichenor's Antiseptic** Dr. G. H. Tichenor	liquid	SDA alcohol 38-B, 70%	oil of peppermint · extract of arnica · water
	Listerine [a] Warner-Lambert Consumer	liquid	alcohol, 26.9% · eucalyptol, 0.092% · thymol, 0.064% · methyl salicylate, 0.06% · menthol, 0.042%	benzoic acid · poloxamer 407 · caramel
	Listerine, Cool Mint or FreshBurst [a] Warner-Lambert Consumer	liquid	alcohol, 21.6% · eucalyptol, 0.092% · thymol, 0.064% · methyl salicylate, 0.06% · menthol, 0.042%	water · sorbitol solution · poloxamer 407 · benzoic acid · flavoring · saccharin sodium · sodium citrate · citric acid · FD&C green#3 · D&C yellow#10 (FreshBurst)
	Mentadent Mouthwash, Cool Mint or Fresh Mint Chesebrough-Pond's	liquid	alcohol, 12%	water · sorbitol · sodium bicarbonate · hydrogen peroxide · poloxamer 407 · sodium lauryl sulfate · flavor · polysorbate 20 · methyl salicylate (Cool Mint) · saccharin sodium · phosphoric acid · blue#1 · yellow#5 (Cool Mint)
	Oral-B Anti-Plaque Rinse § Oral-B Labs	liquid	alcohol, 8% · cetylpyridinium chloride	water · glycerin · saccharin sodium · methylparaben · propylparaben · FD&C blue #1 · D&C yellow #10 · poloxamer 407
	Plax Advanced Formula, Mint Sensation Pfizer Consumer	liquid	alcohol, 8.5%	water · glycerin · tetrasodium pyrophosphate · benzoic acid · flavor · poloxamer 407 · sodium benzoate · sodium lauryl sulfate · saccharin sodium · xanthan gum · FD&C blue#1
	Plax Advanced Formula, Original or SoftMINT Pfizer Consumer	liquid	alcohol, 8.5%	sodium lauryl sulfate · water · glycerin · sodium benzoate · tetrasodium pyrophosphate · benzoic acid · poloxamer 407 · saccharin sodium · SoftMINT only: flavor · xanthan gum · flavor enhancer · FD&C blue#1 · FD&C yellow#5
	S.T.37 Solution Menley & James Labs	solution	hexylresorcinol, 0.1%	glycerin · propylene glycol · citric acid · disodium edetate · sodium bisulfite · sodium citrate
** PU	**Scope, Baking Soda** Procter & Gamble	liquid	SD alcohol 38-F, 9.9% · cethylpyridinium chloride · domiphen bromide	sodium bicarbonate · saccharin sodium · sorbitol · flavor

See Chapter 25, "Oral Health Products," for more information about these products.

ORAL HYGIENE PRODUCTS - continued

	Product Manufacturer/Supplier	Dosage Form	Antiseptic	Other Ingredients
	Scope, Cool Peppermint Procter & Gamble	liquid	SD alcohol 38-F, 14% · cetylpyridinium chloride · domiphen bromide	purified water · glycerin · poloxamer 407 · saccharin sodium · sodium benzoate · N-ethylmethylcarboxamide · benzoic acid · FD&C blue#1
AL GL	**Tech 2000 Antimicrobial Rinse** Care-Tech Labs	liquid	cetylpyridinium chloride	water · glycerin · poloxamer 407 · flavor · FD&C blue#1 · FD&C yellow#5 · nutritive dextrose or sucrose and/or calcium saccharin
AL	**Tom's Natural Mouthwash, Cinnamon or Spearmint** Tom's of Maine	liquid	menthol	water · glycerin · aloe vera juice · witch hazel · poloxamer 335 · spearmint oil · ascorbic acid
	Viadent Oral Rinse Colgate-Palmolive	liquid	alcohol, 10%	zinc chloride, 0.2% · glycerin · polysorbate 80 · flavor · saccharin sodium · poloxamer 237 · citric acid · sanguinaria extract

** New listing
§ Manufacturer/supplier did not confirm information for this edition. Product listing is reprinted from the '96-97 edition.
[a] Carries American Dental Association (ADA) seal indicating safety and efficacy

See Chapter 25, "Oral Health Products," for more information about these products.

TOPICAL FLUORIDE PRODUCTS

	Product Manufacturer/Supplier	Dosage Form	Therapeutic Agent	Other Ingredients
** PE	**Fluoride Foam [a]** Laclede Research Labs	foam	fluoride, 1.23% (from sodium fluoride and hydrogen fluoride)	water · phosphoric acid · poloxamer · saccharin sodium · flavor
DY GL	**Fluorigard Anti-Cavity [a]** Colgate-Palmolive	liquid	sodium fluoride, 0.05%	ethyl alcohol · pluronic F108, F127 · sweetener · flavor · glycerin · sorbitol · preservatives
	Oral-B Anti-Cavity [a] § Oral-B Labs	liquid	sodium fluoride, 0.05%	water · sodium benzoate · potassium sorbate · saccharin sodium · glycerin · PEG-40 · FD&C blue#1 · phosphoric acid
AL	**Reach Act Adult Anti-Cavity Treatment, Cinnamon §** Johnson & Johnson Consumer	liquid	sodium fluoride, 0.05%	cetylpyridinium chloride · D&C red#33 · edetate calcium disodium · FD&C yellow#5 · flavors · glycerin · monobasic sodium phosphate · dibasic sodium phosphate · poloxamer 407 · polysorbate 80 · propylene glycol · sodium benzoate · saccharin sodium · water
AL	**Reach Act Adult Anti-Cavity Treatment, Mint §** Johnson & Johnson Consumer	liquid	sodium fluoride, 0.05%	cetylpyridinium chloride · edetate calcium disodium · FD&C green#3 · FD&C yellow#5 · flavor · glycerin · menthol · methyl salicylate · monobasic sodium phosphate · dibasic sodium phosphate · poloxamer 407 · polysorbate 20 · potassium sorbate · propylene glycol · sodium benzoate · saccharin sodium · water
AL PE	**Reach Act for Kids [a] §** Johnson & Johnson Consumer	liquid	sodium fluoride, 0.05%	cetylpyridinium chloride · D&C red#33 · dibasic sodium phosphate · edetate calcium disodium · flavors · glycerin · monobasic sodium phosphate · poloxamer 407 · polysorbate 80 · propylene glycol · sodium benzoate · saccharin sodium · water

** New listing

§ Manufacturer/supplier did not confirm information for this edition. Product listing is reprinted from the '96-97 edition.

[a] Carries American Dental Association (ADA) seal indicating safety and efficacy

See Chapter 25, "Oral Health Products," for more information about these products.

DENTIFRICE PRODUCTS

Product Manufacturer/Supplier	Dosage Form	Abrasive Ingredient	Therapeutic Ingredient	Foaming Agent	Other Ingredients [b]
Aim Anti Tartar Formula Cheseborough-Pond's	gel	hydrated silica	sodium fluoride, 0.23%	sodium lauryl sulfate	sorbitol and related polyols · water · glycerin · zinc citrate trihydrate · SD alcohol 38B · flavor · xanthan gum · saccharin sodium · sodium benzoate · blue#1 · yellow#10
Aim Baking Soda Cheseborough-Pond's	gel	hydrated silica · sodium bicarbonate	sodium fluoride, 0.23%	sodium lauryl sulfate	sorbitol and related polyols · water · glycerin · SD alcohol 38B · flavor · xanthan gum · saccharin sodium · sodium benzoate · blue#1 · yellow#10
Aim Extra Strength [a] Cheseborough-Pond's	gel	hydrated silica	sodium monofluorophosphate, 1.2%	sodium lauryl sulfate	sorbitol and other related polyols · water · glycerin · SD alcohol 38B · flavor · xanthan gum · saccharin sodium · sodium benzoate · blue #1 · yellow #10
Aim Regular Strength Cheseborough-Pond's	gel	hydrated silica	sodium fluoride, 0.23%	sodium lauryl sulfate	sorbitol and other related polyols · water · glycerin · SD alcohol 38B · flavor · xanthan gum · saccharin sodium · sodium benzoate · blue #1 · yellow #10
Aquafresh Baking Soda SmithKline Beecham	paste	calcium carbonate · hydrated silica · sodium bicarbonate	sodium monofluorophosphate	sodium lauryl sulfate	calcium carrageenan · cellulose gum · colors · flavor · glycerin · PEG-8 · sodium benzoate · saccharin sodium · sorbitol · titanium dioxide · water
Aquafresh Extra Fresh [a] SmithKline Beecham	paste	hydrated silica · calcium carbonate	sodium monofluorophosphate	sodium lauryl sulfate	sorbitol · water · glycerin · PEG-8 · titanium dioxide · cellulose gum · flavor · saccharin sodium · sodium benzoate · calcium carrageenan · colors
Aquafresh for Kids [a] SmithKline Beecham	paste	hydrated silica · calcium carbonate	sodium monofluorophosphate	sodium lauryl sulfate	sorbitol · water · glycerin · PEG-8 · titanium dioxide · cellulose gum · flavor · saccharin sodium · calcium carrageenan · sodium benzoate · colors
** **Aquafresh Gum Care** SmithKline Beecham	paste	calcium carbonate	sodium monofluorophosphate (fluoride, 0.15%)		calcium carrageenan · calcium glycerophosphate
Aquafresh Sensitive SmithKline Beecham	paste	hydrated silica	potassium nitrate · sodium fluoride	sodium lauryl sulfate	colors · flavors · glycerin · sodium benzoate · saccharin sodium · sorbitol · titanium dioxide · water · xanthan gum
Aquafresh Tartar Control [a] SmithKline Beecham	paste	hydrated silica	sodium fluoride	sodium lauryl sulfate	tetrapotassium pyrophosphate · tetrasodium pyrophosphate · sorbitol · glycerin · PEG-8 · flavor · xanthan gum · saccharin sodium · sodium benzoate · D&C red#30 lake · FD&C blue#1 · D&C yellow#10 · titanium dioxide · water

See Chapter 25, "Oral Health Products," for more information about these products.

DENTIFRICE PRODUCTS - continued

Product Manufacturer/Supplier	Dosage Form	Abrasive Ingredient	Therapeutic Ingredient	Foaming Agent	Other Ingredients [b]
Aquafresh Triple Protection [a] SmithKline Beecham	paste	hydrated silica · calcium carbonate	sodium monofluorophosphate	sodium lauryl sulfate	PEG-8 · sorbitol · cellulose gum · sodium benzoate · titanium dioxide · calcium carrageenan · flavor · saccharin sodium · colors · water
Aquafresh Whitening SmithKline Beecham	paste	hydrated silica	sodium fluoride	sodium lauryl sulfate	D&C yellow#10 · FD&C blue#1 · flavor · glycerin · PEG-8 · sodium benzoate · sodium hydroxide · saccharin sodium · sodium tripolyphosphate · sorbitol · titanium dioxide · water · xanthan gum
DY **Arm & Hammer Dental Care §** Church & Dwight	paste	sodium bicarbonate	sodium fluoride	sodium lauryl sulfate	water · glycerin · saccharin sodium · PEG-8 · flavor blend · cellulose gum · sodium lauryl sarcosinate
Arm & Hammer Dental Care § Church & Dwight	gel	hydrated silica · sodium bicarbonate	sodium fluoride	sodium lauryl sulfate	sorbitol · glycerin · water · flavor blend · cellulose gum · sodium lauryl sarcosinate · saccharin sodium · FD&C blue#1 · FD&C yellow#5
Arm & Hammer Dental Care Tartar Control § Church & Dwight	paste	sodium bicarbonate	sodium fluoride	sodium lauryl sulfate	water · glycerin · sodium pyrophosphates · saccharin sodium · PEG-8 · flavor blend · sodium phosphates · cellulose gum · sodium lauryl sarcosinate
Arm & Hammer Dental Care Tartar Control § Church & Dwight	gel	sodium bicarbonate · hydrated silica	sodium fluoride	sodium lauryl sulfate	water · sorbitol · glycerin · sodium pyrophosphates · flavor · cellulose gum · saccharin sodium · sodium lauryl sarcosinate · FD&C blue#1 · FD&C yellow#5
DY **Arm & Hammer Dental Care Toothpowder §** Church & Dwight	powder	sodium bicarbonate	sodium fluoride		mint flavor · saccharin sodium · trisodium phosphate · magnesium oxide · PEG-8
DY SU **Arm & Hammer PeroxiCare §** Church & Dwight	paste	sodium bicarbonate · silica	sodium fluoride	sodium carbonate peroxide · sodium lauryl sulfate	PEG-8 · poloxamer 338 · flavor · water · saccharin sodium · sodium lauryl sarcosinate
** **Biotène Dry Mouth Toothpaste** Laclede Research Labs	paste	hydrated silica · calcium pyrophosphate	sodium monoflourophosphate, 0.76% · glucose oxidase · lysozyme · lactoperoxidase		glycerin · sorbitol · cellulose gum · sodium benzoate · xylitol · flavor · isoceteth-20 · potassium thiocyanate · beta-d-glucose
Caffree Anti-Stain [a] Block Drug	paste	diatomaceous earth · aluminum silicate	sodium monofluorophosphate	sodium lauryl sulfate	water · glycerin · sorbitol · titanium dioxide · hydroxyethyl cellulose · flavor · saccharin sodium · methylparaben · propylparaben

See Chapter 25, "Oral Health Products," for more information about these products.

DENTIFRICE PRODUCTS - continued

	Product Manufacturer/Supplier	Dosage Form	Abrasive Ingredient	Therapeutic Ingredient	Foaming Agent	Other Ingredients [b]
	Close-Up Anti-Plaque Chesebrough-Pond's	gel	hydrated silica	stannous fluoride, 0.41%	sodium lauryl sulfate	sorbitol · water · PEG-32 · SD alcohol 38B · flavor · zinc citrate trihydrate · cellulose gum · saccharin sodium · sodium benzoate · sodium hydroxide · blue #1
	Close-Up Baking Soda Chesebrough-Pond's	paste	hydrated silica · sodium bicarbonate	sodium monofluorophosphate, 0.79% (fluoride, 0.15%)	sodium lauryl sulfate	sorbitol and related polyols · water · glycerin · SD alcohol 38B · flavor · cellulose gum · saccharin sodium · sodium benzoate · red#33 · red#40 · titanium dioxide
	Close-Up Crystal Clear, Mint Chesebrough-Pond's	gel	hydrated silica	sodium monofluorophosphate, 0.79% (fluoride, 0.15%)	sodium lauryl sulfate	sorbitol · water · glycerin · SD alcohol 38B · cellulose gum · saccharin sodium · polysorbate 20 · sodium benzoate · sodium chloride · blue#1 · mica · red#33 · titanium dioxide
	Close-Up Original Chesebrough-Pond's	gel	hydrated silica	sodium fluoride, 0.23%	sodium lauryl sulfate	sorbitol and other related polyols · water · glycerin · SD alcohol 38B · flavor · xanthan gum · saccharin sodium · sodium benzoate · sodium chloride · red #33 · red #40
	Close-Up Tartar Control Chesebrough-Pond's	gel	hydrated silica	sodium monofluorophosphate, 0.79% (fluoride, 0.15%)	sodium lauryl sulfate	sorbitol and related polyols · water · glycerin · zinc citrate trihydrate · SD alcohol 38B · flavor · cellulose gum · saccharin sodium · sodium benzoate · sodium chloride · red#33 · red#40
SU	**Colgate [a]** Colgate-Palmolive	paste	dicalcium phosphate dihydrate	sodium monofluorophosphate, 0.76%	sodium lauryl sulfate	glycerin · cellulose gum · tetrasodium pyrophosphate · saccharin sodium · flavor
SU	**Colgate Baking Soda & Peroxide Tartar Control [a]** Colgate-Palmolive	paste	hydrated silica · sodium bicarbonate	sodium monofluorophosphate, 0.76%	sodium lauryl sulfate	glycerin · propylene glycol · water · potassium triphosphate · tetrasodium pyrophosphate · titanium dioxide · flavor · sodium hydroxide · calcium peroxide · saccharin sodium · carrageenan · cellulose gum · FD&C blue#1 · D&C yellow #10
** SU	**Colgate Baking Soda & Peroxide Whitening** Colgate-Palmolive	paste	hydrated silica · sodium bicarbonate · aluminum oxide	sodium monofluorophosphate, 0.76%	sodium lauryl sulfate	glycerin · propylene glycol · water · potassium triphosphate · tetrasodium pyrophosphate · titanium dioxide · flavor · sodium hydroxide · calcium peroxide · saccharin sodium · carrageenan · cellulose gum · FD&C blue#1 · D&C yellow#10

See Chapter 25, "Oral Health Products," for more information about these products.

DENTIFRICE PRODUCTS - continued

	Product Manufacturer/Supplier	Dosage Form	Abrasive Ingredient	Therapeutic Ingredient	Foaming Agent	Other Ingredients [b]
	Colgate Baking Soda [a] Colgate-Palmolive	gel	hydrated silica · sodium bicarbonate	sodium fluoride, 0.243%	sodium lauryl sulfate	glycerin · water · PEG-12 · cellulose gum · flavor · saccharin sodium · FD&C blue#1 · D&C yellow#10
SU	**Colgate Baking Soda [a]** Colgate-Palmolive	paste	hydrated silica · sodium bicarbonate	sodium fluoride, 0.243%	sodium lauryl sulfate	glycerin · water · PEG-12 · cellulose gum · titanium dioxide · flavor · saccharin sodium
SU	**Colgate Baking Soda Tartar Control** Colgate-Palmolive	gel · paste	hydrated silica · sodium bicarbonate	sodium fluoride, 0.243%	sodium lauryl sulfate	glycerin · tetrasodium pyrophosphate · PVM/MA copolymer · cellulose gum · flavor · saccharin sodium · sodium hydroxide · titanium dioxide (paste) · FD&C blue#1 & D&C yellow#10 (gel)
SU PE	**Colgate Junior [a]** Colgate-Palmolive	gel	hydrated silica	sodium fluoride, 0.243%	sodium lauryl sulfate	sorbitol · water · PEG-12 · cellulose gum · tetrasodium pyrophosphate · flavor · saccharin sodium · mica · titanium dioxide · colorants
	Colgate Platinum Whitening Colgate-Palmolive	paste	silica · aluminum oxide	sodium monofluorophosphate, 0.76%	sodium lauryl sulfate	water · hydrated silica · sorbitol · glycerin · PEG-12 · tetrapotassium pyrophosphate · PVM/MA copolymer · flavor · sodium hydroxide · saccharin sodium · titanium dioxide
**	**Colgate Platinum Whitening with Baking Soda** Colgate-Palmolive	paste	sodium bicarbonate · aluminum oxide	sodium monofluorophosphate	sodium lauryl sulfate	water · glycerin · PEG-12 · tetrapotassium pyrophosphate · PVM/MA copolymer · cellulose gum · flavor · sodium hydroxide · saccharin sodium · titanium dioxide
SU	**Colgate Tartar Control Micro Cleansing Formula [a]** Colgate-Palmolive	gel · paste	hydrated silica	sodium fluoride, 0.243%	sodium lauryl sulfate	water · sorbitol · glycerin · PEG-12 · tetrasodium pyrophosphate · PVM/MA copolymer · cellulose gum · flavor · sodium hydroxide · titanium dioxide (paste) · saccharin sodium · carrageenan · FD&C blue#1 (gel)
SU	**Colgate Winterfresh [a]** Colgate-Palmolive	gel	hydrated silica	sodium fluoride, 0.243%	sodium lauryl sulfate	sorbitol · glycerin · PEG-12 · flavor · tetrasodium pyrophosphate · cellulose gum · saccharin sodium · FD&C blue#1
	Crest Baking Soda Tartar Control, Mint [a] Procter & Gamble	gel · paste	hydrated silica · sodium bicarbonate	sodium fluoride, 0.243%	sodium lauryl sulfate	water · glycerin · sorbitol · tetrasodium pyrophosphate · PEG-6 · sodium carbonate · flavor · cellulose gum · saccharin sodium · titanium dioxide (paste) · FD&C blue#1 (gel)

See Chapter 25, "Oral Health Products," for more information about these products.

DENTIFRICE PRODUCTS - continued

	Product Manufacturer/Supplier	Dosage Form	Abrasive Ingredient	Therapeutic Ingredient	Foaming Agent	Other Ingredients [b]
	Crest Baking Soda, Mint [a] Procter & Gamble	gel · paste	hydrated silica · sodium bicarbonate	sodium fluoride, 0.243%	sodium lauryl sulfate	sorbitol · water · glycerin · sodium carbonate · flavor · cellulose gum · saccharin sodium · titanium dioxide (paste) · FD&C blue#1 (gel)
	Crest Cavity Fighting, Cool Mint [a] Procter & Gamble	gel	hydrated silica	sodium fluoride, 0.243%	sodium lauryl sulfate	sorbitol · water · trisodium phosphate · flavor · sodium phosphate · xanthan gum · saccharin sodium · carbomer 956 · FD&C blue#1
	Crest Cavity Fighting, Icy Mint or Regular [a] Procter & Gamble	paste	hydrated silica	sodium fluoride, 0.243%	sodium lauryl sulfate	sorbitol · water · glycerin · Mint · trisodium phosphate · flavor · sodium phosphate · cellulose gum (Mint) · xanthan gum (Regular) · saccharin sodium · carbomer 956 · titanium dioxide · FD&C blue#1
PE	**Crest for Kids, Sparkle Fun [a]** Procter & Gamble	gel	hydrated silica	sodium fluoride, 0.243%	sodium lauryl sulfate	sorbitol · water · trisodium phosphate · sodium phosphate · xanthan gum · flavor · saccharin sodium · carbomer 956 · mica · titanium dioxide · FD&C blue#1
	Crest Gum Care Procter & Gamble	gel · paste	hydrated silica	stannous fluoride, 0.454%	sodium lauryl sulfate	sorbitol · water · saccharin sodium · sodium gluconate · stannous chloride · titanium dioxide (paste) · sodium hydroxide · hydroxyethyl cellulose · carrageenan · flavor · FD&C blue#1 (gel)
**	**Crest MultiCare** Procter & Gamble	gel/paste	sodium bicarbonate	sodium fluoride		tetrasodium pyrophosphate · xylitol
DY	**Crest Sensitivity Protection, Mild Mint [a]** Procter & Gamble	paste	hydrated silica	potassium nitrate, 5% · sodium fluoride, 0.243%	sodium lauryl sulfate	water · glycerin · sorbitol · trisodium phosphate · cellulose gum · flavor · xanthan gum · saccharin sodium · titanium dioxide
	Crest Tartar Control, Fresh Mint or Smooth Mint [a] Procter & Gamble	gel	hydrated silica	sodium fluoride, 0.243%	sodium lauryl sulfate	water · sorbitol · glycerin · tetrapotassium pyrophosphate · PEG-6 · disodium pyrophosphate · tetrasodium pyrophosphate · flavor · xanthan gum · saccharin sodium · carbomer 956 · FD&C blue#1 · FD&C yellow#5 (Smooth Mint)

See Chapter 25, "Oral Health Products," for more information about these products.

DENTIFRICE PRODUCTS - continued

	Product Manufacturer/Supplier	Dosage Form	Abrasive Ingredient	Therapeutic Ingredient	Foaming Agent	Other Ingredients [b]
	Crest Tartar Control, Original Flavor [a] Procter & Gamble	paste	hydrated silica	sodium fluoride, 0.243%	sodium lauryl sulfate	water · sorbitol · glycerin · tetrapotassium pyrophosphate · PEG-6 · disodium pyrophosphate · tetrasodium pyrophosphate · flavor · xanthan gum · saccharin sodium · carbomer 956 · titanium dioxide · FD&C blue#1
DY	**Dr. Tichenor's Toothpaste** Dr. G. H. Tichenor	paste	hydrated silica	sodium fluoride	sodium lauryl sulfate	sorbitol · water · glycerin · insoluble sodium metaphosphate · peppermint oil · cellulose gum · saccharin sodium · sodium phosphate · titanium dioxide · magnesium aluminum silicate
** PE	**First Teeth Baby Toothpaste** Laclede Research Labs	gel		lactoperoxidase, 0.7 U/gm · lactoferrin · glucose oxidase		glycerin · water ·sorbitol · pectin · xylitol · flavor · aloe vera · propylene glycol
DY	**Gleem** Procter & Gamble	paste	hydrated silica	sodium fluoride, 0.243%	sodium lauryl sulfate	sorbitol · water · trisodium phosphate · flavor · sodium phosphate · xanthan gum · saccharin sodium · carbomer 956 · titanium dioxide
	Interplak Bausch & Lomb	paste	hydrated silica	sodium fluoride	sodium lauryl sulfate	purified water · poloxamer 407 · sorbitol · glycerin · flavor · dibasic sodium phosphate · saccharin sodium · monobasic sodium phosphate · sodium benzoate · D&C yellow#10
**	**Listerine Toothpaste Tartar Control, Cool Mint** Warner-Lambert Consumer	gel · paste	hydrated silica	sodium fluoride	sodium lauryl sulfate	sorbitol · water · glycerin · PEG-32 · tetrapotassium pyrophosphate · flavors (gel) · saccharin sodium · cellulose gum · FD&C blue#1 · D&C yellow#10
	Listerine Toothpaste, Cool Mint Warner-Lambert Consumer	paste	hydrated silica	sodium monofluorophosphate	sodium lauryl sulfate	sorbitol · water · glycerin · flavors · saccharin sodium · cellulose gum · xanthan gum · phosphoric acid · titanium dioxide · sodium phosphate · benzoic acid · FD&C blue#1 · D&C yellow#10
	Listerine Toothpaste, Cool Mint Warner-Lambert Consumer	gel	hydrated silica	sodium monofluorophosphate	sodium lauryl sulfate	sorbitol · glycerin · flavors · saccharin sodium · cellulose gum · xanthan gum · phosphoric acid · sodium phosphate · benzoic acid · FD&C blue#1 · D&C yellow#10 · water
	Mentadent Gum Care Chesebrough-Pond's	gel · paste	hydrated silica · sodium bicarbonate	sodium fluoride, 0.15%	sodium lauryl sulfate · hydrogen peroxide	zinc citrate trihydrate, 2% · water · glycerin · sorbitol · poloxamer 407 · PEG-32 · SD alcohol 38B · menthol · methyl salicylate · cellulose gum · saccharin sodium · phosphoric acid · green#3 · titanium dioxide

See Chapter 25, "Oral Health Products," for more information about these products.

DENTIFRICE PRODUCTS - continued

	Product Manufacturer/Supplier	Dosage Form	Abrasive Ingredient	Therapeutic Ingredient	Foaming Agent	Other Ingredients [b]
	Mentadent Tartar Control Chesebrough-Pond's	gel · paste	hydrated silica · sodium bicarbonate	sodium fluoride, 0.24%	sodium lauryl sulfate · hydrogen peroxide	sorbitol syrup · water · glycerol · poloxamer 407 · PEG-32 · zinc citrate · SD alcohol 38B · flavor · cellulose gum · menthol · saccharin sodium · titanium dioxide · phosphoric acid · FD&C blue#1
	Mentadent with Baking Soda & Peroxide [a] Chesebrough-Pond's	paste	hydrated silica · sodium bicarbonate	sodium fluoride, 0.24% (fluoride, 0.15%)	sodium lauryl sulfate · hydrogen peroxide	water · sorbitol · glycerin · poloxamer 407 · PEG- 32 · SD alcohol 38B · flavor · cellulose gum · saccharin sodium · phosphoric acid · blue#1 · titanium dioxide
SU	**Natural White** Natural White	paste	hydrated silica	sodium fluoride	sodium lauryl sulfate	sorbitol · water · glycerin · titanium dioxide · cellulose gum · flavor · sodium benzoate
** SU	**Natural White Baking Soda** Natural White	paste	calcium carbonate	sodium monofluorophosphate	sodium lauryl sulfate	sorbitol · water · glycerin · sodium bicarbonate · carrageenan · natural flavors
** SU	**Natural White Fights Plaque** Natural White	paste	hydrated silica	sodium fluoride	sodium lauryl sulfate	glycerin · water · sorbitol · titanium dioxide · flavor · cellulose gum · sodium benzoate
** SU	**Natural White Sensitive** Natural White	paste	hydrated silica	sodium monofluorophosphate · potassium nitrate	sodium lauryl sulfate	sorbitol · water · glycerin · flavor · xanthan gum · sodium benzoate · titanium dioxide · saccharin sodium · FD&C red#40
SU	**Natural White Tartar Control** Natural White	paste	hydrated silica	sodium fluoride	sodium lauryl sulfate	sorbitol · water · glycerin · tetrapotassium pyrophosphate · titanium dioxide · cellulose gum · flavor · sodium benzoate · FD&C blue#1 · D&C yellow#10
** SU	**Natural White with Peroxide** Natural White	gel		hydrogen peroxide		water · glycerin · flavor · dipotassium phophate · saccharin sodium · phosphoric acid · poloxamer
PE	**Orajel Baby Tooth & Gum Cleanser** Del Ph'cals	gel				poloxamer 407, 2% · simethicone, 0.12% · Microdent · carboxymethylcellulose · sodium · citric acid · flavor · glycerin · methylparaben · potassium sorbate · propylene glycol · propylparaben · water · saccharin sodium · sorbitol
	Oral-B Sensitive § Oral-B Labs	paste	hydrated silica	potassium nitrate, 5% · sodium fluoride, 0.243%	sodium lauryl sulfate	sorbitol · water · glycerin · PEG-8 · trisodium phosphate · flavor · cellulose gum · titanium dioxide · saccharin sodium

See Chapter 25, "Oral Health Products," for more information about these products.

DENTIFRICE PRODUCTS - continued

Product Manufacturer/Supplier	Dosage Form	Abrasive Ingredient	Therapeutic Ingredient	Foaming Agent	Other Ingredients [b]
Oral-B Sesame Street, Bubblegum or Fruity [a] § Oral-B Labs	paste	hydrated silica	sodium fluoride, 0.248%	sodium lauryl sulfate	sorbitol · water · glycerin · acesulfame K · flavor · xanthan gum · carbomer · sodium hydroxide · FD&C red#3
Oral-B Tooth and Gum Care § Oral-B Labs	paste	calcium pyrophosphate	stannous fluoride, 0.454%	sodium lauryl sulfate	sorbitol · water · glycerin · flavor · xanthan gum · PVM/MA copolymer · PEG-8 · zinc citrate · carbomer · saccharin sodium · sodium hydroxide
DY SU **Pearl Drops Whitening Baking Soda Tartar Control** Carter Products	paste	sodium bicarbonate · hydrated silica	sodium fluoride	sodium lauryl sulfate	water · sorbitol · glycerin · tetrapotassium pyrophosphate · tetrasodium pyrophosphate · PEG-12 · flavor · titanium dioxide · saccharin sodium · cellulose gum
DY SU **Pearl Drops Whitening Extra Strength** Carter Products	paste	hydrated silica · calcium pyrophosphate · dicalcium phosphate	sodium monofluorophosphate	sodium lauryl sulfate	water · sorbitol · glycerin · PEG-12 · flavor · titanium dioxide · cellulose gum · trisodium phosphate · sodium phosphate · saccharin sodium
DY SU **Pearl Drops Whitening Regular Tartar Control** Carter Products	paste	hydrated silica	sodium fluoride	sodium lauryl sulfate	water · sorbitol · glycerin · tetrapotassium pyrophosphate · tetrasodium pyrophosphate · PEG-12 · flavor · titanium dioxide · cellulose gum · saccharin sodium
** SU **Pearl Drops Whitening Toothpolish** Carter Products	gel	hydrated silica	sodium fluoride	sodium lauryl sulfate	water · sorbitol · glycerin · tetrapotassium pyrophosphate · tetrasodium pyrophosphate · PEG-12 · flavor · saccharin · cellulose gum · FD&C blue#1 · D&C yellow#10
** SU **Pearl Drops Whitening Toothpolish, Icy Cool Mint** Carter Products	gel	hydrated silica	sodium fluoride	sodium lauryl sulfate	water · sorbitol · glycerin · tetrapotassium pyrophosphate · tetrasodium pyrophosphate · PEG-12 · flavor · cellulose gum · saccharin sodium · FD&C blue#1 · D&C yellow#10
DY SU **Pearl Drops Whitening Toothpolish, Spearmint** Carter Products	paste	calcium pyrophosphate · hydrated silica · aluminum hydroxide · dicalcium phosphate	sodium monofluorophosphate	sodium lauryl sulfate	water · sorbitol · glycerin · flavor · PEG-12 · titanium dioxide · cellulose gum · trisodium phosphate · sodium phosphate · saccharin sodium
Pepsodent Baking Soda Chesebrough-Pond's	paste	hydrated silica	sodium fluoride, 0.24%	sodium lauryl sulfate	sorbitol · water · sodium bicarbonate · PEG-32 · SD alcohol 38B · flavor · xanthan gum · saccharin sodium · titanium dioxide

See Chapter 25, "Oral Health Products," for more information about these products.

DENTIFRICE PRODUCTS - continued

Product Manufacturer/Supplier	Dosage Form	Abrasive Ingredient	Therapeutic Ingredient	Foaming Agent	Other Ingredients [b]
Pepsodent Original Chesebrough-Pond's	paste	hydrated silica	sodium fluoride, 0.23%	sodium lauryl sulfate	sorbitol and related polyols · water · glycerin · SD alcohol 38B · flavor · xanthan gum · saccharin sodium · sodium benzoate · titanium dioxide
** PE **Pete & Pam Toothpaste Pre-measured Strips** Laclede Research Labs	gel	hydrated silica	sodium monoflourophosphate, 0.76%	sodium lauryl sarcosinate	sorbitol · water · glycerin · xanthan gum · polysorbate 20 · flavor · sodium benzoate · xylitol · pluronic P-84 · FD&C blue#1 · FD&C red#33 · FD&C yellow#5
Promise Block Drug	paste	dicalcium phosphate	potassium nitrate · sodium monofluorophosphate	sodium lauryl sulfate	water · hydroxyethyl cellulose · flavor · saccharin sodium · methylparaben · propylparaben · D&C yellow#10 · FD&C blue#1 · glycerin · sorbitol · silicon dioxide
Rembrandt Whitening Baking Soda Rembrandt	paste	sodium bicarbonate · silica	sodium monofluorophosphate (fluoride, 0.15%)	sodium lauryl sulfate	glycerin · sorbitol · alumina · water · sodium citrate · sodium carrageenan · papain · flavor · sodium hydroxide · FD&C blue#1 · saccharin sodium
DY **Rembrandt Whitening Natural** Rembrandt	paste	dicalcium phosphate · silica	sodium monofluorophosphate		glycerin · xylitol · water · sodium citrate · natural flavors · papain · sodium carrageenan · citric acid
Rembrandt Whitening Sensitive Rembrandt	paste	dicalcium phosphate dihydrate	potassium nitrate, 5% · sodium monofluorophosphate, 0.76%	sodium lauryl sulfate	glycerin · sorbitol · water · alumina · papain · sodium citrate · flavor · carboxymethylcellulose sodium · saccharin sodium · methylparaben · citric acid · FD&C red#40
Rembrandt Whitening, Mint or Original Rembrandt	paste	dicalcium phosphate dihydrate	sodium monofluorophosphate, 0.76%	sodium lauryl sulfate	glycerin · sorbitol · water · alumina · sodium citrate · flavor · sodium carrageenan · papain · saccharin sodium · methylparaben · citric acid · FD&C blue#1 · FD&C yellow#5
Rembrandt with Peroxide Rembrandt	gel		sodium monofluorophosphate	carbamide peroxide · sodium lauryl sulfate	glycerin · sodium citrate · carbomer · titanium dioxide · flavor · triethanolamine
DY **Revelation** Alvin Last	powder	calcium carbonate		vegetable soap powder	methyl salicylate · menthol
DY **Sensodyne Baking Soda** Dentco	paste	silica · sodium bicarbonate	potassium nitrate · sodium fluoride	sodium lauryl sulfate	water · glycerin · flavor · hydroxyethyl cellulose · titanium dioxide · saccharin sodium
** **Sensodyne Original Flavor** Dentco	paste	calcium carbonate · silica	sodium monoflurophosphate · potassium nitrate	sodium methyl cocoyl taurate	water · glycerin · sorbitol · cellulose gum · flavor · PEG-40 stearate · titanium dioxide · sacchrin sodium · D&C red#28

See Chapter 25, "Oral Health Products," for more information about these products.

DENTIFRICE PRODUCTS - continued

	Product Manufacturer/Supplier	Dosage Form	Abrasive Ingredient	Therapeutic Ingredient	Foaming Agent	Other Ingredients [b]
** DY	**Sensodyne Tartar Control** Dentco	paste	hydrated silica · silica · sodium bicarbonate	sodium fluoride · potassium nitrate	cocamidopropyl betaine	water · glycerin · cellulose gum · flavor · saccharin sodium · tetrasodium pyrophosphate · titanium dioxide
	Sensodyne, Cool Gel Dentco	gel	silica	potassium nitrate · sodium fluoride	sodium methyl cocoyl taurate	water · sorbitol · glycerin · sodium carboxyethylcellulose · flavor · saccharin sodium · FD&C blue#1 · trisodium phosphate
	Sensodyne, Fresh Mint [a] Dentco	paste	dicalcium phosphate	potassium nitrate · sodium monofluorophosphate	sodium lauryl sulfate	water · glycerin · sorbitol · hydroxyethyl cellulose · flavor · saccharin sodium · methylparaben · propylparaben · D&C yellow#10 · FD&C blue#1 · silicon dioxide
SU PE	**Slimer** Perio Products	gel	hydrated silica	sodium fluoride, 0.15%		sorbitol · water · glycerin · PEG-32 · flavor · ethyl alcohol · propylene glycol · glyceryl triacetate · cellulose gum · saccharin sodium · sodium benzoate · FD&C blue#1 · FD&C red#33
	Thermodent Lee Consumer	paste	diatomaceous earth · silica	strontium chloride hexahydrate	sodium methyl cocoyl taurate	sorbitol · glycerin · titanium dioxide · guar gum · PEG-40 stearate · hydroxyethyl cellulose · flavor · preservative · water
FL	**Tom's Natural Baking Soda with Propolis & Myrrh** Tom's of Maine	paste	calcium carbonate · sodium bicarbonate		sodium lauryl sulfate	glycerin · water · carrageenan · peppermint oil · myrrh · propolis
PE	**Tom's Natural for Children, with Calcium & Fluoride** Tom's of Maine	paste	calcium carbonate · hydrated silica	sodium monofluorophosphate	sodium lauryl sulfate	glycerin · water · fruit extracts · carrageenan
	Tom's Natural with Baking Soda, Calcium, & Fluoride Tom's of Maine	paste	calcium carbonate · sodium bicarbonate	sodium monofluorophosphate	sodium lauryl sulfate	glycerin · water · carrageenan · xylitol · peppermint oil
	Tom's Natural with Calcium & Fluoride Tom's of Maine	paste	calcium carbonate · hydrated silica	sodium monofluorophosphate	sodium lauryl sulfate	glycerin · water · xylitol · carrageenan · natural wintergreen oil
	Tom's Natural with Calcium & Fluoride [a] Tom's of Maine	paste	calcium carbonate	sodium monofluorophosphate	sodium lauryl sulfate	glycerin · water · xylitol (Spearmint) · carrageenan · either cinnamon, fennel oil or spearmint · peppermint oil (Cinnamon, Spearmint)
FL	**Tom's Natural with Propolis & Myrrh** Tom's of Maine	paste	calcium carbonate		sodium lauryl sulfate	glycerin · water · carrageenan · spearmint, peppermint, cassia, or fennel oil · myrrh · propolis

See Chapter 25, "Oral Health Products," for more information about these products.

DENTIFRICE PRODUCTS - continued

Product Manufacturer/Supplier	Dosage Form	Abrasive Ingredient	Therapeutic Ingredient	Foaming Agent	Other Ingredients [b]
Toothpaste Booster Dental Concepts	paste			hydrogen peroxide · sodium lauryl sulfate	deionized water · corn starch · sorbitol · propylene glycol · carbomer 940 · menthol · sodium benzoate · potassium sorbate
SU **Ultra Brite** Colgate-Palmolive	paste	hydrated silica · alumina	sodium monofluorophosphate, 0.76%	sodium lauryl sulfate	glycerin · sorbitol · cellulose gum · carrageenan gum · titanium dioxide · saccharin sodium · flavor · tetrasodium pyrophosphate
Ultra Brite [a] Colgate-Palmolive	gel	hydrated silica	sodium monofluorophosphate, 0.76%	sodium lauryl sulfate	sorbitol · PEG-12 · flavor · cellulose gum · saccharin sodium · glycerin · FD&C blue#1 · D&C red#33
SU **Ultra Brite Baking Soda** Colgate-Palmolive	paste	hydrated silica · sodium bicarbonate · alumina	sodium monofluorophosphate, 0.76%	sodium lauryl sulfate	glycerin · sorbitol · cellulose gum · flavor · saccharin sodium · titanium dioxide
** SU **Ultra Brite Baking Soda & Peroxide** Colgate-Palmolive	paste	hydrated silica · alumina · sodium bicarbonate	sodium monofluorophosphate, 0.76%	sodium lauryl sulfate	water · glycerin · sorbitol · flavor · cellulose gum · titanium dioxide · saccharin sodium
Viadent Fluoride Colgate-Palmolive	paste	hydrated silica	sodium monofluorophosphate, 0.8%	sodium lauryl sulfate	sorbitol · titanium dioxide · carboxymethylcellulose · flavor · saccharin sodium · citric acid · zinc chloride · sanguinaria extract
Viadent Fluoride Colgate-Palmolive	gel	hydrated silica	sodium monofluorophosphate, 0.8%	sodium lauryl sulfate	saccharin sodium · zinc chloride · teaberry flavor · carboxymethylcellulose sodium · sorbitol · anhydrous sanguinaria extract · citric acid
FL **Viadent Original** Colgate-Palmolive	paste	dicalcium phosphate		sodium lauryl sulfate	glycerin · sorbitol · titanium dioxide · zinc chloride · carrageenan · flavor · saccharin sodium · citric acid · sanguinaria extract
** **Vince** Lee Consumer	powder	calcium carbonate · sodium carbonate · tricalcium phosphate			sodium alum · sodium perborate monohydrate · magnesium trisilicate · saccharin sodium · flavor · D&C red

** New listing

§ Manufacturer/supplier did not confirm information for this edition. Product listing is reprinted from the '96-97 edition.

[a] Carries American Dental Association (ADA) seal indicating safety and efficacy

[b] Sodium bicarbonate can also be considered an abrasive.

See Chapter 25, "Oral Health Products," for more information about these products.

ARTIFICIAL SALIVA PRODUCTS

Product Manufacturer/Supplier	Dosage Form	Viscosity Agent	Preservative	Other Ingredients
Glandosane Mouth Moisturizer; Lemon, Mint, or Unflavored Kenwood Labs	aerosol spray	carboxymethylcellulose sodium, 0.51g		sorbitol, 1.52g · sodium chloride, 0.043g · potassium chloride, 0.061g · calcium chloride dihydrate, 0.007g · magnesium chloride hexahydrate, 0.003g · dipotassium hydrogen phosphate, 0.017g · flavoring · carbon dioxide
Moi-Stir Mouth Moistening Kingswood Labs	pump spray	carboxymethylcellulose sodium		water · sorbitol · methylparaben · propylparaben · potassium chloride · dibasic sodium phosphate · calcium chloride · magnesium chloride · sodium chloride · flavor
Moi-Stir Oral Swabsticks Kingswood Labs	swab	carboxymethylcellulose sodium		water · sorbitol · methylparaben · propylparaben · potassium chloride · dibasic sodium phosphate · calcium chloride · magnesium chloride · sodium chloride · flavor
Mouth Kote Parnell Ph'cals	solution		sodium benzoate	water · xylitol · sorbitol · yerba santa · citric acid · ascorbic acid · natural lemon-lime flavor · saccharin sodium
Optimoist Colgate-Palmolive	liquid	hydroxyethyl cellulose	sodium benzoate	citric acid · malic acid · sodium phosphate monobasic · calcium chloride · sodium monofluorophosphate · sweetener · xylitol · polysorbate 20 · flavor · sodium hydroxide
** **Oralbalance Moisturizing** Laclede Research Labs	gel	hydroxyethyl cellulose · glycerate polyhydrate		glucose oxidase · lactoperoxidase · lysozyme · lactoferrin · hydrogenated starch · xylitol · aloe vera · potassium thiocyamate
Salivart Synthetic Saliva [a] Gebauer	aerosol spray	carboxymethylcellulose sodium, 1%		water, 95.7% · sorbitol, 3% · potassium chloride, 0.12% · sodium chloride, 0.08% · calcium chloride dihydrate · magnesium chloride hexahydrate · potassium phosphate dibasic · nitrogen (as propellant)

** New listing
[a] Carries American Dental Association (ADA) seal indicating safety and efficacy

See Chapter 25, "Oral Health Products," for more information about these products.

DENTURE CLEANSER PRODUCTS

Product Manufacturer/Supplier	Dosage Form	Cleaning/Abrasive Agent	Other Ingredients
Ban-A-Stain Brimms Labs	liquid	phosphoric acid, 25%	deionized water · imidurea · methylparaben · xanthan gum · alkyl phenoxy polyethoxy ethanol · oil of cassis · FD&C red#40
Dentu-Creme Dentco	paste	dicalcium phosphate dihydrate · calcium carbonate · aluminum silicate	propylene glycol · sodium lauryl sulfate · glycerin · hydroxyethyl cellulose · flavor · magnesium aluminum silicate · saccharin sodium · methylparaben · propylparaben
** **Dentu-Gel** Dentco	gel	silica	sorbitol · sodium lauryl sulfate · glycerin · cellulose gum · flavor · PEG-32 · saccharin sodium · methylparaben · propylparaben
Efferdent Antibacterial [a] Warner-Lambert Consumer	tablet	sodium carbonate · sodium bicarbonate · potassium monopersulfate · sodium perborate	fragrance · colors
Efferdent Plus Warner-Lambert Consumer	tablet	sodium bicarbonate · sodium perborate · potassium monopersulfate · detergents	fragrance · colors (including FD&C yellow#5) · saccharin sodium · chelating agents
Efferdent, 2 Layer Warner-Lambert Consumer	tablet	sodium bicarbonate · sodium carbonate · potassium monopersulfate · detergents	fragrance · colors · saccharin sodium · chelating agents
Polident Block Drug	tablet	sodium carbonate · sodium bicarbonate	potassium monopersulfate · sodium perborate monohydrate · surfactant · citric acid · fragrance
** **Polident Double Action** Block Drug	tablet	sodium carbonate · sodium bicarbonate	potassium monopersulfate · sodium perborate monohydrate · surfactant · citric acid · fragrance
** **Polident Overnight** Block Drug	tablet	sodium carbonate · sodium bicarbonate	potassium monopersulfate · sodium perborate monohydrate · surfactant · citric acid · fragrance
Smokers' Polident Block Drug	tablet	sodium carbonate · sodium bicarbonate · potassium monopersulfate · sodium perborate monohydrate · surfactant	citric acid · chelating agents · proteolytic enzyme · fragrance

** New listing
[a] Carries American Dental Association (ADA) seal indicating safety and efficacy

See Chapter 25, "Oral Health Products," for more information about these products.

DENTURE ADHESIVE PRODUCTS

Product Manufacturer/Supplier	Dosage Form	Adhesive Agent	Other Ingredients
Confident Block Drug	cream	carboxymethylcellulose gum, 32% · ethylene oxide polymer, 13%	petrolatum · liquid petrolatum · propylparaben
Corega Block Drug	powder	karaya gum, 94.6% · water-soluble ethylene oxide polymer, 5%	flavor
Cushion Grip Schering-Plough Healthcare	gel		alcohol, 26.2% · triacetin · polyvinyl acetate
** **Dentlock** Lee Consumer	powder	karaya gum	
Dentrol Block Drug	liquid	carboxymethylcellulose sodium · ethylene oxide polymer	mineral oil · polyethylene · flavor · propylparaben
Denturite Brimms Labs	liquid · powder		liquid: butyl phthalyl butyl glycolate · vinyl acetate · SDA alcohol powder: polyethyl methacrylate polymer
Effergrip [a] Warner-Lambert Consumer	cream	carboxymethylcellulose sodium · polyvinylmethylether maleic acid calcium sodium double salt	color · flavor · preservatives · vehicle
Ezo Cushions Medtech	pad		paraffin wax · cotton
Fixodent Procter & Gamble	powder	carboxymethylcellulose sodium	calcium zinc gantrez (PVA/MA copolymer) · corn starch · silicon dioxide · peppermint oil, rectified
Fixodent Procter & Gamble	cream	carboxymethylcellulose sodium	calcium zinc gantrez (PVM/MA copolymer) · mineral oil · petrolatum · silicon dioxide · color
Fixodent Extra Hold Procter & Gamble	powder	carboxymethylcellulose sodium	calcium zinc gantrez (PVM/MA copolymer) · silicon dioxide · peppermint oil, rectified
** **Fixodent Free** Procter & Gamble	cream	carboxymethylcellulose sodium	calcium zinc gantrez (PVM/MA copolymer)
Fixodent Fresh Procter & Gamble	cream	carboxymethylcellulose sodium	calcium zinc gantrez (PVM/MA copolymer) · mineral oil · petrolatum · silicon dioxide · color · peppermint flavor · methyl lactate · menthol
Plasti-Liner Brimms Labs	strip		polyethyl methacrylate polymer · butyl phthalyl butyl glycolate · triacetin
Poli-Grip Block Drug	cream	karaya gum, 51%	petrolatum, 36.7% · liquid petrolatum · magnesium oxide · propylparaben · flavor
** **Poli-Grip Free** Block Drug	cream	carboxymethylcellulose sodium · methyl vinyl ether maleic acid salt	petrolatum · mineral oil
Poli-Grip Super Block Drug	cream	carboxymethylcellulose sodium · methyl vinyl ether maleic acid salt copolymer	petrolatum · mineral oil · flavor · dye
Poli-Grip Super Block Drug	powder	carboxymethylcellulose sodium · methyl vinyl ether maleic acid salt copolymer	flavor
Polident Dentu-Grip Block Drug	powder	carboxymethylcellulose gum, 49% · methyl vinyl ether maleic acid salt copolymer	flavor
Quik-Fix Brimms Labs	liquid · powder		liquid: methyl methacrylate monomer · hydroxyethyl methacrylate monomer · colorsatable concentrate · triacetin powder: polyethyl methacrylate polymer · polymethyl methacrylate polymer

See Chapter 25, "Oral Health Products," for more information about these products.

DENTURE ADHESIVE PRODUCTS - continued

Product Manufacturer/Supplier	Dosage Form	Adhesive Agent	Other Ingredients
Sea-Bond Combe	pad	ethylene oxide polymer	sodium alginate
** **Snug Cushions** Mentholatum	sponge	acrylate resin	propylene glycol monolaurate
Wernet's Block Drug	powder	karaya gum, 94.6% · water-soluble ethylene oxide polymer, 5%	flavor, 0.4%
Wernet's Super [a] Block Drug	powder	carboxymethylcellulose gum · ethylene oxide polymer	dicalcium phosphate · monosodium phosphate · flavor

** New listing
[a] Carries American Dental Association (ADA) seal indicating safety and efficacy

See Chapter 25, "Oral Health Products," for more information about these products.

Dermatologic Product Tables

DERMATITIS PRODUCTS

Product Manufacturer/Supplier	Dosage Form	Hydro-cortisone	Astringent	Other Ingredients
Aquanil HC Person & Covey	lotion	1%	cetyl alcohol · stearyl alcohol	purified water · glycerin · benzyl alcohol · sodium laureth · sulfate · xanthan gum
Bactine Hydrocortisone 1% Bayer Consumer	cream	1%	cetearyl alcohol · hydrocortisone alcohol · aluminum sulfate · calcium acetate	beeswax · dextrin · glycerin · light mineral oil · methylparaben · water · sodium lauryl sulfate · white petrolatum
Caldecort Novartis Consumer	cream	1%		cetostearyl alcohol · sodium lauryl sulfate · white petrolatum · propylene glycol · purified water
Cortaid FastStick Pharmacia & Upjohn	stick	1%	alcohol, 55%	butylated hydroxytoluene · methylparaben · purified water
Cortaid Maximum Strength Pharmacia & Upjohn	spray	1%	alcohol, 55%	glycerin · methylparaben · water
Cortaid Maximum Strength Pharmacia & Upjohn	cream	1%	cetyl alcohol	glycerin · methylparaben · water · aloe · ceteareth-20 · cetyl palmitate · isopropyl myristate · isopropyl pentanoate
Cortaid Maximum Strength Pharmacia & Upjohn	ointment	1%		butylparaben · cholesterol · methylparaben · microcrystalline wax · mineral oil · white petrolatum
Cortaid Sensitive Skin Formula Pharmacia & Upjohn	ointment	0.5%		aloe · butylparaben · cholesterol · methylparaben · mineral oil · white petrolatum · microcrystalline wax
Cortaid Sensitive Skin Formula Pharmacia & Upjohn	cream	0.5%		aloe · butylparaben · cetyl palmitate · glyceryl stearate · methylparaben · propylethylene glycol · stearamidoethyl diethylamine · water
Corticaine UCB Pharma	cream	0.5%		
** **CortiCool Anti-Itch** Tec Labs	gel	1%		
Cortizone-10 Pfizer Consumer	cream	1%	aluminum sulfate · calcium acetate	glycerin · light mineral oil · methylparaben · propylparaben · potato dextrin · sodium lauryl sulfate · water · white petrolatum · white wax · aloe · cetearyl alcohol
Cortizone-10 Pfizer Consumer	ointment	1%		white petrolatum
Cortizone-10 Scalp Itch Pfizer Consumer	liquid	1%	SD alcohol 40	benzyl alcohol · propylene glycol · water
Cortizone-5 Pfizer Consumer	ointment	0.5%		white petrolatum · aloe
Cortizone-5 Pfizer Consumer	cream	0.5%	aluminum sulfate · calcium acetate	glycerin · light mineral oil · methylparaben · propylparaben · potato dextrin · sodium lauryl sulfate · water · white petrolatum · white wax · aloe · cetearyl alcohol
Dermarest DriCort Del Ph'cals	cream	1%		
DermiCort Republic Drug	cream	0.5%		aloe
Hytone Dermik Labs	cream	1%	cetyl alcohol	isopropyl myristate · cholesterol & related sterols · polysorbate 60 · sorbitan monostearate · polyoxyl 40 stearate · glyceryl monostearate SE · propylene glycol · sorbic acid · purified water

See Chapter 26, "Dermatologic Products," for more information about these products.

DERMATITIS PRODUCTS - continued

Product Manufacturer/Supplier	Dosage Form	Hydro-cortisone	Astringent	Other Ingredients
Hytone Dermik Labs	lotion	1%	cetyl alcohol	carbomer 940 · propylene glycol · polysorbate 40 · propylene glycol stearate · cholesterol and related sterols · isopropyl myristate · sorbitan palmitate · triethanolamine · sorbic acid · simethicone · purified water
Kericort 10 Maximum Strength Bristol-Myers Products	cream	1%	stearyl alcohol · cetyl alcohol	citric acid · glyceryl stearate · isopropyl myristate · methylparaben · polyoxyl 40 stearate · polysorbate 60 · propylene glycol · propylparaben · sodium citrate · sorbic acid · sorbitan monostearate · water · white wax
Lanacort Combe	cream	0.5%		
Lanacort 10 Combe	cream · ointment	1%		
Neutrogena T/Scalp Anti-Pruritic Neutrogena Dermatologics	liquid	1%		
Preparation H Hydrocortisone 1% Anti-Itch Whitehall-Robins Healthcare	cream	1%	cetyl alcohol · stearyl alcohol	citric acid · disodium EDTA · glycerin · lanolin · methylparaben · white petrolatum · propylparaben · sodium benzoate · sodium lauryl sulfate · water · tegacid special · arlacel 186 · medical antifoam emulsion · carboxymethylcellulose sodium · rhodigel · Tenox-2
Procort Lee Consumer	cream	1%		glycerin · glyceryl stearate · mineral oil · methylparaben · polysorbate 60 · propylparaben · sorbitan stearate · purified water · aloe vera gel
** **Sarnol-HC** Stiefel Labs	lotion	1%		camphor · menthol
Scalpicin Anti-Itch Combe	liquid	1%	SD alcohol 40	menthol · propylene glycol · water

** New listing

See Chapter 26, "Dermatologic Products," for more information about these products.

DRY SKIN PRODUCTS

Product Manufacturer/Supplier	Dosage Form	Emollient/ Moisturizer	Humectant	Keratin Softener	Other Ingredients
ACID Mantle Doak Dermatologics	cream	light mineral oil · white petrolatum	glycerin	citric acid	aluminum acetate · aluminum sulfate · calcium acetate · cetearyl alcohol · methylparaben · water · sodium lauryl sulfate · synthetic beeswax · white potato dextrin · ammonium hydroxide
ActiBath Soak Oatmeal Treatment Andrew Jergens	effervescent tablet		colloidal oatmeal, 20%		fumaric acid · sodium carbonate · lactose · sodium bicarbonate · PEG-150 · magnesium oxide · sucrose stearate
** FR **Allercreme** Carmé	lotion	mineral oil	sorbitol		purified water · isopropyl palmitate · stearic acid · tiethanolamine · methylparaben · propylparaben · butylparaben
** FR **Allercreme Moisturizer with Sunscreen SPF 8** Carmé	lotion	petrolatum · mineral oil	glycerin · sorbitol		octyl dimethyl PABA · deionized water · glyceryl stearate · PEG-100 stearate · polysorbate 60 · isopropyl palmitate · sodium hyaluronate · collagen · sunflower seed oil · cetyl alcohol · vanillin · carbomer 941 · corn oil · BHT · tetrasodium EDTA · potassium hydroxide · methylparaben · propylparaben · diazolidinyl urea
** **Aloe Grande** Gordon Labs	cream	petrolatum · mineral oil	propylene glycol		vitamin A, 100000 IU/oz · vitamin E, 1500 IU/oz · aloe vera gel · cetyl alcohol · white wax · sodium lauryl sulfate · methylparaben · propylparaben
FR **Alpha Glow Body Care Lotion with SPF 16** Fischer Ph'cals	lotion			glycolic acid, 10%	octyl methoxycinnamate, 7.5% · titanium dioxide, 2%
FR **Alpha Glow Day Cream with SPF 16** Fischer Ph'cals	cream			glycolic acid, 8%	octyl methoxycinnamate, 7.5% · titanium dioxide, 2%
Alpha Keri Moisture Rich Bristol-Myers Products	cleansing bar	mineral oil · lanolin oil	glycerin		sodium tallowate · sodium cocoate · fragrance · PEG-75 · titanium dioxide · sodium chloride · BHT · trisodium HEDTA · D&C green#5 · D&C yellow#10
Alpha Keri Moisture Rich Bristol-Myers Products	oil	mineral oil · lanolin oil			PEG-4-dilaurate · benzophenone-3 · fragrance · D&C green#6
Ambi Cocoa Butter Kiwi Brands	cream	dimethicone, 1% · mineral oil	glycerin · propylene glycol		water · cocoa butter · glyceryl stearate SE · stearic acid · steareth-21 · tocopheryl acetate · retinyl palmitate · cholecalciferol · carbomer · triethanolamine · BHT · corn oil · diazolidinyl urea · methylparaben · propylparaben · quaternium-15 · disodium EDTA · fragrance · FD&C yellow#5 · FD&C red#4

See Chapter 26, "Dermatologic Products," for more information about these products.

DRY SKIN PRODUCTS - continued

Product Manufacturer/Supplier	Dosage Form	Emollient/ Moisturizer	Humectant	Keratin Softener	Other Ingredients
Aqua A Baker Cummins Derm'cals	cream	mineral oil · dimethicone · lecithin			water · caprylic/capric triglyceride · methyl gluceth-10 · glyceryl stearate squalene · PPG-20 methyl glucose ether distearate · stearic acid · PEG-50 stearate · retinyl palmitate · sodium hyaluronate · sodium polyglutamate · magnesium aluminum silicate · carbomer 934 · dichlorobenzyl alcohol · cetyl alcohol · BHT · xanthan gum · menthol · sodium hydroxide · tetrasodium EDTA · diazolidinyl urea
Aqua Care Menley & James Labs	lotion	mineral oil · petrolatum	propylene glycol stearate	urea, 10% · lactic acid	sorbitan stearate · cetyl alcohol · magnesium aluminum silicate · sodium lauryl sulfate · methylparaben · propylparaben · may contain sodium hydroxide
Aqua Care Menley & James Labs	cream	petrolatum · lanolin oil · mineral oil/lanolin alcohol	glycerin	urea, 10%	cetyl esters · DEA-oleth-3 phosphate · triethanolamine · carbomer · benzyl alcohol · fragrance · water
** **Aqua Glycolic Hand & Body** Allergan Skin Care	lotion	mineral oil		glycolic acid, 14%	purified water · ammonium glycolate · cetyl alcohol · glyceryl stearate · PEG-100 stearate · C12-15 alkyl benzoate · magnesium aluminum silicate · stearyl alcohol · xanthan gum · disodium EDTA · methylparaben · propylparaben
** **Aqua Glycolic Shampoo & Body Cleanser** Allergan Skin Care	shampoo; liquid		glycerin · propylene glycol	glycolic acid, 14%	purified water · ammonium laureth sulfate · ammonium glycolate · disodium cocoamphodiacetate · fragrance · diazolidnyl urea · methylparaben · propylparaben
Aquabase Paddock Labs	ointment	petrolatum · mineral oil			mineral wax · wool wax alcohol · cholesterol
Aquaderm Baker Cummins Derm'cals	cream · lotion	dimethicone · petrolatum · mineral oil · lecithin			water · caprylic/capric triglyceride · methyl gluceth-10 · glyceryl stearate · ether distearate · stearic acid · sodium hyaluronate · sodium polyglutamate · magnesium aluminum silicate · carbomer 934 · dichlorobenzyl alcohol · cetyl alcohol · BHT · xanthan gum · menthol · tetrasodium EDTA · sodium hydroxide · diazolidinyl urea
Aquaphilic Medco Lab	ointment	petrolatum	propylene glycol · sorbitol		stearyl alcohol · isopropyl palmitate · methylparaben · propylparaben · water · sodium lauryl sulfate
Aquaphilic with Carbamide Medco Lab	ointment	petrolatum	propylene glycol · sorbitol	urea, 10%; 20% · lactic acid	stearyl alcohol · isopropyl palmitate · methylparaben · propylparaben · water · sodium lauryl sulfate
** **Aquaphor Healing** Beiersdorf	ointment	petrolatum · mineral oil	glycerin		mineral wax · wool wax alcohol · panthenol · bisabolol
** **Aquaphor Original** Beiersdorf	ointment	petrolatum · mineral oil			mineral wax · wool wax alcohol

See Chapter 26, "Dermatologic Products," for more information about these products.

DRY SKIN PRODUCTS - continued

	Product Manufacturer/Supplier	Dosage Form	Emollient/ Moisturizer	Humectant	Keratin Softener	Other Ingredients
FR	**Aveeno Bath Treatment Moisturizing Formula** Rydelle Labs	powder	mineral oil	colloidal oatmeal, 43%		
FR	**Aveeno Bath Treatment Soothing Formula** Rydelle Labs	powder		colloidal oatmeal, 100%		
FR	**Aveeno for Combination Skin** Rydelle Labs	cleansing bar		colloidal oatmeal, 38% · glycerin	lactic acid	sodium cocoyl isethionate · sodium lactate · magnesium aluminum silicate · potassium sorbate · titanium dioxide · PEG-14M · cetyl alcohol · benzaldehyde · C12-14 alkyl benzoate · iodopropynyl butylcarbamate · polyoxymethylene urea
FR	**Aveeno for Dry Skin** Rydelle Labs	cleansing bar		colloidal oatmeal, 38% · glycerin	lactic acid	sodium cocoyl isethionate · hydrogenated vegetable oil · vegetable shortening · PEG-75 · lauramide DEA · sodium lactate · sorbic acid · titanium dioxide · cetyl alcohol · benzaldehyde · polyoxymethylene urea · C12-14 alkyl benzoate
FR	**Aveeno Gentle Skin Cleanser** Rydelle Labs	lotion		oatmeal flour · sodium PCA	citric acid	deionized water · disodium laureth sulfosuccinate · hydrogenated tallow glyceride · potassium cocoyl hydrolyzed collagen · disodium lauroamphodiacetate · ammonium lauryl sulfate · sodium citrate · phenylcarbinol · PEG-150 distearate · diethyl phthalate · phantolid · galaxolid
FR	**Aveeno Moisturizing** Rydelle Labs	cream · lotion	petrolatum · dimethicone	colloidal oatmeal, 1% · glycerin		distearyldimonium chloride · isopropyl palmitate · cetyl alcohol · sodium chloride · benzyl alcohol
FR	**Aveeno Shower & Bath** Rydelle Labs	bath oil	mineral oil	colloidal oatmeal, 4%		laureth-4 · benzaldehyde · quaternium-18 hectorite · phenylcarbinol · silica
	Bagbalm Dairy Assn. Co.	ointment	petrolatum · lanolin			8-hydroxyquinoline sulfate, 0.3%
**	**Boroleum** Sinclair Pharmacal	ointment	petrolatum			camphor · menthol · methyl salicylate · eucalyptol · boric acid
**	**Cameo Oil** Medco Lab	bath oil	mineral oil · lanolin oil			isopropyl myrisate · PEG-400 dioleate
	Candermyl Galderma Labs	cream		glycerin · propylene glycol		oleic/palmitoleic triglycerides · polyamidoacid · sodium lactate methylsilanol · polyglyceryl-3 · hexadecylether · cholesterol
	Care-Creme Antimicrobial Cream Care-Tech Labs	cream	lanolin oil	propylene glycol		chloroxylenol, 0.8% · cetyl alcohol · cod liver oil · lanolin alcohol · vitamins A, D3, and E
	Carmol 10 Doak Dermatologics	lotion			urea, 10%	nonlipid base
	Carmol 20 Doak Dermatologics	cream			urea, 20%	nonlipid base

See Chapter 26, "Dermatologic Products," for more information about these products.

DRY SKIN PRODUCTS - continued

	Product Manufacturer/Supplier	Dosage Form	Emollient/ Moisturizer	Humectant	Keratin Softener	Other Ingredients
	Cetaphil Galderma Labs	cleansing bar				sodium cocoyl isethionate · stearic acid · sodium tallowate
FR	**Cetaphil Gentle Cleanser** Galderma Labs	liquid		propylene glycol		cetyl alcohol · stearyl alcohol · sodium lauryl sulfate
FR	**Cetaphil Moisturizing** Galderma Labs	lotion	dimethicone	glycerin		hydrogenated polyisobutene · cetearyl alcohol · ceteareth-20 · macadamia nut oil · tocopheryl acetate
FR	**Cetaphil Moisturizing** Galderma Labs	cream	petrolatum · dimethicone	polyglycerylmethacry-late · propylene glycol		dicapryl ether · PEG-5 glyceryl stearate · dimethiconol · sweet almond oil
	ChapStick Lip Balm; Cherry, Mint, Orange, or Strawberry Whitehall-Robins Healthcare	stick	petrolatum, 44% · lanolin, 1% · mineral oil			padimate O, 1.5% · isopropyl myristate, 0.5% · cetyl alcohol · arachidyl propionate · camphor (Cherry · Strawberry) · carnauba wax · colors · flavors · isopropyl lanolate · methylparaben · 2-octyl dodecanol · polyphenylmethylsiloxane 556 · propylparaben · saccharin · paraffin wax · white wax · l-menthol (Mint)
	ChapStick Plus Whitehall-Robins Healthcare	ointment	white petrolatum, 99% · lanolin			aloe · butylated hydroxytoluene · flavor · phenonip · fragrance · padimate O
	ChapStick Plus, Cherry Whitehall-Robins Healthcare	ointment	white petrolatum, 98.85% · lanolin			aloe · butylated hydroxytoluene · D&C red#6 barium lake · flavors · phenonip · saccharin · maltol
	ChapStick, Regular/Original Whitehall-Robins Healthcare	stick	petrolatum, 44% · lanolin, 1% · mineral oil			padimate O, 1.5% · isopropyl myristate, 1% · cetyl alcohol, 0.5% · arachidyl propionate · camphor · carnauba wax · D&C red#6 barium lake · FD&C yellow#5 aluminum lake · fragrance · isopropyl lanolate · methylparaben · 2-octyl dodecanol · oleyl alcohol · polyphenylmethylsiloxane 556 · propylparaben · titanium dioxide · paraffin wax · white wax · eugenol · lavender oil
	Clocream Lee Consumer	cream	mineral oil	glycerin		cetyl palmitate · cottonseed oil · glyceryl monostearate · methylparaben · potassium stearate · propylparaben · sodium citrate · vitamins A and D · fragrance · purified water
**	**Cloverine Salve** Medtech	ointment	petrolatum, 97%			rectified turpentine oil · white wax · perfume
FR	**Complex 15 Therapeutic Moisturizing** Schering-Plough Healthcare	cream · lotion		glycerin · lecithin		
	Complex 15 Therapeutic Moisturizing Face Cream Schering-Plough Healthcare	cream		glycerin · lecithin		

See Chapter 26, "Dermatologic Products," for more information about these products.

DRY SKIN PRODUCTS - continued

	Product Manufacturer/Supplier	Dosage Form	Emollient/ Moisturizer	Humectant	Keratin Softener	Other Ingredients
	Corn Huskers Warner-Lambert Consumer	lotion		glycerin		SD alcohol 40 · oleyl sarcosine · methylparaben · guar gum · calcium sulfate · calcium chloride · sodium calcium alginate · triethanolamine · fragrance · fumaric acid · boric acid · water
FR	**Curél Alpha Hydroxy** Bausch & Lomb	lotion	petrolatum · dimethicone	glycerin	lactic acid · glycolic acid	distearyl dimonium chloride · isopropylpalmitate · 1-hexadecanol · ammonium hydroxide · methylparaben · propylparaben
	Curél Nutrient Rich Severe Dry Skin Bausch & Lomb	lotion	petrolatum · dimethicone	glycerin		quaternium-5 · isopropyl palmitate · 1-hexadecanol · nylon 12 · methylparaben · tocopheryl acetate · propylparaben · DL-panthenol · ascorbyl palmitate
FR	**Curél Therapeutic Moisturizing, Fragrance-Free or Scented** Bausch & Lomb	cream · lotion	petrolatum · dimethicone	glycerin		quaternium-5 · isopropyl palmitate · 1-hexadecanol · methylparaben · propylparaben · sodium chloride
	Cutemol Emollient Skin Cream Summers Labs	cream	liquid petrolatum · acetylated lanolin		allantoin	lanolin alcohols extract · isopropyl myristate wax · sorbitan sesquioleate
	Dermabase Paddock Labs	cream	mineral oil · petrolatum	propylene glycol		water · cetostearyl alcohol · sodium lauryl sulfate · isopropyl palmitate · methylparaben · propylparaben · imidazolidinyl urea
FR	**Dermal Therapy Extra Strength Body** Bayer Diagnostics	lotion		propylene glycol	urea · lactic acid	deionized water · hydrogenated polyisobutene · isopropyl myristate · cetyl alcohol · GMS/PEG-100 stearate · triethanolamine · emulsifying wax · silk amino acid · imidazolidinyl urea · carbomer 941 · tetrasodium EDTA · sorbic acid · quaternium-15
	Dermasil Dry Skin Treatment Chesebrough-Pond's	lotion	dimethicone, 1.1% · petrolatum · mineral oil	glycerin		water · stearic acid · sunflower seed oil · glycol stearate · triethanolamine · PEG-40 stearate · acetylated lanolin alcohol · magnesium aluminum silicate · methylparaben · propylparaben · cetyl alcohol · stearamide AMP · cholesterol · carbomer 934 · disodium EDTA · lecithin · ethylene brassylate · palmarosa oil · rose extract · sandalwood oil · sweet almond oil · borage seed oil · DMDM hydantoin · vanilla · ascorbyl palmitate

See Chapter 26, "Dermatologic Products," for more information about these products.

DRY SKIN PRODUCTS - continued

	Product Manufacturer/Supplier	Dosage Form	Emollient/ Moisturizer	Humectant	Keratin Softener	Other Ingredients
	Dermasil Dry Skin Treatment Chesebrough-Pond's	cream	dimethicone, 1.1% · petrolatum	glycerin		water · myreth-3 myristate · sunflower seed oil · cetostearyl alcohol · triethanolamine · carbomer 934 · ceteareth-20 · methylparaben · DMDM hydantoin · propylparaben · cholesterol · stearic acid · lecithin · ethylene brassylate · palmarosa oil · rose extract · sandalwood oil · sweet almond oil · borage seed oil · vanilla
FR	**Dermsol** Parnell Ph'cals	lotion	dimethicone, 1% · mineral oil · lecithin	glycerin · propylene glycol		yerba santa · cetyl alcohol · glyceryl stearate · isopropyl myristate · PEG-40 stearate · squalene · stearic acid · diazolidinyl urea · PEG-12 oleate · benzoic acid · quaternized acetamide MEA · BHT · retinyl palmitate · tocopheryl acetate
**	**Diabetic Pure Skin Therapy Azulene Night Repair** Consumers Choice	cream	dimethicone	propylene glycol dicaprylate/dicaprate · sodium PCA	allantoin	aloe vera gel · methyl gluceth-20 · stearic acid · stearyl alcohol · cetyl alcohol · carpylic/capric triglyceride · magnesium aluminum silicate · birch bark extract · lotus extract · dong quai extract · matricaria oil · bergamot oil · retinyl palmitate · ascorbic acid · tocopherol · wheat germ glycerides · hydrolyzed wheat protein · xanthan gum · disodium EDTA · polysorbate 80 · sodium dehydroacetate · triethanolamine · imidazolidinyl urea · methylparaben · propylparaben · guaiazulene
**	**Diabetic Pure Skin Therapy Day Protection SPF 15** Consumers Choice	cream	dimethicone	glycerin		octyl methoxycinnamate · oxybenzone · deionized water · stearic acid · isodecyl neopentanoate · DEA cetyl phosphate · isostearyl stearoyl stearate · cetyl alcohol · retinyl palmitate · squalane · farnesyl acetate · farnesol · panthenyl triacetate · tocopherol · sodium hyaluronate · carbomer · triethanolamine · methylparaben · propylparaben · DMDM hydantoin

See Chapter 26, "Dermatologic Products," for more information about these products.

DRY SKIN PRODUCTS - continued

	Product Manufacturer/Supplier	Dosage Form	Emollient/ Moisturizer	Humectant	Keratin Softener	Other Ingredients
**	**Diabetic Pure Skin Therapy Diapedic Foot Cream** Consumers Choice	cream	lanolin	propylene glycol · sodium PCA	allantoin	aloe vera · jojoba oil · paraffin · octyl stearate · olive oil · methyl salicylate · beeswax · triethanolamine · emulsifying wax · eucalyptus oil · bergamot oil · evening primrose oil · ascorbyl palmitate · tocopherol · asorbic acid · retinyl palmitate · panthenol · menthol · camphor · linoleic acid · linolenic acid · arachidonic acid · glyceryl stearate · PEG-100 stearate · steareth-2 · steareth-21 · stearic acid · carbomer · hydrolyzed glycosaminoglycans · cetyl alcohol · xanthan gum · imidazolidinyl urea · propylparaben · methylparaben
**	**Diabetic Pure Skin Therapy Hand & Body** Consumers Choice	cream	lanolin	propylene glycol · sodium PCA	allantoin	aloe vera · jojoba oil · octyl stearate · olive oil · beeswax · triethanolamine · emulsyfying wax · steareth-2 · tocopherol · retinyl palmitate · ascorbyl palmitate · evening primrose oil · bergamot oil · panthenol · linoleic acid · linolenic acid · arachidonic acid · glyceryl stearate · PEG-100 stearate · stearic acid · carbomer · steareth-21 · hydrolyzed glycosaminoglycans · cetyl alcohol · xanthan gum · imidazolidinyl urea · methylparaben · propylparaben
FR	**DiabetiDerm** Health Care Products	cream	dimethicone copolymer		urea · lactic acid · allantoin	purified water · cetyl alcohol · hydrogenated apricot kernel oil · glyceryl stearate · PEG-100 stearate · polysorbate 60 · isostearyl alcohol · benzyl alcohol · wheat germ oil · soybean and calendula extract · St. John's Wort · silk protein · carbomer 940 · cosmedia polymer · may contain sodium hydroxide
FR	**DiabetiDerm** Health Care Products	lotion	dimethicone copolymer	glycerin · propylene glycol dipelargonate · propylene glycol	urea · lactic acid	purified water · stearic acid · cetyl alcohol · PEG-8 dioleate · sodium lauryl sulfate · benzyl alcohol · PEG-8 distearate · silk protein · carbomer 940 · xanthan gum · may contain sodium hydroxide
FR	**DML Facial Moisturizer** Person & Covey	cream	petrolatum · dimethicone	propylene glycol dioctanoate · glycerin		octyl methoxycinnamate, 8% · oxybenzone, 4% · water · DEA cetyl phosphate · glyceryl stearate · PEG-100 stearate · stearic acid · hyaluronic acid · benzyl alcohol · PVP/eicosene copolymer · sodium carbomer 941 · disodium EDTA · magnesium aluminum silicate

See Chapter 26, "Dermatologic Products," for more information about these products.

DRY SKIN PRODUCTS - continued

	Product Manufacturer/Supplier	Dosage Form	Emollient/ Moisturizer	Humectant	Keratin Softener	Other Ingredients
FR	**DML Forte** Person & Covey	cream	petrolatum	propylene glycol dioctanoate · glycerin		water · glyceryl stearate · PEG-100 stearate · stearic acid · D-panthenol · DEA-cetyl phosphate · simethicone · PVP/eicosene copolymer · benzyl alcohol · cetyl alcohol · silica · disodium EDTA · magnesium aluminum silicate · sodium carbomer 1542
	DML Lotion Person & Covey	lotion	petrolatum	glycerin		PPG-2 · myristyl ether propionate · glyceryl stearate · simethicone · benzyl alcohol · silica · EDTA · sodium carbomer 1342
	Emollia Gordon Labs	lotion	mineral oil	propylene glycol		cetyl alcohol · white wax · sodium lauryl sulfate · oleic acid · methylparaben · propylparaben
**	**Epilyt Concentrate** Stiefel Labs	lotion		propylene glycol · glycerin	lactic acid	oleic acid · quarternium-26 · BHT
	Eucerin Beiersdorf	cleansing bar				disodium lauryl sulfosuccinate · sodium cocoyl isethionate · cetearyl alcohol · corn starch · glyceryl stearate · water · titanium dioxide · octyldodecanol · cyclopentadecanolide · lanolin alcohol · bisabolol
	Eucerin Beiersdorf	lotion		sorbitol · propylene glycol		water · mineral oil · isopropyl myristate · PEG-40 sorbitan peroleate · lanolin acid glycerin ester · cetyl palmitate · magnesium sulfate · aluminum stearate · lanolin alcohol · BHT · methylchloroisothiazolinone-methylisothiazolinone
	Eucerin Creme Beiersdorf	cream	petrolatum · mineral oil			water · mineral wax · lanolin alcohol · methylchloroisothiazolinone-methylisothiazolinone
**	**Eucerin Light Moisture-Restorative** Beiersdorf	lotion	dimethicone	glycerin · sodium PCA	allantoin	water · sunflower seed oil · cetearyl alcohol · panthenol · octyldodecanol · caprylic/capric triglyceride · stearic acid · vitamin E · glyceryl stearate · triethanolamine · sodium lactate · cholesterol · ceresin · carbomer · disodium EDTA · BHT · methylchloroisothiazolinone · methylisothiazolinone
	Eucerin Plus Beiersdorf	lotion	mineral oil	glycerin	urea	water · PEG-7 hydrogenated castor oil · isohexadecane · sodium lactate · isopropyl palmitate · panthenol · ozokerite · magnesium sulfate · lanolin alcohol · bisabolol · methylchloroisothiazolinone-methylisothiazolinone
	Eucerin Plus Creme Beiersdorf	cream	mineral oil		urea	water · magnesium stearate · polyglyceryl-3 diisostearate · mineral wax · isopropyl palmitate · benzyl alcohol · panthenol · bisabolol · lanolin alcohol · magnesium sulfate · sodium lactate

See Chapter 26, "Dermatologic Products," for more information about these products.

DRY SKIN PRODUCTS - continued

	Product Manufacturer/Supplier	Dosage Form	Emollient/ Moisturizer	Humectant	Keratin Softener	Other Ingredients
	Facial Hydrating Fluid, Oil Free C & M Pharmacal	lotion		glycerin	allantoin	purified water · soluble collagen · hydrolyzed elastin · hydroxyethyl ethylcellulose · sorbic acid · octoxynol-9
	Facial Hydrating Gel, Oil Free C & M Pharmacal	gel		glycerin	allantoin	purified water · soluble collagen · hydrolyzed elastin · carbomer 940 · triethanolamine · disodium EDTA · sorbic acid · octoxynol-9 · hyaluronic acid
**	**Gordon's Vite A Creme** Gordon Labs	cream	petrolatum · mineral oil	propylene glycol		vitamin A, 100000 IU/oz · cetyl alcohol · sodium lauryl sulfate · methylparaben · propylparaben
FR	**Gormel** Gordon Labs	cream	mineral oil	propylene glycol	urea, 20%	cetyl alcohol · white wax · sodium lauryl sulfate
	Hydrisinol Pedinol Pharmacal	cream · lotion				sulfonated hydrogenated castor oil · hydrogenated vegetable oil
	Hydrocream Base Paddock Labs	cream	petrolatum · mineral oil			water · cholesterol · mineral wax · woolwax alcohol · methylparaben · propylparaben · imidazolidinyl urea
**	**Hydrolatum** Denison Ph'cals	cream	petrolatum			purfied water
	Jergens Advanced Therapy Dry Skin Care Andrew Jergens	lotion	dimethicone · lanolin	glycerin		water · cetearyl alcohol · isopropyl myristate · ceteareth-20 · tocopherol · cholesteryl isostearate · C12-15 alkyl benzoate · cyclomethicone · stearic acid · cetyl alcohol · sodium carbomer · methylparaben · propylparaben · DMDM hydantoin · fragrance
FR	**Jergens Advanced Therapy Dual Healing** Andrew Jergens	cream	mineral oil · dimethicone · petrolatum · cetyl dimethicone	glycerin		water · cyclomethicone · isopropyl palmitate · cetyl dimethicone copolyol · cetyl-PG hydroxyethyl palmitamide · sodium lactate · cholesteryl isostearate · isostearyl glyceryl ether · trihydroxystearin · dextrin palmitate · sodium chloride · diazolidinyl urea · pentasodium pentetate · tetrasodium etidronate
FR	**Jergens Advanced Therapy Ultra Healing, Reg. or Frag. Free** Andrew Jergens	lotion	petrolatum · mineral oil · dimethicone	glycerin	allantoin	water · cetearyl alcohol (Reg.) · stearyl alcohol (Frag. Free) · ceteareth-20 · cetyl-PG hydroxyethyl palmitamide · cholesteryl isostearate · cyclomethicone · glyceryl dilaurate · stearic acid (Frag. Free) · aluminum starch octenylsuccinate · cetyl alcohol (Frag. Free) · sodium carbomer · methylparaben · propylparaben · DMDM hydantoin · fragrance (Reg.)
** PE	**Johnson's Baby Lotion §** Johnson & Johnson Consumer	lotion				aloe vera · vitamin E

See Chapter 26, "Dermatologic Products," for more information about these products.

DRY SKIN PRODUCTS - continued

	Product Manufacturer/Supplier	Dosage Form	Emollient/ Moisturizer	Humectant	Keratin Softener	Other Ingredients
FR PE	**Johnson's Ultra Sensitive Baby Cream §** Johnson & Johnson Consumer	cream	mineral oil	glycerin		water · polyethylene · sorbitan isostearate · sodium lactate · methylparaben · propylparaben · ethylparaben · butylparaben · magnesium sulfate
FR PE	**Johnson's Ultra Sensitive Baby Lotion §** Johnson & Johnson Consumer	lotion	mineral oil · PEG-55 lanolin	glycerin		water · carbomer · ceteareth-6 · sodium citrate · methylparaben · stearyl alcohol · butylparaben · ethylparaben · propylparaben
**	**Just Lotion** Care-Tech Labs	lotion	mineral oil	glycerin		water · stearic acid · cetyl alcohol · silicone · triethanolamine · aloe vera gel · DMDM hydantoin · fragrance
**	**Keri Anti-Bacterial Hand** Bristol-Myers Products	lotion	mineral oil · petrolatum · dimethicone · dimethicone copolyol	glycerin		triclosan · water · hydrogenated polyisobutene · stearic acid · cetyl alcohol · tocopheryl acetate · PEG-5 soya sterol · cyclomethicone · glyceryl stearate · triethanolamine · PEG-100 stearate · carbomer · phenoxyethanol · magnesium aluminum silicate · disodium EDTA · methylparaben · propylparaben · titanium dioxide · fragrance · diazolidinyl urea
	Keri Original Formula Therapeutic Dry Skin Bristol-Myers Products	lotion	mineral oil · lanolin oil	propylene glycol		PEG-40 stearate · glyceryl stearate · PEG-100 stearate · PEG-40 dilaurate · laureth-4 · methylparaben · propylparaben · carbomer 934 · triethanolamine · fragrance · sodium dioctyl sulfosuccinate · quarternium-15
FR	**Keri Silky Smooth, Fragrance Free or Sensitive Skin** Bristol-Myers Products	lotion	petrolatum · dimethicone	glycerin		water · steareth-2 · cetyl alcohol · benzyl alcohol · laureth-23 · magnesium aluminium silicate · tocopheryl linoleate or tocopheryl acetate · carbomer 934 · BHT (Fragrance Free) · fragrance (Sensitive Skin) · sodium hydroxide · disodium EDTA · quarternium-15
FR	**Lac-Hydrin Five** Westwood-Squibb Ph'cals	lotion	petrolatum · dimethicone	propylene glycol dioctanoate · glycerin	lactic acid	squalene · steareth-2 · steareth-21 · cetyl alcohol · cetyl palmitate · magnesium aluminum silicate · kathon CG · ammonium hydroxide · water · diazolidinyl urea
	Lacti-Care Stiefel Labs	lotion	mineral oil	sodium PCA	lactic acid	water · isopropyl palmitate · stearyl alcohol · ceteareth-20 · sodium hydroxide · glyceryl stearate · PEG-100 stearate · myristyl lactate · cetyl alcohol · carbomer · DMDM hydantoin · fragrance · methylparaben · propylparaben
	Lanaphilic Medco Lab	ointment	petrolatum · lanolin oil	propylene glycol · sorbitol		stearyl alcohol · isopropyl palmitate · methylparaben · propylparaben · sodium lauryl sulfate · water

See Chapter 26, "Dermatologic Products," for more information about these products.

DRY SKIN PRODUCTS - continued

	Product Manufacturer/Supplier	Dosage Form	Emollient/ Moisturizer	Humectant	Keratin Softener	Other Ingredients
	Lanaphilic with Urea Medco Lab	ointment	petrolatum · lanolin oil	propylene glycol · sorbitol	urea, 10%; 20% · lactic acid	stearyl alcohol · isopropyl palmitate · methylparaben · propylparaben · water · sodium lauryl sulfate
	Lazer Creme Pedinol Pharmacal	cream		propylene glycol		vitamin A, 100000 IU/oz · vitamin E, 3500 IU/oz · stearic acid · isopropyl palmitate · triethanolamine · PEG-2 stearate · PEG-2 stearate SE · borax · carbomer 934 · DMDM hydantoin · methylparaben · propylparaben · diazolidinyl urea
FR PE	**Little Noses Saline Moisturizing** Vetco	gel	dimethicone copolyol	glycerin · propylene glycol · sodium chloride	allantoin · citric acid	water · PEG-100 · hydroxyethyl cellulose · aloe vera gel · methyl gluceth-10 · diazolidinyl urea · methylparaben · vitamin E acetate · olive oil · geranium oil · propylparaben
**	**Loving Lotion** Care-Tech Labs	lotion	mineral oil · lanolin oil · petrolatum ·	propylene glycol		chloroxylenol, 0.8% · water · stearic acid · emulsifying wax · triethanolamine · isostearyl alcohol · glycol stearate · methyl gluceth-20 · methylparaben · cetyl alcohol · stearamide DEA · fragrance · myristyl propionate · propylparaben · carbomer 934 · aloe vera gel · hydrolyzed collagen · FD&C red#40 · FD&C yellow#5
	Lowila Cake Westwood-Squibb Ph'cals	cleansing bar	mineral oil	sorbitol	urea · lactic acid	dextrin · sodium lauryl sulfoacetate · boric acid · PEG-14M · dioctyl sodium sulfosuccinate · cellulose gum · fragrance
**	**Lubrex** Allerderm Labs	lotion	mineral oil · petrolatum	propylene glycol stearate		water · sorbitan stearate · cetyl alcohol · sodium lauryl sulfate · methylparaben · propylparaben
	Lubricating Hand and Body C & M Pharmacal	cream	petrolatum · mineral oil	propylene glycol · glycerin		purified water · cetostearyl alcohol · sodium lauryl sulfate · sorbic acid
	Lubriderm Moisture Recovery GelCreme Warner-Lambert Consumer	cream	mineral oil	glycerin · propylene glycol dicaprylate/dicaprate		cetyl alcohol · cyclomethicone fluid · emulsifying wax · BHT · carbomer 940 · tocopheryl acetate · sodium benzoate · dicaprylate/dicaprate · PEG-40 stearate · isopropyl isostearate · diazolidinyl urea · titanium dioxide · tri (PPG-3 myristyl ether) citrate · disodium edetate · retinyl palmitate · sodium pyruvate · iodopropynyl butylcarbamate · sodium hydroxide · xanthan gum · lecithin · water

See Chapter 26, "Dermatologic Products," for more information about these products.

DRY SKIN PRODUCTS - continued

	Product Manufacturer/Supplier	Dosage Form	Emollient/ Moisturizer	Humectant	Keratin Softener	Other Ingredients
	Lubriderm Seriously Sensitive Warner-Lambert Consumer	lotion	petrolatum · dimethicone · mineral oil	glycerin · propylene glycol dicaprylate/dicaprate		water · carbomer 940 · titanium dioxide · methylparaben · propylparaben · cetyl alcohol · emulsifying wax · glyceryl stearate · butylene glycol · xanthan gum · PEG-40 stearate · C11-C13 isoparaffin · ethylparaben · titanium dioxide · tri (PPG-3 myristyl ether) citrate · DMDM hydantoin · disodium EDTA · sodium hydroxide · butylparaben
	Lubriderm Skin Conditioning Warner-Lambert Consumer	bath oil	mineral oil			PPG-15 stearyl ether · oleth-2 · nonoxynol-5 · fragrance · D&C green#6
	Lubriderm, Scented or Unscented Warner-Lambert Consumer	lotion	mineral oil · petrolatum · lanolin · dimethicone	sorbitol solution · propylene glycol		lanolin alcohol · stearic acid · triethanolamine · cetyl alcohol · fragrance (Scented) · methylparaben · propylparaben · water · tri (PPG-3 myristyl ether) citrate · methyldibromo glutaronitrile · ethylparaben · butylparaben · glyceryl stearate/PEG-100 stearate · disodium EDTA · xanthan gum
	Mammol Abbott Labs	ointment	anhydrous lanolin, 22%			bismuth subnitrate, 40% · castor oil, 30% · ceresin wax, 7% · peruvian balsam, 1%
FR	**Moisturel** Westwood-Squibb Ph'cals	lotion	petrolatum · dimethicone	glycerin		steareth-2 · cetyl alcohol · benzyl alcohol · laureth-23 · carbomer 934 · magnesium aluminum silicate · quaternium-15 · sodium hydroxide · water
FR	**Moisturel** Westwood-Squibb Ph'cals	cream	petrolatum · dimethicone	glycerin		PG dioctanoate · cetyl alcohol · steareth-2 · PVP/hexadecene copolymer · laureth-23 · magnesium aluminum silicate · carbomer 934 · sodium hydroxide · kathon CG · diazolidinyl urea · water
FR	**Moisturel Sensitive Skin** Westwood-Squibb Ph'cals	lotion				sodium laureth sulfate · laureth 6 carboxylic acid · disodium laureth sulfosuccinate · methyl gluceth 20 · cocamidopropyl betaine · kathon CG · diazolidinyl urea · water
	Moisturizing Lotion C & M Pharmacal	lotion	petrolatum	propylene glycol · glycerin		purified water · cetearyl · PEG-40 stearate
	Nephro-Derm R & D Labs	cream	petrolatum · mineral oil			water · eucerin · paraffin wax · Tween · camphor · menthol · methylparaben · propylparaben · vitamin B12 · glyceryl stearate

See Chapter 26, "Dermatologic Products," for more information about these products.

DRY SKIN PRODUCTS - continued

	Product Manufacturer/Supplier	Dosage Form	Emollient/ Moisturizer	Humectant	Keratin Softener	Other Ingredients
**	**Neutrogena Body Lotion** Neutrogena Dermatologics	lotion	dimethicone copolyol	glycerin		purified water · sesame oil · isopropyl myristate · cetyl alcohol · glyceryl stearate · PEG-100 stearate · tetrasodium EDTA · acrylates/C10-30 alkyl acrylate crosspolymer · magesium aluminum silicate · xanthan gum · triethanolamine · methylparaben · ethylparaben · propylparaben · diazolidinyl urea · BHT · fragrance
	Neutrogena Body Oil Neutrogena Dermatologics	body oil				isopropyl myristate · sesame oil · PEG-40 sorbitan peroleate · methylparaben · propylparaben
**	**Neutrogena Daily Moisture Supply** Neutrogena Dermatologics	lotion	dimethicone · hydrogenated lanolin · dimethicone copolyol	glycerin · propylene glycol isoceteth-3 acetate · propylene glycol		purified water · emulsifying wax · octyl isononanoate · cyclomethicone · stearic acid · aloe extract · matricaria extract · tocopheryl acetate · glyceryl laurate · acrylates/C10-30 alkyl acrylate crosspolymer · tetrasodium EDTA · cetearyl alcohol · sodium cetearyl sulfate · sodium sulfate · BHT · triethanolamine · methylparaben · ethylparaben · propylparaben · diazolidinyl urea · benzalkonium chloride · fragrance
	Neutrogena Norwegian Formula Neutrogena Dermatologics	cream		glycerin, 41%		
FR	**Neutrogena Norwegian Formula Emulsion** Neutrogena Dermatologics	emulsion		glycerin, 25%		
	Nivea Creme Ultra Moisturizing Beiersdorf	cream	mineral oil · petrolatum	glycerin		water · isohexadecane · microcrystalline wax · lanolin alcohol · paraffin · panthenol · magnesium sulfate · decyl oleate · octyldodecanol · aluminum stearate · fragrance · methylchloroisothiazolinone-methylisothiazolinone · citric acid · magnesium stearate
**	**Nivea Daily Care for Lips** Beiersdorf	stick	petrolatum			polydecene · paraffin · ceresin · cyclomethicone · isopropyl palmitate · carnauba · polyglyceryl-3 diisostearate · synthetic beeswax · lanolin alcohol · tocopheryl acetate · panthenol · fragrance
	Nivea Moisturizing Extra Enriched Beiersdorf	lotion	mineral oil · petrolatum ·	glycerin		purified water · isohexadecane · PEG-40 · sorbitan peroleate · polyglyceryl-3 diisostearate · isopropyl palmitate · cetyl palmitate · glyceryl lanolate · magnesium sulfate · fragrance · aluminum stearate · lanolin alcohol · phenoxyethanol · methyldibromo glutaronitrile

See Chapter 26, "Dermatologic Products," for more information about these products.

DRY SKIN PRODUCTS - continued

Product Manufacturer/Supplier	Dosage Form	Emollient/ Moisturizer	Humectant	Keratin Softener	Other Ingredients
Nivea Shower & Bath Beiersdorf	cleansing bar	petrolatum	glycerin		sodium tallowate/sodium cocoate · fragrance · titanium dioxide · sodium chloride · octyldodecanol · macadamia nut oil · aloe extract · sodium thiosulfate · purified water · lanolin alcohol · pentasodium pentetate · tetrasodium etidronate · BHT · beeswax
Nivea Skin Original Therapeutic Beiersdorf	body oil	mineral oil · lanolin · petrolatum			water · glyceryl lanolate · lanolin alcohol · fragrance · sodium borate · methylchloroisothiazolinone-methylisothiazolinone
Noncomedogenic Facial Moisturizing Cream C & M Pharmacal	cream		glycerin · sorbitol		purified water · polawax A-31 · isopropyl palmitate · castor oil · benzyl alcohol · polysorbate 20
** **Nose Better** Lee Consumer	gel	lanolin		allantoin	camphor · menthol · eucalyptus oil · vitamin E
Noxzema Original Procter & Gamble	cream		propylene glycol		water · stearic acid · linseed oil · soybean oil · fragrance · ammonium hydroxide · gelatin · camphor · menthol · phenol · clove oil · eucalyptus oil · calcium hydroxide
Noxzema Original Procter & Gamble	lotion		propylene glycol		water · stearic acid · soybean oil · fragrance · linseed oil · gelatin · calcium hydroxide · cetyl alcohol · camphor · menthol · phenol · clove oil · eucalyptus oil · carbomer · triethanolamine
Noxzema Plus Cleansing Procter & Gamble	lotion		glycerin		water · stearic acid · caprylic/capric triglyceride · glycol distearate · cetyl alcohol · PEG-8 · fragrance · cetearyl alcohol · ceteareth-20 · cocamide DEA · castor oil · triethanolamine · methylparaben · imidazolidinyl urea · carbomer · propylparaben · PEG-10 soya sterol · disodium EDTA
Noxzema Plus Cleansing Procter & Gamble	cream		glycerin · propylene glycol		water · stearic acid · linseed oil · soybean oil · gelatin · calcium hydroxide · ammonium hydroxide · fragrance · methylparaben · propylparaben · DMDM hydantoin · disodium EDTA · phenoxyethanol
Noxzema Sensitive Cleansing Procter & Gamble	cream · lotion		glycerin		water · stearic acid · cetyl alcohol · caprylic/capric triglyceride · glycol distearate · PEG-8 · cetearyl alcohol · triethanolamine · carbomer · ceteareth-20 · DMDM hydantoin · iodopropynyl butylcarbamate · PEG-10 soya sterol · disodium EDTA
Nutra Soothe Oatmeal Bath Brimms Labs	powder		colloidal oatmeal, 100%		

See Chapter 26, "Dermatologic Products," for more information about these products.

DRY SKIN PRODUCTS - continued

Product Manufacturer/Supplier	Dosage Form	Emollient/ Moisturizer	Humectant	Keratin Softener	Other Ingredients
Nutraderm Galderma Labs	cream	mineral oil			sorbitan stearate · stearyl alcohol · sodium lauryl sulfate · cetyl alcohol · methylparaben · propylparaben · fragrance
Nutraderm Galderma Labs	bath oil	mineral oil · lanolin oil			bath oil · PEG-4 dilaurate · benzophenone-3 · butylparaben
Nutraderm Galderma Labs	lotion	mineral oil			sorbitan stearate · stearyl and cetyl alcohol · carbomer 940
Nutraderm 30 Galderma Labs	lotion	petrolatum · dimethicone	sodium PCA · glycerin	lactic acid · malic acid	cetearyl alcohol · ceteareth-20 · C10-30 cholesterol/lanosterol esters · cyclomethicone · cetyl alcohol · sodium lactate · cetyl lactate · C12-C15 alcohols lactate · xanthan gum · sodium hydroxide · methylparaben · propylparaben · fragrance · diazolidinyl urea
Nutraplus Healthpoint	lotion	petrolatum		urea, 10%	glyceryl stearate · acetylated lanolin alcohol · isopropyl palmitate · stearic acid · methylparaben · propylparaben · carbomer 940
Nutraplus Healthpoint	cream	mineral oil	propylene glycol	urea, 10%	glyceryl stearate · methylparaben · propylparaben
Oil of Olay Bath Bar, Pink or White Procter & Gamble	cleansing bar				sodium cocoyl isethionate · sodium cetearyl sulfate · paraffin · stearic acid · water · sodium isethionate · coconut acid · sodium stearate · sodium cocoate · fragrance · sodium chloride · titanium dioxide · lauric acid · sodium laurate · trisodium EDTA · trisodium etidronate · colorant (Pink)
Oil of Olay Foaming Face Wash, Regular or Sensitive Procter & Gamble	liquid		glycerin	citric acid	water · sodium myristol sarcosinate · PEG-120 methyl glucose dioleate · sodium lauroamphoacetate · disodium lauroamphodiacetate · glycol distearate · PEG-150 pentaerythritol tetra stearate · sodium trideceth sulfate · polyquaternium-10 · sodium laureth sulfate · phenoxyethanol · cocamide MEA · DMDM hydantoin · disodium EDTA · laureth-9 · fragrance (Regular)
Oil of Olay Sensitive Skin Bath Bar Procter & Gamble	cleansing bar				sodium cocoyl isethionate · sodium cetearyl sulfate · paraffin · stearic acid · water · sodium isethionate · coconut acid · sodium stearate · sodium cocoate · sodium chloride · titanium dioxide · lauric acid · sodium laurate · trisodium EDTA · trisodium etidronate · masking fragrance

See Chapter 26, "Dermatologic Products," for more information about these products.

DRY SKIN PRODUCTS - continued

	Product Manufacturer/Supplier	Dosage Form	Emollient/ Moisturizer	Humectant	Keratin Softener	Other Ingredients
	Oilatum Soap Stiefel Labs	cleansing bar		propylene glycol	citric acid	sodium tallowate · sodium cocoate · water · peanut oil · octyl hydroxystearate · lecithin · fragrance · sodium chloride · PEG-14M · titanium dioxide · o-tolyl biguanide · trisodium HEDTA · sodium borohydride · glyceryl oleate · corn oil · t-butyl hydroquinone · FD&C red#4 · D&C orange#4
	Pacquin Medicated Hand and Body Pfizer Consumer	cream	dimethicone, 1%	glycerin, 12%		water · stearic acid · potassium stearate · sodium stearate · cetyl alcohol · fragrance · diisopropyl sebacate · carbomer 940 · methylparaben · propylparaben
	Pacquin Plus Dry Skin Hand and Body Pfizer Consumer	cream	lanolin anhydrous, 0.5%	glycerin, 12%		water · stearic acid · potassium stearate · sodium stearate · myristyl lactate · cetyl alcohol · cetyl esters · fragrance · diisopropyl sebacate · stearamide DZA · carbomer 940 · methylparaben · propylparaben
	Pacquin Plus with Aloe Pfizer Consumer	cream	dimethicone, 1% · lanolin anhydrous, 0.5% · mineral oil · petrolatum			aloe vera gel, 20% · water · isopropyl palmitate · white synthetic beeswax · cetyl alcohol · triethanolamine · glyceryl stearate · carbomer 934 · stearic acid · fragrance · methylparaben · laureth-23 · quaternium-15 · D&C red#33 · imidazolidinyl urea
**	**Palmer's Cocoa Butter** E. T. Browne Drug	cream	mineral oil			cocoa butter · microcrystalline wax · vitamin E · carotene
**	**Palmer's Cocoa Butter** E. T. Browne Drug	lotion	mineral oil · petrolatum	propylene glycol · glycerin		deionized water · cocoa butter · glyceryl stearate · coconut oil · palm oil · cetyl alcohol · PEG-8 stearate · vitamin E · steapyrium chloride · methylparaben · propylparaben · FD&C yellow#5 · D&C orange #4
**	**Palmer's Cocoa Butter Concentrated Hand Cream SPF 8** E. T. Browne Drug	cream	dimethicone · lecithin	glycerin		octyl methoxycinnamate · water · cetearyl alcohol · cocoa butter · sodium cetearyl sulfate · stearic acid · methylparaben · propylparaben · sodium sulfite · dilauryl thiodipropionate · acetylated lanolin alcohols · isopropyl palmitate · vitamin E · FD&C yellow#5 · FD&C red#4
	Panthoderm Jones Medical	cream				dexpanthenol, 2% · water-miscible base
	Pedi-Vit-A Pedinol Pharmacal	cream				vitamin A, 100000 IU/30mg

See Chapter 26, "Dermatologic Products," for more information about these products.

DRY SKIN PRODUCTS - continued

	Product Manufacturer/Supplier	Dosage Form	Emollient/ Moisturizer	Humectant	Keratin Softener	Other Ingredients
FR	**Pen-Kera** B. F. Ascher	cream	mineral oil	glycerin		octyl palmitate · polysorbate 60 · sorbitan stearate · carbomer 940 · triethanolamine · wheat germ glycerides · polyamino sugar condensate · dehydroacetic acid · DMDMH iodo-propynyl-butylcarbamate · diazolidinyl urea · water
	Perry Shampoo Perry Products	shampoo				water · sodium laureth sulfate · cocamidopropyl betaine · hydrolyzed animal protein · sodium chloride · methylparaben · propylparaben · quaternium-15 · skin esters
** FR	**Physicians Formula Self Defense Moisturizing SPF 15** Pierre Fabre Dermatology	lotion	petrolatum	glycerin · sodium PCA		octyl methoxycinnamate · benzophenone-3 · octyl salicylate · water · glyceryl stearate · PEG-100 stearate · panthenol · TEA-stearate · isocetyl stearate · tridecyl stearate · neopentylglycol dicaprylate/dicaprate tridecyl trimellitate · carbomer · hydrolyzed soy protein · lanolin alcohol · magnesium aluminum silicate · PEG-20 · sodium hyaluronate · xanthan gum · methylparaben · propylparaben · diazolidinyl urea · quarternium-15
	Plexo Hand Alvin Last	cream	mineral oil	propylene glycol · glycerin		water · zinc stearate · stearic acid · lanolin benzyl alcohol · fragrance · potassium hydroxide · cetyl alcohol · butylparaben
FR	**Plexolan Moisturizing** Alvin Last	cream	petrolatum · mineral oil			water · ceresin · lanolin alcohol · methylparaben · propylparaben
	Polysorb Hydrate E. Fougera	cream	petrolatum			sorbitan sesquioleate · wax · water
**	**Pretty Feet & Hands Replenishing Creme** B. F. Ascher	cream	mineral oil			water · glyceryl stearate · cetyl alcohol · aloe vera gel · sodium laureth-sulfate · carbomer 940 · triethanolamine · fragrance · methylparaben propylparaben
**	**Pretty Feet & Hands Rough Skin Remover** B. F. Ascher	cream				water · paraffin · magnesium aluminum silicate · palmitic acid · stearic acid · triethanolamine · methylparaben · propylparaben · fragrance
	Pro-Cute Ferndale Labs	cream		glycerin		water · stearic acid · cetyl alcohol · ceraphyl 230 · forlan-LM · deltyl prime · trolamine · silicone · povidone · dowicil 200 · perfume
	Q.O.D. Bath Additive Perry Products	liquid	petrolatum · lanolin	propylene glycol · sodium PCA		sodium laureth sulfate · water · PEG-7 glyceryl cocoate · lauramide DEA · dioctyl adipate · octyl stearate · octyl palmitate · methylparaben · imidazolidinyl urea · propylparaben · cetyl alcohol · polysorbate 85

See Chapter 26, "Dermatologic Products," for more information about these products.

DRY SKIN PRODUCTS - continued

	Product Manufacturer/Supplier	Dosage Form	Emollient/ Moisturizer	Humectant	Keratin Softener	Other Ingredients
**	**Red Fox Bottle O'Butter** Majestic Drug	lotion	mineral oil · lanolin	glycerin · sorbitol		water · stearic acid · triethanolamine · cocoa butter · hydrogenated vegetable oil · cetyl alcohol · fragrance · methylparaben · propylparaben · FD&C yellow#6 · FD&C red#4
**	**Red Fox Tub O'Butter** Majestic Drug	cream	petrolatum · lanolin			cocoa butter · hydrogenated vegetable oil · propylparaben · fragrance
	Sardo Schering-Plough Healthcare	bath oil	mineral oil			isopropyl palmitate
	Sardoettes Schering-Plough Healthcare	wipe	mineral oil			isopropyl palmitate
	Sarna Stiefel Labs	lotion	emollient base			camphor, 0.5% · menthol, 0.5%
**	**Sayman Salve** Merz Consumer	ointment	petrolatum, 87.3% · lanolin	propylene glycol		zinc oxide · fragrance · quaternium-15
FR	**Shepards Cream Lotion** Dermik Labs	cream/lotion		glycerin · propylene glycol	citric acid	water · sesame oil · SD alcohol 40-B · stearic acid · ethoxydiglycol · triethanolamine · glyceryl stearate · cetyl alcohol · simethicone · methylparaben · propylparaben · vegetable oil · monoglyceride citrate · BHT
FR	**Shepards Skin Cream** Dermik Labs	cream		glycerin · propylene glycol	urea	water · glyceryl stearate · ethoxydiglycol · stearic acid · isopropyl myristate · cetyl alcohol · lecithin · methylparaben · propylparaben
FR	**Silk Solution** Thompson Medical	lotion	dimethicone, 2.0%	glycerin		cetyl alcohol · cyclomethicone · dimethiconol · dioctyl adipate · methyldibromoglutaronitrite · phenoxyethanol · stearic acid · triethanolamine · water
	Skin Cream or Lotion Perry Products	cream · lotion	petrolatum · lanolin	propylene glycol · sodium PCA		water · cetyl alcohol · polysorbate 85 · glyceryl stearate · PEG-100 stearate · sodium lauryl sulfate · methylparaben · imidazolidinyl urea
**	**Skin Magic** Care-Tech Labs	lotion	mineral oil · lanolin oil	propylene glycol		chloroxylenol, 0.4% · water · stearic acid · isostearyl alcohol · glycol stearate · stearamide DEA · triethanolamine · cetyl alcohol · myristyl propionate · fragrance · propylparaben · DMDM hydantoin · methylparaben · carbomer 934
	Sofenol 5 C & M Pharmacal	lotion	petrolatum · dimethicone	glycerin	allantoin	purified water · cetostearyl alcohol · soluble collagen · PEG-40 stearate · kaolin · sunflower seed oil · sorbic acid · carbomer 940 · disodium EDTA · sodium hydroxide
FR	**Soft Sense Alpha Hydroxy Moisturizing** Bausch & Lomb	lotion	petrolatum · dimethicone	glycerin	lactic acid	distearyl dimonium chloride · isopropyl palmitate · l-hexadecanol · ammonium hydroxide · tocopheryl acetate · titanium dioxide · methylparaben · propylparaben

See Chapter 26, "Dermatologic Products," for more information about these products.

DRY SKIN PRODUCTS - continued

	Product Manufacturer/Supplier	Dosage Form	Emollient/ Moisturizer	Humectant	Keratin Softener	Other Ingredients
FR	**Soft Sense Moisturizing, Fragrance Free or Original** Bausch & Lomb	lotion	petrolatum · dimethicone	glycerin		purified water · distearyldimonium chloride · isopropyl palmitate · vitamin E · aloe · keratin protein · titanium dioxide · methylparaben · propylparaben
**	**Soft Skin After Bath Oil** Care-Tech Labs	pump spray	mineral oil			benzophenone-3 · apricot kernel oil · oleth 5 · fragrance · D&C red#17 · D&C yellow#11
	Softlips, Cool Cherry Mentholatum	stick	dimethicone, 2% · lanolin · petrolatum			cetyl octanoate · fragrance · menthol · ozokerite · squalane · vitamin E acetate
	Softlips, Sparkle Mint Mentholatum	stick	dimethicone, 2% · lanolin · petrolatum			padimate O, 3% · cetyl octanoate · fragrance · menthol · ozokerite · squalane · vitamin E acetate
PE	**Stevens Baby** Stevens Skin Softener	cream		glycerin	allantoin	deionized water · glyceryl stearate · stearic acid · jojoba oil · cetyl alcohol · apricot kernel oil · castor oil · sweet almond oil · cetyl palmitate · cetearyl octanoate · squalene · methyl gluceth-20 · magnesium aluminum silicate · panthenol · diazolidinyl urea · propylparaben · avocado oil · methylparaben · butylparaben · tetrasodium EDTA · tocopherol · fragrance · aloe vera gel
**	**Stevens Lip Cream SPF 15** Stevens Skin Softener	cream	dimethicone	glycerin	allantoin	octyl methoxycinnamate · benzophenone-3 · deionized water · glyceryl stearate · PEG-100 stearate · C21-15 alkyl benzoate · jojoba oil · apricot kernel oil · stearic acid · dimethyl stearamine · sweet almond oil · cetearyl octanoate · methyl gluceth-20 · castor oil · acrylates/octylacrylamide copolymer · squalene · panthenol · cetyl alcohol · cetyl palmitate · propylparaben · diazolidinyl urea · triethanolamine · methylparaben · butylparaben · fragrance · tocopherol · tetrasodium EDTA · avocado oil · magnesium aluminum silicate · aloe vera gel
FR	**Stevens Skin Softener** Stevens Skin Softener	cream		glycerin	allantoin	deionized water · glyceryl stearate · stearic acid · jojoba oil · cetyl alcohol · apricot kernel oil · castor oil · sweet almond oil · cetyl palmitate · cetearyl octanoate · squalene · methyl gluceth-20 · magnesium aluminum silicate · panthenol · diazolidinyl urea · propylparaben · avocado oil · methylparaben · butylparaben · tetrasodium EDTA · tocopherol · aloe vera gel
	Sustained Effect Hydrating Lotion C & M Pharmacal	lotion	petrolatum	propylene glycol · glycerin	lactic acid · allantoin	purified water · cetearyl alcohol · PEG-40 storate · potassium hydroxide

See Chapter 26, "Dermatologic Products," for more information about these products.

DRY SKIN PRODUCTS - continued

	Product Manufacturer/Supplier	Dosage Form	Emollient/ Moisturizer	Humectant	Keratin Softener	Other Ingredients
**	**Sweedish-Formula Creme** Palco Labs	cream	mineral oil	glycerin		purified water · cetyl alcohol · carbamide · eucalyptus oil · benzalkonium chloride · cetrimonium bromide · methylparaben · diazolidnyl urea · sodium citrate
FR	**Theraplex Hydrolotion** Medicis Dermatologics	lotion	dimethicone copolyol · special petrolatum fraction			water · cyclomethicone · SD alcohol 40 · benzyl alcohol · sodium chloride · sorbitan laurate
**	**Topifram Traitement Dermatologiste Moisturising** E. T. Browne Drug	lotion		propylene glycol		purified water · stearic acid · cetyl alcohol · octyl methoxycinnamate, 2% · vitamin E · carbomer 941 methylparaben · propylparaben · geranium extract · maleated soybean oil · triethanolamine
FR	**U-Lactin** Allerderm Labs	lotion	mineral oil · petrolatum	propylene glycol stearate	urea, 10% · lactic acid	purified water · sorbitan stearate · cetyl alcohol · sodium lauryl sulfate · magnesium aluminum silicate · methylparaben · propylparaben · quarternium-15
	Ultra Derm Baker Cummins Derm'cals	bath oil	mineral oil · lanolin oil			octoxynol-3
	Ultra Derm Moisturizer Baker Cummins Derm'cals	lotion	mineral oil · petrolatum · lanolin oil	glycerin · propylene glycol · propylene glycol stearate SE		glyceryl stearate · PEG-50-stearate · cetyl alcohol · sorbitan laurate · potassium sorbate · phosphoric acid · tetrasodium EDTA
	Ultra Mide 25 Moisturizer Baker Cummins Derm'cals	lotion			urea, 25%	
	Ureacin-10 Pedinol Pharmacal	lotion			urea, 10% · lactic acid	vegetable oil base
	Ureacin-20 Pedinol Pharmacal	cream			urea, 20% · lactic acid	vegetable oil base
	Vaseline Dermatology Formula Chesebrough-Pond's	lotion	white petrolatum, 5% · mineral oil, 4% · dimethicone, 1%	glycerin		water · stearic acid · glycol stearate · cetyl acetate · glyceryl stearate · triethanolamine · PEG-40 stearate · magnesium aluminum silicate · cetyl alcohol · acetylated lanolin alcohol · methylparaben · fragrance · propylparaben · stearamide AMP · carbomer 934 · disodium EDTA · DMDM hydantoin

See Chapter 26, "Dermatologic Products," for more information about these products.

DRY SKIN PRODUCTS - continued

	Product Manufacturer/Supplier	Dosage Form	Emollient/ Moisturizer	Humectant	Keratin Softener	Other Ingredients
**	**Vaseline Dual Action Alpha Hydroxy Formula** Chesebrough-Pond's	cream	petrolatum · dimethicone	glycerin	lactic acid	water · butylene glycol · potassium lactate · PPG-2 myristyl ether propionate · stearic acid · PEG-100 stearate · glyceryl stearate · stearyl alcohol · sorbitan stearate · sunflower seed oil · vitamin E acetate · lecithin · soya sterol · isocetyl alcohol · magnesium aluminum silicate · xanthan gum · hydroxyethyl cellulose · fragrance · disodium EDTA · simethicone · DMDM hydantoin · iodopropynyl butylcarbamate
	Vaseline Intensive Care Extra Strength Chesebrough-Pond's	lotion	petrolatum · dimethicone, 1.5%	glycerin · sodium PCA	urea · lactic acid	water · stearic acid · C11-13 isoparaffin · glycol stearate · glyceryl stearate · triethanolamine · zinc oxide · cetyl alcohol · potassium cetyl phosphate · carbomer 934 · stearamide AMP · fragrance · sunflower seed oil · soya sterol · lecithin · sodium stearoyl lactylate · tolopherylacetate · retinyl palmitate · potassium lactate · collagen amino acids · magnesium aluminum silicate · corn oil · methylparaben · DMDM hydantoin · iodopropynyl butyl carbamate · disodium EDTA
	Vaseline Medicated Anti-Bacterial Petrolatum Jelly Chesebrough-Pond's	ointment	petrolatum, 98.3%			chloroxylenol, 0.53% · lanolin · beta carotene · phenol
** FR	**Vita-Ray Creme** Gordon Labs	cream	petrolatum · mineral oil	propylene glycol		vitamin A, 200000 IU/oz · vitamin E, 3000 IU/oz · aloe vera gel · cetyl alcohol · white wax · sodium lauryl sulfate · methylparaben · propylparaben
	Vitacel Republic Drug	cream				retinyl palmitate · collagen · elastin · squalene
	Wibi Healthpoint	lotion		glycerin		SD alcohol 40 · PEG-4 · PEG-6-32 · stearate · glycol stearate · carbomer 940 · PEG-75 · methylparaben · triethanolamine · menthol · fragrance

** New listing

§ Manufacturer/supplier did not confirm information for this edition. Product listing is reprinted from the '96-97 edition.

See Chapter 26, "Dermatologic Products," for more information about these products.

DANDRUFF, SEBORRHEA, AND PSORIASIS PRODUCTS

Product [a] Manufacturer/Supplier	Dosage Form	Keratolytic	Cytostatic	Tar Product	Other Ingredients
Balnetar Westwood-Squibb Ph'cals	bath oil			coal tar, 2.5%	mineral oil · lanolin oil · PEG-4-dilaurate · laureth 4 · fragrance · docusate sodium
Brylcreem Anti-Dandruff J. B. Williams	cream		pyrithione zinc, 1%		mineral oil · propylene glycol · paraffin wax · water · triceteareth-4 phosphate · petrolatum · poloxamer 234 and 334 · trolamine · carbomer · fragrance
Creamy Dandruff Shampoo C & M Pharmacal	shampoo	salicylic acid, 2% · sulfur, 2%			sodium lauryl sulfate · purified water · diglycol monostearate · lauramide DEA · cetearyl alcohol · petrolatum · fragrance
Cutar Summers Labs	emulsion			coal tar, 1.5%	
Dandruff Shampoo Maximum Strength C & M Pharmacal	shampoo	sulfur, 5% · salicylic acid, 3%			sodium lauryl sulfate · purified water · diethylene glycol monostearate · lauramide DEA · cetostearyl alcohol · glycerin · fragrance · petrolatum · hydroxyethyl ethylcellulose · FD&C red#40
Dandruff Wash, Medicated C & M Pharmacal	cream	sulfur, 4% · salicylic acid, 2%			water · TEA-dodecylbenzene sulfonate · magnesium aluminum silicate · glycerin · stearic acid · cetearyl alcohol · polysorbate 20 · fragrance · FD&C red#40
Denorex Dandruff for Dry Scalp, Shampoo or Shampoo & Cond. Whitehall-Robins Healthcare	shampoo · conditioner			coal tar extract, 2% (equivalent to 0.5% coal tar)	ammonium laureth sulfate · ammonium lauryl sulfate · avocado oil · citric acid · cocamide MEA · dimethicone copolyol · disodium EDTA · FD&C blue#1 · fragrance · glycol distearate · hydroxypropyl methylcellulose · imidurea · lauramide DEA · lauramidopropyl betaine · laureth-9 · menthol · methylparaben · panthenol · PEG-27 lanolin · quaternium-80 · ricinoleamidopropyl ethyldimonium ethosulfate (Shampoo & Conditioner) · sodium laureth sulfate · trolamine · vitamin E acetate · water
Denorex Medicated Shampoo & Conditioner Whitehall-Robins Healthcare	shampoo · conditioner			coal tar solution, 9% (equivalent to 1.8% coal tar)	alcohol, 7.5% · chloroxylenol · citric acid · fragrance · hydroxypropyl methylcellulose · lauramide DEA · menthol · PEG-27 lanolin · polyquaternium-11 · TEA-lauryl sulfate · water · compound 64.404/NY/D
Denorex Medicated Shampoo & Conditioner, Extra Strength Whitehall-Robins Healthcare	shampoo · conditioner			coal tar solution, 12.5% (equivalent to 2.5% coal tar)	alcohol, 10.4% · avocado oil · chloroxylenol · citric acid · dimethicone copolyol · FD&C red#40 · fragrance · glycol distearate · hydroxypropyl methylcellulose · lauramide DEA · menthol · panthenol · PEG-27 lanolin · quaternium-80 · ricinoleamidopropyl ethyldimonium ethosulfate · TEA-lauryl sulfate · vitamin E acetate · water

See Chapter 26, "Dermatologic Products," for more information about these products.

DANDRUFF, SEBORRHEA, AND PSORIASIS PRODUCTS - continued

Product [a] Manufacturer/Supplier	Dosage Form	Keratolytic	Cytostatic	Tar Product	Other Ingredients
Denorex Medicated, Extra Strength Whitehall-Robins Healthcare	shampoo			coal tar solution, 12.5% (equivalent to 2.5% coal tar)	chloroxylenol · FD&C red#40 · fragrance · glycol distearate · hydroxypropyl methylcellulose · lauramide DEA · menthol · panthenol · TEA-lauryl sulfate · vitamin E acetate · water
Denorex Medicated, Mountain Fresh Scent Whitehall-Robins Healthcare	shampoo			coal tar solution, 9% (equivalent to 1.8% coal tar)	alcohol, 7.5% · chloroxylenol · fragrance · hydroxypropyl methylcellulose · lauramide DEA · menthol · stearic acid · TEA-lauryl sulfate · water · compound 64.404/NY/D
DHS Sal Person & Covey	liquid	salicylic acid, 3%			sodium C14-16 · olefin sulfonate · TEA-lauryl sulfate · cocamidopropyl betaine · cocamide DEA · cocamide MEA · disodium EDTA · PEG-8 distearate · purified water
DHS Tar Person & Covey	shampoo			coal tar, 0.5%	water · TEA-lauryl sulfate · sodium chloride · PEG-8 distearate · cocamide DEA · cocamide MEA · citric acid
DHS Tar Gel Person & Covey	shampoo			coal tar, 0.5%	water · TEA lauryl sulfate · sodium chloride · PEG-8 distearate · cocamide DEA · cocamide MEA · hydroxypropyl methylcellulose · citric acid · fragrance
DHS Zinc Person & Covey	shampoo		pyrithione zinc, 2%		water · TEA lauryl sulfate · PEG-8 distearate · sodium chloride · cocamide DEA · cocamide MEA · magnesium aluminum silicate · hydroxypropyl methylcellulose · fragrance · FD&C yellow#6
Doak Tar Doak Dermatologics	oil			tar distillate, 2% · (equivalent to 0.8% coal tar)	
Doak Tar Doak Dermatologics	lotion			tar distillate, 5% (equivalent to 2% coal tar)	
Doak Tar Doak Dermatologics	shampoo			tar distillate, 3% (equivalent to 1.2% coal tar)	
Doctar Savage Labs	shampoo			tar, 2% (equivalent to 0.5% coal tar)	demineralized water · sodium laureth sulfate · TEA-lauryl sulfate · cocamidopropyl betaine · PEG-30 glyceryl stearate · polysorbate 80 · cocamidopropylamine oxide · cocamide DEA · fragrance
Duplex-T C & M Pharmacal	shampoo			coal tar solution, 10%	purified water · sodium lauryl sulfate · lauramide DEA
Estar Westwood-Squibb Ph'cals	gel			coal tar, 5%	alcohol, 15.6% · alanine · benzyl alcohol · carbomer 940 · glycereth-7 cocoanate · polysorbate 80 · simethicone · sorbitol · water
** **Fototar** ICN Ph'cals	cream			coal tar extract (equivalent to 2% coal tar)	
Glover's Dandruff Control Medicine J. K. Ph'cals	liquid	sulfur, 2.5%		pine tar oil	mineral oil · polysorbate 85 · quaternium-18-hectorite · fragrance

See Chapter 26, "Dermatologic Products," for more information about these products.

DANDRUFF, SEBORRHEA, AND PSORIASIS PRODUCTS - continued

Product [a] Manufacturer/Supplier	Dosage Form	Keratolytic	Cytostatic	Tar Product	Other Ingredients
Glover's Medicated J. K. Ph'cals	shampoo			coal tar solution, 5% (equivalent to 1% coal tar)	water · TEA lauryl sulfate · potassium coco hydrolyzed animal protein · lauramide DEA · TEA coco hydrolyzed animal protein · fragrance · methylparaben · propylparaben
Glover's Medicated Dandruff Soap J. K. Ph'cals	cleansing bar	sulfur, 2.08%		pine tar	sodium tallowate · sodium cocoate · water · petroleum · trisodium HEDTA · BHT
Glover's Medicated for Dandruff J. K. Ph'cals	ointment	sulfur, 5% · salicylic acid, 3%			petrolatum · mineral oil · glyceryl tribehenate · arachidyl propionate · fragrance · polysorbate-20 · propylparaben · iron oxides · talc
Grandpa's Pine Tar Shampooing (liquid) Grandpa Soap	shampoo			pine tar oil, 1%	water · sodium lauryl sulfate · sodium laureth sulfate · sodium chloride · cocamide DEA · dihydrogenated tallow phthalic acid amide · polymethoxy bicyclic oxazolidine · fragrance
Grandpa's Pine Tar Soap Grandpa Soap	cleansing bar			pine tar oil, 2.7%	
Head & Shoulders Dandruff 2-in-1 Procter & Gamble	shampoo		pyrithione zinc, 1%		ammonium laureth sulfate · ammonium lauryl sulfate · sodium lauroyl sarcosinate · glycol distearate · dimethicone · fragrance · DMDM hydantoin · disodium phosphate · sodium phosphate · lauryl alcohol · PEG-600 · polyquaternium-10 · FD&C blue#1
Head & Shoulders Dandruff, Fine or Oily Hair Procter & Gamble	shampoo		pyrithione zinc, 1%		ammonium laureth sulfate · ammonium lauryl sulfate · sodium lauroyl sarcosinate · glycol distearate · sodium sulfate · fragrance · DMDM hydantoin · sodium chloride · disodium phosphate · dimethicone · sodium phosphate · lauryl alcohol · PEG-600 · polyquaternium-10 · FD&C blue#1
Head & Shoulders Dandruff, Normal Hair Procter & Gamble	shampoo		pyrithione zinc, 1%		ammonium laureth sulfate · ammonium lauryl sulfate · sodium lauroyl sarcosinate · glycol distearate · sodium sulfate · fragrance · DMDM hydantoin · sodium chloride · disodium phosphate · dimethicone · sodium phosphate · lauryl alcohol · PEG-600 · polyquaternium-10 · FD&C blue#1
Head & Shoulders Dry Scalp, Regular or 2-in-1 Procter & Gamble	shampoo		pyrithione zinc, 1%		ammonium laureth sulfate · ammonium lauryl sulfate · sodium lauroyl sarcosinate · glycol distearate · dimethicone · sodium sulfate · sodium chloride · fragrance · DMDM hydantoin · disodium phosphate · sodium phosphate · lauryl alcohol · PEG-600 · polyquaternium-10 · FD&C blue#1

See Chapter 26, "Dermatologic Products," for more information about these products.

DANDRUFF, SEBORRHEA, AND PSORIASIS PRODUCTS - continued

Product [a] Manufacturer/Supplier	Dosage Form	Keratolytic	Cytostatic	Tar Product	Other Ingredients
Head & Shoulders Intensive Treatment, Regular or 2-in-1 Procter & Gamble	shampoo		selenium sulfide, 1%		ammonium laureth sulfate · ammonium lauryl sulfate · cocamide MEA · glycol distearate · ammonium xylensulfonate · fragrance · dimethicone · tricetylmonium chloride · cetyl alcohol · stearyl alcohol · DMDM hydantoin · sodium chloride · hydroxypropyl methylcellulose · FD&C red#4
Ionil Healthpoint	shampoo	salicylic acid, 2%			polyoxyethylene ethers · benzalkonium chloride · alcohol · tetrasodium edetate
Ionil Plus Healthpoint	shampoo	salicylic acid, 2%			sodium laureth sulfate · lauramide DEA · quaternium-22 · talloweth-60 · myristyl glycol · laureth-23 · TEA lauryl sulfate · glycol distearate · laureth-4 · TEA abietoyl hydrolyzed collagen · DMDM hydantoin · tetrasodium EDTA · sodium hydroxide · fragrance · FD&C blue#1
Ionil T Healthpoint	shampoo			coal tar solution, 5%	alcohol, 12% · isopropyl alcohol, 4% · benzalkonium chloride, 0.2% · polyoxyethylene ethers · EDTA
Ionil T Plus Healthpoint	shampoo			crude coal tar	sodium laureth sulfate · lauramide DEA · quaternium-22 · laureth-23 · talloweth-60 · myristyl glycol · TEA lauryl sulfate · glycol distearate · laureth-4 · TEA-abietoyl hydrolyzed collagen · DMDM hydantoin · EDTA · fragrance · FD&C blue#1 · FD&C yellow#7
** **Medotar** Medco Lab	ointment			coal tar, 1%	white petrolatum · zinc oxide · starch · octoxynol-9 · polysorbate 80
Meted GenDerm	shampoo	sulfur, 5% · salicylic acid, 3%			
** **MG217 for Psoriasis** Triton Consumer	shampoo			coal tar solution, 15%	
MG217 for Psoriasis Triton Consumer	ointment			coal tar solution, 10%	
MG217 for Psoriasis Triton Consumer	lotion			coal tar solution, 5%	
MG217 for Psoriasis Sal-Acid Triton Consumer	ointment	salicylic acid, 3%			
** **MG217 Tar-Free for Dandruff** Triton Consumer	shampoo	sulfur, 5% · salycylic acid, 3%			
Neutrogena Healthy Scalp Anti-Dandruff Neutrogena Dermatologics	shampoo	salicylic acid, 1.8%			
Neutrogena T/Derm Neutrogena Dermatologics	body oil			tar, 5% (equivalent to 1.2% coal tar)	

See Chapter 26, "Dermatologic Products," for more information about these products.

DANDRUFF, SEBORRHEA, AND PSORIASIS PRODUCTS - continued

Product [a] Manufacturer/Supplier	Dosage Form	Keratolytic	Cytostatic	Tar Product	Other Ingredients
Neutrogena T/Gel Extra Strength Therapeutic Neutrogena Dermatologics	shampoo			tar, 4% (equivalent to 1% coal tar)	
Neutrogena T/Gel Shampoo or Conditioner Neutrogena Dermatologics	shampoo · conditioner			tar, 2% (equivalent to 0.5% coal tar)	
Neutrogena T/Sal Maximum Strength Therapeutic Neutrogena Dermatologics	shampoo	salicylic acid, 3%			
Oxipor VHC Medtech	lotion			coal tar solution, 25% (equivalent to 5% coal tar)	alcohol, 79% · citric acid · PEG-8 · water
P&S Shampoo Baker Cummins Derm'cals	shampoo	salicylic acid, 2%			
Pentrax GenDerm	shampoo			coal tar, 4.3%	
Pentrax Gold GenDerm	shampoo			coal tar, 2%	
Polytar Stiefel Labs	cleansing bar			tar, 2.5% (equivalent to 0.5% coal tar)	
Polytar Stiefel Labs	shampoo			tar, 4.5% (equivalent to 0.5% coal tar)	
Poslam Psoriasis Alvin Last	ointment	sulfur, 5% · salicylic acid, 2%			petrolatum · corn starch · lanolin · zinc oxide · ozokerite · phenol · menthol · fragrance · talc · iron oxides
Psor-A-Set Hogil Ph'cal	lotion	salicylic acid, 2%			hydrogenated coconut oil · glycerin · beeswax · glyceryl stearate · laureth-23 · polysorbate 60 · polysorbate 80 · squalene · stearic acid · tocopheryl nicotinate · cetyl alcohol · PEG-40 stearate · fish liver oil · isopropyl myristate · pyridoxine · niacin · lecithin · potassium hydroxide · methylparaben · propylparaben
Psor-A-Set Hogil Ph'cal	cleansing bar	salicylic acid, 2%			tocopheryl acetate · titanium dioxide · alpha bisabolol · octylhydroxy stearate
Psor-A-Set Hogil Ph'cal	shampoo	salicylic acid, 2%			sodium laureth sulfate · ammonium myreth sulfate · cocamide DEA · magnesium aluminum silicate · cocamidopropyl betaine · tocopheryl nicotinate · sodium PCA · TEA cocoylglutamate · acetamide MEA · hydroxypropyl methylcellulose · PEG-14M · disodium EDTA · sodium hydroxide · methylchloroisothiazolinone · methylisothizolinone · FD&C blue#1 · fragrance
Psoriasin Alva-Amco Pharmacal	gel			coal tar, 1.25%	isopropyl alcohol, 50% · polyethylene glycol · vitamin E · aloe vera

See Chapter 26, "Dermatologic Products," for more information about these products.

DANDRUFF, SEBORRHEA, AND PSORIASIS PRODUCTS - continued

Product [a] Manufacturer/Supplier	Dosage Form	Keratolytic	Cytostatic	Tar Product	Other Ingredients
Psoriasis Tar C & M Pharmacal	lotion			coal tar solution, 5%	purified water · propylene glycol · ceto stearyl alcohol · petrolatum · glycerin · PEG-40 stearate
Psorigel Healthpoint	gel			coal tar solution, 8.8%	alcohol · laureth-4 · fragrance · propylene glycol · hydroxyethylcellulose
Salicylic Acid & Sulfur Soap Stiefel Labs	cleansing bar	precipitated sulfur, 5% · salicylic acid, 3%			
Scalpicin Maximum Strength Combe	foam	salicylic acid, 3%			emulsifying wax · isobutane · menthol · propylene glycol · SD alcohol 40 · water
Scalpicin Maximum Strength Combe	liquid	salicylic acid, 3%			menthol · propylene glycol · SD alcohol 40 · water
Sebucare Westwood-Squibb Ph'cals	lotion	salicylic acid, 1.8%			laureth-4, 4.5% · alcohol, 61% · PPG-40 · butyl ether · dihydroabietyl alcohol · fragrance
Sebulex Conditioning with Protein Westwood-Squibb Ph'cals	shampoo	salicylic acid, 2% · sulfur, 2%			sodium octoxynol-3 sulfonate · sodium lauryl sulfate · lauramide DEA · acetamide MEA · amphoteric-2 · hydrolyzed animal protein · magnesium aluminum silicate · propylene glycol · methylcellulose · PEG-14M · fragrance · disodium EDTA · FD&C blue#1 · D&C yellow#10 · dioctyl sodium sulfosuccinate · water
Sebulex Medicated Westwood-Squibb Ph'cals	shampoo	sulfur, 2% · salicylic acid, 2%			sodium octoxynol-2 ethane sulfonate · sodium dodecyl benzene sulfonate · PEG-6 lauramide · sodium dioctyl sulfosuccinate · PEG-14M · fragrance · EDTA · FD&C blue#1 · D&C yellow#10 · water
Sebulon Westwood-Squibb Ph'cals	shampoo		pyrithione zinc, 2%		acetamide MEA · benzyl alcohol · cocamide DEA · D&C green#5 · disodium oleamido PEG-2 sulfosuccinate · FD&C green#3 · fragrance · guar gum · magnesium aluminum silicate · TEA lauryl sulfate · quaternium-15 · water
Sebutone Westwood-Squibb Ph'cals	shampoo	sulfur, 1.5% · salicylic acid, 1.5%		coal tar, 0.5%	sodium dodecyl benzene sulfonate · sodium octoxynol-2-ethane sulfonate · PEG-6 lauramide · sodium dioctyl sulfosuccinate · titanium dioxide · sodium chloride · PEG-90M · fragrance · lanolin oil · EDTA · FD&C blue#1 · D&C yellow#10 · water
Sebutone Cream Westwood-Squibb Ph'cals	shampoo	sulfur, 1.5% · salicylic acid, 1.5%		coal tar, 0.5%	sodium octoxynol-2 ethane sulfonate · PEG-6 lauramide · sodium dodecyl benzene sulfonate · dextrin · stearyl alcohol · sodium dioctyl sulfosuccinate · titanium dioxide · magnesium aluminum silicate · PEG-14M · fragrance · lanolin oil · FD&C blue#1 · D&C yellow#10 · EDTA · water

See Chapter 26, "Dermatologic Products," for more information about these products.

DANDRUFF, SEBORRHEA, AND PSORIASIS PRODUCTS - continued

	Product [a] Manufacturer/Supplier	Dosage Form	Keratolytic	Cytostatic	Tar Product	Other Ingredients
**	**Selsun Blue 2-in-1 Treatment** Ross Products/Abbott Labs	shampoo		selenium sulfide, 1%		
	Selsun Blue Medicated Treatment Ross Products/Abbott Labs	shampoo		selenium sulfide, 1%		
**	**Selsun Blue Moisturizing Treatment** Ross Products/Abbott Labs	shampoo		selenium sulfide, 1%		
**	**Skin Miracle** Breckenridge Ph'cal	pump spray		pyrithione zinc, 0.25%		ethyl alcohol · zinc sulfate
	SLT Lotion C & M Pharmacal	lotion			liquid coal tar distillate, 2.5%	isopropyl alcohol · purified water · lactic acid · glycolic acid · fragrance · benzalkonium chloride
	Sulfoam Medicated Antidandruff Doak Dermatologics	shampoo	sulfur, 2%			
	Sulray Alvin Last	cleansing bar	sulfur, 5%			fragrance free natural soap base · aloe vera · trisodium HEDTA
	Sulray Dandruff Alvin Last	shampoo	sulfur, 2%			aloe vera gel · sodium lauryl sulfate · lauramide DEA · glycol stearate · methylparaben · propylparaben · citric acid
	Tar Scalp Solution C & M Pharmacal	lotion			liquid coal tar distillate, 2.5%	isopropyl alcohol · purified water · lactic acid · glycolic acid · fragrance · benzalkonium chloride
	Tar Shampoo Maximum Strength C & M Pharmacal	shampoo			coal tar solution, 25%	purified water · sodium lauryl sulfate · glycerin · citric acid · lauramide DEA · fragrance · hydroxyethyl ethylcellulose
	Taraphilic Medco Lab	ointment			coal tar distillate, 1%	white petrolatum · stearyl alcohol · sorbitol · propylene glycol · polysorbate 20 · sodium lauryl sulfate · methylparaben · propylparaben · isopropyl palmitate
	Tarsum Shampoo/Gel Summers Labs	shampoo			coal tar solution, 10%	
	Tegrin Block Drug	cream			coal tar solution, 5%	acetylated lanolin alcohol · alcohol · carbomer 934P · ceteth-2 · cetyl alcohol · 5-chloro-4 isothiazolin-2 methyl-3-one · D&C red#28 · fragrance · glyceryl tribehenate · laureth 16 · laureth 23 · methyl gluceth 20 · mineral oil · octyldodecanol · petrolatum · potassium hydroxide · stearyl alcohol · titanium dioxide · water
	Tegrin Block Drug	cleansing bar			coal tar extract, 2%	chromium hydroxide green · D&C yellow#10 lake · fragrance · glycerin · soap · titanium dioxide · water

See Chapter 26, "Dermatologic Products," for more information about these products.

DANDRUFF, SEBORRHEA, AND PSORIASIS PRODUCTS - continued

Product [a] Manufacturer/Supplier	Dosage Form	Keratolytic	Cytostatic	Tar Product	Other Ingredients
Tegrin Block Drug	shampoo			coal tar solution, 7% (equivalent to 1.1% coal tar)	water · sodium laureth sulfate · ammonium lauryl sulfate · alcohol · glycol stearate · hexylene · citric acid · lauramide DEA · fragrance · hydroxypropyl methylcellulose · guar hydroxypropyl triamonium chloride · methylparaben · propylparaben · FD&C blue#1
** **Tiseb** Allerderm Labs	shampoo	salicylic acid			water · TEA lauryl · sulfate cocamide DEA · acetylated lanolin · alcohol · cetyl acetate · polysorbate 80 · propylene glycol · PEG-120 · methyl glucose dioleate · methylparaben · propylparaben · chloroxylenol · disodium EDTA
** **Tiseb-T** Allerderm Labs	shampoo			tar, 2% (equivalent to 0.5% coal tar)	water · laureth-4 · DEA-lauryl sulfate · laureth-23 · PEG-6 lauramide · DEA lauraminopropionate · tetrasodium EDTA · sodium lauraminoproprionate
X-Seb Baker Cummins Derm'cals	shampoo		pyrithione zinc, 1%		
X-Seb Plus Baker Cummins Derm'cals	shampoo		pyrithione zinc, 1%		
X-Seb T Pearl Baker Cummins Derm'cals	shampoo			coal tar solution, 10% (crude coal tar, 2%)	
X-Seb T Plus Baker Cummins Derm'cals	shampoo			coal tar solution, 10% (crude coal tar, 2%)	
Zetar Dermik Labs	shampoo			whole coal tar, 1%	parachlorometaxylenol, 0.5% · cocoamphocarboxyglycinate EDTA · fragrance · hexylene glycol · lauramide DEA · linoleamide DEA · magnesium aluminum silicate · PEG-75 lanolin · polysorbate 20 · polysorbate 80 · purified water · sodium polynaphthalene sulfonate
Zincon Medtech	shampoo		pyrithione zinc, 1%		water · sodium methyl cocoyl taurate · cocamide MEA · sodium chloride · magnesium aluminum silicate · sodium cocoyl isethionate · fragrance · glutaraldehyde · D&C green#5 · may contain: citric acid · sodium hydroxide
ZNP Bar Stiefel Labs	cleansing bar		pyrithione zinc, 2%		

** New listing

[a] Topical hydrocortisone may also be used to relieve the itching associated with seborrhea. See the Dermatitis Products table for products containing hydrocortisone.

See Chapter 26, "Dermatologic Products," for more information about these products.

TOPICAL ANTIFUNGAL PRODUCTS

Product [a] Manufacturer/Supplier	Dosage Form	Antifungal	Other Ingredients
Aerodine Graham-Field	aerosol spray	povidone-iodine	propellant nitrogen
Aftate Schering-Plough Healthcare	aerosol spray powder	tolnaftate, 1%	SD alcohol 40-2, 14% · BHT · isobutane · PPG-12-buteth-16 · talc
Aftate Spray Liquid Schering-Plough Healthcare	aerosol spray	tolnaftate, 1%	SD alcohol 40-2, 36% · BHT · isobutane · PPG-12-buteth-16
Betadine Purdue Frederick	douche · gel · ointment	povidone-iodine, 10%	
Betadine First Aid Purdue Frederick	aerosol spray · cream	povidone-iodine, 5%	
Blis-To-Sol Oakhurst	liquid	tolnaftate, 1%	acetone · D&C red#22 · PEG-8 · thymol
Blis-To-Sol Oakhurst	powder	zinc undecylenate, 12%	bentonite · talc · thymol · zinc oxide
Cruex Novartis Consumer	aerosol spray powder	total undecylenate, 19% (as undecylenic acid and zinc undecylenate)	fragrance · isobutane · isopropyl myristate · menthol · talc · trolamine
Cruex Novartis Consumer	cream	total undecylenate, 20% (as undecylenic acid and zinc undecylenate)	fragrance · glycol stearate SE · lanolin · methylparaben · PEG-8 laurate · PEG-6 stearate · propylparaben · sorbitol solution · stearic acid · trolamine · water · white petrolatum
** **Cruex Prescription Strength** Novartis Consumer	aerosol spray powder	miconazole nitrate, 2%	aloe vera gel · aluminum starch · octenyl succinate · isopropyl myristate · propylene carbonate · SD alcohol 40B · sorbitan monooleate · stearalkonium hectorite · isobutane/propane
** **Cruex Prescription Strength AF** Novartis Consumer	cream	clotrimazole, 1%	cetostearyl alcohol · cetyl ester wax · 2-oxtyldodecanol · polysorbate 60 · sorbitan monostearate · purified water · benzyl alcohol
Cruex Squeeze Powder Novartis Consumer	powder	calcium undecylenate, 10%	talc · colloidal silicon dioxide · fragrance · isopropyl myristate
Desenex Antifungal Spray Liquid Novartis Consumer	aerosol spray	tolnaftate, 1%	BHT · fragrance · isobutane · PEG-400 · SD alcohol 40-B
Desenex Prescription Strength AF Novartis Consumer	cream	clotrimazole, 1%	cetostearyl alcohol · cetyl ester wax · 2-oxtyldodecanol · polysorbate 60 · sorbitan monostearate · purified water · benzyl alcohol
Desenex Prescription Strength AF Novartis Consumer	aerosol spray powder	miconazole nitrate, 2%	aloe vera gel · aluminum starch octenylsuccinate · isopropyl myristate · propylene carbonate · SD alcohol 40B · sorbitan monooleate · stearalkonium hectorite · isobutane/propane
Desenex Prescription Strength AF Spray Liquid Novartis Consumer	aerosol spray	miconazole nitrate, 2%	polyethylene glycol 300 · polysorbate 20 · SD alcohol 40-B · dimethyl ether
** **Fungi Nail** Kramer Labs	solution	undecylenic acid, 25%	

See Chapter 26, "Dermatologic Products," for more information about these products.

TOPICAL ANTIFUNGAL PRODUCTS - continued

Product [a] Manufacturer/Supplier	Dosage Form	Antifungal	Other Ingredients
FungiCure Alva-Amco Pharmacal	liquid	undecylenic acid, 10%	isopropyl alcohol, 70% · aloe vera gel · vitamin E
FungiCure Alva-Amco Pharmacal	gel	tolnaftate, 1%	isopropyl alcohol · vitamin E · aloe vera gel
** **Fungoid AF** Pedinol Pharmacal	solution	undecylenic acid, 25%	PEG-8 · benzalkonium chloride · chloroxylenol
Fungoid Tincture Pedinol Pharmacal	solution	miconazole nitrate, 2%	benzyl alcohol · isopropyl alcohol · water · acetic acid (glacial) · laureth-4
** **Gordochom** Gordon Labs	solution	undecylenic acid, 25%	chloroxylenol, 3%
Lotrimin AF Schering-Plough Healthcare	solution	clotrimazole, 1%	benzyl alcohol, 1% · PEG
Lotrimin AF Schering-Plough Healthcare	powder	miconazole nitrate, 2%	talc
Lotrimin AF Schering-Plough Healthcare	cream	clotrimazole, 1%	benzyl alcohol, 1%
Lotrimin AF Schering-Plough Healthcare	aerosol spray powder	miconazole nitrate, 2%	SD alcohol 40, 10% · talc
Lotrimin AF Schering-Plough Healthcare	lotion	clotrimazole, 1%	benzyl alcohol, 1%
Lotrimin AF Spray Liquid Schering-Plough Healthcare	aerosol spray	miconazole nitrate, 2%	SD alcohol 40, 17%
Micatin § Johnson & Johnson Consumer	cream · powder	miconazole nitrate, 2%	
Micatin § Johnson & Johnson Consumer	aerosol spray powder	miconazole nitrate, 2%	SD alcohol 40, 10% · sorbitan sesquioleate · stearalkonium hectorite · talc · isobutane · propane
** **Micatin Cooling Action Spray Liquid §** Johnson & Johnson Consumer	aerosol spray	miconazole nitrate, 2%	dimethyl ether · lactic acid · menthol · polysorbate 60 · polysorbate 65 · SD alcohol 40-B · sodium hydroxide · sorbitan stearate · water
** **Micatin Jock Itch §** Johnson & Johnson Consumer	cream	miconazole nitrate, 2%	benzoic acid · BHA · mineral oil · peglicol 5 oleate · pegoxol 7 stearate · purified water
Micatin Spray Liquid § Johnson & Johnson Consumer	aerosol spray	miconazole nitrate, 2%	SD alcohol 40, 16.8% · benzyl alcohol · cocamide DEA · sorbitan sesquioleate · tocopherol · isobutane · propane
Minidyne Pedinol Pharmacal	solution	povidone-iodine, 10%	
NP-27 Cream Thompson Medical	cream	tolnaftate, 1%	aloe · polyethylene glycol · carbopol · titanium dioxide · butylated hydroxytoluene · monoamylamine · propylene glycol · cocoa butter · fragrance
NP-27 Solution Thompson Medical	solution	tolnaftate, 1%	polyethylene glycol · butylated hydroxytoluene · propylene glycol
NP-27 Spray Powder Thompson Medical	aerosol spray powder	tolnaftate, 1%	alcohol, 14% · aloe · cocoa butter · isobutane · isopropyl myristate · fragrance

See Chapter 26, "Dermatologic Products," for more information about these products.

TOPICAL ANTIFUNGAL PRODUCTS - continued

Product [a] Manufacturer/Supplier	Dosage Form	Antifungal	Other Ingredients
** **Ony-Clear** Pedinol Pharmacal	spray	tolnaftate, 1%	SD alcohol 40B, 45% · dimethyl ether · PEG-6 · benzalkonium chloride · chloroxylenol
** **Podactin Antifungal** Reese Chemical	cream	miconazole nitrate, 2%	benzoic acid · BHA · mineral oil · peglicol 7 stearate · glyceryl monstearate · purified water
Polydine Century Ph'cals	solution	povidone-iodine, 10%	
Tinactin Jock Itch Schering-Plough Healthcare	cream	tolnaftate, 1%	BHT
Tinactin Spray Liquid Schering-Plough Healthcare	aerosol spray	tolnaftate, 1%	SD alcohol 40-2, 36% · BHT
Tinactin, Deodorant or Regular Schering-Plough Healthcare	aerosol spray powder	tolnaftate, 1%	SD alcohol 40-2, 14% · BHT
Ting Novartis Consumer	powder	tolnaftate, 1%	corn starch · fragrance · talc
Ting Novartis Consumer	cream	tolnaftate, 1%	BHT · PEG-400 · PEG-3350 · titanium dioxide · white petrolatum
Ting Novartis Consumer	aerosol spray powder	miconazole nitrate, 2%	aloe vera gel · aluminum starch · octenylsuccinate · isoproopyl myristate · propylene carbonate · SD alcohol 40B · sorbitan monooleate · stearalkonium hectorite · isobutane/propane
Ting Spray Liquid Novartis Consumer	aerosol spray	tolnaftate, 1%	SD alcohol 40-B · BHT · fragrance · isobutane · PEG-400
Undelenic Gordon Labs	ointment	undecylenic acid · zinc undecylenate	
Undelenic Gordon Labs	tincture	undecylenic acid	isopropyl alcohol, 79% · propylene glycol · triethanolamine · chloroxylenol
Zeasorb-AF Stiefel Labs	powder	miconazole nitrate, 2%	

** New listing

§   Manufacturer/supplier did not confirm information for this edition. Product listing is reprinted from the '96-97 edition.

[a] For products used to treat fungal infections of the feet, see the Athlete's Foot Products table.

See Chapter 26, "Dermatologic Products," for more information about these products.

HYPERPIGMENTATION PRODUCTS

Product Manufacturer/Supplier	Dosage Form	Hydro-quinone	Other Ingredients
Ambi Skin Discoloration Fade Cream, Dry Skin Kiwi Brands	cream	2%	padimate O · water · stearic acid · glycerin · isopropyl myristate · cetyl alcohol · DEA-cetyl phosphate · glyceryl stearate · PEG-100 stearate · BHA · sodium metabisulfite · tocopheryl acetate · methyl-, ethyl-, propyl-, and butylparaben · disodium EDTA · fragrance
Ambi Skin Discoloration Fade Cream, Normal Skin Kiwi Brands	cream	2%	padimate O · water · stearic acid · isopropyl myristate · stearyl alcohol · glycerin · emulsifying wax · glyceryl stearate · myrtrimonium bromide · PEG-8 stearate · BHA · sodium metabisulfite · tocopheryl acetate · methyl-, ethyl-, propyl-, and butylparaben · disodium EDTA · fragrance
Ambi Skin Discoloration Fade Cream, Oily Skin Kiwi Brands	cream	2%	padimate O · water · stearic acid · PPG-2 myristyl ether propionate · PEG-8 · isopropyl myristate · glyceryl myristate · stearyl alcohol · glyceryl stearate · emulsifying wax · myrtrimonium bromide · PEG-8 stearate · BHA · sodium metabisulfite · tocopheryl acetate · methyl-, ethyl-, propyl-, and butylparaben · disodium EDTA · fragrance
Eldopaque ICN Ph'cals	cream	2%	
Eldoquin ICN Ph'cals	cream	2%	
Esotérica Facial Formula Medicis Dermatologics	cream	2%	padimate O, 3.3% · oxybenzone, 2.5% · water · isopropyl myristate · stearyl alcohol · glyceryl monostearate · propylene glycol · ceresin · poloxamer 188 · steareth-20 · ceteareth-3 · dimethicone · fragrance · sodium bisulfite · methylparaben · propylparaben · sodium lauryl sulfate · BHA · citric acid · trisodium EDTA
Esotérica Regular Formula Medicis Dermatologics	cream	2%	water · glyceryl stearate · isopropyl palmitate · ceresin · mineral oil · propylene glycol · stearyl alcohol · PEG-6-32 stearate · poloxamer 188 · propylene glycol monostearate · steareth-20 · laureth-23 · sodium bisulfite · sodium lauryl sulfate · citric acid · dimethicone · fragrance · methylparaben · propylparaben · trisodium EDTA · BHA
Nudit Fade Cream Medtech	cream	2%	
** **Palmer's Skin Success Fade Cream, Dry Skin** E. T. Browne Drug	cream	2%	octyl salicylate, 3% · purified water · mineral oil · glyceryl stearate · cetearyl alcohol · cetearyth-20 · isopropyl myristate · stearyl stearate · propylene glycol · PEG-75 · lanolin · dimethicone · PEG-100 stearate · vitamin E · magnesium aluminum silicate · xanthan gum · tetrasodium EDTA · corn oil · glyceryl oleate · BHA · BHT · citric acid · ascorbic acid · sodium lauryl sulfate · sodium sulfite · sodium metabisulfite · imidazolidinyl urea · methylparaben · propylparaben · fragrance
** **Palmer's Skin Success Fade Cream, Normal Skin** E. T. Browne Drug	cream	2%	octyl salicylate, 3% · purified water · glyceryl stearate · cetearyl alcohol · ceteareth-20 · isopropyl myristate · stearyl stearate · propylene glycol · mineral oil · PEG-75 · lanolin · PEG-100 stearate · vitamin E · dimethicone · magnesium aluminum silicate · xanthan gum · tertrasodium EDTA · corn oil · glyceryl oleate · BHA · BHT · t-butyl hydroquinone · citric acid · ascorbic acid · sodium lauryl sulfate · sodium sulfite · sodium metabisulfite · imidazolinyl urea · methylparaben · propylparaben · fragrance
** **Palmer's Skin Success Fade Cream, Oily Skin** E. T. Browne Drug	cream	2%	octyl salicylate, 3% · glyceryl stearate · cetearyl alcohol · ceteareth-20 · isopropyl myristate · stearyl stearate · propylene glycol · PPG-9 · PEG-75 · lanolin · PEG-100 stearate · vitamin E · dimethicone · magnesium aluminum silicate · xanthan gum · tertrasodium EDTA · corn oil · glyceryl oleate · BHA · BHT · t-butyl hydroquinone · citric acid · ascorbic acid · sodium lauryl sulfate · sodium sulfite · sodium metabisulfite · imidazolinyl urea · methylparaben · propylparaben · fragrance

See Chapter 26, "Dermatologic Products," for more information about these products.

HYPERPIGMENTATION PRODUCTS - continued

Product Manufacturer/Supplier	Dosage Form	Hydro- quinone	Other Ingredients
** **Palmer's Skin Success Fade Serum** E. T. Browne Drug	liquid	2%	octyl methoxycinnamate · water · cyclomethicone · diisodecyl adipate · dimethicone copolyol · ethylene/VA copolymer · dimethicone · leaf extract · sugar cane extract · sugar maple, orange, and lemon extracts · vitamin E · hexanediol beeswax · mineral oil · propylene glycol · diazolidinyl urea · methylparaben · propylparaben · sodium metabisulfite · FD&C red#17 · FD&C yellow#11 · citric acid · sodium chloride · decyl polyglucose · sodium sulfite
** **Phade** Alva-Amco Pharmacal	gel	2%	extracts of bilberry, sugar cane, sugar maple, orange, and lemon · aloe vera gel · panthenol
Porcelana Original Formula § Dep	cream	2%	water · mineral oil · glyceryl stearate · PEG-50 stearate · isopropyl palmitate · cetyl alcohol · propylene glycol · stearic acid · hydroxyethyl cellulose · citric acid · sodium metabisulfite · disodium EDTA · BHA · propylparaben · methylparaben · diazolidinyl urea · fragrance
Porcelana Sunscreen Formula § Dep	cream	2%	octyl methoxycinnamate, 2.5% · water · mineral oil · cetyl alcohol · propylene glycol · ceteth-2 · stearic acid · magnesium aluminum silicate · PEG-40 stearate · citric acid · hydroxyethyl cellulose · fragrance · sodium sulfite · imidazolidinyl urea · sodium metabisulfite · disodium EDTA · methylparaben · BHA
Solaquin ICN Ph'cals	cream	2%	
** **Topifram Age Spot Fade Cream** E. T. Browne Drug	cream	2%	octyl salicylate, 3% · purified water · glyceryl stearate · cetearyl alcohol · ceteareth-20 · isopropyl myristate · stearyl stearate · propylene glycol · mineral oil · PEG-75 · lanolin · PEG-100 stearate · vitamin E · dimethicone · magnesium aluminum silicate · xanthan gum · tetrasodium EDTA · corn oil · glyceryl oleate · BHA · BHT · t-butyl hydroquinone · citric acid · ascorbic acid · sodium lauryl sulfite · sodium sulfite · sodium metabisulfite · imidazolidinyl urea · methylparaben · propylparaben · fragrance

** New listing

§ Manufacturer/supplier did not confirm information for this edition. Product listing is reprinted from the '96-97 edition.

See Chapter 26, "Dermatologic Products," for more information about these products.

HAIR REGROWTH PRODUCTS

Product Manufacturer/Supplier	Dosage Form	Minoxidil	Other Ingredients
** **Consort Hair Regrowth Treatment for Men** Alberto Culver	solution	2%	alcohol, 60% · propylene glycol · purified water
** **HealthGuard Minoxidil Topical Solution for Men** Bausch & Lomb Ph'cal	solution	2%	alcohol, 60% · propylene glycol · purified water · packaged with two applicators: sprayer and child-resistant dropper
** **HealthGuard Minoxidil Topical Solution for Women** Bausch & Lomb Ph'cal	solution	2%	alcohol, 60% · propylene glycol · purified water · packaged with extender spray applicator (helps direct spray through hair onto scalp)
** **Minoxidil Topical Solution for Men** Copley Ph'cal	solution	2%	alcohol 60% · propylene glycol · purified water
Minoxidil Topical Solution for Men Alpharma	solution	2%	alcohol, 60% · propylene glycol · purified water
Minoxidil Topical Solution for Men Lemmon	solution	2%	alcohol, 60% · propylene glycol · purified water
Rogaine for Men Pharmacia & Upjohn	solution	2%	alcohol, 60% · propylene glycol · purified water · packaged with two applicators: sprayer and child-resistant dropper
Rogaine for Women Pharmacia & Upjohn	solution	2%	alcohol, 60% · propylene glycol · purified water · packaged with extender spray applicator (helps direct spray through hair onto scalp)

** New listing

See Chapter 26, "Dermatologic Products," for more information about these products.

Acne Product Table

ACNE PRODUCTS

Product Manufacturer/Supplier	Dosage Form	Benzoyl Peroxide	Sulfur	Resorcinol/ Salicylic Acid	Other Ingredients
Acne Treatment Cleanser C & M Pharmacal	liquid			salicylic acid, 2%	purified water · sodium lauryl sulfate · propylene glycol · lauramide DEA · fragrance · chloroxylenol · hydroxyethyl ethylcellulose
Acne Treatment Wash C & M Pharmacal	liquid		4%	resorcinol, 2%	purified water · magnesium aluminum silicate · TEA-dodecyl benzene sulfonate · glycerin · stearic acid · cetostearyl alcohol · polysorbate 20 · fragrance · FD&C red#40
Acne Treatment, Tinted C & M Pharmacal	lotion		8%	resorcinol, 2%	purified water · isopropyl alcohol · propylene glycol · titanium dioxide · acetone · magnesium aluminum silicate · iron oxide yellow · octoxynol 9 · chloroxylenol · iron oxide brown · iron oxide red · xanthan gum · fragrance
Acne Treatment, Vanishing C & M Pharmacal	lotion		10%		purified water · glycerin · magnesium aluminum silicate · sorbic acid · fragrance · FD&C red#40
Acno Baker Cummins Derm'cals	lotion		3%	salicylic acid, 2%	
Acnomel Menley & James Labs	cream		8%	resorcinol, 2%	alcohol, 15% · bentonite · titanium dioxide · fragrance · iron oxide · potassium hydroxide · propylene glycol · water
Acnotex C & M Pharmacal	lotion		8%	resorcinol, 2%	purified water · isopropyl alcohol · propylene glycol · titanium dioxide · acetone · magnesium aluminum silicate · iron oxide yellow · octoxynol 9 · chloroxylenol · iron oxide brown · iron oxide red · xanthan gum · fragrance
AMBI 10 Acne Medication Kiwi Brands	cream	10%			aluminum hydroxide · bentonite · carbomer 940 · glyceryl stearate SE · isopropyl myristate · methylparaben · PEG-12 · potassium hydroxide · propylene glycol · propylparaben · purified water
Aveeno Medicated Cleanser Rydelle Labs	liquid			salicylic acid, 2%	water · sodium laureth sulfosuccinate · disodium lauroamphoacetate · ammonium lauryl sulfate · hydrogenated tallow glyceride · potassium cocoyl hydrolyzed collagen · benzyl alcohol · guar hydroxypropyl ammonium chloride · oatmeal flour · sodium PCA · sodium citrate · citric acid phantolid · galaxolide · PEG-150 distearate

See Chapter 27, "Acne Products," for more information about these products.

ACNE PRODUCTS - continued

Product Manufacturer/Supplier	Dosage Form	Benzoyl Peroxide	Sulfur	Resorcinol/ Salicylic Acid	Other Ingredients
Benoxyl 5 Stiefel Labs	lotion	5%			
Benoxyl 10 Stiefel Labs	lotion	10%			
Clean & Clear Invisible Blemish Treatment § Johnson & Johnson Consumer	gel			salicylic acid, 2%	butylene glycol · glycerin · hydroxyethyl cellulose · propylene glycol · SD alcohol 40B, 28% · sodium citrate · water
Clean & Clear Invisible Blemish Treatment, Sensitive Skin § Johnson & Johnson Consumer	gel			salicylic acid, 0.5%	butylene glycol · citric acid · glycerin · hydroxyethyl cellulose · propylene glycol · SD alcohol 40B, 28% · sodium citrate · water
Clean & Clear Oil Controlling Astringent § Johnson & Johnson Consumer	liquid			salicylic acid, 2%	water · alcohol, 42% · eucalyptus oil · benzoic acid · camphor · peppermint oil · clove oil · FD&C red#4 · denatonium benzoate
Clean & Clear Oil Controlling Astringent Sensitive Skin § Johnson & Johnson Consumer	liquid			salicylic acid, 0.5%	water · alcohol, 36.5% · glycerin · PPG-5-ceteth 20 · eucalyptus oil · benzoic acid · camphor · peppermint oil · clove oil · benzophenone-4 · denatonium benzoate · FD&C blue#1
Clean & Clear Persa-Gel Extra Strength § Johnson & Johnson Consumer	gel	5%			water · carbomer · laureth-4 · hydroxypropyl methylcellulose · sodium hydroxide
Clean & Clear Persa-Gel Maximum Strength § Johnson & Johnson Consumer	gel	10%			water · carbomer · laureth-4 · hydroxypropyl methylcellulose · sodium hydroxide
** **Clean & Clear Pore Prep Clarifier §** Johnson & Johnson Consumer	liquid			salicylic acid, 2%	aloe barbadensis extract · chamomile extract · fragrance · glycol stearate · matricaria extract · panthenol · PEG-32 · propylene glycol · PVM/MA decadiene crosspolymer · water
Clearasil Adult Care Procter & Gamble	cream		3% · 8%	resorcinol, 2%	alcohol, 10% · water · bentonite · glyceryl stearate SE · propylene glycol · isopropyl myristate · sodium bisulfite · dimethicone · methylparaben · propylparaben · fragrance · iron oxides

See Chapter 27, "Acne Products," for more information about these products.

ACNE PRODUCTS - continued

Product Manufacturer/Supplier	Dosage Form	Benzoyl Peroxide	Sulfur	Resorcinol/ Salicylic Acid	Other Ingredients
Clearasil Clearstick Maximum Strength Procter & Gamble	liquid			salicylic acid, 2%	alcohol, 39% · water · aloe vera gel · triethanolamine · menthol · disodium EDTA · fragrance
Clearasil Clearstick Regular Strength Procter & Gamble	liquid			salicylic acid, 1.25%	alcohol, 39% · water · aloe vera gel · triethanolamine · menthol · disodium EDTA · fragrance
Clearasil Clearstick Sensitive Skin Procter & Gamble	liquid			salicylic acid, 2%	alcohol, 39% · water · glycerin · aloe vera gel · triethanolamine · menthol · disodium EDTA
Clearasil Double Textured Maximum Strength Procter & Gamble	pad			salicylic acid, 2%	alcohol, 40% · water · isoceteth-20 · aloe vera gel · triethanolamine · fragrance · menthol · disodium EDTA
Clearasil Double Textured Reg. Strength with Skin Soothers Procter & Gamble	pad			salicylic acid, 2%	alcohol, 40% · water · glycerin · aloe vera gel · triethanolamine · disodium EDTA
Clearasil Maximum Strength, Tinted or Vanishing Procter & Gamble	cream	10%			water · propylene glycol · bentonite · aluminum hydroxide · glyceryl stearate SE · PEG-12 · isopropyl myristate · carbomer · dimethicone · methylparaben · propylparaben · titanium dioxide (Tinted) · iron oxides (Tinted)
Clearasil Maximum Strength, Vanishing Procter & Gamble	lotion	10%			water · aluminum hydroxide · isopropyl stearate · PEG-100 stearate · glyceryl stearate · cetyl alcohol · glycereth-26 · isocetyl stearate · glycerin · dimethicone copolyol · sodium citrate · citric acid · methylparaben · propylparaben · fragrance
Clearasil Medicated Deep Cleanser Procter & Gamble	liquid			salicylic acid, 0.5%	alcohol, 42% · water · aloe vera gel · menthol · allantoin · fragrance · sorbitol · sodium lactate · proline · sodium PCA · hydrolyzed collagen · PEG-40 hydrogenated castor oil · disodium EDTA
Drytex C & M Pharmacal	liquid			salicylic acid, 2%	purified water · isopropyl alcohol · acetone · polysorbate 20 · benzalkonium chloride · fragrance · FD&C red#40 · FD&C yellow#5

See Chapter 27, "Acne Products," for more information about these products.

ACNE PRODUCTS - continued

Product Manufacturer/Supplier	Dosage Form	Benzoyl Peroxide	Sulfur	Resorcinol/ Salicylic Acid	Other Ingredients
ExACT Adult Medication Premier Consumer	cream	2.5%			water · glycerin · acrylates copolymer · sorbitol · cetyl alcohol · glyceryl dilaurate · stearyl alcohol · sodium lauryl sulfate · magnesium aluminum silicate · sodium citrate · silica · citric acid · methylparaben · xanthan gum · propylparaben
ExACT Pore Treatment Premier Consumer	gel			salicylic acid, 2%	purified water · dimethicone · PEG-32 · polyacrylamide · C13-14 isoparaffin · laureth-7 · aloe vera gel · acrylates copolymer · polysorbate 80 · propylene glycol · diazolidinyl urea · methylparaben · propylparaben · triethanolamine · panthenol · allantoin · disodium EDTA
** **ExACT Tinted** Premier Consumer	cream	5%			water · acrylates copolymer · glycerin · titanium dioxide · sorbitol · cetyl alcohol · glyceryl dilaurate · stearyl alcohol · sodium laurel sulfate · magnesium aluminum sulfate · sodium citrate · silica · iron oxides · citric acid · methyparaben · xanthan gum · propylparaben
ExACT Vanishing Premier Consumer	cream	5%			water · acrylates copolymer · glycerin · sorbitol · cetyl alcohol · glyceryl dilaurate · stearyl alcohol · sodium lauryl sulfate · magnesium aluminum silicate · sodium citrate · silica · citric acid · methylparaben · xanthan gum · propylparaben
Exfoliating Astringent for Oily Skin C & M Pharmacal	liquid			salicylic acid, 2%	purified water · isopropyl alcohol · acetone · polysorbate 20 · benzalkonium chloride · fragrance · FD&C red#40 · FD&C yellow#5
Fostex 10% BPO Bristol-Myers Products	gel	10%			carbomer 940 · diisopropanolamine · disodium EDTA · laureth-4 · water
Fostex 10% BPO Bristol-Myers Products	cleansing bar	10%			boric acid · cellulose gum · dextrin · disodium EDTA · docusate sodium · lactic acid · PEG-14M · sodium lauryl sulfoacetate · sorbitol · urea · water
Fostex 10% BPO Wash Bristol-Myers Products	liquid	10%			citric acid · disodium EDTA · docusate sodium · magnesium aluminum silicate · methylcellulose · sodium chloride · sodium laureth sulfate · water

See Chapter 27, "Acne Products," for more information about these products.

ACNE PRODUCTS - continued

Product Manufacturer/Supplier	Dosage Form	Benzoyl Peroxide	Sulfur	Resorcinol/ Salicylic Acid	Other Ingredients
Fostex Medicated Bristol-Myers Products	cleansing bar			salicylic acid, 2%	boric acid · carboxymethylcellulose sodium · dextrin · docusale sodium · disodium edetate · fragrance · iron oxides · lactic acid · PEG-14M · sodium lauryl sulfoacetate · sodium octoxynol-2 ethane sulfonate · sorbitol · urea · water
Fostex Medicated Cleansing Bristol-Myers Products	cream			salicylic acid, 2%	ceteareth-20 · D&C yellow#10 · docusate sodium · edetic acid · fragrance · methylcellulose · modified starch · poloxomer 188 · sodium chloride · sodium dodecyl benzene sulfonate · sodium octoxynol-2 ethane sulfonate · stearyl alcohol · water
Fostril Westwood-Squibb Ph'cals	lotion		2%		laureth-4 · zinc oxide · talc · PEG-40 stearate · magnesium · aluminum silicate · PEG-8 stearate · bentonite · iron oxides · methylcellulose · methylparaben · citric acid · EDTA · fragrance · quaternium-15 · simethicone · water
Ionax Astringent Skin Cleanser Healthpoint	liquid			salicylic acid	isopropyl alcohol, 48% · allantoin · acetone · polyoxyethylene ethers
Liquimat Summers Labs	lotion		4%		alcohol, 22% · tinted bases
Loroxide Summers Labs	lotion	5.5%			BHA · BHT · caprylic/capric triglyceride · caramel · cetyl alcohol · decyl oleate · disodium phosphate · edetic acid · hydroxyethylcellulose · kaolin · methylparaben · mineral oil · lanolin alcohol · monoglyceride citrate · sodium phosphate · talc · tetrasodium EDTA · titanium dioxide · vegetable oil · polysorbate 20 · propylene glycol · propylene glycol stearate · propyl gallate · propylparaben · purified water · simethicone · stearyl heptanoate · sodium hydroxide
Neutrogena Acne Neutrogena Dermatologics	mask	5%			
Neutrogena Clear Pore Treatment Neutrogena Dermatologics	gel			salicylic acid, 2%	purified water · PEG-32 · PVM/MA decadiene crospolymer · sodium hydroxide · fragrance
** **Neutrogena Multi-Vitamin Acne Treatment** Neutrogena Dermatologics	cream			salicylic acid, 1.5%	

See Chapter 27, "Acne Products," for more information about these products.

ACNE PRODUCTS - continued

Product Manufacturer/Supplier	Dosage Form	Benzoyl Peroxide	Sulfur	Resorcinol/ Salicylic Acid	Other Ingredients
Neutrogena Oil-Free Wash Neutrogena Dermatologics	liqui-gel			salicylic acid, 2%	
Noxzema 2 in 1 Maximum Strength Procter & Gamble	pad			salicylic acid, 2%	alcohol, 63% · water · PEG-4 · PPG-11 stearyl ether · camphor · clove oil · eucalyptus oil · menthol · fragrance · disodium EDTA
Noxzema 2 in 1 Regular Strength Procter & Gamble	pad			salicylic acid, 0.5%	alcohol, 63% · water · PPG-11 stearyl ether · clove oil · eucalyptus oil · menthol · fragrance · PEG-4 · disodium EDTA
Noxzema Oily Astringent Procter & Gamble	liquid			salicylic acid, 2%	alcohol, 49% · water · triethanolamine · fragrance · menthol · disodium EDTA · FD&C yellow#5 · FD&C blue#1
On-the-Spot, Tinted or Vanishing Neutrogena Dermatologics	lotion	2.5%			
Oxy Balance Deep Action Night Formula SmithKline Beecham	gel	2.5%			acrylates copolymer · carbomer 940 · citric acid · diazolidinyl urea · dimethicone · dioctyl sodium sulfosuccinate · edetate disodium · glycerin · propylene glycol · silica · sodium citrate · sodium hydroxide · water · xanthan gum
Oxy Balance Deep Pore Cleanser SmithKline Beecham	liquid			salicylic acid, 0.5%	alcohol, 43% · citric acid · menthol · sodium lauryl sulfate · fragrance · glycerin · propylene glycol · water
Oxy Balance Deep Pore Cleansing SmithKline Beecham	pad			salicylic acid, 0.5%	alcohol, 43% · citric acid · fragrance · glycerin · menthol · sodium lauryl sulfate · water · propylene glycol
Oxy Balance Gentle Deep Pore Cleansing SmithKline Beecham	pad			salicylic acid, 0.5%	alcohol, 22% · disodium lauryl sulfosuccinate · fragrance · glycerin · menthol · PEG-4 · sodium lauryl sarcosinate · sodium PCA · trisodium EDTA · water
Oxy Balance Maximum Deep Pore Cleansing SmithKline Beecham	pad			salicylic acid, 2%	alcohol, 50% · citric acid · fragrance · glycerin · menthol · sodium lauryl sulfate · water · propylene glycol · polyethylene glycol

See Chapter 27, "Acne Products," for more information about these products.

ACNE PRODUCTS - continued

Product Manufacturer/Supplier	Dosage Form	Benzoyl Peroxide	Sulfur	Resorcinol/ Salicylic Acid	Other Ingredients
Oxy Balance Maximum Medicated Face Wash SmithKline Beecham	liquid	10%			citric acid · cocamidopropyl betaine · diazolidinyl urea · methylparaben · propylparaben · sodium citrate · sodium cocoyl isethionate · sodium laureth sulfate sarcosinate · water · xanthan gum
Oxy-10 Balance Emergency Spot Treatment Cover-Up Formula SmithKline Beecham	lotion	10%			carbomer 940 · dioctyl sulfosuccinate · edetate disodium · iron oxides · sodium hydroxide · titanium dioxide · water
Oxy-10 Balance Emergency Spot Treatment Invisible Formula SmithKline Beecham	lotion	10%			acrylates copolymer · carbomer 940 · citric acid · diazolidinyl urea · dimethicone · dioctyl sodium sulfosuccinate · edetate disodium · glycerin · propylene glycol · silica · sodium citrate · sodium hydroxide · water · xanthan gum
** **Palmer's Skin Success Acne Medication Cleanser** E. T. Browne Drug	liquid			salicylic acid, 0.5%	SD alcohol 40B, 69% · water · propylene glycol · PEG-40 hydrogenated castor oil · PPG-2 isodeceth-12 · aloe vera gel · vitamin E · fragrance · menthol
** **Palmer's Skin Success Invisible Acne Medication** E. T. Browne Drug	cream	10%			water · cetearyl alcohol · ceteareth-20 · silica · vitamin E · aloe vera gel · propylene glycol · citric acid · sodium citrate · sodium lauryl sulfoacetate · methylparaben · propylparaben
Pan Oxyl 5 Stiefel Labs	cleansing bar	5%			mild surfactant base
Pan Oxyl 10 Stiefel Labs	cleansing bar	10%			mild surfactant base
Pernox Westwood-Squibb Ph'cals	lotion		2%	salicylic acid, 1.5%	polyethylene granules · sodium octoxynol-2 · ethane sulfonate · sodium dodecylbenzene sulfonate · fragrance · docusate sodium · modified starch · magnesium aluminum · silicate · methylcellulose · EDTA · water

See Chapter 27, "Acne Products," for more information about these products.

ACNE PRODUCTS - continued

Product Manufacturer/Supplier	Dosage Form	Benzoyl Peroxide	Sulfur	Resorcinol/ Salicylic Acid	Other Ingredients
Pernox, Lemon or Regular Westwood-Squibb Ph'cals	abrasive		2%	salicylic acid, 1.5%	polyethylene granules · sodium octoxynol-2 · ethane sulfonate · sodium dodecylbenzene sulfonate · poloxamer 184 · docusate sodium · methylcellulose · food starch · fragrance · EDTA · D&C yellow#10 · FD&C blue#1 (Regular) · water
Propa pH Astringent Cleanser Del Ph'cals	lotion			salicylic acid, 0.5%	aloe vera gel · benzophenone-4 · disodium EDTA · fragrance · menthol · citric acid · green tea extract · lactic acid · malic acid · peppermint oil · SD alcohol 40-A · sodium citrate · sodium laureth-12 sulfate · triclosan · water
Propa pH Astringent Cleanser Maximum Strength Del Ph'cals	lotion			salicylic acid, 2%	aloe vera gel · benzophenone-4 · disodium EDTA · fragrance · menthol · citric acid · green tea extract · lactic acid · malic acid · peppermint oil · polysorbate 20 · SD alcohol 40-A · sodium citrate · triclosan · water
Propa pH Foaming Face Wash Del Ph'cals	liquid			salicylic acid, 2%	aloe vera gel · disodium EDTA · fragrance · glycol distearate · citric acid · green tea extract · lactic acid · malic acid · polyol alkoxy esters · polyoxyethylene-15-cocoamine phosphate/oleate complex · menthol · quaternium-15 · sodium laureth sulfate · sodium lauryl sarcosinate · water
Propa pH Peel-off Del Ph'cals	mask			salicylic acid, 2%	aloe vera gel · FD&C red#4 · FD&C yellow#5 · fragrance · methylparaben · citric acid · green tea extract · lactic acid · malic acid · polyethylene glycol · polysorbate 80 · polyvinyl alcohol · PPG-5-ceteth-20 · propylparaben · purified water · SD alcohol 40 · sodium carbonate · tocopheryl acetate
Rezamid Acne Lotion Summers Labs	liquid		5%	resorcinol, 2%	
SalAc Cleanser GenDerm	liquid			salicylic acid, 2%	
SAStid Soap Stiefel Labs	cleansing bar		10%		
Seales Lotion-Modified C & M Pharmacal	lotion		6.4%		purified water · acetone · zinc oxide · sodium borate · bentonite

See Chapter 27, "Acne Products," for more information about these products.

ACNE PRODUCTS - continued

Product Manufacturer/Supplier	Dosage Form	Benzoyl Peroxide	Sulfur	Resorcinol/ Salicylic Acid	Other Ingredients
Sebasorb Summers Labs	liquid			salicylic acid, 2%	attapulgite, 10% · polysorbate 80
Stri-Dex Clear Blistex	gel			salicylic acid, 2%	SD alcohol, 9.3% · glycerin
Stri-Dex Maximum Strength, Single or Dual Textured Blistex	pad			salicylic acid, 2%	SD alcohol, 44%
Stri-Dex Regular Strength, Dual Textured Blistex	pad			salicylic acid, 0.5%	SD alcohol, 28%
Stri-Dex Sensitive Skin, Dual Textured Blistex	pad			salicylic acid, 0.5%	SD alcohol, 28% · aloe vera gel
Stri-Dex Super Scrub Blistex	pad			salicylic acid, 2%	SD alcohol, 54%
Sulforcin Healthpoint	lotion		5%	resorcinol, 2%	alcohol, 11.65%
Sulmasque C & M Pharmacal	mask		6.4%		purified water · bentonite · kaolin · isopropyl alcohol · zinc oxide · calcium oxide · sodium lauryl sulfate · lauramide DEA · fragrance · methylparaben
Sulpho-Lac Doak Dermatologics	cream		5%		
Sulpho-Lac Medicated Soap Doak Dermatologics	cleansing bar		5%		
Sulray Acne Treatment Alvin Last	cream		3%		water · kaolin · glyceryl stearate · laureth-23 · PEG-8 stearate · aloe vera gel · glycerin · PEG-8 distearate · silica · methylparaben · propylparaben · caramel
Sulray Facial Cleanser Alvin Last	liquid		3%		aloe vera gel · sodium lauryl sulfate · lauramide DEA · glycol stearate · methylparaben · propylparaben · citric acid
Sulray Soap Alvin Last	cleansing bar		5%		fragrance free natural soap base · aloe vera · trisodium HEDTA
Therac C & M Pharmacal	lotion		10% (colloidal)	salicylic acid, 2.35%	purified water · glycerin · magnesium aluminum silicate · sorbic acid · fragrance · FD&C red#40
Thylox Acne Treatment Soap C. S. Dent	cleansing bar		3%		sodium tallowate · sodium cocoate · water · glycerin · fragrance · titanium dioxide · tetrasodium etidronate · pentasodium pentetate · cosmetic orange oxide

See Chapter 27, "Acne Products," for more information about these products.

ACNE PRODUCTS - continued

Product Manufacturer/Supplier	Dosage Form	Benzoyl Peroxide	Sulfur	Resorcinol/ Salicylic Acid	Other Ingredients
Vanoxide Dermik Labs	lotion	5%			calcium phosphate · silica · BHA · BHT · caprylic/capric triglyceride · cetyl alcohol · decyl oleate · disodium phosphate · edetic acid · hydroxyethylcellulose · laureth-10 acetate · methylparaben · mineral oil · lanolin alcohol · monoglyceride citrate · polysorbate 20 · propylene glycol · propylene glycol stearate · propyl gallate · propylparaben · purified water · simethicone · sodium hydroxide · sodium phosphate · stearyl heptanoate · tetrasodium EDTA · vegetable oil

** New listing

§ Manufacturer/supplier did not confirm information for this edition. Product listing is reprinted from the '96-97 edition.

See Chapter 27, "Acne Products," for more information about these products.

First-Aid Products and
Minor Wound Care Table

FIRST-AID ANTIBIOTIC AND ANTISEPTIC PRODUCTS

Product Manufacturer/Supplier	Dosage Form	Antibiotic	Antiseptic	Other Ingredients
B·F·I· Powder Menley & James Labs	powder		bismuth formic iodide, 16%	bismuth subgallate · boric acid · magnesium carbonate · potassium alum · talc · zinc phenylsulfonate · eucalyptol · menthol · thymol
Baciguent Lee Consumer	ointment	bacitracin, 500 IU/g		white petroleum · mineral oil
Bactine Bayer Consumer	spray		benzalkonium chloride, 0.13%	lidocaine HCl, 2.5% · disodium edetate · fragrance · octoxynol-9 · propylene glycol · water
Bagbalm Dairy Assn. Co.	ointment		8-hydroxyquinoline sulfate, 0.3%	petrolatum · lanolin
Benzalkonium Chloride Multisource	liquid		benzalkonium chloride, 17% · bismuth formic iodide, 16%	
Betadine First Aid Antibiotics + Moisturizer Purdue Frederick	ointment	polymyxin B sulfate, 10000 IU/g · bacitracin zinc, 500 IU/g		cholesterolized base
Betadine Skin Cleanser Purdue Frederick	liquid		povidone-iodine, 7.5%	
Buro-Sol Antiseptic Doak Dermatologics	powder		sodium diacetate, 0.23% · benzethonium chloride, 4.4%	aluminum acetate, 46.8%
Campho-phenique Pain Relieving Antiseptic Bayer Consumer	gel · liquid		camphor, 10.8% · phenol, 4.7%	eucalyptus oil
Campho-phenique Triple Antibiotic Bayer Consumer	ointment	polymyxin B sulfate, 10000 IU/g · bacitracin zinc, 500 IU/g · neomycin sulfate, 5mg/g (equivalent to neomycin base, 3.5mg)		lidocaine HCl, 40mg
Castellani Paint, Modified Pedinol Pharmacal	liquid		phenol, 1.5% · SD alcohol 40B	water · resorcinol · acetone · basic fuschin (color)
** **Clinical Care Antimicrobial Wound Cleanser** Care-Tech Labs	pump spray		benzethonium chloride, 0.1%	water · amphoteric 2 · aloe vera gel · DMDM hydantoin · citric acid
Clomycin Lee Consumer	cream	polymyxin B sulfate, 5000 IU/g · bacitracin, 500 IU/g · neomycin sulfate, 3.5mg/g		lidocaine, 40mg/g · yellow petrolatum · anhydrous lanolin · mineral oil
Dakins 1/2 Strength Century Ph'cals	solution		sodium hypochlorite, 0.25%	
Dakins Full Strength Century Ph'cals	solution		sodium hypochlorite, 0.5%	
Dr. Tichenor's Antiseptic Dr. G. H. Tichenor	liquid		SDA alcohol 38B, 70%	oil of peppermint · extract of arnica · water
Efodine E. Fougera	ointment		available iodine, 1%	anhydrous carbowax base

See Chapter 28, "First-Aid Products and Minor Wound Care," for more information about these products.

FIRST-AID ANTIBIOTIC AND ANTISEPTIC PRODUCTS - continued

Product Manufacturer/Supplier	Dosage Form	Antibiotic	Antiseptic	Other Ingredients
First Aid Cream § Johnson & Johnson Consumer	cream		cetylpyridinium chloride	water · cetyl alcohol · glyceryl stearate · isopropyl palmitate · stearyl alcohol · benzyl alcohol · synthetic beeswax · lapyrium chloride · hydroxypropyl methylcellulose · trisodium phosphate
** **Hibistat** Zeneca Ph'cals	liquid		chlorhexidine gluconate, 0.5%	
Hibistat Towelette Zeneca Ph'cals	wipe		chlorhexidine gluconate, 0.5%	
Hydrogen Peroxide Multisource	solution		hydrogen peroxide, 3%	
** **Iodex Anti-Infective** Lee Consumer	ointment		iodine, 4.7%	petrolatum · oleic acid · paraffin
Iodine Topical Multisource	solution		sodium iodide, 2.5% · iodine, 2%	
Lanabiotic Combe	ointment	polymyxin B sulfate, 10000 IU/g · bacitracin, 500 IU/g · neomycin sulfate, 5mg/g		
Mercurochrome Multisource	solution		merbromin, 2%	
Mersol Century Ph'cals	liquid · ointment		alcohol, 52.5% · thimerosal, 0.1%	
Myciguent Lee Consumer	cream	neomycin sulfate, 3.5mg/g		anhydrous lanolin · mineral oil · white petroleum
Mycitracin McNeil Consumer	ointment	polymyxin B sulfate, 10000 IU/g · bacitracin zinc, 500 IU/g · neomycin sulfate, 5mg (equivalent to neomycin, 3.5mg)		butylparaben · cholesterol · methylparaben · microcrystalline wax · mineral oil · white petrolatum
Mycitracin Plus McNeil Consumer	ointment	polymyxin B sulfate, 10000 IU/g · bacitracin zinc, 500 IU/g · neomycin sulfate (equivalent to neomycin, 3.5mg)		lidocaine, 40mg · butylparaben · cholesterol · methylparaben · microcrystalline wax · mineral oil · white petrolatum
Neosporin Warner-Lambert Consumer	ointment	polymyxin B sulfate, 5000 IU/g · bacitracin zinc, 400 IU/g · neomycin base, 3.5mg/g		white petrolatum
Neosporin Plus Maximum Strength Warner-Lambert Consumer	cream	polymyxin B sulfate, 10000 IU/g · neomycin base, 3.5mg/g		pramoxine HCl, 10mg · methylparaben, 0.25% · emulsifying wax · mineral oil · poloxamer 188 · purified water · white petrolatum · propylene glycol
Neosporin Plus Maximum Strength Warner-Lambert Consumer	ointment	polymyxin B sulfate, 10000 IU/g · bacitracin zinc, 500 IU/g · neomycin base, 3.5mg/g		pramoxine HCl, 10mg · white petrolatum
New Skin Liquid Bandage Medtech	liquid		8-hydroxyquinoline, 1%	alcohol, 6.7% · proxylin solution · clove oil

See Chapter 28, "First-Aid Products and Minor Wound Care," for more information about these products.

FIRST-AID ANTIBIOTIC AND ANTISEPTIC PRODUCTS - continued

Product Manufacturer/Supplier	Dosage Form	Antibiotic	Antiseptic	Other Ingredients
New Skin Liquid Bandage Medtech	spray		8-hydroxyquinoline, 1%	proxylin (collodion), 98% · clove oil, 1% · isobutane propane (propellant) · acetone ACS
Oxyzal Wet Dressing Gordon Labs	solution		benzalkonium chloride, 0.05%	oxyquinoline sulfate
Polysporin Warner-Lambert Consumer	ointment · powder	polymyxin B sulfate, 10000 IU/g · bacitracin zinc, 500 IU/g		white petrolatum (ointment) · lactose (powder)
Povidone-Iodine Multisource	ointment · solution		povidone-iodine, 10%	
S.T.37 Solution Menley & James Labs	solution		hexylresorcinol, 0.1%	glycerin · propylene glycol · citric acid · disodium edetate · sodium bisulfite · sodium citrate
** **Tri-Biozene** Reese Chemical	ointment	polymyxin B sulfate, 10000 IU/g · bacitracin zinc, 500 IU/g · neomycin sulfate, 5mg/g (equivalent to neomycin base, 3.5mg)		pramoxine HCl, 10mg/g · white petrolatum
Tribiotic Plus Thompson Medical	ointment	polymyxin B sulfate, 5500 IU/g · bacitracin, 600 IU/g · neomycin sulfate, 3.85mg/g		lidocaine, 40mg/g · petrolatum · anhydrous lanolin · light mineral oil
Unguentine Mentholatum	ointment		phenol, 1%	eucalyptus oil · oleostearine · petrolatum · thyme oil · zinc oxide
Unguentine Plus Mentholatum	cream		phenol, 0.5%	lidocaine HCl, 2% · fragrance · glyceryl stearate · isoceteth-20 · isopropyl palmitate · methylparaben · mineral oil · poloxamer 407 · propylparaben · quaternium-15 · sorbitan stearate · tetrasodium EDTA · water

** New listing
§ Manufacturer/supplier did not confirm information for this edition. Product listing is reprinted from the '96-97 edition.

See Chapter 28, "First-Aid Products and Minor Wound Care," for more information about these products.

Diaper Rash, Prickly Heat, and Adult Incontinence Product Tables

DIAPER RASH AND PRICKLY HEAT PRODUCTS

	Product Manufacturer/Supplier	Dosage Form	Protectant	Powder Base	Antimicrobial	Other Ingredients
PE	**A + D Ointment with Zinc Oxide** Schering-Plough Healthcare	ointment	zinc oxide, 1% · dimethicone, 10% · cod liver oil (contains vitamins A and D) · light mineral oil			aloe extract · benzyl alcohol · fragrance · glyceryl oleate · ozokerite · paraffin · propylene glycol · sorbitol · synthetic beeswax · water
	A + D Original Ointment Schering-Plough Healthcare	ointment	petrolatum, 80% · lanolin, 15.5% · cod liver oil (contains vitamins A and D) · light mineral oil			fragrance · paraffin
	ActiBath Soak Oatmeal Treatment Andrew Jergens	effervescent tablet	colloidal oatmeal, 20%	sodium bicarbonate		fumaric acid · sodium carbonate · lactose · PEG-150 · magnesium oxide · sucrose stearate
**	**Ammens Extra Medicated** Bristol-Myers Products	powder	zinc oxide, 12%	talc · corn starch	8-hydroxyquinoline sulfate	eucalyptol · fragrance · methyl salicylate · thymol · tribasic calcium phosphate
	Ammens Medicated Original Fragrance Bristol-Myers Products	powder	zinc oxide, 9.1%	talc · corn starch	8-hydroxyquinoline · 8-hydroxyquinoline sulfate	fragrance · isostearic acid · PPG-20 methyl glucose ether
	Ammens Medicated Shower Fresh Scent Bristol-Myers Products	powder	zinc oxide, 9.1%	talc · corn starch		fragrance · isostearic acid · PPG-20 methyl glucose ether
	Aveeno Bath Treatment Moisturizing Formula Rydelle Labs	powder	colloidal oatmeal, 43% · mineral oil			
	Aveeno Bath Treatment Soothing Formula Rydelle Labs	powder	colloidal oatmeal, 100%			
	Bagbalm Dairy Assn. Co.	ointment	petrolatum		8-hydroxyquinoline sulfate, 0.3%	lanolin
PE	**Balmex** Block Drug	ointment	zinc oxide			beeswax · silicone · synthetic white wax · purified water · balsam · benzoic acid · bismuth subnitrate · mineral oil · others
PE	**Caldesene Medicated** Novartis Consumer	powder	talc		calcium undecylenate, 10%	fragrance
	Care-Creme Antimicrobial Cream Care-Tech Labs	cream	petrolatum · cod liver oil · lanolin oil · vitamins A and D		chloroxylenol, 0.8%	cetyl alcohol · lanolin alcohol · propylene glycol · vitamin E
	Clocream Lee Consumer	cream	vitamins A and D			cetyl palmitate · glycerin · cottonseed oil · glyceryl monostearate · methylparaben · mineral oil · potassium stearate · propylparaben · sodium citrate · fragrance · purified water
	Delazinc Mericon	ointment	zinc oxide, 25% · mineral oil · white petrolatum			synaceti · beeswax · sodium borate · water

See Chapter 29, "Diaper Rash, Prickly Heat, and Adult Incontinence Products," for more information about these products.

DIAPER RASH AND PRICKLY HEAT PRODUCTS - continued

	Product Manufacturer/Supplier	Dosage Form	Protectant	Powder Base	Antimicrobial	Other Ingredients
**	**Dermi-Heal** Quality Formulations	ointment	zinc oxide · allantoin · peruvian balsam oil · petrolatum			castor oil
PE	**Desitin** Pfizer Consumer	ointment	zinc oxide, 40% · cod liver oil · petrolatum · lanolin	talc		water · methylparaben · BHA · fragrance
PE	**Desitin Cornstarch Baby Powder** Pfizer Consumer	powder	zinc oxide, 10%	corn starch, 88.2%		fragrance · tribasic calcium phosphate
PE	**Desitin Daily Care** Pfizer Consumer	ointment	zinc oxide, 10% · dimethicone · petrolatum · mineral oil			water · white wax · cyclomethicone · sorbitan sesquioleate · sodium borate · fragrance · methylparaben · propylparaben
PE	**Diapa-Kare** Perry Products	powder		corn starch · sodium bicarbonate	methylbenzethonium chloride	fragrance
PE	**Diaparene Cornstarch Baby Powder** Personal Care Group	powder		corn starch, 88%		aloe vera extract · chamomile · evening primrose extract · tricalcium phosphate · fragrance
PE	**Diaparene Diaper Rash** Personal Care Group	ointment	zinc oxide, 15.8%		methylparaben · propylparaben · imidazolidinyl urea	trihydroxystearin · bisabolol · petrolatum
PE	**Diaper Guard** Del Ph'cals	ointment	white petrolatum, 66% · dimethicone, 1% · cocoa butter · colloidal oatmeal · cholecalciferol · zinc oxide		benzalkonium chloride	colloidal silicon dioxide · fragrance · magnesium silicate · methylparaben · paraffin · propylparaben · retinyl palmitate · d-alpha tocopheryl acetate
PE	**Dyprotex** Blistex	ointment · pad	micronized zinc oxide, 40% · petrolatum, 31.1% dimethicone, 2.5% · cod liver oil (Norwegian)	zinc stearate		aloe extract
PE	**Flanders Buttocks Ointment** Flanders	ointment	zinc oxide · white petrolatum ·			castor oil · peruvian balsam
PE	**Gold Bond Baby Powder** Chattem	powder	zinc oxide, 10%	talc		fragrance
** PE	**Gold Bond Cornstarch Plus Medicated Baby Powder** Chattem	powder	zinc oxide, 15% · kaolin, 4%	corn starch, 7%		fragrance · silica
	Gold Bond Medicated, Extra Strength Chattem	powder	zinc oxide, 5%	talc		menthol, 0.8% · eucalyptol · methyl salicylate · salicylic acid · thymol · zinc stearate
	Gold Bond Medicated, Regular Strength Chattem	powder	zinc oxide, 1%	talc		menthol, 0.15% · eucalyptol · methyl salicylate · salicylic acid · thymol · zinc stearate

See Chapter 29, "Diaper Rash, Prickly Heat, and Adult Incontinence Products," for more information about these products.

DIAPER RASH AND PRICKLY HEAT PRODUCTS - continued

	Product Manufacturer/Supplier	Dosage Form	Protectant	Powder Base	Antimicrobial	Other Ingredients
	Hydropel C & M Pharmacal	ointment	silicone, 30% · petrolatum			aluminum starch octenyl succinate
PE	**Johnson's Baby Cream §** Johnson & Johnson Consumer	cream	dimethicone, 2% · lanolin · mineral oil			fragrance · glyceryl stearate · paraffin · propylparaben · sodium borate · water
PE	**Johnson's Baby Powder §** Johnson & Johnson Consumer	powder		talc		fragrance
PE	**Johnson's Baby Powder Cornstarch §** Johnson & Johnson Consumer	powder		corn starch, 95%		tricalcium phosphate · fragrance
PE	**Johnson's Baby, Medicated §** Johnson & Johnson Consumer	powder	zinc oxide	corn starch		fragrance
PE	**Johnson's Diaper Rash Ointment §** Johnson & Johnson Consumer	ointment	petrolatum · zinc oxide		benzethonium chloride	trihydroxystearin · bisabolol · fragrance
PE	**Little Bottoms** Vetco	ointment	zinc oxide, 15%· balsam peru · mineral oil · petrolatum · dimethicone			aloe · PEG-40 · sorbitan peroleate · beeswax · titanium dioxide · bismuth subnitrate · benzoic acid · deionized water
	Lobana Derm-ADE Lobana Labs	cream	vitamins A, D, and E · silicone			
	Lobana Peri-Gard Lobana Labs	ointment	petrolatum · vitamins A and D		chloroxylenol	
	Mexsana Medicated Schering-Plough Healthcare	powder	zinc oxide, 10.8%	corn starch · kaolin	benzethonium chloride	camphor · eucalyptus oil
	Nutra Soothe Medicated Brimms Labs	powder	colloidal oatmeal · zinc oxide	corn starch · oat starch		tricalcium phosphate · fragrance
	Panthoderm Jones Medical	lotion	dexpanthenol, 2%			water-miscible base
	Plexolan Lanolin Alvin Last	cream	petrolatum, 23.7% · mineral oil · zinc oxide			water · lanolin wax · PEG-400 distearate · fragrance · methylparaben
	Protective Barrier C & M Pharmacal	ointment	silicone, 30% · petrolatum			aluminum starch octenyl succinate
PE	**Resinol Diaper Rash** Mentholatum	ointment	zinc oxide, 12% · calamine			lanolin · petrolatum · starch
	Schamberg's Anti-itch C & M Pharmacal	lotion	zinc oxide			purified water · refined peanut oil · propylene glycol · magnesium aluminum silicate · phenol · cellulose gum · calcium oxide · octoxynol-9 · menthol
	Spectro-Jel Recsei Labs	gel			cetylpyridinium chloride, 0.1%	isopropyl alcohol, 5% · methylcellulose, 1.5% · glycol- polysiloxane, 1%
	Triple Paste Summers Labs	ointment	white petrolatum, 52% · zinc oxide ·			aluminum acetate solution

See Chapter 29, "Diaper Rash, Prickly Heat, and Adult Incontinence Products," for more information about these products.

DIAPER RASH AND PRICKLY HEAT PRODUCTS - continued

	Product Manufacturer/Supplier	Dosage Form	Protectant	Powder Base	Antimicrobial	Other Ingredients
	Vaseline Pure Petroleum Jelly Chesebrough-Pond's	ointment	white petrolatum, 100%			
	Velvet Fresh Powder Care-Tech Labs	powder		corn starch		tricalcium phosphate · fragrance
PE	**ZBT Baby Powder** Glenwood	powder	mineral oil	talc · magnesium stearate		BHT · fragrance · Arlacel 186
	Zeasorb Stiefel Labs	powder		talc · microporous cellulose	chloroxylenol	carbohydrate acrylic copolymer · imidazolidinyl urea · aldioxa · fragrance

** New listing

§ Manufacturer/supplier did not confirm information for this edition. Product listing is reprinted from the '96-97 edition.

See Chapter 29, "Diaper Rash, Prickly Heat, and Adult Incontinence Products," for more information about these products.

ADULT INCONTINENCE GARMENTS

Product Manufacturer/Supplier	Product Form	Absorbency	Comments
Attends Briefs Procter & Gamble	brief	heavy	sizes S, M, L · refastenable tapes
Attends Guards Procter & Gamble	pad	light · moderate (super)	curved
Attends Pads Procter & Gamble	pad	light	
Attends Undergarments Procter & Gamble	undergarment	moderate (regular) · heavy (super)	reusable elastic belts
Depend Fitted Briefs § Kimberly-Clark	brief	heavy/complete (regular · overnight)	regular absorbency in sizes S, M, L · overnight absorbency (absorbs 30% more) size M · each has six refastenable tapes plus elastic leg and waist
Depend Guards for Men § Kimberly-Clark	pad	light/moderate	one size · anatomical design with elasticized pouch · cup-like fit
Depend Poise § Kimberly-Clark	pad	light (thin · regular · extra · extra plus)	maxi pad size · elasticized sides
Depend Poise Guards § Kimberly-Clark	pad	light/moderate (super · super plus)	thermo-formed shell creates a reservoir
Depend Poise Shields § Kimberly-Clark	pad	light (regular · extra)	one size · cup-shaped design
Depend Undergarments § Kimberly-Clark	undergarment	moderate (EasyFit: regular, extra · Elastic Leg: regular, extra · Non-Elastic Leg: extra)	soft, cloth-like outer cover · three styles, each in one size: EasyFit with reusable strap tabs, Elastic Leg with reusable button strap tabs, and Non-Elastic Leg with reusable button strap tabs
** **Dignity Lites** Humanicare	pad	light (liner · stackable insert) · moderate (extra-long)	
** **Dignity Pads** Humanicare	pad	light (regular) · mild/moderate (natural) · mild/heavy (extra)	
** **Dignity Plus Briefmates Guards** Humanicare	pad	moderate	curved
** **Dignity Plus Briefmates Pads** Humanicare	pad	light	curved
** **Dignity Plus Briefmates Undergarments** Humanicare	undergarment	moderate/heavy	curved · beltless or belted
** **Dignity Plus Fitted Briefs** Humanicare	brief	moderate	sizes S, M, L, XL · four refastenable tapes, elastic leg, wetness indicator
** **Dignity Plus Liners** Humanicare	pad	mild/moderate	
** **Free & Active Pads** Humanicare	pad	light/moderate (regular) · moderate/heavy (super)	
** **Rejoice Liners** Caring Products	pad	light	ultra thin · may be used by women within their own underpants · to be used by men or women with Rejoice Pants
** **Rejoice Pants** Caring Products	undergarment	moderate	men's and women's pull-on or side-closing styles · sizes S, M, L, XL, XXL · cotton, washable and dryable · fabric side walls within the pant crotch help prevent side-seepage

See Chapter 29, "Diaper Rash, Prickly Heat, and Adult Incontinence Products," for more information about these products.

ADULT INCONTINENCE GARMENTS - continued

	Product Manufacturer/Supplier	Product Form	Absorbency	Comments
	Stayfree Serenity Curved Pads § Johnson & Johnson Consumer	pad	light/moderate (extra) · moderate (extra plus)	curved
	Stayfree Serenity Guards § Johnson & Johnson Consumer	pad	moderate (regular) · moderate/heavy (super) · heavy (super plus)	
	Stayfree Serenity Pads § Johnson & Johnson Consumer	pad	light (thin) · light/moderate	
**	**Wearever Reusable, Washable Briefs (Universal)** Wearever Health Care	brief	light/severe	sizes S, M, L, XL, XXL · built-in pad system and waterproof liner
**	**Wearever Reusable, Washable Briefs For Men** Wearever Health Care	brief	light	sizes S, M, L, XL, XXL · built-in pad system and waterproof liner · fly-front design
**	**Wearever Reusable, Washable Briefs For Women** Wearever Health Care	brief	light	sizes 6-10 · built-in pad system and waterproof liner · three styles: Julia (lace panels), LadyFem (cotton/polyester blend), and Virginia (acetate)

** New listing

§   Manufacturer/supplier did not confirm information for this edition. Product listing is reprinted from the '96-97 edition.

See Chapter 29, "Diaper Rash, Prickly Heat, and Adult Incontinence Products," for more information about these products.

Sunscreen and Suntan Product Table

SUNSCREEN AND SUNTAN PRODUCTS

	Product Manufacturer/Supplier	Dosage Form	SPF Value	Sunscreen	Other Ingredients
	A-Fil GenDerm	cream	8 · 15	menthyl anthranilate, 5% · titanium dioxide, 5%	
	Aquaderm Sunscreen Moisturizer Baker Cummins Derm'cals	cream	15	octyl methoxycinnamate, 7.5% · oxybenzone, 6%	
PE	**Bain de Soleil All Day for Kids Waterproof Sunblock** Pfizer Consumer	lotion	30	octyl methoxycinnamate · octocrylene · oxybenzone · titanium dioxide	water · PVP/eicosene copolymer · isohexadecane · butylene glycol · dimethicone · cyclomethicone · panthenol · triethanolamine · cetyl palmitate · tribehenin · stearoxytrimethylsilane · stearyl alcohol · tocopheryl acetate · DEA-cetyl phosphate · carbomer · acrylates/C10-30 alkyl acrylate crosspolymer · disodium EDTA · DMDM hydantoin · iodopropynyl butylcarbamate
	Bain de Soleil All Day Six Hour Waterproof Sunfilter Pfizer Consumer	lotion	4 · 8	octocrylene · octyl methoxycinnamate · titanium dioxide	water · PVP/eicosene copolymer · isohexadecane · butylene glycol · dimethicone · cyclomethicone · panthenol · triethanolamine · cetyl palmitate · tribehenin · stearoxytrimethylsilane · stearyl alcohol · tocopheryl acetate · DEA-cetyl phosphate · carbomer · acrylates/C10-30 alkyl acrylate crosspolymer · disodium EDTA · DMDM hydantoin · iodopropynyl butylcarbamate
	Bain de Soleil All Day Waterproof Sunblock Pfizer Consumer	lotion	15	octyl methoxycinnamate · octocrylene · oxybenzone · titanium dioxide	water · PVP/eicosene copolymer · isohexadecane · butylene glycol · dimethicone · cyclomethicone · panthenol · triethanolamine · cetyl palmitate · tribehenin · stearoxytrimethylsilane · stearyl alcohol · tocopheryl acetate · DEA-cetyl phosphate · carbomer · acrylates/C10-30 alkyl acrylate crosspolymer · disodium EDTA · DMDM hydantoin · iodopropynyl butylcarbamate
**	**Bain de Soleil Le Sport** Pfizer Consumer	lotion	30	octyl methoxycinnamate, 7.5% · octocrylene, 4% · oxybenzone, 2% · titanium dioxide, 2%	
**	**Bain de Soleil Le Sport** Pfizer Consumer	lotion	15	octyl methoxycinnamate, 7.5% · octocrylene, 5% · titanium dioxide, 2% · oxybenzone, 1%	
**	**Bain de Soleil Mademoiselle** Pfizer Consumer	lotion	4 · 8 · 15	octyl methoxycinnamate, 7.5% · octocrylene, 4% · titanium dioxide, 2% · oxybenzone, 1% (SPF 15)	
	Bain de Soleil Mega Tan Pfizer Consumer	lotion	4	octyl methoxycinnamate · octocrylene	water · dihydroxyacetone · cyclomethicone · butylene glycol · PVP/eicosene copolymer · isohexadecane · fragrance · polyquarternium-37 · mineral oil · PPG-1- trideceth-6 · cetyl palmitate · tribehenin · extracts of aloe, lanolin, cocoa butter, palm, chamomile, eucalyptus, and guava · cetyl alcohol · cetyl hydroxyethyl cellulose · distearyldimonium chloride · DMDM hydantoin · iodopropynyl butylcarbamate · disodium EDTA

See Chapter 30, "Sunscreen and Suntan Products," for more information about these products.

SUNSCREEN AND SUNTAN PRODUCTS - continued

Product Manufacturer/Supplier	Dosage Form	SPF Value	Sunscreen	Other Ingredients
Bain de Soleil Orange Gelee Pfizer Consumer	gel	4	octyl methoxycinnamate · octyl salicylate	mineral oil · petrolatum · paraffin · ozokerite · isopropyl myristate · fragrance · propylparaben · butylparaben · D&C red#17 · D&C yellow#10 aluminum lake
Bain de Soleil Sand Buster Pfizer Consumer	oil	2	octyl methoxycinnamate · octyl salicylate	mineral oil · cyclomethicone · polybutene · coconut oil · lanolin oil · fragrance · extracts of aloe, lanolin, cocoa butter, eucalyptus, palm, chamomile, and guava · propylparaben · D&C red#17 · D&C violet#2
Bain de Soleil SPF+Color Pfizer Consumer	lotion	8 ·15 · 30	octyl methoxycinnamate · octocrylene · oxybenzone	dihydroxyacetone
Bain de Soleil Tropical Deluxe Tanning Pfizer Consumer	lotion	4	octyl methoxycinnamate · octyl salicylate	water · mineral oil · stearic acid · cyclomethicone · butylene glycol · cetyl alcohol · fragrance · myristyl myristate · shea butter · triethanolamine · extracts of aloe, lanolin, cocoa butter, palm oil, chamomile, eucalyptus, and guava · glycol stearate · DMDM hydantoin · iodopropynyl butylcarbamate · carbomer · acrylates/C10-30 alkyl acrylate crosspolymer · disodium EDTA
Banana Boat Faces Sunblock Spot Stick Sun Ph'cals	stick	30	octocrylene · homosalate · octyl methoxycinnamate · oxybenzone · octyl salicylate	
FR **Banana Boat Maximum Sunblock** Sun Ph'cals	lotion	50	octyl methoxycinnamate · octocrylene · oxybenzone · octyl salicylate · titanium dioxide	
FR **Banana Boat Sport Sunblock** Sun Ph'cals	lotion	15 · 50	octyl methoxycinnamate · octocrylene (SPF50) · oxybenzone · octyl salicylate · titanium dioxide (SPF50)	
Banana Boat Sunscreen or Sunblock Sun Ph'cals	lotion	8 (Sunscreen) · 15 (Sunblock)	padimate O · oxybenzone · octyl methoxycinnamate (Sunblock)	
Banana Boat Tanning Sun Ph'cals	oil	4 · 8	padimate O · octyl methoxycinnamate	
** **Bio Sun** Playtex Products	lotion	15 · 30 · 45	octyl methoxycinnamate · octocrylene (SPF 45) · oxybenzone · octyl salicylate	
** PE **Bio Sun Children** Playtex Products	lotion	30	octyl methoxycinnamate · oxybenzone · octyl salicylate	
** **Bio Sun Faces** Playtex Products	lotion	25	octyl methoxycinnamate · oxybenzone · octyl salicylate	

See Chapter 30, "Sunscreen and Suntan Products," for more information about these products.

SUNSCREEN AND SUNTAN PRODUCTS - continued

	Product Manufacturer/Supplier	Dosage Form	SPF Value	Sunscreen	Other Ingredients
** FR	**BioShield Facial Sunblock for Normal or for Sensitive Skin** Hawaiian Tropic	lotion	15 · 30	octyl methoxycinnamate · octyl salicylate · titanium dioxide · octocrylene · fragrance (Normal Skin)	
	Blistex DCT Daily Conditioning Treatment for Lips Blistex	ointment	20	octyl methoxycinnamate, 7.3% · benzophenone-3, 4.5%	petrolatum, 56.26% · aloe extract · cetyl alcohol · cocoa butter · flavor · lanolin · mixed waxes · phenol · vitamins A and E
	Blistex Lip Balm; Berry, Mint, or Regular Blistex	stick	10	padimate O, 6.6% · oxybenzone, 2.5%	dimethicone, 2% · cocoa butter · color (Berry, Regular) · flavor · isopropyl esters · lanolin · methylparaben · mineral oil · mixed waxes · petrolatum · propylparaben
	Blistex Lip Tone Lip Balm Blistex	stick	15	octyl methoxycinnamate, 7.3% · menthyl anthranilate, 4%	dimethicone, 2% · aloe extract · arginine · glycine · mixed waxes · petrolatum · vitamins A and E · color
	Blistex Ultra Protection Lip Balm Blistex	stick	30	octyl methoxycinnamate, 7.4% · oxybenzone, 5.2% · octyl salicylate, 5% · menthyl anthranilate, 4.8% · homosalate, 4.5%	dimethicone, 3% · flavors · isopropyl myristate · mixed waxes · myristyl myristate
	Bull Frog Chattem	stick	18	octyl methoxycinnamate, 7.5% · benzophenone-3, 2.5%	aloe extract · carotene · fragrance · hydrogenated vegetable oil · isostearyl alcohol · microcrystalline wax · ozokerite · tocopheryl acetate
	Bull Frog Chattem	gel	36	octyl methoxycinnamate, 7.5% · octocrylene, 10% · benzophenone-3, 3%	aloe extract · beeswax · caprylic/capric triglyceride · cyclomethicone · fragrance · isostearyl alcohol · silica · tocopheryl acetate
PE	**Bull Frog for Kids** Chattem	gel	36	octyl methoxycinnamate, 7.5% · octocrylene, 10% · benzophenone-3, 3%	aloe extract · beeswax · caprylic/capric triglyceride · cyclomethicone · fragrance · isostearyl alcohol · silica · tocopheryl acetate
**	**Bull Frog Quik** Chattem	gel	36	octorylene, 10% · methoxycinnamate, 7.5% · benzophenone-3, 5% · octyl salicylate, 5%	acrylates/octylacrylamide copolymer · aloe extract · C12-15 alkyl benzoate · fragrance · hydroxypropyl cellulose · SD alcohol 40 · tocopheryl acetate
	Bull Frog Quik Chattem	gel	18	octyl methoxycinnamate, 7.5% · octyl salicylate, 5% · benzophenone-3, 5%	acrylates/octylacrylamide copolymer · aloe extract · C12-15 alkyl benzoate · fragrance · hydroxypropyl cellulose · SD alcohol 40 · tocopheryl acetate
	Bull Frog Sport Chattem	lotion	18	octyl methoxycinnamate, 7.5% · octocrylene, 7% · octyl salicylate, 5% · benzophenone-3, 4% · titanium dioxide, 2%	
	Bull Frog Sunblock Chattem	gel	18	octyl methoxycinnamate, 7.5% · octocrylene, 7% · benzophenone-3, 2%	aloe extract · beeswax · cyclomethicone · fragrance · isostearyl alcohol · panthenol · silica · tocopheryl acetate

See Chapter 30, "Sunscreen and Suntan Products," for more information about these products.

SUNSCREEN AND SUNTAN PRODUCTS - continued

Product Manufacturer/Supplier	Dosage Form	SPF Value	Sunscreen	Other Ingredients
ChapStick Lip Moisturizer Whitehall-Robins Healthcare	ointment · stick	15	octyl methoxycinnamate, 7.5% · oxybenzone, 3.5%	petrolatum, 40.7% (stick) or 33% (ointment) · aloe vera oil · carnauba wax (stick) · cetyl alcohol (stick) · fragrance · isocetyl stearate · isopropyl lanolate (stick) · isopropyl myristate (stick) · lanolin · methylparaben · paraffin wax (stick) · propylparaben · vitamin E acetate · vitamin E linoleate · white wax (stick)
ChapStick Sunblock 15 Whitehall-Robins Healthcare	stick	15	padimate O, 7% · oxybenzone, 3% · titanium dioxide	petrolatum, 44% · cetyl alcohol, 0.5% · lanolin, 0.5% · isopropyl myristate, 0.5% · camphor · carnauba wax · D&C red#6 barium lake · FD&C yellow#5 aluminum lake · fragrance · isopropyl lanolate · methylparaben · mineral oil · propylparaben · paraffin wax · white wax
ChapStick Sunblock 15 Petroleum Jelly Plus Whitehall-Robins Healthcare	ointment	15	padimate O, 7% · oxybenzone, 3%	white petrolatum, 89% · aloe · butylated · hydroxytoluene · flavor · lanolin · phenonip
ChapStick Ultra Whitehall-Robins Healthcare	stick	30	octocrylene, 10% · octyl methoxycinnamate, 7.5% · octyl salicylate, 5% · oxybenzone, 5% · titanium dioxide	white petrolatum, 30% · aloe vera oil · arachidyl propionate · carnauba wax · cetyl alcohol · fragrance · isopropyl lanolate · isopropyl myristate · lanolin · methylparaben · octyldodecanol · oleyl alcohol · paraffin wax · propylparaben · vitamin E acetate · vitamin E linoleate · white wax · polyphenyl · methylsiloxane
** **Coppertone Aloe & Vitamin E Lip Balm with Sunscreen** Schering-Plough Healthcare	stick	15	octyl methoxycinnamate · oxybenzone ·	
Coppertone Dry Schering-Plough Healthcare	oil	2	homosalate	
** **Coppertone Gold Dark Tanning** Schering-Plough Healthcare	oil	4	homosalate · oxybenzone	vitamin E · aloe
** **Coppertone Gold Dry** Schering-Plough Healthcare	oil	2	homosalate	vitamin E · aloe
** **Coppertone Gold Tan Magnifier** Schering-Plough Healthcare	oil	2	triethanolamine salicylate	tyrosine · vitamin E · aloe
** PE **Coppertone Kids Colorblock Disappearing Purple Sunblock** Schering-Plough Healthcare	lotion	30	octyl methoxycinnamate · oxybenzone · octyl salicylate · homosalate	
PE **Coppertone Kids Sunblock** Schering-Plough Healthcare	lotion	40	octyl methoxycinnamate · octyl salicylate · oxybenzone · homosalate	
PE **Coppertone Kids Sunblock** Schering-Plough Healthcare	lotion	15 · 30	octyl methoxycinnamate · oxybenzone · octyl salicylate · homosalate (SPF 15)	
** PE **Coppertone Kids Sunblock** Schering-Plough Healthcare	stick	30	octyl methoxycinnamate · oxybenzone · octyl salicylate · homosalate	

See Chapter 30, "Sunscreen and Suntan Products," for more information about these products.

SUNSCREEN AND SUNTAN PRODUCTS - continued

	Product Manufacturer/Supplier	Dosage Form	SPF Value	Sunscreen	Other Ingredients
	Coppertone LipKote Sunblock Lip Balm Schering-Plough Healthcare	stick	15	octyl methoxycinnamate · oxybenzone	
PE	**Coppertone Little Licks Sunblock Lip Balm** Schering-Plough Healthcare	stick	30	octyl methoxycinnamate · oxybenzone · octyl salicylate	
	Coppertone Moisturizing Sunblock Schering-Plough Healthcare	lotion	45	octyl methoxycinnamate · octyl salicylate · octocrylene · oxybenzone	
	Coppertone Moisturizing Sunblock Schering-Plough Healthcare	lotion	30	octyl methoxycinnamate · oxybenzone · octyl salicylate · homosalate	
	Coppertone Moisturizing Sunblock or Suntan Schering-Plough Healthcare	lotion	4 (Suntan) · 15 (Sunblock)	octyl methoxycinnamate · oxybenzone	
	Coppertone Moisturizing Sunscreen Schering-Plough Healthcare	lotion	6 · 8	octyl methoxycinnamate · oxybenzone	
**	**Coppertone Natural Fruit Flavor Lip Balm with Sunscreen** Schering-Plough Healthcare	stick	15	octyl methoxycinnamate · oxybenzone	
	Coppertone Oil-Free Sunblock Schering-Plough Healthcare	lotion	4 · 8 · 15	octyl methoxycinnamate · oxybenzone	
**	**Coppertone Oil-Free Sunblock** Schering-Plough Healthcare	lotion	30	homosalate · octyl methoxycinnamate · octyl salicylate · oxybenzone ·	
	Coppertone Protect & Tan Schering-Plough Healthcare	lotion	15	octyl methoxycinnamate · octyl salicylate · oxybenzone · homosalate	
	Coppertone Skin Selects Dry Skin Sunblock Schering-Plough Healthcare	lotion	15	octyl methoxycinnamate · oxybenzone	
	Coppertone Skin Selects Oily Skin Sunblock Schering-Plough Healthcare	lotion	15	octyl methoxycinnamate · oxybenzone	
	Coppertone Skin Selects Sensitive Skin Sunblock Schering-Plough Healthcare	lotion	15	titanium dioxide · octyl methoxycinnamate	
	Coppertone Sport Schering-Plough Healthcare	lotion	4 · 8 · 15 · 30	octyl methoxycinnamate · oxybenzone · octyl salicylate (SPF30)	

See Chapter 30, "Sunscreen and Suntan Products," for more information about these products.

SUNSCREEN AND SUNTAN PRODUCTS - continued

	Product Manufacturer/Supplier	Dosage Form	SPF Value	Sunscreen	Other Ingredients
FR	**Dermsol-30** Parnell Ph'cals	lotion	30	octyl methoxycinnamate, 7.5% · oxybenzone, 6.0% · octyl salicylate, 5.0%	octyldodecyl neopentanoate · glycerin · TEA stearate · DEA-cetyl phosphate · ceteth-25 · cetyl alcohol · laneth-25 · oleth-25 · steareth-25 · diazolidinyl urea · methylparaben · propylparaben · yerba santa · hyaluronic acid · hydrolyzed collagen · sodium PCA · carbomer
FR	**DuraScreen** Pierre Fabre Dermatology	lotion	15	octyl methoxycinnamate · octyl salicylate · benzophenone-3 · titanium dioxide	water · octyldodecyl neopentanoate · PPG-12/SMDI copolymer · propylene glycol · stearic acid · DEA-cetyl phosphate · algae extract · aluminum stearate · carbomer · cetyl alcohol · chamomile oil · dimethicone · sodium dehydroacetate · stearyl alcohol · triethanolamine · imidazolidinyl urea · methylparaben · propylparaben
FR	**DuraScreen** Pierre Fabre Dermatology	lotion	30	octyl methoxycinnamate · octyl salicylate · benzophenone-3 · phenylbenzimidazole sulfonic acid · titanium dioxide	water · PPG-12/SMDI copolymer · octyldodecyl neopentanoate · dimethicone · triethanolamine · cetearyl alcohol · acrylates/C10-30 alkyl acrylate crosspolymer · aluminum stearate · ceteareth-20 · fluoroalkyldimethicone · propylene glycol · shea butter · trifluoromethyl C1-4 alkyl dimethicone · xanthan gum · phenoxyethanol · diazolidinyl urea · methylparaben · propylparaben
	Facial Moisturizing Sunscreen C & M Pharmacal	cream	20	octyl methoxycinnamate, 7.5% · benzophenone-4, 5% · titanium dioxide micronized	purified water · dioctyl maleate · emulsifying wax · propylene glycol · glycerin · sodium lauryl sulfate · soluble collagen · DEA-cetyl phosphate · PVP/eicosene copolymer · benzyl alcohol · hydrolyzed elastin · magnesium aluminum silicate · xanthan gum
	Full Body Sunscreen C & M Pharmacal	lotion	15	octyl methoxycinnamate, 7.5% · benzophenone-4	purified water · dioctyl maleate · glycerin · PVP/eicosene · stearic acid · DEA-cetyl phosphate · cetyl alcohol · titanium dioxide · fragrance · methylparaben · carbomer 940 · triethanolamine · propylparaben
**	**Hawaiian Tropic 45 Plus Lip Balm** Hawaiian Tropic	stick	45	octocrylene · octyl methoxycinnamate · benzophenone-3 · octyl salicylate · menthyl anthranilate	
PE	**Hawaiian Tropic Baby Faces Sunblock** Hawaiian Tropic	lotion	35 · 50	octyl methoxycinnamate · octyl salicylate · titanium dioxide	
**	**Hawaiian Tropic Clear Sense** Hawaiian Tropic	lotion	4 · 8	octyl methoxycinnamate · octyl salicylate · titanium dioxide	benzoyl peroxide · vitamins A, C, and E
**	**Hawaiian Tropic Clear Sense Sunblock** Hawaiian Tropic	lotion	15	octyl methoxycinnamate · octyl salicylate · titanium dioxide · octocrylene	benzoyl peroxide · vitamins A, C, and E

See Chapter 30, "Sunscreen and Suntan Products," for more information about these products.

SUNSCREEN AND SUNTAN PRODUCTS - continued

	Product Manufacturer/Supplier	Dosage Form	SPF Value	Sunscreen	Other Ingredients
**	**Hawaiian Tropic Dark Tanning with Extra Sunscreen** Hawaiian Tropic	oil	4	2-octyl methoxycinnamate · octyl dimethyl ABA	
	Hawaiian Tropic Dark Tanning with Sunscreen Hawaiian Tropic	lotion	4	2-octyl p-methoxycinnamate · menthyl anthranilate	
**	**Hawaiian Tropic Dark Tanning with Sunscreen** Hawaiian Tropic	oil	2	octyl methoxycinnamate · octyl dimethyl ABA	
**	**Hawaiian Tropic Golden Tanning** Hawaiian Tropic	lotion	6	titanium dioxide	
**	**Hawaiian Tropic Herbal Tanning** Hawaiian Tropic	lotion	4	octyl methoxycinnamate · benzophenone-3	extracts of: Hawaiian white ginger, aloe vera, chamomile, ginseng
**	**Hawaiian Tropic Herbal Tanning Mist** Hawaiian Tropic	pump spray	2	phenylbenzimidazole sulfonic acid · benzophenone-4	water · extracts of: Hawaiian white ginger, aloe vera, chamomile, ginseng
** AL PE	**Hawaiian Tropic Just for Kids Sunblock** Hawaiian Tropic	lotion	30 · 45	octyl methoxycinnamate · octyl salicylate · titanium dioxide	
**	**Hawaiian Tropic Protection Plus** Hawaiian Tropic	lotion	15 · 30 · 45	octyl methoxycinnamate · octyl salicylate · titanium dioxide	vitamins A, C, and E
**	**Hawaiian Tropic Protection Plus** Hawaiian Tropic	lotion	10	octyl methoxycinnamate · menthyl anthranilate · benzophenone-3	vitamins A, C, and E
**	**Hawaiian Tropic Protective Tanning Dry Oil** Hawaiian Tropic	pump spray	6	2-octyl methoxycinnamate · homosalate · menthyl anthranilate	
**	**Hawaiian Tropic Protective Tanning Dry Oil** Hawaiian Tropic	lotion	8	octyl methoxycinnamate · benzophenone-3	
**	**Hawaiian Tropic Sport Sunblock** Hawaiian Tropic	lotion	15 · 45	octyl methyoxycinnamate · octyl salicylate · titanium dioxide	
**	**Hawaiian Tropic Tan Amplifier** Hawaiian Tropic	lotion	4	octyl methoxycinnamate · benzophenone-3	
	Hawaiian Tropic Tan Amplifier Hawaiian Tropic	gel	2	phenylbenzimidazole sulfonic acid	

See Chapter 30, "Sunscreen and Suntan Products," for more information about these products.

SUNSCREEN AND SUNTAN PRODUCTS - continued

	Product Manufacturer/Supplier	Dosage Form	SPF Value	Sunscreen	Other Ingredients
	Herpecin-L Cold Sore Lip Balm Chattem	stick	15	padimate O, 7% · titanium dioxide	allantoin, 0.5% · beeswax · cetyl esters · flavoring · octyldodecanol · paraffin · petrolatum · sesame oil · vitamins B6, C, and E
	Mentholatum Lipbalm Mentholatum	stick	14	padimate O, 8%	dimethicone, 1% · petrolatum · fragrance · lanolin · menthol · mineral oil · ozokerite ·
	Mentholatum Lipbalm, Cherry Ice Mentholatum	stick	11	padimate O, 8%	dimethicone, 1% · fragrance · lanolin · menthol · mineral oil · ozokerite · petrolatum
** PE	**Neutrogena Kids Sunblock** Neutrogena Dermatologics	lotion	30	homosalate · octyl methoxycinnamate · benzophenone-3 · octyl salicylate	
	Neutrogena Lip Moisturizer Neutrogena Dermatologics	stick	15	octyl methoxycinnamate, 7.5% · benzophenone-3, 4%	castor oil · corn oil · ozokerite · petrolatum · beeswax · octyl palmitate · paraffin · stearyl alcohol · carnauba · BHT
	Neutrogena Moisture for the Face, Tinted and Untinted Neutrogena Dermatologics	lotion	15	octyl methoxycinnamate, 7.5 % · oxybenzone, 5%	
**	**Neutrogena Oil Free Sunblock** Neutrogena Dermatologics	lotion	30	homosalate · octyl · methoxycinnamate · benzophenone-3 · octyl salicylate	
	Neutrogena Sensitive Skin Sunblocker Neutrogena Dermatologics	lotion	17	titanium dioxide	
**	**Neutrogena Sunblock** Neutrogena Dermatologics	pump spray	20	homosalate · octyl methoxycinnamate · octyl salicylate · menthyl anthranilate	
	Neutrogena Sunblock Neutrogena Dermatologics	cream	30	octocrylene · octyl methoxycinnamate · menthyl anthranilate	
	Neutrogena Sunblock Neutrogena Dermatologics	cream	15	octyl methoxycinnamate · octyl salicylate · menthyl anthranilate	
	Neutrogena Sunblock Neutrogena Dermatologics	stick	25	octyl methoxycinnamate · benzophenone-3 · octyl salicylate	
**	**Neutrogena Sunless Tanning Lotion; Light/Med, Med/Deep, Deep** Neutrogena Dermatologics	cream	8	octyl methoxycinnamate	
	Nivea Hand Therapy Beiersdorf	lotion	15	octyl methoxycinnamate · phenylbenzimidazole sulfonic acid · oxybenzone	

See Chapter 30, "Sunscreen and Suntan Products," for more information about these products.

SUNSCREEN AND SUNTAN PRODUCTS - continued

	Product Manufacturer/Supplier	Dosage Form	SPF Value	Sunscreen	Other Ingredients
	Nivea Sun Beiersdorf	lotion	15	octyl methoxycinnamate · octyl salicylate · benzophenone-3 · phenoxylbenzimidazole sulfonic acid	
** FR PE	**Nivea Sun Kids** Beiersdorf	lotion	30	octocrylene · octyl methoxycinnamate · octyl salicylate · oxybenzone · titanium dioxide	
**	**Nivea UV Care Lip Balm** Beiersdorf	stick	18	octyl methoxycinnamate, 7.5% · octocrylene, 7.5% · benzophenone-3, 2%	petrolatum · octyldodecanol · polydecene · paraffin · ceresin · polyisobutene · carnauba · synthetic beeswax · shea butter · tocopheryl acetate · fragrance
	Oil of Olay Daily UV Protectant Fragrance Free Procter & Gamble	cream · lotion	15	octyl methoxycinnamate · phenylbenzimidazole sulfonic acid · titanium dioxide	water · isohexadecane · butylene glycol · triethanolamine · glycerin · stearic acid · cetyl alcohol · cetyl palmitate · DEA-cetyl phosphate · aluminum starch octenylsuccinate · imidazolidinyl urea · methylparaben · propylparaben · carbomer · acrylates/C10-30 alkyl acrylate crosspolymer · PEG-10 soya sterol · disodium EDTA · castor oil
	Oil of Olay Daily UV Protectant Original Procter & Gamble	cream · lotion	15	octyl methoxycinnamate · phenylbenzimidazole sulfonic acid · titanium dioxide	water · isohexadecane · butylene glycol · triethanolamine · glycerin · stearic acid · cetyl alcohol · cetyl palmitate · DEA-cetyl phosphate · aluminum starch octenylsuccinate · imidazolidinyl urea · methylparaben · propylparaben · carbomer · acrylates/C10-30 alkyl acrylate crosspolymer · PEG-10 soya sterol · disodium EDTA · castor oil · fragrance · FD&C red#4 · FD&C yellow#5
**	**Palmer's Aloe Vera Formula Medicated Lip Balm** E. T. Browne Drug	stick	15	octyl methoxycinnamate, 7.5% · oxybenzone, 4.5%	dimethicone
**	**Palmer's Cocoa Butter Formula Moisturizing Lip Balm** E. T. Browne Drug	stick	15	octyl methoxycinnamate, 7.5% · oxybenzone, 4.5%	dimethicone
**	**Palmer's Skin Success Anti-Darkening** E. T. Browne Drug	cream	30	octocrylene, 9% · octyl methoxycinnamate, 7.5% · oxybenzone, 6% · octyl salicylate, 5%	water · propylene glycol · tricontanyl PVP · cetearyl alcohol · aloe vera gel · lilial · leaf extract · hedione · vitamin E · diazolidinyl urea · methylparaben · propylparaben · sorbitan oleate · triethanolamine · carbomer · acrylates/C10-30 alkyl acrylate crosspolymer
	PreSun 15 or 30 Active Westwood-Squibb Ph'cals	gel	15 · 30	benzophenone-3 · octyl methoxycinnamate · octyl salicylate	SD alcohol · PPG-15 stearyl ether · acrylates/t-octylpropenamide · hydroxypropylcellulose
	PreSun 15 Sensitive Skin Westwood-Squibb Ph'cals	lotion	15 · 29	octyl methoxycinnamate · benzophenone-3 · oxybenzone (29) · octyl salicylate	carbomer 940 · cetyl alcohol · DEA-cetyl phosphate · diazolidinyl urea · dimethicone · isopropyl myristate · isodecyl neopentanoate · kathon CG · PG dioctanoate · PVP/eicosene copolymer · stearic acid · triethanolamine · water

See Chapter 30, "Sunscreen and Suntan Products," for more information about these products.

SUNSCREEN AND SUNTAN PRODUCTS - continued

	Product Manufacturer/Supplier	Dosage Form	SPF Value	Sunscreen	Other Ingredients
	PreSun 21 Westwood-Squibb Ph'cals	lotion	21	titanium dioxide	phenyl trimethicone · C12-15 alcohol benzoate · polyglyceryl-4-isostearate · cetyl dimethicone copolyol · hexyl laurate · isopropyl myristate · octyl dodecyl neopentanoate · propylene glycol · magnesium stearate · magnesium sulfate · sodium chloride · dioctyl sodium sulfosuccinate · diazolidinyl urea · dichlorobenzyl alcohol · BHT · aluminum hydroxide · lauric acid · water
	PreSun 23 Westwood-Squibb Ph'cals	spray	23	octyl dimethyl ABA · octyl methoxycinnamate · benzophenone-3 · octyl salicylate	cyclomethicone · SD alcohol · C12-15 alcohol benzoate · PG dioctanoate · PVP/hexadecene copolymer
	PreSun 25 Moisturizing Westwood-Squibb Ph'cals	lotion	25	octyl methoxycinnamate · benzophenone-3 · octyl salicylate	dimethicone · diazolidinyl urea · carbomer 940 · triethanolamine · kathon CG · petrolatum · isopropyl myristate · PG dioctanoate · isodecyl neopentanoate · DEA-cetyl phosphate · PVP/eicosene copolymer · stearic acid · cetyl alcohol
FR	**PreSun 46 Moisturizing** Westwood-Squibb Ph'cals	lotion	46	octyl dimethyl ABA · benzophenone	carbomer 940 · cetyl alcohol · DEA-cetyl phosphate · diazolidinyl urea · dimethicone · isopropyl myristate · isodecyl neopentanoate · kathon CG · PG dioctanoate · PVP/eicosene copolymer · stearic acid · triethanolamine · water
PE	**PreSun for Kids** Westwood-Squibb Ph'cals	spray	23	octyl dimethyl ABA · octyl methoxycinnamate · benzophenone-3 · octyl salicylate	cyclomethicone · SD alcohol · C12-15 alcohol benzoate · PG dioctanoate · PVP/hexadecene copolymer
PE	**PreSun for Kids** Westwood-Squibb Ph'cals	lotion	29	octyl methoxycinnamate · octyl salicylate · benzophenone-3	carbomer 940 · cetyl alcohol · DEA-cetyl phosphate · diazolidinyl urea · dimethicone · isopropyl myristate · isodecyl neopentanoate · kathon CG · PG dioctanoate · PVP/eicosene copolymer · stearic acid · triethanolamine · water
**	**Reflect** Wisconsin Pharmacal	lotion	8 · 15 · 30	octyl methoxycinnamate · octyl salicylate	
**	**Reflect Sun Stick** Wisconsin Pharmacal	stick	22	padimate O · benzophenone-3	mineral oil · petrolatum · ozokerite · paraffin · carnauba · candelilla · beeswax
	RV Paque ICN Ph'cals	cream	24	octyl methoxycinnamate, 7% · zinc oxide, 20%	
	Shade Sunblock Schering-Plough Healthcare	stick	30 · 45	octyl methoxycinnamate · octyl salicylate · oxybenzone · homosalate (SPF 30) · octocrylene (SPF 45)	
	Shade Sunblock Oil-Free Schering-Plough Healthcare	gel	30	octyl methoxycinnamate · homosalate · oxybenzone	SD alcohol 40, 73%
	Shade UVAGuard Schering-Plough Healthcare	lotion	15	octyl methoxycinnamate, 7.5% · avobenzone, 3% · oxybenzone, 3%	
** PE	**Snoopy Sunblock** Minnetonka Brands	pump spray	30	padimate O · octyl salicylate · octyl methoxycinnamate · benzophenone-3	

See Chapter 30, "Sunscreen and Suntan Products," for more information about these products.

SUNSCREEN AND SUNTAN PRODUCTS - continued

Product Manufacturer/Supplier	Dosage Form	SPF Value	Sunscreen	Other Ingredients
** PE **Snoopy Sunblock** Minnetonka Brands	pump spray	15	padimate O · oxybenzone · octyl salicylate	
Softlips, Sparkle Mint Mentholatum	stick	7	padimate O, 3%	cetyl octanoate · dimethicone, 2% · fragrance · lanolin · menthol · ozokerite · petrolatum · squalane · vitamin E acetate
Softlips, UV Mentholatum	stick	17	octyl methoxycinnamate, 7.5% · padimate O, 7% · oxybenzone, 3%	butylated hydroxytoluene · dimethicone, 2% · lanolin · menthol · ozokerite · petrolatum · squalane · vitamin E acetate
** **Solar** Minnetonka Brands	pump spray	30	padimate O · octyl salicylate · octyl methoxycinnmate · benzophenone-3	
** **Solar** Minnetonka Brands	pump spray	15	padimate O · oxbenzone · octyl salicylate	
** **Solar** Minnetonka Brands	pump spray	8	padimate O · oxybenzone	
Solbar PF 30 Person & Covey	gel	30	octocrylene, 10% · octyl methoxycinnamate, 7.5% · oxybenzone, 6%	SD alcohol 40
Solbar PF 50 Person & Covey	cream	50	oxybenzone · octyl methoxycinnamate · octocrylene	
Stay Moist Moisturizing Lip Conditioner Stanback	stick	15	padimate O, 7% · oxybenzone, 3%	petrolatums · isopropyl myristate · aloe vera oil · wax · flavor
Stevens Sun Block Stevens Skin Softener	cream	15	octyl methoxycinnamate · benzophenone-3	deionized water · glyceryl stearate · PEG-100 stearate · C21-15 alkyl benzoate · glycerin · jojoba oil · apricot kernel oil · stearic acid · dimethyl stearamine · sweet almond oil · cetearyl octanoate · methyl gluceth-20 · castor oil · acrylates/octylacrylamide copolymer · squalene · dimethicone · panthenol · cetyl alcohol · cetyl palmitate · propylparaben · diazolidinyl urea · triethanolamine · methylparaben · butylparaben · fragrance · tocopherol · allantoin · tetrasodium EDTA · avocado oil · magnesium aluminum silicate · aloe vera gel
** **Sun Ban 30 Moisturizing Lip Conditioner** Stanback	stick	30	octocrylene, 10% · octyl methoxycinnamate, 7.5% · oxybenzone, 6%	
** **Sun Stuff** Wisconsin Pharmacal	stick	20	padimate O · benzophenone-3	mineral oil · petrolatum · ozokerite · paraffin · carnauba · candelilla · beeswax
** **Sun Stuff** Wisconsin Pharmacal	lotion	15	octyl methoxycinnamate · octyl salicylate	
** **Super Sunblock** ICN Ph'cals	cream	25	octyl methoxycinnamate, 7.5% · menthyl anthranilate, 5% · octyl salicylate, 5% · titanium dioxide, 3%	
FR PE **TI-Baby Natural Sunblock** Pedinol Pharmacal	lotion	16	titanium dioxide, 5%	

See Chapter 30, "Sunscreen and Suntan Products," for more information about these products.

SUNSCREEN AND SUNTAN PRODUCTS - continued

	Product Manufacturer/Supplier	Dosage Form	SPF Value	Sunscreen	Other Ingredients
**	**TI-Screen Cooling** Pedinol Pharmacal	spray	23	octyl methoxycinnamate, 7.5% · octocrylene, 4% · menthyl anthranilate, 3.5% · benzophenone-3, 3%	SD alcohol 40, 57% · C12-15 alkyl benzoate · water · cyclomethicone · acrylates/octylacrylamide copolymer · tocopheryl acetate · fragrance
FR	**TI-Screen Moisturizing** Pedinol Pharmacal	lotion	15	octyl methoxycinnamate, 7.5% · benzophenone-3, 5%	
FR	**TI-Screen Moisturizing** Pedinol Pharmacal	lotion	30	octyl methoxycinnamate, 7.5% · octocrylene, 7.5% · benzophenone-3, 6% · octyl salicylate, 5%	
FR	**TI-Screen Moisturizing Lip Protectant** Pedinol Pharmacal	stick	15	octyl methoxycinnamate, 7.5% · benzophenone-3	
FR	**TI-Screen Natural Sunblock** Pedinol Pharmacal	lotion	16	titanium dioxide, 5%	
FR	**TI-Screen Sports** Pedinol Pharmacal	gel	20	octyl methoxycinnamate, 7.5% · benzophenone-3, 6% · octyl salicylate, 5%	
**	**TI-Screen Sunless Tanning Creme** Pedinol Pharmacal	cream	17	octyl methoxycinnamate, 7.5% · benzophenone-3, 3%	water · mineral oil · dihydroxyacetone · cetearyl stearate · sorbitol · glycercyl stearate · PEG-100 stearate · glyceryl stearate · isopropyl myristate · propylene glycol · walnut extract · dimethicone · fragrance · tocopheryl acetate · phenethyl alcohol · methylparaben · citric acid · propylparaben
	Vaseline Lip Therapy Balm, Advanced or Cherry Chesebrough-Pond's	stick	8	octyl methoxycinnamate · oxybenzone	white petrolatum · paraffin · hydrogenated castor oil · triisostearin esters · dimethicone · borage seed oil · sunflower seed oil · nylon-12 · tocopheryl acetate · bisabolol · retinyl palmitate · panthenol · aloe extract · kukui nut oil · lecithin · stearic acid · soya sterol · carnauba · corn oil · zinc sulfate · saccharin sodium · flavor
	Vaseline Lip Therapy, Advanced or Cherry Chesebrough-Pond's	ointment	8	octyl methoxycinnamate · oxybenzone	white petrolatum · borage seed oil · sunflower seed oil · tocopheryl acetate · bisabolol · retinyl palmitate · panthenol · aloe extract · kukui nut oil · lecithin · stearic acid · soya sterol · corn oil · zinc sulfate · flavor
PE	**Water Babies UVA/UVB Sunblock** Schering-Plough Healthcare	lotion	30	octyl methoxycinnamate · octyl salicylate · homosalate	
PE	**Water Babies UVA/UVB Sunblock** Schering-Plough Healthcare	lotion	45	octyl methoxycinnamate · octyl salicylate · oxybenzone · octocrylene	
	Zilactin Lip Balm Zila Ph'cals	stick	24	octyl methoxycinnamate, 7% · homosalate, 4% · oxybenzone, 3%	dimethicone, 1.5% · menthol, 0.5%

See Chapter 30, "Sunscreen and Suntan Products," for more information about these products.

Burn and Sunburn Product Table

BURN AND SUNBURN PRODUCTS

	Product Manufacturer/Supplier	Dosage Form	Anesthetic	Antimicrobial	Other Ingredients
**	**A + D Ointment with Zinc Oxide** Schering-Plough Healthcare	ointment			dimethicone, 10% · zinc oxide, 1% · cod liver oil (contains vitamin A&D) · aloe extract · paraffin
	A + D Original Ointment Schering-Plough Healthcare	ointment			petrolatum 80.5% · lanolin 15.5% · cod liver oil (contains vitamins A&D) · paraffin
	ActiBath Soak Oatmeal Treatment Andrew Jergens	effervescent tablet			colloidal oatmeal, 20% · fumaric acid · sodium carbonate · lactose · sodium bicarbonate · PEG-150 · magnesium oxide · sucrose stearate
	Anti-Itch Blistex	lotion	pramoxine HCl, 1%	benzethonium chloride	dimethicone, 1% · glyceryl stearate · PEG-100 stearate · petrolatum · polysorbate 60 · polyquaternium-24 · water · sesame oil · stearic acid · stearyl alcohol
	Aveeno Bath Treatment Moisturizing Formula Rydelle Labs	powder			colloidal oatmeal, 43% · mineral oil
	Aveeno Bath Treatment Soothing Formula Rydelle Labs	powder			colloidal oatmeal, 100%
	Bactine First Aid Bayer Consumer	liquid · spray	lidocaine HCl, 2.5%	benzalkonium chloride, 0.13%	disodium edetate · fragrance · octoxynol 9 · propylene glycol · water
	Bicozene External Analgesic Creme Novartis Consumer	cream	benzocaine, 6%	resorcinol, 1.67%	stearic acid · glycerin · glyceryl monostearate · castor oil · triglycerol diisostearate · parachlorometaxylenol · sodium borate · ethanolamine stearates · polysorbate 80 · chlorothymol · fragrance · water
	Boil Ease Del Ph'cals	ointment	benzocaine, 5%		anhydrous lanolin · camphor · eucalyptus oil · ichthammol · juniper tar · menthol · paraffin · petrolatum · precipitated sulfur · rosin · sexadecyl alcohol · thymol · yellow wax · zinc oxide
	Burntame Otis Clapp & Son	spray	benzocaine, 20%	8-hydroxyquinoline	
	Butesin Picrate Abbott Labs	ointment	butamben picrate, 1%		anhydrous lanolin · ceresin wax · mineral oil · mixed triglycerides · methylparaben · propylparaben · potassium chloride · sodium borate · white wax
**	**CalaGel Medicated Anti-Itch** Tec Labs	gel		benzethonium chloride, 0.15%	diphenhydramine HCl, 1.8% · zinc acetate, 0.21% · purified water · polysorbate 20 · hydroxypropyl methylcellulose · disodium EDTA · fragrance
	Clomycin Lee Consumer	cream	lidocaine, 40mg/g	polymyxin B sulfate, 5000IU/g · bacitracin, 500IU/g · neomycin sulfate, 3.5mg/g	yellow petrolatum · anhydrous lanolin · mineral oil
	Delazinc Mericon	ointment			zinc oxide, 25% · mineral oil · white petrolatum · synaceti · beeswax · sodium borate · water

See Chapter 31, "Burn and Sunburn Products," for more information about these products.

BURN AND SUNBURN PRODUCTS - continued

Product Manufacturer/Supplier	Dosage Form	Anesthetic	Antimicrobial	Other Ingredients
Dermoplast Medtech	spray	benzocaine, 20%		menthol, 0.5% · acetylated lanolin alcohol · aloe vera gel · butane · cetyl acetate · hydrofluorocarbon · methylparaben · PEG-8 laurate · polysorbate 85
Dibucaine Multisource	ointment	dibucaine, 1%		
Family Medic Tender	liquid · pump spray · wipe	lidocaine HCl, 2.5%	benzalkonium chloride, 0.13%	aloe vera gel, 80% · fragrance, 0.05%
Family Medic Afterburn Tender	gel	lidocaine HCl, 0.5%		aloe vera gel, 80%
First Aid Cream § Johnson & Johnson Consumer	cream		cetylpyridinium chloride	water · cetyl alcohol · glyceryl stearate · isopropyl palmitate · stearyl alcohol · benzyl alcohol · synthetic beeswax · lapyrium chloride · hydroxypropyl methylcellulose · trisodium phosphate
Foille Medicated First Aid Blistex	aerosol	benzocaine, 5%	chloroxylenol, 0.6%	corn oil · fragrance · lecithin · water · benzyl alcohol
Foille Medicated First Aid Blistex	ointment	benzocaine, 5%	chloroxylenol, 0.1%	calcium disodium EDTA · corn oil · fragrance · mixed waxes · water · benzyl alcohol
Foille Plus Blistex	aerosol	benzocaine, 20%	benzethonium chloride, 0.15%	water-washable base
Foille Plus Medicated First Aid Blistex	cream	benzocaine, 5%	chloroxylenol, 0.4%	BHA · carbomer 934 · cetyl alcohol · fragrance · isopropyl myristate · isopropyl palmitate · isopropyl stearate · methylparaben · mineral oil · polysorbate 60 · propylparaben · water · stearic acid · sorbitan tristearate · triethanolamine
Gold Bond Medicated Anti-Itch Chattem	cream	lidocaine, 4%		menthol, 1% · cetearyl alcohol · DMDM hydantoin · eucalyptol · glyceryl stearate · methyl salicylate · methylparaben · petrolatum · propylene glycol · simethicone · sorbic acid · sorbitol · thymol · tocopherol · water · zinc oxide
Itch-X B. F. Ascher	gel · pump spray	benzyl alcohol, 10% · pramoxine HCl, 1%		aloe vera gel
Lagol Alvin Last	ointment	benzocaine, 5%		petrolatum · corn starch · allantoin
Lanacane Combe	aerosol spray	benzocaine, 20%	benzethonium chloride, 0.1%	ethanol, 36% · aloe extract · cyclomethicone · dipropylene glycol · fragrance · isobutane
Lanacane Creme Combe	cream	benzocaine, 6%	benzethonium chloride, 0.1%	aloe · chlorothymol · dioctyl sodium sulfosuccinate · ethoxydiglycol · fragrance · glycerin · glyceryl stearate SE · isopropyl alcohol · methylparaben · propylparaben · sodium borate · stearic acid · sulfated castor oil · triethanolamine - water · zinc oxide · pyrithione zinc

See Chapter 31, "Burn and Sunburn Products," for more information about these products.

BURN AND SUNBURN PRODUCTS - continued

	Product / Manufacturer/Supplier	Dosage Form	Anesthetic	Antimicrobial	Other Ingredients
**	**Lanacane Maximum Strength** / Combe	cream	benzocaine, 20%	benzethonium chloride, 0.2%	acetylated lanolin alcohol · aloe · cetyl acetate · cetyl alcohol · dimethicone · fragrance · glycerin · glyceryl stearate · isopropyl myristate · methylparaben · mineral oil · PEG-100 stearate · propylparaben · sorbitan stearate · stearamidopropyl PG-dimonium chloride phosphate · water · pyrithione zinc
	Medi-Quik First Aid / Mentholatum	aerosol spray	lidocaine, 2%	benzalkonium chloride, 0.13%	benzyl alcohol · BHA · isobutane · isopropyl palmitate · methyl gluceth-20 sesquistearate · methyl glucose sesquistearate · phosphoric acid · polyglyceryl-6 distearate · water
	Medicated First Aid Burn / Blistex	cream	benzocaine, 5%	chloroxylenol, 0.4%	BHA · carbomer 934 · cetyl alcohol · fragrance · isopropyl myristate · isopropyl palmitate · isopropyl stearate · methylparaben · mineral oil · polysorbate 60 · propylparaben · water · stearic acid · sorbitan tristearate · triethanolamine
**	**Palmer's Medicated Aloe Vera Formula** / E. T. Browne Drug	gel	lidocaine HCl, 0.5%		aloe vera gel · infusion of chamomile · butylene glycol · carbomer-940 · vitamin E · glycerin, 96% · DMDM hydantoin · benzophenone-4 · PPG-2-isodeceth-12 · disodium EDTA · triethanolamine · polysorbate-80 · fragrance · FD&C blue #1
**	**Palmer's Skin Success** / E. T. Browne Drug	ointment	benzocaine, 5%		petrolatum · microcrystalline wax · isopropyl alcohol · fragrance · D&C green#6 · D&C yellow#11
	Pramegel / GenDerm	gel	pramoxine HCl, 1% · benzyl alcohol		menthol, 0.5% · carbomer 940 · methyl gluceth-20 · SD alcohol 40 · sodium hydroxide · water
	Prax / Ferndale Labs	lotion	pramoxine HCl, 1%		hydrophilic base
	Solarcaine Aloe Extra Burn Relief / Schering-Plough Healthcare	cream	lidocaine, 0.5%		aloe extract
	Solarcaine Aloe Extra Burn Relief Gel or Mist / Schering-Plough Healthcare	gel · pump spray	lidocaine HCl, 0.5%		aloe vera gel · isopropyl alcohol, 0.05%
	Solarcaine Medicated First Aid / Schering-Plough Healthcare	aerosol spray	benzocaine, 20%		SD alcohol, 35% · triclosan, 0.13% · propellants
	Tronothane Hydrochloride / Abbott Labs	cream	pramoxine HCl, 1%		cetyl alcohol · glycerin sodium · lauryl sulfate · methylparaben · propylparaben · cetyl esters wax
	Unguentine / Mentholatum	ointment		phenol, 1%	eucalyptus oil · oleostearine · petrolatum · thyme oil · zinc oxide
	Unguentine Plus / Mentholatum	cream	lidocaine HCl, 2%	phenol, 0.5%	fragrance · glyceryl stearate · isoceteth-20 · isopropyl palmitate · methylparaben · mineral oil · poloxamer 407 · propylparaben · quaternium-15 · sorbitan stearate · tetrasodium EDTA · water

See Chapter 31, "Burn and Sunburn Products," for more information about these products.

BURN AND SUNBURN PRODUCTS - continued

Product Manufacturer/Supplier	Dosage Form	Anesthetic	Antimicrobial	Other Ingredients
Vaseline Medicated Anti-Bacterial Petroleum Jelly Chesebrough-Pond's	ointment		chloroxylenol, 0.53% · phenol	petrolatum, 98.3% · lanolin · beta carotene

** New listing

§ Manufacturer/supplier did not confirm information for this edition. Product listing is reprinted from the '96-97 edition.

See Chapter 31, "Burn and Sunburn Products," for more information about these products.

Poison Ivy, Oak, and Sumac
Product Table

POISON IVY, OAK, AND SUMAC PRODUCTS

Product Manufacturer/Supplier	Dosage Form	Hydro- cortisone	Antipruritic/ Anesthetic	Antihistamine	Astringent	Other Ingredients
ActiBath Soak Oatmeal Treatment Andrew Jergens	effervescent tablet		colloidal oatmeal, 20%			fumaric acid · sodium carbonate · lactose · sodium bicarbonate · PEG-150 · magnesium oxide · sucrose stearate
Anti-Itch Blistex	lotion		pramoxine HCl, 1%			dimethicone, 1% · benzethonium chloride · glyceryl stearate · PEG-100 stearate · petrolatum · polysorbate 60 · polyquaternium-24 · water · sesame oil · stearic acid · stearyl alcohol
Aveeno Anti-Itch Rydelle Labs	cream · lotion		pramoxine HCl, 1% · camphor, 0.3% · oatmeal flour		calamine, 3%	glycerin · distearyldimonium chloride · petrolatum · isopropyl palmitate · 1-hexadecanol · dimethicone · sodium chloride
Aveeno Bath Treatment Moisturizing Formula Rydelle Labs	powder		colloidal oatmeal, 43%			mineral oil
Aveeno Bath Treatment Soothing Formula Rydelle Labs	powder		colloidal oatmeal, 100%			
Aveeno Moisturizing Rydelle Labs	cream · lotion		colloidal oatmeal, 1% · benzyl alcohol			glycerin · distearyldimonium chloride · petrolatum · isopropyl palmitate · dimethicone · sodium chloride · cetyl alcohol
Bactine Hydrocortisone 1% Bayer Consumer	cream	1%			aluminum sulfate · cetearyl alcohol	beeswax · calcium acetate · dextrin · glycerin · hydrocortisone alcohol · light mineral oil · methylparaben · water · sodium lauryl sulfate · white petrolatum
Benadryl Itch Relief Extra Strength Warner-Lambert Consumer	stick			diphenhydramine HCl, 2%	alcohol, 73.5% · zinc acetate, 0.1%	glycerin · povidone · tromethamine · purified water
PE **Benadryl Itch Stopping Children's Formula** Warner-Lambert Consumer	gel		camphor	diphenhydramine HCl, 1%	zinc acetate, 1% · SD alcohol 38B	citric acid · diazolidinyl urea · glycerin · hydroxypropyl methylcellulose · methylparaben · propylene glycol · propylparaben · sodium citrate · purified water

See Chapter 32, "Poison Ivy, Oak, and Sumac Products," for more information about these products.

POISON IVY, OAK, AND SUMAC PRODUCTS - continued

Product Manufacturer/Supplier	Dosage Form	Hydro- cortisone	Antipruritic/ Anesthetic	Antihistamine	Astringent	Other Ingredients
Benadryl Itch Stopping Extra Strength Warner-Lambert Consumer	cream			diphenhydramine HCl, 2%	zinc acetate, 0.1% · cetyl alcohol	diazolidinyl urea · methylparaben · polyethylene glycol monostearate 1000 · propylene glycol · propylparaben · purified water
Benadryl Itch Stopping Extra Strength Warner-Lambert Consumer	spray			diphenhydramine HCl, 2%	alcohol, 73.5% · zinc acetate, 0.1%	glycerin · povidone · tromethamine · purified water
Benadryl Itch Stopping Extra Strength Warner-Lambert Consumer	gel		camphor	diphenhydramine HCl, 2%	zinc acetate, 1% · SD alcohol 38B	citric acid · diazolidinyl urea · glycerin · hydroxypropyl methylcellulose · methylparaben · propylene glycol · propylparaben · sodium citrate · purified water
Benadryl Itch Stopping Original Strength Warner-Lambert Consumer	cream			diphenhydramine HCl, 1%	zinc acetate, 0.1% · cetyl alcohol	diazolidinyl urea · methylparaben · polyethylene glycol monostearate 1000 · propylene glycol · propylparaben · purified water
Benadryl Itch Stopping Regular Strength Warner-Lambert Consumer	spray			diphenhydramine HCl, 1%	alcohol, 73.6% · zinc acetate, 0.1%	glycerin · povidone · tromethamine · purified water
Bluboro Allergan	powder				aluminum sulfate, 53.9%	calcium acetate, 43% · boric acid · FD&C blue#1
Blue Star Quaker House Products	ointment		camphor			salicylic acid · benzoic acid · methyl salicylate · lanolin oil · petrolatum
Buro-Sol Antiseptic Doak Dermatologics	powder				aluminum acetate, 0.23%	sodium diacetate, 48.8% · benzethonium chloride, 4.4%
Caladryl Warner-Lambert Consumer	lotion		pramoxine HCl, 1%		calamine, 8% · SD alcohol 38B	propylene glycol · polysorbate 80 · xanthan gum · hydroxypropyl methylcellulose · fragrance · diazolidinyl urea · methylparaben · propylparaben · camphor · water

See Chapter 32, "Poison Ivy, Oak, and Sumac Products," for more information about these products.

POISON IVY, OAK, AND SUMAC PRODUCTS - continued

Product Manufacturer/Supplier	Dosage Form	Hydro-cortisone	Antipruritic/ Anesthetic	Antihistamine	Astringent	Other Ingredients
Caladryl Warner-Lambert Consumer	cream		pramoxine HCl, 1%		calamine, 8% · cetyl alcohol	propylene glycol · polysorbate 60 · sorbitan stearate · soya sterol · cyclomethicone · fragrance · diazolidinyl urea · methylparaben · camphor · propylparaben · purified water
Caladryl Clear Warner-Lambert Consumer	lotion		pramoxine HCl, 1%		zinc acetate, 0.1% · SD alcohol 38B	camphor · polysorbate 40 · glycerin · fragrance · sodium citrate · citric acid · diazolidinyl urea · hydroxypropyl methylcellulose · methylparaben · propylene glycol · propylparaben · purified water
** **CalaGel Medicated Anti-Itch** Tec Labs	gel			diphenhydramine HCl, 1.8%	zinc acetate, 0.21%	benzethonium chloride, 0.15% · purified water · polysorbate 20 · hydroxypropyl methylcellulose · disodium EDTA · fragrance
CaldeCORT Novartis Consumer	cream	1%				cetostearyl alcohol · sodium lauryl sulfate · white petrolatum · propylene glycol · purified water
Care-Creme Antimicrobial Cream Care-Tech Labs	cream				cetyl alcohol	chloroxylenol 0.8% · cod liver oil · lanolin oil · lanolin alcohol · propylene glycol · vitamins A, D3, and E
Cortaid FastStick Pharmacia & Upjohn	stick	1%			alcohol, 55%	butylated hydroxytoluene · methylparaben · purified water
Cortaid Maximum Strength Pharmacia & Upjohn	spray	1%			alcohol, 55%	glycerin · methylparaben · water
Cortaid Maximum Strength Pharmacia & Upjohn	cream	1%				glycerin · methylparaben · water · aloe · ceteareth-20 · cetyl palmitate · isopropyl myristate · isopropyl pentanoate · cetyl alcohol
Cortaid Sensitive Skin Formula Pharmacia & Upjohn	ointment	0.5%				aloe · butylparaben · cholesterol · methylparaben · mineral oil · white petrolatum · microcrystalline wax

See Chapter 32, "Poison Ivy, Oak, and Sumac Products," for more information about these products.

POISON IVY, OAK, AND SUMAC PRODUCTS - continued

	Product Manufacturer/Supplier	Dosage Form	Hydro- cortisone	Antipruritic/ Anesthetic	Antihistamine	Astringent	Other Ingredients
	Cortaid Sensitive Skin Formula Pharmacia & Upjohn	cream	0.5%				aloe · butylparaben · cetyl palmitate · glyceryl stearate · methylparaben · polyethylene glycol · stearamidoethyl diethylamine · water
**	**CortiCool Anti-Itch** Tec Labs	gel	1%				
	Cortizone-10 Pfizer Consumer	ointment	1%				white petrolatum
	Cortizone-10 Pfizer Consumer	cream	1%			aluminum sulfate	calcium acetate · glycerin · light mineral oil · methylparaben · propylparaben · potato dextrin · sodium lauryl sulfate · water · white petrolatum · white wax · aloe · cetyl alcohol
	Cortizone-5 Pfizer Consumer	ointment	0.5%				white petrolatum · aloe
	Cortizone-5 Pfizer Consumer	cream	0.5%			aluminum sulfate	glycerin · mineral oil · white petrolatum · propylparaben · methylparaben · calcium acetate · potato dextrin · sodium lauryl sulfate · water · white wax · aloe · cetyl alcohol
PE	**Cortizone-5 for Kids** Pfizer Consumer	cream	0.5%			aluminum sulfate	aloe vera gel · calcium acetate · cetearyl alcohol · glycerin · light mineral oil · methylparaben · potato dextrin · propylparaben · sodium C12-15 alcohols sulfate · sodium lauryl sulfate · water · white petrolatum
**	**Delacort** Mericon	lotion	1%				stearic acid · propylene glycol · lanolin alcohol · mineral oil · isopropyl myristate · cetyl alcohol · monoglyceride · diglyceride · polysorbate 80 · sobitan monoleate · scent · purified water · methylparaben · propylparaben
	Dermapax Recsei Labs	spray		benzyl alcohol, 1%	diphenhydramine HCl, 0.5%	isopropyl alcohol, 35%	chlorobutanol, 1%
	Dermarest Del Ph'cals	gel			diphenhydramine HCl, 2%		

See Chapter 32, "Poison Ivy, Oak, and Sumac Products," for more information about these products.

POISON IVY, OAK, AND SUMAC PRODUCTS - continued

Product Manufacturer/Supplier	Dosage Form	Hydro-cortisone	Antipruritic/ Anesthetic	Antihistamine	Astringent	Other Ingredients
Dermarest DriCort Del Ph'cals	cream	1%				
Dermarest Plus Del Ph'cals	gel		menthol, 1%	diphenhydramine HCl, 2%		
Dermatox Reese Chemical	lotion		pramoxine HCl, 1%		zinc acetate, 0.1%	
DermiCort Republic Drug	cream	1%				greaseless base
Dermoplast Medtech	spray		benzocaine, 20% · menthol, 0.5%		alcohol	acetylated lanolin · aloe vera gel · butane · cetyl acetate · hydrofluorocarbon · methylparaben · PEG-8 laurate · polysorbate 85
Di-Delamine Del Ph'cals	gel · spray		menthol, 0.1%	diphenhydramine HCl, 1% · tripelennamine HCl, 0.5%		benzalkonium chloride, 0.12%
Dickinson's Witch Hazel Formula Hampton Essex	liquid				witch hazel distillate · witch hazel extract · alcohol, 14%	water
Domeboro Bayer Consumer	powder				aluminum sulfate, 1191mg	calcium acetate, 938mg · dextrin
FoilleCort Blistex	cream	0.5%				BHA · carbomer 934 · fragrance · isopropyl palmitate · isopropyl myristate · isopropyl stearate · methylparaben · mineral oil · polysorbate 60 · propylparaben · purified water · stearic acid · sorbitan tristearate · triethanolamine · cetyl alcohol
Gold Bond Medicated Anti-Itch Chattem	cream		lidocaine, 4% · menthol, 1%	methyl salicylate	cetearyl alcohol · zinc oxide	DMDM hydantoin · eucalyptol · glyceryl stearate · methylparaben · petrolatum · propylene glycol · simethicone · sorbic acid · sorbitol · thymol · tocopherol · water
Gold Bond Medicated, Extra Strength Chattem	powder		menthol, 0.8%		zinc oxide, 5%	eucalyptol · methyl salicylate · salicylic acid · talc · thymol · zinc stearate
Gold Bond Medicated, Regular Strength Chattem	powder		menthol, 0.15%		zinc oxide, 1%	eucalyptol · methyl salicylate · salicylic acid · talc · thymol · zinc stearate

** *(Dermatox)*

See Chapter 32, "Poison Ivy, Oak, and Sumac Products," for more information about these products.

POISON IVY, OAK, AND SUMAC PRODUCTS - continued

Product Manufacturer/Supplier	Dosage Form	Hydro-cortisone	Antipruritic/ Anesthetic	Antihistamine	Astringent	Other Ingredients
HC-DermaPax Recsei Labs	spray	0.5%	benzyl alcohol, 1%	diphenhydramine HCl, 0.5%		isopropanol, 35%
Hydrosal Hydrosal	ointment			diphenhydramine HCl, 1%	zinc oxide	aloe · D&C red#33 · lanolin · mineral oil · petrolatum · water · sorbitan sesquioleate · ceresin wax
Itch-X B. F. Ascher	gel · pump spray		benzyl alcohol, 10% · pramoxine HCl, 1%			aloe vera gel
Ivarest 8-Hour Medicated Blistex	cream			diphenhydramine HCl, 2%	calamine, 14%	fragrance · hydroxyethylcellulose · lanolin oil · petrolatum · polysorbate 60 · propylene glycol · purified water · sorbitan stearate
Ivy Dry Chilton Labs	cream		benzyl alcohol, 10mg/g	camphor, 6mg/g · menthol, 4mg/g	zinc acetate, 20mg/g	
Ivy Dry Chilton Labs	liquid				isopropyl alcohol, 12.5% · zinc acetate, 20mg/ml	glycerin · acetic acid · methlparaben · propylparaben
Ivy Super Dry Chilton Labs	liquid		benzyl alcohol, 0.1mg/g	camphor, 4mg/g · menthol, 2mg/g	isopropyl alcohol, 35% · zinc acetate, 20mg/ml	methylparaben, 0.01mg/ml · propylparaben, 0.1mg/ml · acetic acid
** **IvyBlock** EnviroDerm Ph'cals	lotion		benzyl alcohol		SDA alcohol 40, 25%	bentoquatum (quaternium-18 bentonite), 5% · diisopropyl adipate · bentonite · methylparaben · purified water
Kericort 10 Maximum Strength Bristol-Myers Products	cream	1%			stearyl alcohol · cetyl alcohol	citric acid · glyceryl stearate · isopropyl myristate · methylparaben · polyoxyl 40 stearate · polysorbate 60 · propylene glycol · propylparaben · sodium citrate · sorbic acid · sorbitan monostearate · water · white wax
Lanacane Combe	aerosol spray		benzocaine, 20%			ethanol, 36% · benzethonium chloride, 0.1% · aloe extract · cyclomethicone · dipropylene glycol · fragrance · isobutane

POISON IVY, OAK, AND SUMAC PRODUCTS - continued

Product Manufacturer/Supplier	Dosage Form	Hydro- cortisone	Antipruritic/ Anesthetic	Antihistamine	Astringent	Other Ingredients
Lanacane Creme Combe	cream		benzocaine, 6%		zinc oxide · isopropyl alcohol	benzethonium chloride, 0.1% · aloe · chlorothymol · dioctyl sodium sulfosuccinate · ethoxydiglycol · fragrance · glycerin · glyceryl stearate SE · methylparaben · propylparaben · sodium borate · stearic acid · sulfated castor oil · triethanolamine - water · pyrithione zinc
** **Lanacane Maximum Strength** Combe	cream		benzocaine, 20%		cetyl alcohol	benzethonium chloride, 0.2% · acetylated lanolin alcohol · aloe · cetyl acetate · dimethicone · fragrance · glycerin · glyceryl stearate · isopropyl myristate · methylparaben · mineral oil · PEG-100 stearate · propylparaben · sorbitan stearate · stearamidopropyl PG-dimonium chloride phosphate · water · pyrithione zinc
Lanacort 10 Combe	cream · ointment	1%				
Lanacort 5 Combe	cream	0.5%				aloe · methylparaben · propylparaben
Lanacort 5 Combe	ointment	0.5%				lanolin alcohols · aloe · petrolatum
Nutra Soothe Oatmeal Bath Brimms Labs	powder		colloidal oatmeal, 100%			
Ostiderm Pedinol Pharmacal	paste		phenol · camphor		aluminum sulfate · zinc oxide	water · glycerin · sorbitol · magnesium carbonate · bentonite 670 · cabosil · acetic acid · kelcoloid HVF · Tween 20 · calcium carbonate · fragrance · Thomasett Nu color blend
Ostiderm Roll-on Pedinol Pharmacal	lotion		phenol · camphor		SD alcohol 40 · aluminum chlorohydrate · aluminum sulfate	water · glycerin · sorbitol · propylene glycol · calcium carbonate · bentonite · hydroxypropyl cellulose · polysorbate 20 · fragrance · EDTA · diazolidinyl urea · sodium benzoate · potassium sorbate

See Chapter 32, "Poison Ivy, Oak, and Sumac Products," for more information about these products.

POISON IVY, OAK, AND SUMAC PRODUCTS - continued

Product Manufacturer/Supplier	Dosage Form	Hydro-cortisone	Antipruritic/ Anesthetic	Antihistamine	Astringent	Other Ingredients
** **Palmer's Medicated Aloe Vera Formula** E. T. Browne Drug	gel		lidocaine HCl, 0.5%			aloe vera gel · infusion of chamomile · butylene glycol · carbomer 940 · vitamin E · glycerin, 96% · DMDM hydantoin · benzophenone-4 · PPG-2-isodeceth-12 · disodium EDTA · triethanolamine · polysorbate 80 · fragrance · FD&C blue#1
** **Palmer's Skin Success** E. T. Browne Drug	ointment		benzocaine, 5%		isopropyl alcohol	petrolatum · microcrystalline wax · fragrance · D&C green#6 · D&C yellow#11
Pedi-Boro Soak Paks Pedinol Pharmacal	powder				aluminum sulfate	calcium acetate
Pramegel GenDerm	gel		pramoxine HCl, 1% · menthol, 0.5% · benzyl alcohol		SD alcohol 40	carbomer 940 · methyl gluceth-20 · sodium hydroxide · water
Preparation H Hydrocortisone 1% Anti-Itch Whitehall-Robins Healthcare	cream	1%				citric acid · disodium EDTA · glycerin · lanolin · methylparaben · white petrolatum · propylparaben · cetyl alcohol · stearyl alcohol · sodium benzoate · sodium lauryl sulfate · water · tegacid special · Arlacel 186 · medical antifoam emulsion · carboxymethylcellulose sodium · rhodigel · Tenox-2
Procort Lee Consumer	cream	1%				glycerin · glyceryl stearate · mineral oil · methylparaben · polysorbate 60 · propylparaben · sorbitan stearate · purified water · aloe vera gel
Resinol Medicated Mentholatum	ointment		resorcinol, 2%		zinc oxide, 12% · calamine, 6%	lanolin · petrolatum · starch
Rhuli Rydelle Labs	spray		benzocaine, 5% · camphor, 0.7% · benzyl alcohol		alcohol, 70% · calamine, 13.8%	hydrated silica · isobutane · isopropyl · sorbitan trioleate · oleyl alcohol
Rhuli Rydelle Labs	gel		benzyl alcohol, 2% · menthol, 0.3% · camphor, 0.3%		SD alcohol 23A, 31%	propylene glycol · carbomer 940 · triethanolamine · benzophenone-4 · EDTA
Sarna Stiefel Labs	lotion		camphor, 0.5% · menthol, 0.5%			

See Chapter 32, "Poison Ivy, Oak, and Sumac Products," for more information about these products.

POISON IVY, OAK, AND SUMAC PRODUCTS - continued

	Product Manufacturer/Supplier	Dosage Form	Hydro- cortisone	Antipruritic/ Anesthetic	Antihistamine	Astringent	Other Ingredients
**	**Sarnol-HC** Stiefel Labs	lotion	1%				
	Tronothane Hydrochloride Abbott Labs	cream		pramoxine HCl, 1%			glycerin · sodium lauryl sulfate · methylparaben · propylparaben · cetyl esters wax · cetyl alcohol
	Witch Hazel T. N. Dickinson					distilled witch hazel extract, 86% · alcohol, 14%	

** New listing

See Chapter 32, "Poison Ivy, Oak, and Sumac Products," for more information about these products.

Insect Sting and Bite Product Tables

PEDICULICIDE PRODUCTS

Product Manufacturer/Supplier	Dosage Form	Active Ingredients	Other Ingredients
A-200 Lice Killing Hogil Ph'cal	shampoo	piperonyl butoxide, 4% · pyrethrum extract, 0.33%	benzyl alcohol · C13-C14 isoparaffin · isopropyl alcohol · fragrance · octylphenoxypolyethoxyenthanol · water · packaged with patented nit comb
A-200 Lice Killing Hogil Ph'cal	gel	piperonyl butoxide, 4% · pyrethrum extract, 0.33%	
A-200 Lice Treatment Kit Hogil Ph'cal	shampoo · aerosol spray	piperonyl butoxide, 4% (shampoo) · pyrethrum extract, 0.33% (shampoo) · permethrin, 0.5% (spray)	packaged with patented nit comb
End-Lice Thompson Medical	liquid	piperonyl butoxide, 4% · pyrethrins, 0.33%	benzyl alcohol · C13-C14 isoparaffin · polyoxyethylene (1,1,3,3,-tetramethylbutylphenyl ether) · water
InnoGel Plus Hogil Ph'cal	gel	piperonyl butoxide, 4% · pyrethrum extract, 0.33%	carbomer 934 · D&C red#33 · FD&C blue#1 · water · benzyl alcohol · C13-C14 isoparaffin · isopropyl alcohol
Licetrol Republic Drug	shampoo	piperonyl butoxide technical, 4% · pyrethrum extract, 0.33%	inert, 95.67%
Licetrol 600 Republic Drug	liquid	piperonyl butoxide, 3% · pyrethrins, 0.3%	
Licide Reese Chemical	shampoo	piperonyl butoxide, 4% · pyrethrins, 0.33%	
Licide Reese Chemical	spray	piperonyl butoxide, 1% · pyrethrins, 0.2%	
Licide Blue Reese Chemical	gel	pyrethrins, 0.2%	
Nix Warner-Lambert Consumer	cream rinse	permethrin, 1%	isopropyl alcohol, 20% · balsam canada · cetyl alcohol · citric acid · FD&C yellow#6 · fragrance · hydrolyzed animal protein · hydroxyethylcellulose · polyoxyethylene 10 cetyl ether · propylene glycol · stearalkonium chloride · methylparaben · propylparaben · packaged with nit comb
Pronto Lice Killing Del Ph'cals	shampoo	piperonyl butoxide, 4% · pyrethrins, 0.33%	
Pronto Lice Killing Del Ph'cals	aerosol spray	pyrethrins, 0.4%	inert, 99.6%
R&C Shampoo/Conditioner Block Drug	shampoo	piperonyl butoxide, 3% · pyrethrins, 0.33%	C-13-14 isoparaffin · fragrance · isocetyl alcohol · isopropyl alcohol · lauramine oxide · laureth-4 · laureth-23 · petroleum distillate · polyquaternium · TEA-lauryl sulfate · water
R&C Spray Block Drug	spray	sumithrin, 0.4%	inert, 99.6%
RID Lice Elimination Kit Pfizer Consumer	aerosol spray · shampoo	permethrin, 0.5% (spray) · piperonyl butoxide, 4% · pyrethrum, 0.33% (shampoo)	spray: inert, 99.5% · shampoo: C13-C14 isoparaffin · fragrance · isopropyl alcohol · PEG-25 hydrogenated castor oil · water · xanthan gum
RID Lice Killing Pfizer Consumer	shampoo	piperonyl butoxide, 4% · pyrethrum, 0.33%	C13-C14 isoparaffin · fragrance · isopropyl alcohol · PEG-25 hydrogenated castor oil · water · xanthan gum

See Chapter 33, "Insect Sting and Bite Products," for more information about these products.

Product Manufacturer/Supplier	Dosage Form	Active Ingredients	Other Ingredients
Tegrin-LT Lice Treatment Block Drug	shampoo · conditioner	piperonyl butoxide, 3% · pyrethrum extract, 0.33%	inert, 96.67% · C-13-14 isoparaffin · fragrance · isocetyl alcohol · isopropyl alcohol · lauramine oxide · laureth-4 · laureth-23 · petroleum distillate · polyquaternium-11 · TEA-lauryl sulfate · water · packaged with nit comb

See Chapter 33, "Insect Sting and Bite Products," for more information about these products.

INSECT STING AND BITE PRODUCTS

Product [a] Manufacturer/Supplier	Dosage Form	Antipruritic/Anesthet- ic/Counterirritant	Hydrocortisone	Other Ingredients
ActiBath Soak Oatmeal Treatment Andrew Jergens	effervescent tablet	colloidal oatmeal, 20%		fumaric acid · sodium carbonate · lactose · sodium bicarbonate · PEG-150 · magnesium oxide · sucrose stearate
After-Bite Tender	liquid · wipe	ammonia, 3.6%		
Anti-Itch Blistex	lotion	pramoxine HCl, 1%		dimethicone, 1% · glyceryl stearate · PEG-100 stearate · petrolatum · polysorbate 60 · polyquaternium-24 · water · sesame oil · stearic acid · stearyl alcohol · benzethonium chloride
Aveeno Anti-Itch Rydelle Labs	cream · lotion	pramoxine HCl, 1% · camphor, 0.3% · oatmeal flour		calamine, 3% · glycerin · distearyldimonium chloride · petrolatum · isopropyl palmitate · 1-hexadecanol · dimethicone · sodium chloride
Bactine Antiseptic/Anesthetic First Aid Bayer Consumer	spray	lidocaine HCl, 2.5%		benzalkonium chloride, 0.13% · disodium edetate · fragrance · octoxynol 9 · propylene glycol · water
Bactine Hydrocortisone 1% Bayer Consumer	cream		1%	aluminum sulfate · beeswax · calcium acetate · cetearyl alcohol · dextrin · glycerin · hydrocortisone alcohol · light mineral oil · methylparaben · water · sodium lauryl sulfate · white petrolatum
Bicozene External Analgesic Creme Novartis Consumer	cream	benzocaine, 6% · resorcinol, 1.67%		stearic acid · glycerin · glyceryl monostearate · castor oil · triglycerol diisostearate · parachlorometaxylenol · sodium borate · ethanolamine stearates · polysorbate 80 · chlorothymol · fragrance · water
Bluboro Allergan	powder			aluminum sulfate, 53.9% · calcium acetate, 43% · boric acid · FD&C blue#1
Blue Star Quaker House Products	ointment	camphor		salicylic acid · benzoic acid · methyl salicylate · lanolin oil · petrolatum
Buro-Sol Antiseptic Doak Dermatologics	powder	aluminum acetate, 46.8%		sodium diacetate, 0.23% · benzethonium chloride, 4.4%
Caladryl [b] Warner-Lambert Consumer	cream	pramoxine HCl, 1%		calamine, 8% · cetyl alcohol · propylene glycol · polysorbate 60 · sorbitan stearate · soya sterol · cyclomethicone · diazolidinyl urea · methylparaben · fragrance · camphor
Caladryl [b] Warner-Lambert Consumer	lotion	pramoxine HCl, 1%		calamine, 8% · propylene glycol · polysorbate 80 · SD alcohol 38B · xanthan gum · hydroxypropyl methylcellulose · fragrance · diazolidinyl urea · methylparaben · propylparaben · camphor
Caladryl Clear [b] Warner-Lambert Consumer	lotion	pramoxine HCl, 1%		SD alcohol 38B, 2.5% · zinc acetate, 0.1% · camphor · polysorbate 40 · glycerin · fragrance · sodium citrate · citric acid · diazolidinyl urea · hydroxypropyl methylcellulose · methylparaben · propylene glycol · propylparaben · purified water

See Chapter 33, "Insect Sting and Bite Products," for more information about these products.

INSECT STING AND BITE PRODUCTS - continued

	Product [a] Manufacturer/Supplier	Dosage Form	Antipruritic/Anesthet- ic/Counterirritant	Hydrocortisone	Other Ingredients
**	CalaGel Medicated Anti-Itch Tec Labs	gel	diphenhydramine HCl, 1.8%		zinc acetate, 0.21% · benzethonium chloride, 0.15% · purified water · polysorbate 20 · hydroxypropyl methylcellulose · disodium EDTA · fragrance
	Chigger-Tox Scherer Labs	liquid	benzocaine, 2.1%		isopropyl alcohol · benzyl benzoate · soft soap
	Chiggerex Scherer Labs	ointment	benzocaine, 2%		pegosperse 100 · camphor · olive oil · menthol · peppermint oil · methylparaben · clove oil · aloe vera
	Cortaid FastStick Pharmacia & Upjohn	stick		1%	alcohol, 55% · butylated hydroxytoluene · glycerin · methylparaben · purified water
	Cortaid Maximum Strength Pharmacia & Upjohn	cream		1%	cetyl alcohol · glycerin · methylparaben · purified water · aloe · ceteareth-20 · cetyl palmitate · isopropyl myristate · isopropyl pentanoate
	Cortaid Maximum Strength Pharmacia & Upjohn	spray		1%	alcohol, 55% · glycerin · methylparaben · water
	Cortaid Maximum Strength Pharmacia & Upjohn	ointment		1% (as acetate)	butylparaben · cholesterol · methylparaben · microcrystalline wax · mineral oil · white petrolatum
	Cortaid Sensitive Skin Formula Pharmacia & Upjohn	ointment		0.5% (as acetate)	aloe · butylparaben · cholesterol · methylparaben · mineral oil · white petrolatum · microcrystalline wax
	Cortaid Sensitive Skin Formula Pharmacia & Upjohn	cream		0.5% (as acetate)	aloe · butylparaben · cetyl palmitate · glyceryl stearate · methylparaben · polyethylene glycol · stearamidoethyl diethylamine · water
**	CortiCool Anti-Itch Tec Labs	gel		1%	
	Dermarest Del Ph'cals	gel	diphenhydramine HCl, 2%		
	Dermarest DriCort Del Ph'cals	cream		1%	
	Dermarest Plus Del Ph'cals	gel	diphenhydramine HCl, 2% · menthol, 1%		
	Dermoplast Medtech	spray	benzocaine, 20% · menthol, 0.5%		acetylated lanolin alcohol · aloe vera gel · butane · cetyl acetate · hydrofluorocarbon · methylparaben · PEG-8 laurate · polysorbate 85
	Di-Delamine Double Antihistamine Del Ph'cals	gel · spray	diphenhydramine HCl, 1% · menthol, 0.1%		tripelennamine HCl, 0.5% · benzalkonium chloride, 0.12%
	Domeboro Bayer Consumer	powder	aluminum sulfate, 1191mg		calcium acetate, 938mg · dextrin

See Chapter 33, "Insect Sting and Bite Products," for more information about these products.

INSECT STING AND BITE PRODUCTS - continued

Product [a] Manufacturer/Supplier	Dosage Form	Antipruritic/Anesthetic/Counterirritant	Hydrocortisone	Other Ingredients
Gold Bond Medicated Anti-Itch Chattem	cream	lidocaine · menthol		cetearyl alcohol · DMDM hydantoin · eucalyptol · glyceryl stearate · methyl salicylate · methylparaben · petrolatum · propylene glycol · simethicone · sorbic acid · sorbitol · thymol · tocopherol · water · zinc oxide
Gold Bond Medicated, Extra Strength Chattem	powder	menthol, 0.8%		zinc oxide, 5% · eucalyptol · methyl salicylate · salicylic acid · talc · thymol · zinc stearate
Gold Bond Medicated, Regular Strength Chattem	powder	menthol, 0.15%		zinc oxide, 1% · eucalyptol · methyl salicylate · salicylic acid · talc · thymol · zinc stearate
HC-DermaPax Recsei Labs	spray	benzyl alcohol, 1% · diphenhydramine HCl, 0.5%	0.5%	isopropanol, 35%
Itch-X B. F. Ascher	gel · pump spray	benzyl alcohol, 10% · pramoxine HCl, 1%		aloe vera gel
Kericort 10 Maximum Strength Bristol-Myers Products	cream		1%	citric acid · glyceryl stearate · isopropyl myristate · methylparaben · polyoxyl 40 stearate · polysorbate 60 · propylene glycol · propylparaben · sodium citrate · sorbic acid · sorbitan monostearate · water · white wax
Lanacane Combe	aerosol spray	benzocaine, 20%		ethanol, 36% · benzethonium chloride, 0.17% · aloe extract · cyclomethicone · dipropylene glycol · fragrance · isobutane
Lanacane Creme Combe	cream	benzocaine, 6%		benzethonium chloride, 0.1% · aloe · chlorothymol · dioctyl sodium sulfosuccinate · ethoxydiglycol · fragrance · glycerin · glyceryl stearate SE · isopropyl alcohol · methylparaben · propylparaben · sodium borate · stearic acid · sulfated castor oil · triethanolamine - water · zinc oxide · pyrithione zinc
** **Lanacane Maximum Strength** Combe	cream	benzocaine, 20%		benzethonium chloride, 0.2% · acetylated lanolin alcohol · aloe · cetyl acetate · cetyl alcohol · dimethicone · fragrance · glycerin · glyceryl stearate · isopropyl myristate · methylparaben · mineral oil · PEG-100 stearate · propylparaben · sorbitan stearate · stearamidopropyl PG-dimonium chloride phosphate · water · pyrithione zinc
Lanacort 10 Combe	cream · ointment		1%	
Nupercainal Novartis Consumer	ointment	dibucaine, 1%		acetone sodium bisulfite · lanolin · light mineral oil · white petrolatum · purified water
** **Palmer's Skin Success** E. T. Browne Drug	ointment	benzocaine, 5%		petrolatum · microcrystalline wax · isopropyl alcohol · fragrance · D&C green#6 · D&C yellow#11
Pedi-Boro Soak Paks Pedinol Pharmacal	powder	aluminum sulfate		calcium acetate

See Chapter 33, "Insect Sting and Bite Products," for more information about these products.

INSECT STING AND BITE PRODUCTS - continued

Product [a] Manufacturer/Supplier	Dosage Form	Antipruritic/Anesthet-ic/Counterirritant	Hydrocortisone	Other Ingredients
** Peterson's Ointment Lee Consumer	ointment	phenol · camphor		tannic acid · zinc oxide
Pramegel GenDerm	gel	pramoxine HCl, 1% · menthol, 0.5% · benzyl alcohol		carbomer 940 · methyl gluceth-20 · SD alcohol 40 · sodium hydroxide · water
Preparation H Hydrocortisone 1% Anti-Itch Whitehall-Robins Healthcare	cream		1%	cetyl alcohol · citric acid · disodium EDTA · glycerin · lanolin · methylparaben · white petrolatum · propylparaben · sodium benzoate · sodium lauryl sulfate · stearyl alcohol · water · tegacid special · Arlacel 186 · medical anti-foam emulsion · carboxymethylcellulose sodium · rhodigel · Tenox-2
Procort Lee Consumer	cream		1%	glycerin · glyceryl stearate · mineral oil · methylparaben · polysorbate 60 · propylparaben · sorbitan stearate · purified water · aloe vera gel
Rhuli Rydelle Labs	gel	benzyl alcohol, 2% · menthol, 0.3% · camphor, 0.3%		SD alcohol 23A, 31% · propylene glycol · carbomer 940 · triethanolamine · benzophenone-4 · EDTA
Rhuli Rydelle Labs	spray	benzocaine, 5% · camphor, 0.7% · benzyl alcohol		isopropyl alcohol, 70% (concentrate) · calamine, 13.8% · hydrated silica · isobutane · oleyl alcohol · sorbitan trioleate
Rhuli Bite-Aid Rydelle Labs	stick	benzocaine, 10% · benzyl alcohol, 10%		propylene glycol · sodium stearate · polyoxyethylene 20 isohexadecyl ether
Sarna Stiefel Labs	lotion	camphor, 0.5% · menthol, 0.5%		emollient base
** Sarnol-HC Stiefel Labs	lotion		1%	
Skeeter Stik Triton Consumer	liquid	menthol, 1% · pramoxine HCl, 0.5%		
Solarcaine Medicated First Aid Schering-Plough Healthcare	aerosol spray	benzocaine, 20%		SD alcohol 40, 35% · triclosan, 0.13% · isobutane
Sting-Eze Wisconsin Pharmacal	drops	diphenhydramine HCl · camphor · phenol · benzocaine		eucalyptol · propylene glycol

** New listing
[a] For additional hydrocortisone products, see Poison Ivy, Oak, and Sumac Products table.
[b] This product is labeled for use on insect bites but not insect stings.

See Chapter 33, "Insect Sting and Bite Products," for more information about these products.

INSECT REPELLENT PRODUCTS

Product Manufacturer/Supplier	Dosage Form	Active Ingredients	Other Ingredients
Ben's Backyard Tender	lotion · pump spray	n,n-diethyl-meta-toluamide, 23%	
Ben's Max Tender	lotion · pump spray	n,n-diethyl-meta-toluamide, 95%	
Ben's Wilderness Tender	aerosol spray	n,n-diethyl-meta-toluamide, 27.5% · other isomers, 10.5%	inert ingredients, 62%
** **Bug Stuff IPF 20** Wisconsin Pharmacal	lotion	n,n-diethyl-meta-toluamide, 20%	
** PE **Camp Lotion for Kids** Wisconsin Pharmacal	lotion	n,n-diethyl-meta-toluamide, 10%	
** **Coppertone Bug & Sun Adult Formula SPF 15** Schering-Plough Healthcare	lotion	n,n diethyl-meta-tolumide, 9.5% · other isomers, 0.5% · octyl methoxycinnamate · oxybenzone · octyl salicylate · homosalate	inert ingredients, 90%
** PE **Coppertone Bug & Sun Kids Formula SPF 30** Schering-Plough Healthcare	lotion	n,n diethyl-meta-tolumide, 9.5% · other isomers, 0.5% · octocrylene · octyl methoxycinnamate · oxybenzone	inert ingredients, 90%
** **Cutter Backwoods** Spectrum	aerosol spray	n,n-diethyl-meta-toluamide, 21.85% · other isomers, 1.15%	inert ingredients, 77%
** **Cutter Outdoorsman** Spectrum	lotion · stick	n,n-diethyl-meta-toluamide, 28.5% · other isomers, 1.5%	
Cutter Pleasant Protection Spectrum	pump spray	n,n-diethyl-meta-toluamide, 6.65% · other isomers, 0.35%	inert ingredients, 93%
** **Cutter Pleasant Protection** Spectrum	aerosol spray	n,n-diethyl-meta-toluamide, 6.65%	
Cutter with Sunscreen Spectrum	lotion	n,n-diethyl-meta-toluamide, 9.5% · other isomers, 0.5%	inert ingredients, 90%
Muskol Schering-Plough Healthcare	aerosol spray	n,n-diethyl-meta-toluamide, 23.75% · other isomers, 1.25%	inert ingredients, 75%
Muskol Maximum Strength Schering-Plough Healthcare	lotion · pump spray	n,n-diethyl-meta-toluamide, 95% · other isomers, 5%	
Muskol Ultra Extra Strength Schering-Plough Healthcare	aerosol spray	n,n-diethyl-meta-toluamide, 38% · other isomers, 2%	inert ingredients, 60%
Natrapel Tender	lotion · pump spray	citronella oil, 10%	aloe vera gel, 89%
Off! Deep Woods Formula S. C. Johnson & Son	aerosol spray	n,n-diethyl-meta-toluamide, 23.75% · other isomers, 1.25%	inert ingredients, 75%
Off! Deep Woods Formula for Sportsmen S. C. Johnson & Son	aerosol spray	n,n-diethyl-meta-toluamide, 28.5% · other isomers, 1.5%	inert ingredients, 70%
** **Off! Deep Woods with Sunscreen** S. C. Johnson & Son	liquid · lotion	n,n diethyl-meta-toluamide, 19% · related isomers, 1% · octyl methoxycinnamate · benzophenone-3 · octyl salicylate	

See Chapter 33, "Insect Sting and Bite Products," for more information about these products.

INSECT REPELLENT PRODUCTS - continued

Product Manufacturer/Supplier	Dosage Form	Active Ingredients	Other Ingredients
PE **Off! Skintastic for Kids** S. C. Johnson & Son	pump spray	n,n-diethyl-meta-toluamide, 4.75% · related isomers, 0.25%	inert ingredients, 95% · fragrance
** **Off! Skintastic with Sunscreen** S. C. Johnson & Son	lotion	n,n diethyl-meta-toluamide, 9.5% · related isomers, 0.5% · octocrylene · octyl methoxycinnamate · benzophenone-3	
Off! Skintastic, Fresh Scent or Unscented S. C. Johnson & Son	lotion	n,n-diethyl-meta-toluamide, 7.125% · related isomers, 0.375%	inert ingredients, 92.5%
Off! Skintastic, Unscented S. C. Johnson & Son	pump spray	n,n-diethyl-meta-toluamide, 6.65% · related isomers, 0.35%	inert ingredients, 93%
Off! Spring Fresh or Unscented S. C. Johnson & Son	aerosol spray	n,n-diethyl-meta-toluamide, 14.25% · other isomers, 0.75%	inert ingredients, 85%
** **Repel 100** Wisconsin Pharmacal	pump spray	n,n-diethyl-meta-toluamide, 100%	
** **Repel Classic Sportsmen Formula Unscented** Wisconsin Pharmacal	aerosol spray	n,n-diethyl-meta-toluamide, 40%	
Repel Family Formula Scented IPF 15 Wisconsin Pharmacal	aerosol spray	n,n-diethyl-meta-toluamide, 14.25% · other isomers, 0.75%	inert ingredients, 85%
** **Repel Family Formula Scented IPF 18** Wisconsin Pharmacal	pump spray	n,n-diethyl-meta-toluamide, 18%	
** **Repel Natural Citronella Towelettes** Wisconsin Pharmacal	wipe	citronella	
Repel Scented IPF 18 Wisconsin Pharmacal	pump spray	n,n-diethyl-meta-toluamide, 16.62% · n-octylbicycloheptene dicarboximide, 5% · di-n-propyl isocinchomeronate, 2.5% · other isomers, 0.88%	inert ingredients, 75%
Repel Scented IPF 7 Wisconsin Pharmacal	gel	n,n-diethyl-meta-toluamide, 6.65% · n-octylbicycloheptene dicarboximide, 2.5% · related toluamides, 0.35%	inert ingredients, 90.5%
** **Repel Sportsmen Formula IPF 18** Wisconsin Pharmacal	pump spray	n,n-diethyl-meta-toluamide, 18%	
** **Repel Sportsmen Formula IPF 20** Wisconsin Pharmacal	lotion	n,n-diethyl-meta-toluamide, 20%	
Repel Sportsmen Formula Unscented IPF 27 Wisconsin Pharmacal	aerosol spray	n,n-diethyl-meta-toluamide, 25.5% · n-octylbicycloheptene dicarboximide, 7.67% · di-n-propyl isocinchomeronate, 3.84% · other isomers, 1.35%	inert ingredients, 61.64%
Repel Unscented IPF 20 Wisconsin Pharmacal	lotion	n,n-diethyl-meta-toluamide, 19% · other isomers, 1%	inert ingredients, 80%

See Chapter 33, "Insect Sting and Bite Products," for more information about these products.

INSECT REPELLENT PRODUCTS - continued

Product Manufacturer/Supplier	Dosage Form	Active Ingredients	Other Ingredients
** **Repel Unscented IPF 20, SPF 15** Wisconsin Pharmacal	lotion	n,n-diethyl-meta-toluamide, 19% · other isomers, 1% · octyl methoxycinnamate · oxybenzone	inert ingredients, 80%
** **Skedaddle!** Minnetonka Brands	lotion	n,n-diethyl-meta-toluamide, 10%	
PE **Skedaddle! for Children** Minnetonka Brands	lotion	n,n-diethyl-meta-toluamide, 6.5%	inert ingredients, 93.5%
** PE **Skedaddle! for Children SPF 15** Minnetonka Brands	lotion	n,n-diethyl-meta-toluamide, 6.5% · titanium dioxide	
** PE **Snoopy Sunblock SPF 15 Plus Insect Protection** Minnetonka Brands	lotion	n,n-diethyl-meta-toluamide, 6.5% · titanium dioxide	
** **Solar Gel SPF 15 Plus Insect Protection** Minnetonka Brands	lotion	n,n-diethyl-meta-toluamide, 6.5% · titanium dioxide	
** **Sun & Bug Stuff IPF 20, SPF 15** Wisconsin Pharmacal	lotion	n,n-diethyl-meta-toluamide, 20%	

** New listing

Foot Care Product Tables

CALLUS, CORN, WART, AND INGROWN TOENAIL PRODUCTS

	Product Manufacturer/Supplier	Dosage Form	Salicylic Acid	Other Ingredients
**	**Calicylic Creme** Gordon Labs	cream	5%	urea, 10%
	Clear Away One Step Wart Remover System Schering-Plough Healthcare	disc	40%	
	Clear Away Plantar Wart Remover System Schering-Plough Healthcare	disc	40%	
**	**Compound-W Wart Remover** Medtech	pad	40%	
	Compound-W Wart Remover Medtech	gel	17%	alcohol, 67.5% · camphor · castor oil · collodion · colloidal silicon dioxide · hydroxypropyl cellulose · hypophosphorous acid · polysorbate 80
	Compound-W Wart Remover Medtech	liquid	17%	ether, 63.5% · alcohol, 21.2% · camphor · castor oil · collodion · ethylcellulose · hypophosphorous acid · menthol · polysorbate 80
	Corn Fix Alvin Last	liquid	12%	ether, 65.5% · alcohol, 33% · collodion
	Dr. Scholl's Callus Removers Schering-Plough Healthcare	disc · pad	40% (disc)	
	Dr. Scholl's Corn Removers, Regular or Waterproof Schering-Plough Healthcare	disc · pad	40% (disc)	
	Dr. Scholl's Corn/Callus Remover Schering-Plough Healthcare	liquid	12.6%	ether, 55% · alcohol, 18% (from SD alcohol 32)
	Dr. Scholl's Cushlin Gel Callus Removers Schering-Plough Healthcare	disc · pad	40% (disc)	
	Dr. Scholl's Cushlin Gel Corn Removers Schering-Plough Healthcare	disc · pad	40% (disc)	
	Dr. Scholl's Moisturizing Corn Remover Kit Schering-Plough Healthcare	cream · disc	40% (disc)	
	Dr. Scholl's One Step Callus Remover Schering-Plough Healthcare	disc	40%	
	Dr. Scholl's One Step Corn Removers Schering-Plough Healthcare	strip	40%	
	Dr. Scholl's Wart Remover Kit Schering-Plough Healthcare	liquid	17%	ether, 52% · alcohol, 17% (from SD alcohol 32)
	DuoFilm Liquid Wart Remover Schering-Plough Healthcare	liquid	17%	ether, 42.6% · alcohol, 15.8%
** PE	**DuoFilm Wart Remover Patch for Kids** Schering-Plough Healthcare	disc	40%	rubber-based vehicle
	DuoPlant Plantar Wart Remover Schering-Plough Healthcare	gel	17%	alcohol, 57.6% · ether, 16.42%

See Chapter 34, "Foot Care Products," for more information about these products.

CALLUS, CORN, WART, AND INGROWN TOENAIL PRODUCTS - continued

Product Manufacturer/Supplier	Dosage Form	Salicylic Acid	Other Ingredients
Freezone Corn and Callus Remover Medtech	liquid	13.6%	ether, 64.8% · alcohol, 20.5% · balsam oregon · castor oil · hypophosphorous acid · zinc chloride
Gordofilm Gordon Labs	solution	16.7%	flexible collodion
Mosco Corn & Callus Remover Medtech	liquid	17.6%	ether, 65.5% · alcohol, 33% · flexible collodion
Mosco-Cain Medtech	liquid		SDA alcohol, 40-60% · benzocaine, 20% · PEG-6
Occlusal HP GenDerm	liquid	17%	ethyl acetate · isopropyl alcohol · butyl acetate · polyvinyl butyl · dibutyl phthalate · acrylates copolymer · nitrocellulose
OFF·Ezy Corn and Callus Remover Kit Del Ph'cals	liquid	17%	
OFF·Ezy Wart Remover Kit Del Ph'cals	liquid	17%	flexible collodion
Outgro Pain Relieving Medtech	liquid		benzocaine, 20% · alcohol, 61.3% · D&C yellow#10 · FD&C blue#1 · FD&C red#40 · PEG-8
Trans-Ver-Sal 12mm "Adult Patch" Wart Remover Kit Doak Dermatologics	patch	15%	karaya gum base
Trans-Ver-Sal 20mm "PlantarPatch" Wart Remover Kit Doak Dermatologics	patch	15%	karaya gum base
Trans-Ver-Sal 6mm "PediaPatch" Wart Remover Kit Doak Dermatologics	patch	15%	karaya gum base
Wart Fix Alvin Last	liquid	17%	ether, 65.5% · alcohol, 33% · collodion
Wart-Off Pfizer Consumer	liquid	17%	flexible collodion · alcohol · ether · propylene glycol dipelargonate

** New listing

See Chapter 34, "Foot Care Products," for more information about these products.

ATHLETE'S FOOT PRODUCTS

Product Manufacturer/Supplier	Dosage Form	Antifungal	Other Ingredients
Absorbine Jr. Athlete's Foot W. F. Young	cream · powder	tolnaftate, 1%	water · cetyl alcohol · glyceryl stearate · diazolidinyl urea · methylparaben · propylene glycol · propylparaben
Absorbine Jr. Athlete's Foot Spray Liquid W. F. Young	pump spray	tolnaftate, 1%	acetone · water · polysorbate 80 · chloroxylenol · menthol · wormwood oil · FD&C blue#1
Desenex Novartis Consumer	powder	total undecylenate, 25% (as undecylenic acid and zinc undecylenate)	fragrance · talc
Desenex Novartis Consumer	cream · ointment	total undecylenate, 25% (as undecylenic acid and zinc undecylenate)	fragrance · glycol stearate SE · lanolin · methylparaben · PEG-8 laurate · PEG-6 stearate · propylparaben · purified water · sorbitol solution · stearic acid · trolamine · white petrolatum
Desenex Novartis Consumer	aerosol spray powder	total undecylenate, 25% (as undecylenic acid and zinc undecylenate)	fragrance · isobutane · isopropyl myristate · menthol · talc · trolamine
Desenex Foot & Sneaker Deodorant Plus Novartis Consumer	powder	calcium undecylenate, 10%	fragrance · talc
Dr. Scholl's Athlete's Foot Schering-Plough Healthcare	aerosol spray powder	tolnaftate, 1%	SD alcohol 40, 14% · BHT · propellants · talc
Dr. Scholl's Athlete's Foot Schering-Plough Healthcare	powder	tolnaftate, 1%	talc
Dr. Scholl's Athlete's Foot Spray Liquid Schering-Plough Healthcare	aerosol spray	tolnaftate, 1%	SD alcohol, 36% · BHT · propellants
** **Odor-Eaters Antifungal** Combe	powder	tolnaftate, 1%	benzethonium chloride · corn starch · fragrance · magnesium stearate · silica · talc
Odor-Eaters Antifungal Combe	aerosol spray powder	tolnaftate, 1%	ethanol, 14.9% · isobutane · isopropyl myristate
** **Odor-Eaters Foot & Sneaker** Combe	aerosol spray powder	tolnaftate, 1%	fragrance · isobutane · isopropyl myristate · quarternium-18 hectorite · SD alcohol 40-B · sodium bicarbonate
Rid-Itch Thomas & Thompson	liquid	benzoic acid, 2% · chlorothymol, 1% · resorcinol, 1%	salicylic acid, 7% · boric acid, 5% · alcohol · glycerin
Tinactin Schering-Plough Healthcare	cream	tolnaftate, 1%	BHT · PEG-8
Tinactin Schering-Plough Healthcare	solution	tolnaftate, 1%	PEG · BHT
Tinactin Schering-Plough Healthcare	powder	tolnaftate, 1%	corn starch · talc

** New listing

See Chapter 34, "Foot Care Products," for more information about these products.

Herbs and Phytomedicinal Product Table

HERBAL AND PHYTOMEDICINAL PRODUCTS

Product Manufacturer/Supplier	Dosage Form [a]	Ingredients
BILBERRY (Vaccinium myrtillus)		
** **Bilberry** Natrol	capsule	anthocyanosides, 25% (40mg 100:1 extract) · rice powder
** DY GL **Bilberry Extract** NaturPharma	280 mg capsule	anthocyanocides, 25% (60mg standardized extract)
Bilberry Extract PhytoPharmica	80 mg capsule	anthocyanosides, 25% (standardized extract)
** **Bilberry Extract** Nature's Resource/Pharmavite	60 mg capsule	anthocyanosides, 25%
DY GL **Bilberry-Power** Nature's Herbs	475 mg capsule	anthocyanosides, 25% (40mg standardized extract) · citrus bioflavonoids · rutin · quercetin
DY GL **Ultra Active Bilberry** NaturaLife	300 mg capsule	anthocyanosides, 25% (60mg standardized extract)
CAPSICUM (Capsicum species)		
** DY GL **Cayenne** NaturPharma	455 mg capsule	cayenne, 40000 STU (455mg standardized)
Cayenne Nature's Resource/Pharmavite	450 mg capsule	capsaicin, not less than 0.25%
** **Cayenne** Natrol	capsule	cayenne seed pod, 90000 STU · ginger root, 50mg · prickly ash bark, 50mg · Virginia snake root, 50mg
DY GL **Cayenne Extract** Herb Pharm	tincture	alcoholic extract of dried mature fruit
** DY GL **Cayenne Pepper** NaturaLife	450 mg capsule	capsaicin, 40000 STU (whole herb)
** DY GL **Cayenne Power-Herb** Nature's Herbs	450 mg capsule	cayenne, 100000 STU (450mg standardized)
CHASTE TREE BERRY (Vitex agnus-castus)		
** DY GL **Chaste Tree Berry Extract** Herb Pharm	tincture	alcoholic extract
** **Chasteberry-Power** Nature's Herbs	566 mg capsule	glycosides, 0.9-1.1% (100mg standardized) · dong quai root · siberian ginseng
DY GL **Ultra Active Vitex** NaturaLife	290 mg capsule	agnuside, 0.15% (175mg standardized extract)
** DY GL **Vitex Extract** NaturPharma	560 mg capsule	agnusides, 0.5mg (100mg standardized extract) · dong quai root · siberian ginseng powder
CRANBERRY (Vaccinium macrocarpon)		
** **Azo-Cranberry** PolyMedica Ph'cals	450 mg capsule	juice concentrate, 60% · food grade cellulose, 38% · magnesium stearate, 2%
** **Cranberry** Natrol	capsule	cranberry, 250mg (extract) · corn silk, 75mg · uva ursi leaf, 50mg · parsley leaf, 50mg · marshmallow root, 25mg

See Chapter 35, "Herbs and Phytomedicinal Products," for more information about these products.

HERBAL AND PHYTOMEDICINAL PRODUCTS - continued

Product Manufacturer/Supplier	Dosage Form [a]	Ingredients
DY GL	**Cranberry** NaturaLife	530 mg capsule	juice concentrate, 90% (380mg)
**	**Cranberry Fruit** Nature's Resource/Pharmavite	405 mg capsule	juice concentrate, 70% (25:1)
** DY GL	**Cranberry-Power** Nature's Herbs	505 mg capsule	organic acids, 80mg (400mg standardized extract) · vitamin C · freeze-dried cranberries

ECHINACEA (Echinacea species)

Botalia Gold Echinacea Extract Celestial Seasonings	125 mg capsule	total phenols, 4% (standardized Echinacea angustifolia and purpurea extract)
EchinaCare PhytoPharmica	tincture	fresh juice of Echinacea purpurea stems, leaves, and flowers in 22% alcohol (not less than 2.4% soluble beta-1,2-D-fructofuranosides calculated on basis of juice solids)
** DY GL · **Echinacea** NaturaLife	380 mg capsule	whole herb
Echinacea Complex Shaklee	tablet	Echinacea angustifolia root and Echinacea purpurea root and herb, 335mg · hyssop · peppermint · thyme
DY GL · **Echinacea-Power** Nature's Herbs	505 mg capsule	echinacoside, 3.2-4.8% (125mg standardized Echinacea angustifolia extract) · parthenium root · unstandardized Echinacea angustifolia · Echinacea purpurea root
DY GL · **Super Echinacea Extract** Herb Pharm	500 mg tablet	juice of root, leaf, and flower with dried root and seed of Echinacea purpurea and Echinacea angustifolia
DY GL · **Super Echinacea Liquid Extract** Herb Pharm	tincture	fresh juice of seed, plant, and root of Echinacea purpurea and Echinacea angustifolia in alcohol

ELEUTHRO (Eleutherococcus senticosus)

** DY GL · **Siberian Ginseng** MMS Professional	418 mg capsule	eleutheroside E, 0.8%
DY GL · **Siberian Ginseng Extract** Herb Pharm	tincture	extract of dried root (2:1)
** DY GL · **Siberian Ginseng Power-Herb** Nature's Herbs	404 mg capsule	eleutheroside D, 400mcg; eleutheroside B, 300mcg (100mg standardized extract) · siberian ginseng root

EVENING PRIMROSE OIL (Oenothera biennis)

** DY GL · **Evening Primrose Oil** NaturPharma	softgel	cis-linoleic acid, 370mg · gamma-linolenic acid, 50mg
DY GL · **Evening Primrose Oil** NaturaLife	500 mg capsule	cis-linoleic acid, 365mg · gamma-linoleic acid, 45mg
** **Evening Primrose Oil** Natrol	softgel	cis-linoleic acid, 350 mg · oleic acid, 50mg · cis-gamma-linolenic acid, 45mg
** DY GL · **Primrose-Power** Nature's Herbs	softgel	cis-linoleic acid, 962mg · gamma-linolenic acid, 130mg
Royal Brittany Evening Primrose Oil American Health	500 mg softgel	cis-linoleic acid, 365mg · gamma-linoleic acid, 45mg

FEVERFEW (Tanacetum parthenium)

See Chapter 35, "Herbs and Phytomedicinal Products," for more information about these products.

HERBAL AND PHYTOMEDICINAL PRODUCTS - continued

Product Manufacturer/Supplier	Dosage Form [a]	Ingredients
Botalia Gold Feverfew Extract Celestial Seasonings	125 mg capsule	parthenolides, 1.2% (standardized extract)
** DY GL **Feverfew** NaturaLife	380 mg capsule	whole herb
DY GL **Feverfew Extract** Herb Pharm	tincture	alcohol extract of dried leaf and flower
** DY GL **Feverfew-Power** Nature's Herbs	softgel	sesquiterpene lactones, 100mcg (standardized extract) · vitamin E · vegetable oil

GARLIC (Allium sativum)

Product Manufacturer/Supplier	Dosage Form [a]	Ingredients
** DY GL **Daily Garlic** NaturPharma	tablet	allicin total potential, 3mg (400mg standardized extract)
Garlic Shaklee	tablet	garlic equivalent to 0.5 fresh clove · rosemary · spearmint
** **Garlic Enteric Coated** Natrol	tablet	allicin potential, 5000mcg
** DY GL **Garlic-Power** Nature's Herbs	tablet	allicin total potential, 3mg (400mg standardized extract)
Garlique Enteric Coated Sunsource	400 mg tablet	allicin yield, 1800mcg
Garlitrin 4000 Enteric Coated PhytoPharmica	320 mg tablet	allicin yield, 5000mcg
Kwai Coated Lichtwer Pharma	100 mg tablet	allicin yield, 600mcg
One-A-Day Garlic Bayer Consumer	600 mg softgel	oil macerate standardized to yield allicin, not less than 1440mcg
DY GL **Ultra Active Garlic Enteric Coated** NaturaLife	259 mg tablet	allicin yield, 2500mcg

GINGER (Zingiber officinale)

Product Manufacturer/Supplier	Dosage Form [a]	Ingredients
DY GL **Ginger Extract** Herb Pharm	tincture	alcoholic extract of dried rhizome
DY GL **Ginger Root** Nature's Resource/Pharmavite	550 mg capsule	volatile oil, 1.5%
** DY GL **Ginger-Power** Nature's Herbs	480 mg capsule	gingerois, 5% (100mg standardized extract) · ginger root

GINKGO (Ginkgo biloba)

Product Manufacturer/Supplier	Dosage Form [a]	Ingredients
Botalia Gold Ginkgo Biloba Extract Celestial Seasonings	60 mg capsule	ginkgo flavone glycosides, 24% (standardized extract) · ginkgolides, 6%
** **Ginkai** Lichtwer Pharma	50 mg tablet	ginkgo flavonoids, 25% (standardized extract) · terpenoids, 6% (50:1)
** **Ginkgo Biloba** Natrol	capsule	ginkgo flavone glycosides, 24% (60mg 50:1 extract) · terpene lactones, 6%

See Chapter 35, "Herbs and Phytomedicinal Products," for more information about these products.

HERBAL AND PHYTOMEDICINAL PRODUCTS - continued

	Product Manufacturer/Supplier	Dosage Form [a]	Ingredients
	Ginkgo Biloba Extract Hudson	30 mg tablet	ginkgo flavone glycosides, 24% (as quercetin, kaempferol, and isorhamnetin standardized extract)
	Ginkgo Biloba Leaf Extract Nature's Resource/Pharmavite	40 mg capsule	ginkgo flavone glycosides, 24% (standardized extract)
DY GL	**Ginkgo Extract** Herb Pharm	tincture	alcoholic extract of fresh leaf
** DY GL	**Ginkgo Extract** NaturPharma	389 mg capsule	gingko flavone glycosides, 24% (40mg standardized extract) · ginkgo biloba leaf
	Ginkgo Phytosome PhytoPharmica	80 mg capsule	ginkgoheterosides bound to phosphatidylcholine, 24% (standardized extract)
** DY GL	**Ginkgo-Power** Nature's Herbs	389 mg capsule	ginkgo flavone glycosides, 24% (40mg standardized extract) · ginkgolic acid-free ginkgo biloba leaf
	Ginkgolidin PhytoPharmica	40 mg capsule	ginkgoheterosides, 24% (standardized extract)
**	**Liquid Ginkgo Biloba** Natrol	one full dropper	ginkgo flavone glycosides, 24% (60mg 50:1 extract) · terpene lactones, 6% · purified water · natural flavorings · glycerin · citric acid
DY GL	**Ultra Active Ginkgo Biloba** NaturaLife	260 mg tablet	ginkgo flavone glycosides, 24% (40mg standardized extract) · terpene lactones, 6%
	GINSENG (Panax ginseng)		
DY	**Asian Ginseng Complex** Shaklee	tablet	blend of red and white Asian ginseng, 335mg · licorice root · red jujube date
	Botalia Gold Panax Ginseng Extract Celestial Seasonings	100 mg capsule	ginsenosides, 7% (standardized extract, Rg1:Rb1 = 2:1)
**	**Celestial Herbal Extracts Ginseng Plus** Celestial Seasonings	softgel	ginsenosides, 7% (standardized extract, Rg1:Rb1 = 2:1) · zinc, 7.6mg · coenzyme Q10, 10mg
** DY GL	**Daily Ginseng** NaturPharma	495 mg capsule	ginsenosides, 7% (standardized extract) · eleutheroside B1 (standardized) · eleutheroside D (standardized) · siberian ginseng root
	Ginsai Lichtwer Pharma	100 mg capsule	ginsenosides, 7% (standardized extract)
** DY GL	**Ginseng Extract** NaturPharma	270 mg capsule	ginsenosides, 7% (150mg standardized) · Korean panax ginseng powder
	Ginseng Root - Korean White Nature's Resource/Pharmavite	560 mg capsule	ginsenoside, 1.5%
** DY GL	**Korean Ginseng Power-Herb** Nature's Herbs	535 mg capsule	ginsenosides, 7% (100mg standardized) · Korean panax ginseng powder
	Panaxin PhytoPharmica	100 mg capsule	saponins, 7% (calculated as ginsenoside Rg1; standardized extract)
	Ultra Active Ginseng NaturaLife	324 mg softgel	ginsenosides, 5% (110mg standardized extract)
	LEMON BALM (Melissa officinalis)		
	Herpalieve PhytoPharmica	cream	melissa (70:1 extract) · allantoin, 1%

See Chapter 35, "Herbs and Phytomedicinal Products," for more information about these products.

HERBAL AND PHYTOMEDICINAL PRODUCTS - continued

Product Manufacturer/Supplier	Dosage Form [a]	Ingredients
** DY GL **Lemon Balm Extract** Herb Pharm	tincture	alcoholic extract of fresh flowering plant

MILK THISTLE (Silybum marianum)

Product Manufacturer/Supplier	Dosage Form [a]	Ingredients
DY GL **Milk Thistle Extract** Herb Pharm	tincture	alcoholic extract of dried mature seed
** DY GL **Milk Thistle Extract** NaturPharma	540 mg capsule	silymarin, 80% (175mg standardized extract) · turmeric · artichoke
** **Milk Thistle Seed Extract** Nature's Resource/Pharmavite	140 mg capsule	silymarin, 70% (extract)
DY GL **Milk-Thistle Power** Nature's Herbs	540 mg capsule	silymarin, 80% (175mg standardized extract) · turmeric · artichoke
Sil-150 PhytoPharmica	150 mg capsule	silymarin, 70% (standardized extract)
DY GL **Ultra Active Milk Thistle** NaturaLife	310 mg capsule	silymarin, 140mg; including 60mg of silybinin and isosilybinin (180mg standardized extract)

OLIGOMERIC PROANTHOCYANIDINS

Product Manufacturer/Supplier	Dosage Form [a]	Ingredients
** **Grape Seed Extract** Natrol	capsule	proanthocyanidins, 95% (50mg extract)
** **Grape Seed Extract** Nature's Resource/Pharmavite	25 mg capsule	anhydrous procyanidolic value, not less than 95% (extract from vitis vinifera) · anhydrous polyphenols, 90-100%
** DY GL **Grape Seed-Power 100** Nature's Herbs	227 mg capsule	oligomeric proanthocyanidins, 95% (100mg standardized extract) · polyphenols, 14% (standardized grape skin extract)
** DY GL **Grape Seed-Power 50** Nature's Herbs	227 mg capsule	oligomeric proanthocyanidins, 95% (50mg standardized extract) · polyphenols, 14% (standardized grape skin extract)
PCO Phytosome PhytoPharmica	50 mg tablet	procyanidolic oligomers (from Vitis vinifera seed coat bound to phosphatidylcholine)
** **Preferred Pycnogenol Plus** Reese Chemical	capsule	30mg pycnogenol proanthocyanidin complex, 85% (from French Maritime pine tree) · 25mg grape seed extract, leucocyanidin value 90 · 300mg bioflavonoids
** **Pycnogenol** American Health	30 mg capsule	oligomeric proanthocynidins, 85% (extracted from pine tree bark) · citrus bioflavonoids, 300mg
** **Pycnogenol** Natrol	capsule	proanthocyanidins, 85% (50mg Pinus maritima bark extract)
Ultra Active Hawthorn NaturaLife	160 mg tablet	oligomeric proanthocyanadins, 14.5mg (from Crataegus species) · standardized extract

ST. JOHN'S WORT (Hypericum perforatum)

Product Manufacturer/Supplier	Dosage Form [a]	Ingredients
Botalia Gold St. John's Wort Extract Celestial Seasonings	150 mg capsule	hypericin, 0.3% (standardized extract)
Hypericum Extract PhytoPharmica	300 mg capsule	hypericin, 0.3% (standardized extract)
** **Kira** Lichtwer Pharma	300 mg tablet	hypericin, 0.3% (standardized extract)

See Chapter 35, "Herbs and Phytomedicinal Products," for more information about these products.

HERBAL AND PHYTOMEDICINAL PRODUCTS - continued

	Product Manufacturer/Supplier	Dosage Form [a]	Ingredients
**	**St. John's Wort** Natrol	capsule	hypericin, 0.3% (extract) · reishi mushroom mycelia, 100mg · sweet Annie herb, 50mg · wild oats herb, 50mg · lavender flower, 50mg
DY GL	**St. John's Wort** NaturaLife	375 mg capsule	hypericin, 0.15% (0.562mg standardized extract)
** DY GL	**St. John's Wort Extract** NaturPharma	375 mg capsule	hypericin, 0.3% (200mg standardized extract) · St. John's wort powder
DY GL	**St. John's Wort Extract** Herb Pharm	tincture	alcoholic extract of fresh flowering and budding top
**	**St. John's Wort Extract** Nature's Resource/Pharmavite	150 mg capsule	hypericin, not less than 0.3% (extract)
** DY GL	**St. John's-Power** Nature's Herbs	424 mg capsule	hypericin, 0.14% (250mg standardized extract) · St. John's wort powder
** DY GL	**St. John's-Power 0.3%** Nature's Herbs	424 mg capsule	hypericin, 0.3% (250mg standardized extract) · St. John's wort powder
	SAW PALMETTO (Serenoa repens)		
	Botalia Gold Saw Palmetto Extract Celestial Seasonings	80 mg softgel	free fatty acids, 85-95% (standardized extract)
**	**Saw Palmetto Complex** American Health	95 mg softgel	berry extract, 80mg · Pygeum africanum extract, 10mg · bearberry extract, 5mg · pumpkin seed oil extract, 40mg
DY GL	**Saw Palmetto Extract** Herb Pharm	tincture	alcoholic extract of dried mature berry
** DY GL	**Saw Palmetto Extract** NaturPharma	softgel	fatty acids and sterols, 85-95% (160mg standardized extract) · olive oil
**	**Saw Palmetto Plus** Shaklee	160 mg capsule	fatty acids and sterols, 85-95% (standardized extract) · beta-sitosterol, 15mg · pumpkin seed oil · soybean oil · beeswax · soy lecithin · ascorbyl palmitate · mixed tocopherol concentrate · rosemary extract
** DY GL	**Saw Palmetto-Power** Nature's Herbs	softgel	fatty acids and sterols, 85-95% (80mg standardized extract)
** DY GL	**Saw Palmetto-Power 160** Nature's Herbs	softgel	fatty acids and sterols, 85-95% (160mg standardized extract) · pumpkin seed oil
** DY GL	**Saw Palmetto-Power 320** Nature's Herbs	softgel	fatty acids and sterols, 85%-95% (320mg standardized extract)
	Super Saw Palmetto-160 PhytoPharmica	160 mg capsule	fatty acids and sterols, 85-95% (standardized extract)
**	**Ultra Active Saw Palmetto** PhytoPharmica	160 mg softgel	free fatty acids, 80% (standardized extract)
	VALERIAN (Valeriana officinalis)		
	Botalia Gold Valerian Extract Celestial Seasonings	150 mg capsule	valerenic acid, 0.8% (standardized extract)
** DY GL	**Ultra Active Valerian & Passion Flower** NaturaLife	495 mg tablet	100mg valerian root (standardized extract) · 45mg passion flower (standardized extract)

See Chapter 35, "Herbs and Phytomedicinal Products," for more information about these products.

HERBAL AND PHYTOMEDICINAL PRODUCTS - continued

	Product Manufacturer/Supplier	**Dosage Form [a]**	**Ingredients**
	Valer-A-Som PhytoPharmica	150 mg capsule	valerenic acids, 0.2-0.8% (standardized extract)
**	**Valerian Evening Formula** Natrol	capsule	valerenic acid, 0.8% (250mg extract) · hops flowers, 80mg · catnip herb, 30mg · kava kava root, 30mg · lemon balm herb, 30mg · skullcap herb, 30mg
DY GL	**Valerian Extract** Herb Pharm	tincture	alcoholic extract of fresh rhizome and roots
DY	**Valerian Plus** Shaklee	tablet	valerenic acid, 0.8% (75mg standardized valerian root extract) · passion flower · German chamomile
** DY GL	**Valerian-Power** Nature's Herbs	455 mg capsule	valerenic acids, 0.8% (250mg standardized extract) · valerian root powder

** New listing

[a] Quantities specified in this column refer to the total weight of the solid dosage form, not the weight of the active ingredient.

See Chapter 35, "Herbs and Phytomedicinal Products," for more information about these products.

Smoking Cessation Product Table

SMOKING CESSATION PRODUCTS

	Product Manufacturer/Supplier	Dosage Form	Active Ingredient	Other Ingredients
**	**NicoDerm CQ** SmithKline Beecham	transdermal patch	nicotine polacrilex, 7mg; 14mg; 21mg	ethylene vinyl acetate copolymer · polyisobutylene · high intensity polyethylene · polyester backings
	Nicorette SmithKline Beecham	gum	nicotine polacrilex, 2mg	flavors · glycerin · gum base · sodium carbonate · sorbitol · sodium bicarbonate
	Nicorette DS SmithKline Beecham	gum	nicotine polacrilex, 4mg	flavors · glycerin · gum base · sodium carbonate · sorbitol · D&C yellow#10
**	**Nicotrol** McNeil Consumer	transdermal patch	nicotine polacrilex, 15mg	polyisobutylenes · polybutene non-woven polyester · polyester backings

** New listing

See Chapter 36, "Smoking Cessation Products," for more information about these products.

Nonprescription Product Manufacturers/Suppliers

The following companies are manufacturers and/or suppliers of products listed in *Nonprescription Products: Formulations & Features* '97-98. Although this directory is a comprehensive listing of the companies that produce or supply nonprescription products, it should not be considered an all-inclusive listing of such companies.

A&D Medical
1555 McCandless Dr.
Milpitas, CA 95035
800-726-3364

Abbott Laboratories
Pharmaceutical Products Div.
1 Abbott Park Rd.
Abbott Park, IL 60064-3500
800-633-9110

Advanced Care Products Personal Products Co.
Div. of McNeil-PPC, Inc.
199 Grandview Rd.
Skillman, NJ 08558-9418
800-582-6097

Aero Assemblies, Inc.
Dist. for CPC (United Kingdom) Ltd.
Esher, Surrey, KT109PN
800-932-0177

Akorn, Inc.
100 Akorn Dr.
Abita Springs, LA 70420
800-535-7155

AkPharma Inc.
P.O. Box 111
Pleasantville, NJ 08232
800-257-8650

Alberto Culver Co.
2525 Armitage Ave.
Melrose Park, IL 60160
708-450-3000

Alcon Laboratories, Inc.
P.O. Box 6600
Fort Worth, TX 76115
817-293-0450

Allerderm Laboratories, Inc.
P.O. Box 2070
Petaluma, CA 94953-2070
800-365-6868

Allergan Inc.
P.O. Box 19534
Irvine, CA 92623-9534
800-347-4500

Allergan Skin Care
Div. of Allergan, Inc.
P.O. Box 19534
Irvine, CA 92623-9534
800-347-4500

Alpharma
7205 Windsor Blvd.
Baltimore, MD 21244-2654
800-638-9096

Alva-Amco Pharmacal Companies, Inc.
6625 N. Avondale Ave.
Chicago, IL 60631
773-792-0200

Alvin Last, Inc.
19 Babcock Pl.
Yonkers, NY 10701-2714
914-376-1000

American Health
Div. of NBTY
4320 Veterans' Memorial Hwy.
Holbrook, NY 11741
800-445-7137

Andrew Jergens Co.
P.O. Box 145444
Cincinnati, OH 45250-5444
800-222-3553

Ansell Inc.
446 State Hwy. 35
Eatontown, NJ 07724
800-524-1377

Apothecary Products, Inc.
11531 Rupp Dr.
Burnsville, MN 55337-1295
800-328-2742

Apothecon
Div. of Bristol-Myers Squibb Co.
P.O. Box 4500
Princeton, NJ 08543-4500
609-897-2470

Apothecus Pharmaceutical Corp.
20 Audrey Ave.
Oyster Bay, NY 11771-1532
516-624-8200

Atwater Carey Ltd.
5505 Central Ave.
Boulder, CO 80301
800-359-1646

B. F. Ascher & Company, Inc.
P.O. Box 717
Shawnee Mission, KS 66201-0717
913-888-1880

Baker Cummins Dermatologicals
Div. of Baker Norton Pharmaceuticals
4400 Biscayne Blvd.
Miami, FL 33137-3227
305-575-6000

Bard Medical Care
Div. of C. R. Bard, Inc.
8195 Industrial Blvd.
Covington, GA 30209
800-526-4930

Bausch & Lomb Personal Products
Div. of Bausch & Lomb, Inc.
1400 N. Goodman St.
Rochester, NY 14692-0450
800-553-5340

Bausch & Lomb Pharmaceutical
Div. of Bausch & Lomb, Inc.
8500 Hidden River Pkwy.
Tampa, FL 33637
813-975-7700

Bayer Corp., Consumer Care Div.
Subs. of Bayer AG
Morristown, NJ 07960
800-800-4793

Bayer Corp., Diagnostics Div.
Subs. of Bayer AG
511 Benedict Ave.
Tarrytown, NY 10591-5097
800-431-1970

BDI Pharmaceuticals, Inc.
P.O. Box 78610
Indianapolis, IN 46278-0610
800-428-1717

Becton Dickinson and Co.
Consumer Products Div.
1 Becton Dr.
Franklin Lakes, NJ 07417-1883
800-526-4650

Beiersdorf Inc.
P.O. Box 5529
Norwalk, CT 06856-5529
800-233-2340

Beutlich, L.P. Pharmaceuticals
1541 Shields Dr.
Waukegan, IL 60085-8304
800-238-8542

Biocare International, Inc.
2643 Grand Ave.
Bellmore, NY 11710
800-224-0001

Biofilm, Inc.
3121 Scott St.
Vista, CA 92083-8323
800-848-5900

Biomerica, Inc.
1533 Monrovia Ave.
Newport Beach, CA 92663
800-854-3002

Bio-Oxidation Inc.
120 E. Grant St.
Greencastle, PA 17225
888-4-MED-WASTE

BIRA Corp.
2525 Quicksilver Rd.
McDonald, PA 15057
412-796-1820

Bird Products Corp.
1100 Bird Center Dr.
Palm Springs, CA 92262
619-778-7200

Blaine Company, Inc. Pharmaceuticals
1465 Jamike Ln.
Erlanger, KY 41018
606-283-9437

Blair Laboratories, Inc.
Div. of The Purdue Frederick Co.
see Purdue Frederick

Blairex Laboratories, Inc.
P.O. Box 2127
Columbus, IN 47202-2127
800-252-4739

Blanchard Ostomy Products
1510 Raymond Ave.
Glendale, CA 91201
818-242-6789

Blistex Inc.
1800 Swift Dr.
Oak Brook, IL 60521-1574
800-837-1800

Block Drug Co., Inc.
257 Cornelison Ave.
Jersey City, NJ 07302-3198
800-365-6500

Boehringer Mannheim Corp.
P.O. Box 50100
Indianapolis, IN 46250-0100
800-428-5074

Breckenridge Pharmaceutical, Inc.
Subs. of Breckenridge, Inc.
P.O. Box 206
Boca Raton, FL 33429
561-367-8512

Brimms Laboratories
Div. of Brimms Inc.
425 Fillmore Ave.
Tonawanda, NY 14150
800-828-7669

Bristol-Myers Products
Div. of Bristol-Myers Squibb Co.
345 Park Ave.
New York, NY 10154
800-468-7746

Buffington
Div. of Otis Clapp & Son, Inc.
see Otis Clapp

C & M Pharmacal, Inc.
1721 Maplelane
Hazel Park, MI 48030-1215
800-423-5173

C. B. Fleet Co., Inc.
P.O. Box 11349
Lynchburg, VA 24506-1349
800-999-9711

C. S. Dent & Co.
Div. of Grandpa Brands Co.
317 E. 8th St.
Cincinnati, OH 45202
513-241-1677

Can-Am Care Corp.
Cimetra Industrial Park, Box 98
Chazy, NY 12921-0098
800-461-7448

Caraco Pharmaceutical Laboratories, Ltd.
1150 Elijah McCoy Dr.
Detroit, MI 48202
800-818-4555

Care-Tech Laboratories, Inc.
3224 S. Kingshighway Blvd.
St. Louis, MO 63139-1183
800-325-9681

Caring Products International Inc.
200 First Ave. W., Ste. 200
Seattle, WA 98119
800-FEEL-DRY

Carma Laboratories, Inc.
5801 W. Airways Ave.
Franklin, WI 53132
414-421-7707

Carmé International
84 Galli Dr.
Novato, CA 94949
800-227-2628

Carnation Nutritional Products
Div. of Nestlé Food Co.
800 N. Brand Blvd.
Glendale, CA 91203
800-628-2229

Carnrick Laboratories, Inc.
65 Horse Hill Rd.
Cedar Knolls, NJ 07927
201-267-2670

Carter Products
Div. of Carter-Wallace, Inc.
1345 Ave. of the Americas
New York, NY 10105
212-339-5000

Cascade Medical
10180 Viking Dr.
Eden Prairie, MN 55344
800-525-6718

CCA Industries, Inc.
200 Murray Hill Pkwy.
E. Rutherford, NJ 07073
201-330-1400

Celestial Seasonings
4600 Sleepy Time Dr.
Boulder, CO 80301-3292
800-525-0347

Century Pharmaceuticals, Inc.
10377 Hague Rd.
Indianapolis, IN 46256-3399
317-849-4210

Chattem, Inc.
1715 W. 38th St.
Chattanooga, TN 37409-1248
800-366-6833

ChemTrak, Inc.
929 E. Arques Ave.
Sunnyvale, CA 94086-4520
800-927-7776

Chesebrough-Pond's USA Co.
40 Merritt Blvd.
Trumbull, CT 06611
800-786-5135

Chilton Labs
23 Fairfield Pl.
W. Caldwell, NJ 07006-0596
800-443-8856

Chronimed, Inc.
13911 Ridgedale Dr., Ste. 250
Minnetonka, MN 55305
800-888-5957

Church & Dwight Co., Inc.
469 N. Harrison St.
Princeton, NJ 08543-5297
609-683-5900

CIBA Vision Corp.
A Novartis Company
11460 Johns Creek Pkwy.
Duluth, GA 30097
800-227-1524

Clement Clarke, Inc.
3128-D E. 17th Ave.
Columbus, OH 43219
800-848-8923

Clinical Diagnostics, Inc.
117C Spratt St.
Fort Mill, SC 29715
800-860-9937

CNS, Inc.
4400 W. 78th St.
Bloomington, MN 55435
612-820-6696

Colgate-Palmolive Co.
300 Park Ave.
New York, NY 10022
800-221-4607

Coloplast Corp.
1955 W. Oak Cir.
Marietta, GA 30062-2249
800-533-0464

Columbia Laboratories, Inc.
2665 S. Bayshore Dr.
Miami, FL 33133
305-860-1670

Combe, Inc.
1101 Westchester Ave.
White Plains, NY 10604
800-873-7400

Consumers Choice Systems, Inc.
2370 130th Ave. NE, #101
Bellevue, WA 98005
800-479-5232

ConvaTec
Div. of Bristol-Myers Squibb Co.
P.O. Box 5254
Princeton, NJ 08543-5254
800-422-8811

Copley Pharmaceutical Inc.
Canton Commerce Center
25 John Rd.
Canton, MA 02021-2897
800-325-6111

Cymed, Inc.
c/o Eastman Medical
2000 Powell St., Ste. 1540
Emeryville, CA 94608
510-652-2961

Dairy Association Co., Inc.
16 Williams St.
Lyndonville, VT 05851
800-232-3610

Del Pharmaceuticals, Inc.
Subs. of Del Laboratories, Inc.
565 Broad Hollow Rd.
Farmingdale, NY 11735
516-844-2020

Denison Pharmaceuticals, Inc.
P.O. Box 1305
Pawtucket, RI 02862
401-723-5500

Dental Concepts Inc.
100 Clearbrook Rd.
Elmsford, NY 10523
800-592-6661

Dentco, Inc.
Subs. of Block Drug Co., Inc.
see Block

Dep Corp.
2101 E. Via Arado
Rancho Dominguez, CA 90220
800-326-2855

Dermik Laboratories, Inc.
A Rhône-Poulenc Rorer Co.
P.O. Box 1727
Fort Washington, PA 19034
800-523-6674

Dey Laboratories
A Lipha Americas Co.
2751 Napa Valley Corp. Dr.
Napa, CA 94558
800-755-5560

Direct Access Diagnostics
Div. of Ortho Pharmaceutical Corp.
440 Rt. 22 E.
Bridgewater, NJ 08807
908-218-7300

Doak Dermatologics
Subs. of Bradley Pharmaceuticals, Inc.
see Bradley

Dover Pharmaceutical, Inc.
P.O. Box 809
Islington, MA 02090
617-821-5400

Dr. G. H. Tichenor Antiseptic Co.
P.O. Box 53374
New Orleans, LA 70153
504-588-9131

Durex Consumer Products
Div. of London Int'l U.S. Holdings, Inc.
4725 Peachtree Corners Cir., Ste. 150
Norcross, GA 30092
770-582-2222

E. Fougera & Co.
Div. of Altana Inc.
60 Baylis Rd.
Melville, NY 11747-3816
800-645-9833

E. T. Browne Drug Co., Inc.
P.O. Box 1613
Englewood Cliffs, NJ 07632
201-947-3050

Effcon Inc.
P.O. Box 7499
Marietta, GA 30065-1499
800-722-2428

Eli Lilly and Co.
Lilly Corp. Center
Indianapolis, IN 46285
800-545-5979

Entry 21, Ltd.
1830 E. Elliot Rd., Ste. 103
Tempe, AZ 85284
800-400-5027

EnviroDerm Pharmaceuticals, Inc.
Subs. of United Catalyst
P.O. Box 32370
Louisville, KY 40232
502-634-7700

The Female Health Co.
875 N. Michigan Ave., Ste. 3660
Chicago, IL 60611
800-635-0844

Ferndale Laboratories, Inc.
780 W. Eight Mile Rd.
Ferndale, MI 48220-1218
313-548-0900

The Fielding Co.
P.O. Box 2186
Maryland Heights, MO 63043
314-567-5462

Fischer Pharmaceuticals, Inc.
165 Gibraltar Ct.
Sunnyvale, CA 94089
800-782-0222

Flanders, Inc.
Northbridge Station
P.O. Box 39143
Charleston, SC 29414
803-571-3363

Fleming & Co.
1600 Fenpark Dr.
Fenton, MO 63026
314-343-8200

Forest Pharmaceuticals, Inc.
Subs. of Forest Laboratories, Inc.
13622 Lakefront Dr.
St. Louis, MO 63045
800-678-1605

Fox Pharmacal, Inc.
6420 N.W. 5th Way
Ft. Lauderdale, FL 33309-6112
954-772-7487

Freeda Vitamins, Inc.
36 E. 41st St.
New York, NY 10017-6203
800-777-3737

Gainor Medical USA Inc.
P.O. Box 353
McDonough, GA 30253-0353
800-825-8282

Galderma Laboratories, Inc.
P.O. Box 331329
Ft. Worth, TX 76163-1329
817-263-2600

Gebauer Co.
9410 St. Catherine Ave.
Cleveland, OH 44104-5599
800-321-9348

GenDerm Corp.
600 Knightsbridge Pkwy.
Lincolnshire, IL 60069-3657
800-533-3376

Gerber Products Co.
445 State St.
Freemont, MI 49413-0001
800-828-9119

Glenwood Inc.
82 N. Summit St.
Tenafly, NJ 07670
201-569-0050

Goldware
P.O. Box 22335
San Diego, CA 92192
800-669-7311

Goody's Pharmaceuticals, Inc.
Div. of Block Drug Co., Inc.
see Block

Gordon Laboratories
6801 Ludlow St.
Upper Darby, PA 19082
800-356-7870

Graham-Field, Inc.
400 Rabro Dr. E.
Hauppauge, NY 11788
800-645-1023

Grandpa Soap Co.
Div. of Grandpa Brands Co.
317 E. 8th St.
Cincinnati, OH 45202
513-241-1677

GumTech International, Inc.
P.O. Box 36195
Phoenix, AZ 85067-6195
800-676-4769

Hampton Essex Corp.
see Merz Consumer

Hawaiian Tropic
Div. of Tanning Research Laboratories
P.O. Box 265111
Daytona Beach, FL 32126-5111
904-677-9559

Health Care Products
Div. of Hi-Tech Pharmacal Co., Inc.
369 Bayview Ave.
Amityville, NY 11701
800-262-9010

Health-Mark Diagnostics, L.L.C.
Subs. of TCPI
P.O. Box 6186
Ft. Lauderdale, FL 33310
954-984-8881

Healthpoint, Ltd.
2400 Handley-Ederville Rd.
Ft. Worth, TX 76118
800-441-8227

HealthScan Products Inc.
Div. of Healthdyne Technologies
908 Pompton Ave.
Cedar Grove, NJ 07009-1292
800-962-1266

HealthWare
P.O. Box 1693
Idyllwild, CA 92549-1693
800-682-9375

Herb Pharm, Inc.
P.O. Box 116
Williams, OR 97544
800-348-4372

Hershey Foods Corp.
Div. of Hershey Chocolate
19 E. Chocolate Ave.
Hershey, PA 17033-0815
800-468-1714

Hogil Pharmaceutical Corp.
2 Manhattanville Rd.
Purchase, NY 10577-2118
914-696-7600

Hollister Inc.
2000 Hollister Dr.
Libertyville, IL 60048
847-680-1000

Home Access Health Corp.
2401 W. Hassell Rd., Ste. 1510
Hoffman Estates, IL 60195-5200
800-HIV-TEST

Home Diagnostics, Inc.
2300 N.W. 55th Ct.
Ft. Lauderdale, FL 33309
800-342-7226

The Hudson Corp.
Div. of NBTY
90 Orville Dr.
Bohemia, NY 11716-2599
516-567-9500

Humanicare International Inc.
1471 Jersey Ave.
N. Brunswick, NJ 08902
800-631-5270

Hydrosal Company
Div. of Merchandise, Inc.
P.O. Box 10
Miamitown, OH 45041-0010
513-353-2200

Hyrex Pharmaceuticals
3494 Democrat Rd.
Memphis, TN 38118-1542
800-238-5282

ICN Pharmaceuticals, Inc.
3300 Hyland Ave.
Costa Mesa, CA 92626
800-322-1515

Identi-Find
P.O. Box 567
Canton, NC 28716-0567
704-648-6768

ITA Software, Inc.
P.O. Box 448
Cascade, ID 83611
800-510-1024

J. B. Williams Co., Inc.
65 Harristown Rd.
Glen Rock, NJ 07452
800-254-8656

J. K. Pharmaceuticals, Inc.
1645 Oak St.
Lakewood, NJ 08701
908-905-5252

**Johnson & Johnson Consumer
Products, Inc.**
199 Grandview Rd.
Skillman, NJ 08558-9418
800-526-3967

**Johnson & Johnson•Merck Consumer
Pharmaceuticals Co.**
Div. of Johnson & Johnson
7050 Camp Hill Rd.
Ft. Washington, PA 19034
215-233-7700

Jones Medical Industries, Inc.
P.O. Box 46903
St. Louis, MO 63146-6903
314-576-6100

Jordan Medical Enterprises, Inc.
202 Oaklawn Ave.
S. Pasadena, CA 91030
800-541-1193

Kenwood Laboratories
Div. of Bradley Pharmaceuticals, Inc.
see Bradley

Kerr, Frank W. Chemical Co.
P.O. Box 8026
Novi, MI 48376-8026
800-624-7509

Kimberly-Clark Corp.
2001 Marathon Ave.
Neenah, WI 54956
800-558-6423

Kingswood Laboratories, Inc.
10375 Hague Rd.
Indianapolis, IN 46256-3316
317-849-9513

Kiwi Brands
Div. of Sara Lee Corp.
Rt. 662 N.
Douglassville, PA 19518
610-385-3041

KLI Corp.
P.O. Box 567
Carmel, IN 46032
317-846-7452

Konsyl Pharmaceuticals, Inc.
4200 S. Hulen St.
Ft. Worth, TX 76109
817-763-8011

Kramer Laboratories, Inc.
8778 S.W. 8th St.
Miami, FL 33174-9990
800-824-4894

Laclede Research Laboratories
Div. of Laclede Professional Products
15011 Staff Ct.
Gardena, CA 90248
800-922-5856

Lake Consumer Products
625 Forest Edge Dr.
Vernon Hills, IL 60061
800-635-3696

Lavoptik Company, Inc.
661 Western Ave. N.
St. Paul, MN 55103-1667
612-489-1351

Lederle Consumer Health/Whitehall-Robins
Div. of Whitehall-Robins Healthcare
401 N. Middletown Rd.
Pearl River, NY 10965
800-282-8805

Lee Consumer Products
P.O. Box 3836
S. El Monte, CA 91733
800-950-5337

Legere Pharmaceuticals
7326 E. Evans Rd.
Scottsdale, AZ 85260
800-528-3144

Lemmon Co.
Div. of Teva Ph'cal Industries, Inc.
1510 Delp Dr.
Kulpsville, PA 19443
800-545-8800

Lichtwer Pharma U.S., Inc.
Foster Plaza 9
750 Holiday Dr.
Pittsburgh, PA 15220
800-837-3203

LifeScan, Inc.
Subs. of Johnson & Johnson
1000 Gilbraltar Dr.
Milpitas, CA 95035-6312
800-227-8862

LLW Enterprises
P.O. Box 591353
Houston, TX 77259-1353
713-480-1506

Lobana Laboratories
Div. of Ulmer Pharmacal Co.
see Ulmer

Lukens Medical Corp.
3820 Academy Pkwy. North NE
Albuquerque, NM 87109
800-431-8233

Lumiscope Co., Inc.
400 Raritan Center Pkwy.
Edison, NJ 08837
800-422-LUMI

Majestic Drug Co., Inc.
711-717 E. 134th St.
Bronx, NY 10454
800-238-0220

Martin Himmel Inc.
P.O. Box 5479
Lake Worth, FL 33466-5479
800-535-3823

McNeil Consumer Products Co.
Div. of McNeil-PPC, Inc.
7050 Camp Hill Rd.
Fort Washington, PA 19034-2299
800-962-5357

Mead Johnson Nutritionals
Div. of Bristol-Myers Squibb Co.
2400 W. Lloyd Expwy.
Evansville, IN 47721-0001
800-222-9123

Medco Lab, Inc.
P.O. Box 864
Sioux City, IA 51102-0864
712-255-8770

MedData Interactive
1603 Deventer Ridge Dr.
Knoxville, TN 37919-8907
800-792-2966

Medeva Pharmaceuticals, Inc.
755 Jefferson Rd.
Rochester, NY 14623
800-932-1950

Medic Alert
2323 Colorado Ave.
Turlock, CA 95382
800-432-5378

MediCheck International Foundation, Inc.
8320 Ballard Rd.
Niles, IL 60714
847-299-0620

Medicis Dermatologics, Inc.
4343 E. Camelback Rd., Ste. 250
Phoenix, AZ 85018
800-550-5115

Medicool, Inc.
23761 Madison St.
Torrance, CA 90505
800-433-2469

Medicore, Inc.
P.O. Box 4826
Hialeah, FL 33016
800-327-8894

MediLife
30 Monument Sq.
Concord, MA 01742
888-656-5656

MediSense, Inc.
Subs. of Abbott Laboratories
4A Crosby Dr.
Bedford, MA 01730
800-527-3339

Medport Inc.
23 Acorn St.
Providence, RI 02903
800-299-5704

Medtech Inc.
P.O. Box 1108
Jackson Hole, WY 83001
800-443-4908

Menley & James Laboratories, Inc.
Commonwealth Corp. Center
100 Tournament Dr., Ste. 210
Horsham, PA 19044-3697
215-441-6500

Mentholatum Co., Inc.
1360 Niagara St.
Buffalo, NY 14213
716-882-7660

Mericon Industries, Inc.
8819 N. Pioneer Rd.
Peoria, IL 61615-1561
800-242-6464

Merrick Medicine Co.
P.O. Box 1489
Waco, TX 76703
817-753-3461

Merz Consumer Products
4215 Tudor Ln.
Greensboro, NC 27410
910-856-2003

MetaMedix, Inc.
735 E. Ohio Ave., Ste. 202
Escondido, CA 92025
800-455-4105

Milex Products, Inc.
5915 Northwest Hwy.
Chicago, IL 60631
773-631-6484

Minnetonka Brands, Inc.
7665 Commerce Way
Eden Prairie, MN 55344
800-699-6852

Mission Pharmacal Co.
P.O. Box 786099
San Antonio, TX 78278-6099
800-531-3333

Multisource
Manufacturers/suppliers of generic and/or private-label products—including, but not limited to, the following companies:

Goldline Laboratories
Subs. of Zenith Goldline
Pharmaceuticals
1900 W. Commercial Blvd.
Ft. Lauderdale, FL 33309
800-327-4114

Major Pharmaceuticals Corp.
355 N. Ashland Ave.
Chicago, IL 60607
800-688-9696

Pfeiffer Pharmaceuticals, Inc.
Subs. of The S.S.S. Company
P.O. Box 4447
Atlanta, GA 30302-4447
404-521-0857

Roxane Laboratories, Inc.
Div. of Boehringer Ingelheim Corp.
P.O. Box 16532
Columbus, OH 43216-6532
800-848-0120

Rugby Laboratories, Inc.
900 Orlando Ave.
W. Hempstead, NY 11552
800-645-2158

Schein Pharmaceutical, Inc.
100 Campus Dr.
Florham Park, NJ 07932
800-548-6236

Muro Pharmaceutical, Inc.
890 East St.
Tewksbury, MA 01876
800-225-0974

Mustang Enterprises, Inc.
P.O. Box 748
Geneva, IL 60134-0748
630-232-1373

Natrol, Inc.
20731 Marilla St.
Chatsworth, CA 91311
800-326-1520

Natural White, Inc.
15449 Yonge St.
Aurora, Ontario, L4G1P3
905-841-9229

NaturaLife
Murdock Madaus Schwabe Group
1375 N. 1100 West
P.O. Box 4000
Springville, UT 84663
800-926-8883

Nature's Herbs
Div. of Twinlab
600 E. Quality Dr.
American Fork, UT 84003
800-437-2257

**Nature's Resource Products/
Pharmavite Corp.**
15451 San Fernando Mission Blvd.
Mission Hills, CA 91345
800-423-2405

NaturPharma
Div. of Twinlab
600 E. Quality Dr.
American Fork, UT 84003
800-437-2257

Nestlé Clinical Nutrition
P.O. Box 760
Deerfield, IL 60015
800-422-ASK2

Neutrogena Dermatologics
Div. of Neutrogena Corp.
5760 W. 96th St.
Los Angeles, CA 90045
800-421-6857

Nion Laboratories
15501 First St.
Irwindale, CA 91706
800-227-8526

Northampton Medical, Inc.
see UCB Pharma

Novartis Consumer Health, Inc.
560 Morris Ave.
Summit, NJ 07901-1312
800-452-0051

Novartis Nutrition Corporation
5320 W. 23rd St.
P.O. Box 370
Minneapolis, MN 55440
800-999-9978

Novo Nordisk Pharmaceuticals Inc.
Subs. of Novo Nordisk A/S
100 Overlook Center, Ste. 200
Princeton, NJ 08540-7810
800-727-6500

Nu-Hope Laboratories, Inc.
P.O. Box 331150
Pacoima, CA 91333-1150
800-899-5017

Numark Laboratories, Inc.
P.O. Box 6321
Edison, NJ 08818
800-338-8079

Oakhurst Co.
3000 Hempstead Tnpk.
Levittown, NY 11756
800-831-1135

Ocurest Laboratories, Inc.
4400 PGA Blvd., Ste. 300
Palm Beach Gardens, FL 33410
561-627-8121

Omron Healthcare, Inc.
300 Lakeview Pkwy.
Vernon Hills, IL 60061
800-231-4030

Oral-B Laboratories
Div. of Gillette Company, Inc.
1 Lagoon Dr.
Redwood City, CA 94065-1561
800-446-7252

Otis Clapp & Son, Inc.
P.O. Box 9160
Canton, MA 02021-9160
617-821-5400

Owen Mumford, Inc.
849 Pickens Industrial Dr., Ste. 14
Marietta, GA 30062-3165
800-421-6936

Paddock Laboratories, Inc.
P.O. Box 27286
Minneapolis, MN 55427
800-328-5113

Palco Labs
8030 Soquel Ave., Ste. 104
Santa Cruz, CA 95062-2032
800-346-4488

Parnell Pharmaceuticals, Inc.
P.O. Box 5130
Larkspur, CA 94977-5130
800-45-PHARM

The Parthenon Co., Inc.
3311 W. 2400 South
Salt Lake City, UT 84119
800-453-8898

Pascal Company, Inc.
P.O. Box 1478
Bellevue, WA 98009-1478
206-827-4694

Pedinol Pharmacal, Inc.
30 Banfi Plaza N.
Farmingale, NY 11735
800-PEDINOL

Perio Products
6156 Wilcox Rd.
Dublin, OH 43016
614-791-1207

Perry Products
Div. of Health Care Marketing, Inc.
3803 E. Lake St.
Minneapolis, MN 55406-2298
612-722-4783

Persön & Covey, Inc.
P.O. Box 25018
Glendale, CA 91221-5018
800-423-2341

Personal Care Group, Inc.
1 Paragon Dr.
Montvale, NJ 07645
800-816-5742

Personal Health and Hygiene, Inc.
2 N. Charles St.
Baltimore, MD 21201
410-539-5325

Pfizer Inc
Consumer Health Care Group
235 E. 42nd St.
New York, NY 10017-5755
212-573-3131

Pharmacia & Upjohn, Inc.
7000 Portage Rd.
Kalamazoo, MI 49001
800-253-8600

Pharmacy Counter
2655 W. Central Ave.
Toledo, OH 43606
800-984-1137

PhytoPharmica
P.O. Box 1745
Greenbay, WI 54305
800-553-2370

Pierre Fabre Dermatology, Inc.
1055 W. Eighth St.
Azusa, CA 91702
800-788-7891

Playtex Products, Inc.
Consumer Products Div.
300 Nyala Farms Rd.
Westport, CT 06880
888-224-6786

PolyMedica Pharmaceuticals (USA), Inc.
2 Constitution Way
Woburn, MA 01801
617-933-2020

Premier Consumer Products, Inc.
106 Grand Ave.
Englewood, NJ 07631
201-568-9700

The Procter & Gamble Co.
P.O. Box 599
Cincinnati, OH 45201
800-262-1637

Psychemedics Corp.
1280 Massachusetts Ave.
Cambridge, MA 02138
800-628-8073

PTS Labs, LLC
711 S. Dearborn St., Ste. 205
Chicago, IL 60605
312-922-8437

The Purdue Frederick Co.
100 Connecticut Ave.
Norwalk, CT 06850-3590
203-853-0123

Quaker House Products, Inc.
P.O. Box 21088
Houston, TX 77226
713-526-1248

Quality Formulations, Inc.
P.O. Box 827
Zachary, LA 70791
800-259-3376

Quality Health Products, Inc.
P.O. Box 31
Yaphank, NY 11980
800-233-7672

Quidel Corp.
10165 McKellar Ct.
San Diego, CA 92121
619-646-8052

R & D Laboratories, Inc.
4640 Admiralty Way, Ste. 710
Marina del Rey, CA 90292
800-338-9066

Randob Laboratories, Ltd.
P.O. Box 440
Cornwall, NY 12518
914-534-2197

Recsei Laboratories
Goleta, CA 93117
805-964-2912

Reese Chemical Co.
P.O. Box 1957
Cleveland, OH 44106
800-321-7178

Rembrandt
Div. of Den-Mat Corp.
2727 Skyway Dr.
Santa Maria, CA 93455
800-433-6628

Republic Drug Company, Inc.
175 Great Arrow
Buffalo, NY 14027
716-874-5060

Requa, Inc.
P.O. Box 4008
Greenwich, CT 06830
203-661-0995

Rexall Sundown, Inc.
851 Broken Sound Pkwy., N.W.
Boca Raton, FL 33487
800-344-8482

Rhône-Poulenc Rorer Pharmaceuticals, Inc.
P.O. Box 1200
Collegeville, PA 19426-0107
800-340-7502

Ricola USA, Inc.
51 Gibraltar Dr.
Morris Plains, NJ 07950
201-984-6811

Roberts Pharmaceutical Corp.
4 Industrial Way W.
Eatontown, NJ 07724-2274
800-828-2088

Ross Products/Abbott Laboratories
625 Cleveland Ave.
Columbus, OH 43215-1724
614-624-7677

Rydelle Laboratories
Div. of S. C. Johnson & Son, Inc.
see S. C. Johnson

S. C. Johnson & Son, Inc.
1525 Howe St.
Racine, WI 53403-2236
800-558-5252

Savage Laboratories
Div. of Altana Inc.
60 Baylis Rd.
Melville, NY 11747
800-231-0206

Scandipharm, Inc.
22 Inverness Ctr. Pkwy., Ste. 310
Birmingham, AL 35242
800-950-8085

Scherer Laboratories, Inc.
Subs. of Scherer Healthcare, Inc.
2301 Ohio Dr., Ste. 234
Plano, TX 75093
972-612-6225

Schering-Plough Healthcare Products
Div. of Schering-Plough Corp.
3030 Jackson Ave.
Memphis, TN 38151
901-320-2998

Schwarz Pharma
A Kremers Urban Co.
P.O. Box 2038
Milwaukee, WI 53201
800-558-5114

Science Products
Box 888
Southeastern, PA 19399
800-888-7400

Scot-Tussin Pharmacal Co., Inc.
P.O. Box 8217
Cranston, RI 02920-0217
800-638-7268

Selfcare, Inc.
200 Prospect St.
Waltham, MA 02154
800-899-SELF

Shaklee Corp.
Div. of Yamanovchi Pharmaceutical Co.
444 Market St.
San Francisco, CA 94111-5325
415-954-2080

Sinclair Pharmacal, Inc.
Drawer D
Fishers Island, NY 06390
516-780-7210

Slim Fast Foods Co.
P.O. Box 3345
W. Palm Beach, FL 33401
561-835-9199

Smith & Nephew United, Inc.
P.O. Box 1970
Largo, FL 33779-1970
800-876-1261

SmithKline Beecham Consumer Healthcare, L.P.
1500 Littleton Rd.
Parsippany, NJ 07054-3884
800-245-1040

Solvay Pharmaceuticals
901 Sawyer Rd.
Marietta, GA 30062
404-578-5540

Spectrum
Div. of United Industries, Corp.
P.O. Box 15842
St. Louis, MO 63114-0842
800-767-9927

Stanback Co.
P.O. Box 1669
Salisbury, NC 28144-1669
800-338-5428

Stat Medical Devices, Inc.
1835 NE 146th St.
N. Miami, FL 33181
888-STAT-911

Stellar Health Products, Inc.
71 College Dr.
Orange Park, FL 32065
800-635-8372

Stevens Skin Softener, Inc.
Div. of Stevens Products Corp.
4406 S. Century Dr.
Murray, UT 84123
800-678-7546

Stiefel Laboratories, Inc.
255 Alhambra Cir., Ste. 1000
Coral Gables, FL 33134
305-443-3800

Summers Labs, Inc.
103 G.P. Clement Dr.
Collegeville, PA 19426
800-533-SKIN

Sun Pharmaceuticals Corp.
Div. of Playtex Products, Inc.
P.O. Box 2260
Del Ray Beach, FL 33447
800-SAFESUN

Sunbeam Consumer Products
1615 S. Congress Ave., Ste. 200
Delray Beach, FL 33445
561-243-2100

Sunsource International
535 Lipoa Pwy., Ste. 110
Kihei, HI 96753
800-666-6505

Systems Design Associates, Inc.
P.O. Box 30
Beverly Hills, CA 90213
800-272-8423

T. N. Dickinson Co.
P.O. Box 319
E. Hampton, CT 06424
860-267-2279

Tec Laboratories, Inc.
P.O. Box 1958
Albany, OR 97321
800-ITCHING

Tender Corp.
Littleton Industrial Park
P.O. Box 290
Littleton, NH 03561-0290
800-258-4696

Terumo Medical Corp.
Consumer Products Div.
2100 Cottontail Ln.
Somerset, NJ 08873
800-283-7866

Thomas & Thompson Co.
3927 Falls Rd.
Baltimore, MD 21211
410-889-2960

Thompson Medical Company, Inc.
222 Lakeview Ave.
W. Palm Beach, FL 33401
407-820-9900

3M Health Care
3M Center
St. Paul, MN 55144-1000
800-328-0255

3M Pharmaceuticals
see 3M Health

Tom's of Maine, Inc.
Lafayette Center
P.O. Box 710
Kennebunk, ME 04043
207-985-2944

Torbot Group Inc.
P.O. Box 6008
Warwick, RI 02887-6008
800-545-4254

Transfer-Ease, Inc.
P.O. Box 108
Emerson, NJ 07630-0108
201-357-0114

Triton Consumer Products, Inc.
561 W. Golf Rd.
Arlington Heights, IL 60005
800-942-2009

UCB Pharma, Inc.
1950 Lake Park Dr.
Atlanta, GA 30080
800-477-7877

Ulmer Pharmacal Co.
2440 Fernbrook Ln.
Plymouth, MN 55447
800-848-5637

Unico Holding Co.
1830 Second Ave. N.
Lakeworth, FL 33461
800-367-4477

Unipath Diagnostics, Inc.
390 Park Ave.
New York, NY 10022
800-883-EASY

Upsher-Smith Laboratories, Inc.
14905 23rd Ave. N.
Minneapolis, MN 55447-4709
800-654-2299

Vetco, Inc.
105 Baylis Rd.
Melville, NY 11747
800-754-8853

VPI
P.O. Box 266
Spencer, IN 47460-0266
800-843-4851

W. F. Young, Inc.
P.O. Box 14
Springfield, MA 01102-0014
800-628-9653

W. K. Buckley Ltd.
5230 Orbitor Dr.
Mississauga, Ontario, L4W 5G7
800-434-1034

Walker, Corp. and Co., Inc.
P.O. Box 1320
Syracuse, NY 13201
315-463-4511

**Warner-Lambert Consumer
Health Care**
201 Tabor Rd.
Morris Plains, NJ 07950
201-540-2000

Wearever Health Care Products, L.L.C.
202 Red Mountain Rd.
Rougemont, NC 27572
800-307-4968

Westwood-Squibb Pharmaceuticals
Div. of Bristol-Myers Squibb Co.
100 Forest Ave.
Buffalo, NY 14213-1091
800-333-0950 x7667

Whitehall-Robins Healthcare
Div. of American Home Products Corp.
5 Giralda Farms
Madison, NJ 07940-0871
800-322-3129

Whittier Medical Inc.
865 Turnpike St.
N. Andover, MA 01845
800-645-1115

Wisconsin Pharmacal Co.
P.O. Box 198
Jackson, WI 53037
800-558-6614

Wyeth-Ayerst Laboratories
Div. of American Home Products Corp.
240 Radnor-Chester Rd.
St. Davids, PA 19087
610-902-7113

Wyeth-Ayerst/Lederle
Div. of American Home Products Corp.
401 N. Middletown Rd.
Pearl River, NY 10965
800-533-3753

Young Again Products
43 Randolph Rd., Ste. 125
Silver Spring, MD 20904
301-622-1073

Zeneca Pharmaceuticals
A Business Unit of Zeneca Inc.
P.O. Box 15437
Wilmington, DE 19850-5437
302-886-3000

Zila Pharmaceuticals, Inc.
5227 N. 7th St.
Phoenix, AZ 85014-2800
602-266-6700

Index

Boldface entries designate product table titles.

Entries in regular lightface type designate product ingredients, therapeutic drug classes, or product categories.

Italic entries in which all major words are capitalized designate product trade names, including phytomedicinal products.

Other italic entries designate the genus and species of plants from which phytomedicinal products are derived.

H

I

J

K

O

S

W

X

Z

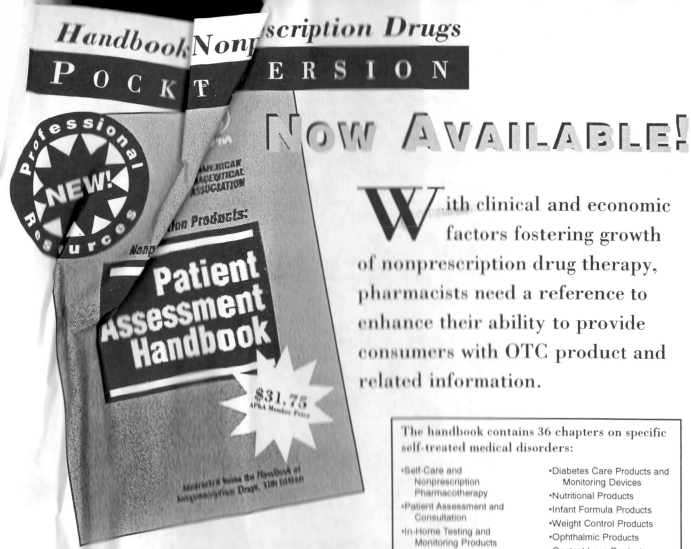